Board Review Series

Pathology

3rd Edition

BOARD REVIEW SERIES

PATHOLOGY

3RD EDITION

Arthur S. Schneider, M.D.
Professor and Chair
Department of Pathology
The Chicago Medical School
Rosalind Franklin University of Medicine and Science
North Chicago, Illinois

Philip A. Szanto, M.D.
Associate Professor of Pathology
The Chicago Medical School
Rosalind Franklin University of Medicine and Science
North Chicago, Illinois

WITH SPECIAL CONTRIBUTIONS BY

Sandra I. Kim, M.D., Ph.D.
Beth Israel Deaconess Medical Center
Harvard Medical School
Boston, Massachusetts
and

Todd A. Swanson, M.D., Ph.D.
William Beaumont Hospital
Royal Oak, Michigan

LIPPINCOTT WILLIAMS & WILKINS
A **Wolters Kluwer** Company
Philadelphia • Baltimore • New York • London
Buenos Aires • Hong Kong • Sydney • Tokyo

Acquisitions Editor: Betty Sun
Developmental Editor: Stacey Sebring
Associate Production Manager: Kevin P. Johnson
Production Services: Maryland Composition
Printer: Courier-Kendalville

530 Walnut Street
Philadelphia, Pennsylvania 19106 USA

351 West Camden Street
Baltimore, Maryland 21201-2436 USA

Printed in the United States of America

Library of Congress Cataloging-in-Publication Data

Schneider, Arthur S.
Pathology / Arthur S. Schneider, Philip A. Szanto, with special contributions by Sandra I. Kim and Todd A. Swanson. — 3rd ed.
p. ; cm. — (Board review series)
Includes index.
ISBN 0-7817-6022-4
1. Pathology—Outlines, syllabi, etc. 2. Pathology—Examinations, questions, etc. I. Szanto, Philip A. II. Title. III. Series.
[DNLM: 1. Pathology—Examination Questions. QZ 18.2 S358p 2006]
RB32.S36 2006
616.07076—dc22

2005027555

10 9 8 7 6 5 4 3 2 1
05 06 07 08 09 10

Dedication

As always,

To Edie

To Anne

with love

Contents

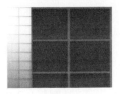

Preface to the Third Edition

While attempting to keep the third edition as short as possible, we have added what we consider to be significant material needed for updating. The most obvious change is that the entire set of end-of-chapter study questions and the comprehensive examination at the end of the book have been entirely recast in vignette format. This should be helpful for students preparing for similar examinations administered by national accrediting groups.

All material is appropriately updated. Of special note, updates or additions include coverage of:

- Apoptosis
- Bacterial vaginosis
- Balanced polymorphisms
- B-type natriuretic peptide as an indicator of heart failure
- Deficiency of vWF metalloprotease in thrombotic thrombocytopenic purpura (TTP)
- Diagnostic criteria for celiac disease
- Heparin-induced thrombocytopenia (HIT) syndrome
- Human androgen receptor gene (*HUMARA*) as a marker of clonality
- Maternal PKU
- Metabolic syndrome
- Newer classification of Niemann-Pick disease
- Newer interpretations of genetic abnormalities in hereditary hemochromatosis
- Relative immunity to AIDS as mediated by coreceptors of HIV cell entry
- Role of dihydrotestosterone (DHT) in nodular prostatic hyperplasia
- Role of *GNAS*1 gene in McCune-Albright syndrome and pseudohypoparathyroidism
- Severe acute respiratory syndrome (SARS)
- Ubiquitin-proteosome system in atrophy and in genetic imprinting

Format

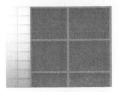

First, as indicated by the series title, Board Review Series, one of the prime purposes of the book is to serve as a source of review material for questions encountered on the USMLE and similar qualifying examinations. A certain part of such preparation consists of recognition of "key associations" that serve as the basis for many such examination questions. Accordingly, in this edition, we have again indicated such associations throughout the text with a symbol resembling a key. Even though we are strongly committed to the view that pathology is a conceptual field consisting of much more than "buzz words," we also believe that recognition of such material is part of learning and that it helps students gain confidence in dealing with voluminous material such as the content of standard pathology courses. The graphic designator used here should serve to identify these "high-yield" items and should be useful to the student in final preparation for board-type examinations.

Organization

The chapter organization continues to parallel that of most major texts, beginning with an initial 8 chapters covering basic or general pathology, followed by 15 chapters covering the pathology of the organ systems. A final chapter deals with statistical concepts of laboratory medicine. Each chapter ends with a set of review questions, and the text concludes with a Comprehensive Examination designed to emulate the content of national licensing examinations.

How to Use This Book

We recommend that this book not be used as a primary text but rather, as the series title suggests, as a supplement for study and for review. Following the initial study of a unit in a pathology course, many students will find that review of the corresponding material in this book will aid in the identification of major concepts that deserve special emphasis. Also, this book can serve as a source for end-of-year review and review for national examinations.

Special attention is again directed to the Answers and Explanations that follow the end-of-chapter Review Test questions and the Comprehensive Examination questions at the end of the text. Much of the teaching material is emphasized in these discussions, and it is recommended that these sections be reviewed carefully as part of examination preparation.

Arthur S. Schneider, M.D.
Philip A. Szanto, M.D.

Acknowledgments

We welcome and thank our new associates and former students, Drs. Sandra I. Kim and Todd A. Swanson, who contributed much to the newly reconstituted vignette style sample question sections throughout this edition. Also, we express appreciation to our students and our many readers throughout the world who have used the preceding editions of this book over the past years. Their overwhelming response and helpful comments have been immensely gratifying and deeply appreciated. We again quote William Osler, who pointed out many years ago that "to study the phenomena of disease without books is to sail an uncharted sea," and "it is easier to buy books than to read them." Our gratification is increased since we have repeatedly heard from our readers that our book has not only been bought but has also been thoroughly read, annotated, and read again.

Again, Ms. Susan Grimm, our editorial assistant, has emerged from "retirement" to help us finalize the manuscript of this third edition. Our debt to her is considerable.

We again acknowledge the continuing contributions of the editorial staff at Lippincott Williams & Wilkins, especially those of Ms. Stacey Sebring, managing editor during the development of this edition; Ms. Betty Sun, acquisitions editor; and Kevin Johnson, production manager. We would also like to thank Martha Cushman and Dvora Konstant, both of whom did much of the copy editing. We thank them all for their hard work and patience. The final product owes a great deal to their efforts.

We thank colleagues who provided illustrations. These include Drs. Jae O. Ro, Deborah E. Powell, Juan Rosai, and John B. Walter.

And again, we thank our respective wives, Edith Schneider and Anne Szanto, for their patience, forbearance, and support. It goes without saying that none of this would have happpened without them.

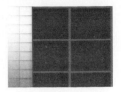

Acknowledgments

CHAPTER 1

Cellular Reaction to Injury

I. Adaptation to Environmental Stress

A. Hypertrophy

1. Hypertrophy is an **increase in the size of an organ or tissue due to an increase in the size of cells.**
2. Other characteristics include an increase in protein synthesis and an increase in the size or number of intracellular organelles.
3. A cellular adaptation to increased workload results in hypertrophy, as exemplified by the increase in skeletal muscle mass associated with exercise and the enlargement of the left ventricle in hypertensive heart disease.

B. Hyperplasia

1. Hyperplasia is an **increase in the size of an organ or tissue caused by an increase in the number of cells.**
2. It is exemplified by glandular proliferation in the breast during pregnancy.
3. In some cases, hyperplasia occurs together with hypertrophy. During pregnancy, uterine enlargement is caused by both hypertrophy and hyperplasia of the smooth muscle cells in the uterus.

C. Aplasia

1. Aplasia is a **failure of cell production.**
2. During fetal development, aplasia results in **agenesis,** or absence of an organ due to failure of production.
3. Later in life, it can be caused by permanent loss of precursor cells in proliferative tissues, such as the bone marrow.

D. Hypoplasia

1. Hypoplasia is a **decrease in cell production is that is less extreme than in aplasia.**
2. It is seen in the partial lack of growth and maturation of gonadal structures in Turner syndrome and Klinefelter syndrome.

E. Atrophy

1. Atrophy is **decrease in the size of an organ or tissue results from a decrease in the mass of preexisting cells.**
2. Most often, causal factors are disuse, nutritional or oxygen deprivation, diminished endocrine stimulation, aging, and denervation (lack of nerve stimulation in peripheral muscles caused by injury to motor nerves).
3. Characteristic features often include the presence of **autophagic granules,** which are intracytoplasmic vacuoles containing debris from degraded organelles.

4. In some instances, atrophy is thought to be mediated in part by the ubiquitin-proteosome pathway of protein degradation. In this pathway, ubiquitin-linked proteins are degraded within the proteosome, a large cytoplasmic protein complex.

F. **Metaplasia** is the **replacement of one differentiated tissue by another.**

1. **Squamous metaplasia**
   a. Squamous metaplasia is exemplified by the replacement of columnar epithelium at the squamocolumnar junction of the cervix by squamous epithelium.
   b. It can also occur in the respiratory epithelium of the bronchus, in the endometrium, and in the pancreatic ducts.
   c. Associated conditions include chronic irritation (e.g., squamous metaplasia of the bronchi with long-term use of tobacco) and vitamin A deficiency.
   d. This process is often reversible.
2. **Osseous metaplasia**
   a. Osseous metaplasia is the formation of new bone at sites of tissue injury.
   b. Cartilaginous metaplasia may also occur.
3. **Myeloid metaplasia** (extramedullary hematopoiesis) is proliferation of hematopoietic tissue at sites other than the bone marrow, such as the liver or spleen.

II. Hypoxic Cell Injury

A. **Causes.** Hypoxic cell injury results from cellular **anoxia** or **hypoxia,** which, in turn, results from various mechanisms, including:

1. **Ischemia** (obstruction of arterial blood flow), the most common cause
2. **Anemia,** a reduction in the number of oxygen-carrying red blood cells
3. **Carbon monoxide poisoning,** which results in diminution in the oxygen-carrying capacity of red blood cells by chemical alteration of hemoglobin
4. **Decreased perfusion of tissues by oxygen-carrying blood,** which occurs in cardiac failure, hypotension, and shock
5. **Poor oxygenation of blood** secondary to pulmonary disease

B. **Early stage.** Hypoxic cell injury first affects the mitochondria, with resultant decreased oxidative phosphorylation and adenosine triphosphate (ATP) synthesis. Consequences of **decreased ATP availability** include:

1. **Failure of the cell membrane pump** (ouabain-sensitive Na^+-K^+-ATPase) results in increased intracellular Na^+ and water and decreased intracellular K^+. This process causes cellular swelling and swelling of organelles.
   a. Cellular swelling, or **hydropic change,** is characterized by the presence of large vacuoles in the cytoplasm.
   b. **Swelling of the endoplasmic reticulum** is one of the first ultrastructural changes evident in reversible injury.
   c. **Swelling of the mitochondria** progresses from reversible, low-amplitude swelling to irreversible, high-amplitude swelling, which is characterized by marked dilation of the inner mitochondrial space.
2. **Disaggregation of ribosomes leads to failure of protein synthesis.** Ribosomal disaggregation is also promoted by membrane damage.
3. **Stimulation of phosphofructokinase activity** results in increased glycolysis, accumulation of lactate, and decreased intracellular pH. Acidification causes reversible clumping of nuclear chromatin.

C. **Late stage**

1. Hypoxic cell injury eventually results in **membrane damage** to plasma and to lysosomal and other organelle membranes, with loss of membrane phospholipids.

2. Reversible morphologic signs of damage include the formation of:
   a. **Myelin figures,** whorl-like structures probably originating from damaged membranes
   b. **Cell blebs,** a cell surface deformity most likely caused by disorderly function of the cellular cytoskeleton

D. **Cell death.** Finally, **cell death** is caused by severe or prolonged injury.
1. The **point of no return** is marked by **irreversible damage to cell membranes,** leading to **massive calcium influx, extensive calcification of the mitochondria,** and cell death.
2. **Intracellular enzymes and various other proteins are released** from necrotic cells into the circulation as a consequence of the loss of integrity of cell membranes. This phenomenon is the basis of a number of useful laboratory determinations as indicators of necrosis.
   a. **Myocardial enzymes in serum.** These are discussed in more depth in Chapter 10.
      (1) Enzymes that have been useful in the diagnosis of myocardial infarction ("heart attack," see Chapters 3 and 10) include the following:
         (a) **Aspartate aminotransferase (AST,** previously known as **SGOT)**
         (b) **Lactate dehydrogenase (LDH)**
         (c) **Creatine kinase (CK,** also known as **CPK)**
      (2) These markers of myocardial necrosis vary in specificity for heart damage, as well as in the time period after the necrotic event in which elevations in the serum appear and persist. The delineation of isoenzyme forms of LDH and CK has been a useful adjunct in adding specificity to these measures.
      (3) The foregoing enzymes are beginning to be replaced by other myocardial proteins in serum as indicators of myocardial necrosis. Important examples include the **troponins** (troponin I [TnI] and troponin T [TnT]) and **myoglobin.**
   b. **Liver enzymes in serum.** These enzymes are discussed in more detail in Chapter 16. Enzymes of special interest include the transaminases **(AST** and **alanine aminotransferase [ALT]), alkaline phosphatase,** and **γ-glutamyltransferase (GGT).**
3. The **vulnerability of cells to hypoxic injury varies** with the tissue or cell type. Hypoxic injury becomes irreversible after:
   a. **3–5 minutes for neurons.** Purkinje cells of the cerebellum and neurons of the hippocampus are more susceptible to hypoxic injury than are other neurons.
   b. **1–2 hours for myocardial cells and hepatocytes.**
   c. **many hours for skeletal muscle cells.**

III. Free Radical Injury

A. **Free radicals**
1. These molecules have a single unpaired electron in the outer orbital.
2. Examples include the activated products of oxygen reduction, such as the superoxide ($O_2^{\bullet -}$) and the hydroxyl ($OH^{\bullet}$) radicals.

B. **Mechanisms that generate free radicals**
1. **Normal metabolism**
2. **Oxygen toxicity,** such as in the alveolar damage that can cause the adult respiratory distress syndrome or as in retrolental fibroplasia (retinopathy of prematurity), an ocular disorder of premature infants that leads to blindness
3. **Ionizing radiation**
4. **Ultraviolet light**
5. **Drugs and chemicals,** many of which promote both proliferation of the smooth endoplasmic reticulum (SER) and induction of the P-450 system of mixed function oxidases of the SER. Proliferation and hypertrophy of the SER of the hepatocyte are classic ultrastructural markers of barbiturate intoxication.
6. **Reperfusion after ischemic injury**

C. **Mechanisms that degrade free radicals**

1. **Intracellular enzymes,** such as glutathione peroxidase, catalase, or superoxide dismutase
2. **Exogenous and endogenous antioxidants,** such as vitamin A, vitamin C, vitamin E, cysteine, glutathione, selenium, ceruloplasmin, or transferrin
3. **Spontaneous decay**

IV. Chemical Cell Injury

- is illustrated by **the model of liver cell membrane damage induced by carbon tetrachloride** (CCl_4).

A. In this model, CCl_4 is processed by the P-450 system of mixed function oxidases within the SER, producing the **highly reactive free radical $CCl_3\cdot$.**

B. $CCl_3\cdot$ diffuses throughout the cell, initiating **lipid peroxidation of intracellular membranes.** Widespread injury results, including:

1. **Disaggregation of ribosomes,** resulting in **decreased protein synthesis.** Failure of the cell to synthesize the apoprotein moiety of lipoproteins causes an accumulation of intracellular lipids (**fatty change**).
2. **Plasma membrane damage,** caused by products of lipid peroxidation in the smooth endoplasmic reticulum, resulting in **cellular swelling** and **massive influx of calcium,** with resultant mitochondrial damage, denaturation of cell proteins, and cell death

V. Necrosis (Table 1-1)

A. **General considerations**

1. **Necrosis** is one of two contrasting morphologic patterns of tissue death. The other is apoptosis (see VI).
2. **Necrosis** is the sum of the degradative and inflammatory reactions occurring after tissue death caused by injury (e.g., hypoxia, exposure to toxic chemicals); it **occurs within living organisms.** In pathologic specimens, fixed cells with well-preserved morphology are dead but not necrotic.
3. **Autolysis** refers to degradative reactions in cells caused by intracellular enzymes indigenous to the cell. **Postmortem autolysis** occurs after the death of the entire organism and is not necrosis.
4. **Heterolysis** refers to cellular degradation by enzymes derived from sources extrinsic to the cell (e.g., bacteria, leukocytes).

B. **Types of necrosis**

1. **Coagulative necrosis**
   a. Coagulative necrosis results most often from a sudden cutoff of blood supply to an organ (ischemia), particularly the heart and kidney.
   b. General **preservation of tissue architecture** is characteristic in the early stages.
   c. **Increased cytoplasmic eosinophilia** occurs because of protein denaturation and loss of cytoplasmic RNA.
   d. **Nuclear changes,** the morphologic hallmark of irreversible cell injury and necrosis, are characteristic. These include:
      (1) **Pyknosis,** chromatin clumping and shrinking with increased basophilia
      (2) **Karyorrhexis,** fragmentation of chromatin
      (3) **Karyolysis,** fading of chromatin material
      (4) **Disappearance of stainable nuclei**

TABLE 1-1 *Types of Necrosis*

Types	Mechanism	Pathologic Changes
Coagulative necrosis	Most often results from interruption of blood supply, resulting in denaturation of proteins; best seen in organs supplied by end arteries with limited collateral circulation, such as the heart and kidney	General architecture well preserved, except for nuclear changes; increased cytoplasmic binding of acidophilic dyes
Liquefactive necrosis	Enzymatic liquefaction of necrotic tissue, most often in the CNS, where it is caused by interruption of blood supply; also occurs in areas of bacterial infection	Necrotic tissue soft and liquefied
Caseous necrosis	Shares features of both coagulation and liquefaction necrosis; most commonly seen in tuberculous granulomas	Architecture not preserved but tissue not liquefied; gross appearance is soft and cheese-like; histologic appearance is amorphous, with increased affinity for acidophilic dyes
Gangrenous necrosis	Most often results from interruption of blood supply to a lower extremity or the bowel	Changes depend on tissue involved and whether gangrene is dry or wet
Fibrinoid necrosis	Characterized by deposition of fibrin-like proteinaceous material in walls of arteries; often observed as part of immune-mediated vasculitis	Smudgy pink appearance in vascular walls; actual necrosis may or may not be present
Fat necrosis	Liberation of pancreatic enzymes with autodigestion of pancreatic parenchyma; trauma to fat cells	Necrotic fat cells, acute inflammation, hemorrhage, calcium soap formation, clustering of lipid-laden macrophages (in the pancreas)

2. **Liquefactive necrosis**
   a. **Ischemic injury to the central nervous system (CNS)** characteristically results in liquefactive necrosis. After the death of CNS cells, liquefaction is caused by autolysis.
   b. Digestion, softening, and liquefaction of tissue are characteristic.
   c. **Suppurative infections** characterized by the formation of pus (liquefied tissue debris and neutrophils) by heterolytic mechanisms involve liquefactive necrosis.
3. **Caseous necrosis**
   a. This type of necrosis occurs as **part of granulomatous inflammation** and is a manifestation of partial immunity caused by the interaction of T lymphocytes (CD4+, CD8+, and CD4−CD8−), macrophages, and probably cytokines, such as interferon-γ, derived from these cells.
   b. **Tuberculosis** is the leading cause of caseous necrosis.
   c. Caseous necrosis combines features of both coagulative necrosis and liquefactive necrosis.
   d. On gross examination, caseous necrosis has a cheese-like (caseous) consistency.
   e. On histologic examination, caseous necrosis has an **amorphous eosinophilic appearance**.
4. **Gangrenous necrosis**
   a. This type of necrosis most often affects the lower extremities or bowel and is secondary to vascular occlusion.
   b. When complicated by infective heterolysis and consequent liquefactive necrosis, gangrenous necrosis is called **wet gangrene**.

c. When characterized primarily by coagulative necrosis without liquefaction, gangrenous necrosis is called **dry gangrene**.

5. **Fibrinoid necrosis**
   a. This **deposition of fibrin-like proteinaceous material in the arterial walls** appears smudgy and acidophilic.
   b. Fibrinoid necrosis is often associated with immune-mediated vascular damage.
6. **Fat necrosis** occurs in two forms.
   a. **Traumatic fat necrosis,** which occurs after a severe injury to tissue with high fat content, such as the breast.
   b. **Enzymatic fat necrosis,** which is a complication of **acute hemorrhagic pancreatitis,** a severe inflammatory disorder of the pancreas.
      (1) Proteolytic and lipolytic pancreatic enzymes diffuse into inflamed tissue and literally digest the parenchyma.
      (2) Fatty acids liberated by the digestion of fat form calcium salts (saponification, or **soap formation**).
      (3) Vessels are eroded, with resultant hemorrhage.

VI. Apoptosis (Table 1-2)

A. **General considerations**
   1. Apoptosis is a second morphologic pattern of tissue death. (The other is necrosis; see V.) It is often referred to as programmed cell death.

TABLE 1-2 *Comparison of Necrosis and Apoptosis*

Characteristics	Necrosis	Apoptosis
Etiology	Gross irreversible cellular injury	Subtle cellular damage, physiologic programmed cell removal
Morphologic changes	Involves many contiguous cells Increased cytoplasmic eosinophilia due to denaturation of proteins Progressive nuclear condensation and fragmentation with eventual disappearance of nuclei Preservation of tissue architecture in early stages of coagulative necrosis	Involves single cells or small clusters of cells Cytoplasmic shrinking and increased eosinophilic staining Chromatin condensation and fragmentation Fragmentation into membrane-bound apoptotic bodies
Biochemical changes	Passive form of cell death not requiring gene involvement or new protein synthesis DNA fragmentation is haphazard rather than regular, resulting in an electrophoretic smudge pattern	Active form of cell death requiring gene expression, protein synthesis, and energy consumption DNA fragmentation is regular at nucleosomal boundaries, resulting in an electrophoretic "laddered" pattern
Inflammatory reaction	Marked inflammatory reaction, liberation of lysosomal enzymes, digestion of cell membranes, and disruption of cells Influx of macrophages due to release of chemotactic factors Removal of debris by phagocytic macrophages	No inflammatory reaction Apoptotic bodies engulfed by neighboring macrophages and epithelial cells

2. This is an important mechanism for the removal of cells. Examples include apoptotic removal of cells with irreparable DNA damage (from free radicals, viruses, cytotoxic immune mechanisms), protecting against neoplastic transformation.
3. In addition, apoptosis is an important mechanism for physiologic cell removal during embryogenesis and in programmed cell cycling (e.g., endometrial cells during menstruation).
4. This involutional process is similar to the physiologic loss of leaves from a tree; *apoptosis* is a Greek term for "falling away from."

B. **Morphologic features**
1. A tendency to involve single isolated cells or small clusters of cells within a tissue
2. Progression through a series of changes marked by a lack of inflammatory response
   a. Blebbing of plasma membrane, cytoplasmic shrinkage, chromatin condensation
   b. Budding of cell and separation of apoptotic bodies (membrane-bound segments)
   c. Phagocytosis of apoptotic bodies
3. **Involution and shrinkage** of affected cells and cell fragments, resulting in small round eosinophilic masses often containing chromatin remnants, exemplified by Councilman bodies in viral hepatitis

C. **Biochemical events**
1. Diverse injurious stimuli (e.g., free radicals, radiation, toxic substances, withdrawal of growth factors or hormones), trigger a variety of stimuli, including cell surface receptors such as FAS, mitochondrial response to stress, and cytotoxic T cells.
2. The **extrinsic pathway of initiation** is mediated by cell surface receptors exemplified by FAS, a member of the tumor necrosis factor receptor family of proteins. This pathway is initiated by signaling by molecules such as the FAS ligand, which in turn signals a series of events that involve activation of caspases. Caspases are aspartate-specific cysteine proteases that have been referred to as "major executioners" or "molecular guillotines." The death signals are conveyed in a proteolytic cascade, through activation of a chain of caspases and other targets. The initial activating caspases are caspase-8 and caspase-9, and the terminal caspases (executioners) include caspase-3 and caspase 6 (among other proteases).
3. The **intrinsic, or mitochondrial, pathway,** which is initiated by the loss of stimulation by growth factors and other adverse stimuli, results in the inactivation and loss of bcl-2 and other antiapoptotic proteins from the inner mitochondrial membrane. This loss results in increased mitochondrial permeability, the release of cytochrome c, and the stimulation of proapoptotic proteins such as bax and bak. Cytochrome c interacts with Apaf-1 causing self-cleavage and activation of caspase-9. Downstream caspases are activated by upstream proteases and act themselves to cleave cellular targets.
4. **Cytotoxic T-cell activation** is characterized by direct activation of caspases by granzyme B, a cytotoxic T-cell protease that perhaps directly activates the caspase cascade. The entry of granzyme B into target cells is mediated by perforin, a cytotoxic T-cell protein.
5. Degradation of DNA by endonucleases into nucleosomal chromatin fragments that are multiples of 180–200 base pairs results in the typical "**laddering**" appearance of DNA on electrophoresis. This phenomenon is characteristic of, but not entirely specific for, apoptosis.
6. Activation of **transglutaminases** crosslinks apoptotic cytoplasmic proteins.

D. **Regulation of apoptosis** is mediated by a number of genes and their products.
1. *bcl*-2: Gene product inhibits apoptosis.
2. *bax:* Gene product facilitates apoptosis.
3. *p53:* Gene product facilitates apoptosis by decreasing transcription of *bcl*-2 and increasing transcription of *bax*.

VII. Reversible Cellular Changes and Accumulations

A. **Fatty change** (fatty metamorphosis, steatosis)
1. **General considerations**
   a. Fatty change is characterized by the **accumulation of intracellular parenchymal triglycerides** and is observed most frequently in the **liver, heart,** and **kidney.** For example, in the liver, fatty change may be secondary to alcoholism, diabetes mellitus, malnutrition, obesity, or poisonings.
2. **Imbalance among the uptake, utilization, and secretion of fat** is the cause of fatty change, and this can result from any of the following mechanism:
   a. **Increased transport of triglycerides or fatty acids** to affected cells
   b. **Decreased mobilization of fat from cells,** most often mediated by decreased production of apoproteins required for fat transport. Fatty change is thus linked to the disaggregation of ribosomes and consequent decreased protein synthesis caused by failure of ATP production in CCl_4-injured cells.
   c. **Decreased use of fat by cells**
   d. **Overproduction of fat in cells**

B. **Hyaline change**
1. This term denotes a characteristic (homogeneous, glassy, eosinophilic) appearance in hematoxylin and eosin sections.
2. It is caused most often by nonspecific accumulations of proteinaceous material.

C. **Accumulations of exogenous pigments**
1. **Pulmonary accumulations of carbon, silica, and iron dust**
2. **Plumbism** (lead poisoning)
3. **Argyria** (silver poisoning), which may cause a permanent gray discoloration of the skin and conjunctivae

D. **Accumulations of endogenous pigments**
1. **Melanin**
   a. This pigment is formed from tyrosine by the action of tyrosinase, synthesized in melanosomes of melanocytes within the epidermis, and transferred by melanocytes to adjacent clusters of keratinocytes and also to macrophages (melanophores) in the subjacent dermis.
   b. **Increased melanin pigmentation** is associated with suntanning and with a wide variety of disease conditions.
   c. **Decreased melanin pigmentation** is observed in albinism and vitiligo.
2. **Bilirubin**
   a. This pigment is a catabolic product of the heme moiety of hemoglobin and, to a minor extent, myoglobin.
   b. In various pathologic conditions, bilirubin accumulates and stains the blood, sclerae, mucosae, and internal organs, producing a yellowish discoloration called jaundice.
      (1) **Hemolytic jaundice,** which is associated with destruction of red cells, is discussed in more depth in Chapter 11.
      (2) **Hepatocellular jaundice,** which is associated with parenchymal liver damage, and **obstructive jaundice,** which is associated with intra- or extrahepatic obstruction of the biliary tract, are discussed more fully in Chapter 16.
3. **Hemosiderin**
   a. This **iron-containing pigment** consists of aggregates of ferritin. It appears in tissues as golden brown amorphous aggregates and can be positively identified by its staining reaction (blue color) with Prussian blue dye. It exists normally in small amounts as physiologic iron stores within tissue macrophages of the bone marrow, liver, and spleen.

TABLE 1-3 *Abnormal Deposition of Hemosiderin*

Type	Pathologic Features	Mechanisms
Local hemosiderosis	Local deposition of hemosiderin	Most often results from hemorrhage into tissue; hemosiderin derived from breakdown of hemoglobin
Systemic hemosiderosis	Generalized hemosiderin deposition without tissue or organ damage	May result from hemorrhage, multiple blood transfusions, hemolysis, and excessive dietary intake of iron, often accompanied by alcohol consumption
Hemochromatosis	Damage to many tissues and organs; scarring and organ dysfunction manifested as hepatic cirrhosis and fibrosis of pancreas, leading to diabetes mellitus; increased melanin pigmentation in skin	More extensive accumulation than hemosiderosis; can result from any of the causes of systemic hemosiderosis; most often a hereditary disorder characterized by increased iron absorption (hereditary hemochromatosis)

b. It accumulates pathologically in tissues in excess amounts (sometimes massive) **(Table 1-3).**

(1) **Hemosiderosis** is defined by accumulation of hemosiderin, primarily within tissue macrophages, without associated tissue or organ damage.

(2) **Hemochromatosis** is more extensive accumulation of hemosiderin, often within parenchymal cells, with accompanying tissue damage, scarring, and organ dysfunction. This condition occurs in both hereditary (primary) and secondary forms.

(a) **Hereditary hemochromatosis** is most often caused by a mutation in the *Hfe* gene on chromosome 6.

(i) Hemosiderin deposition and organ damage in the liver, pancreas, myocardium, and multiple endocrine glands is characteristic, as well as melanin deposition in the skin.

(ii) This results in the triad of **micronodular cirrhosis, diabetes mellitus,** and **skin pigmentation.** This set of findings is referred to as **"bronze diabetes."** Laboratory abnormalities of note include marked elevation of the serum transferrin saturation because of the combination of **increased serum iron** and **decreased total iron-binding capacity (TIBC).**

(b) **Secondary hemochromatosis** is most often caused by **multiple blood transfusions** administered to subjects with hereditary hemolytic anemias such as β-thalassemia major.

4. **Lipofuscin**

a. This yellowish, fat-soluble pigment is an end product of membrane lipid peroxidation.

b. It is sometimes referred to as "wear-and-tear" pigment.

c. It commonly accumulates in elderly patients, in whom the pigment is found most often within hepatocytes and at the poles of nuclei of myocardial cells. The combination of lipofuscin accumulation and atrophy of organs is referred to as **brown atrophy.**

E. **Pathologic calcifications**

1. **Metastatic calcification**

a. **The cause of metastatic calcification is hypercalcemia**

b. Hypercalcemia most often results from any of the following causes:
(a) hyperparathyroidism.
(b) osteolytic tumors with resultant mobilization of calcium and phosphorus.
(c) hypervitaminosis D.
(d) excess calcium intake, such as in the milk-alkali syndrome (nephrocalcinosis and renal stones caused by milk and antacid self-therapy.

2. **Dystrophic calcification**
   a. Dystrophic calcification is **defined as calcification in previously damaged tissue,** such as areas of old trauma, tuberculosis lesions, scarred heart valves, and atherosclerotic lesions.
   b. The cause is not hypercalcemia; typically, the serum calcium concentration is normal.

VIII. Disorders Characterized by Abnormalities of Protein Folding

A. These disorders involve failure of protein structural stabilization or degradation by specialized proteins known as chaperones. Important chaperones include heat shock proteins induced by stress, one of which is ubiquitin, which marks abnormal proteins for degradation.

B. Two known pathogenetic mechanisms include:
1. **Abnormal protein aggregation,** which is characteristic of amyloidosis; a number of neurodegenerative diseases, such as Alzheimer disease, Huntington disease, and Parkinson disease; and perhaps prion diseases, such as "mad cow" disease.
2. **Abnormal protein transport and secretion,** which is characteristic of cystic fibrosis and α_1-antitrypsin deficiency.

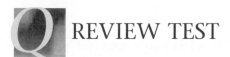

REVIEW TEST

Directions: *Each of the numbered items or incomplete statements in this section is followed by answers or by completions of the statement. Select the* ***one*** *lettered answer or completion that is best in each case.*

1. The illustration shows a section of the heart from a 45-year-old African-American man with long-standing hypertension who died of a "stroke." Which of the following adaptive changes is exemplified in the illustration?

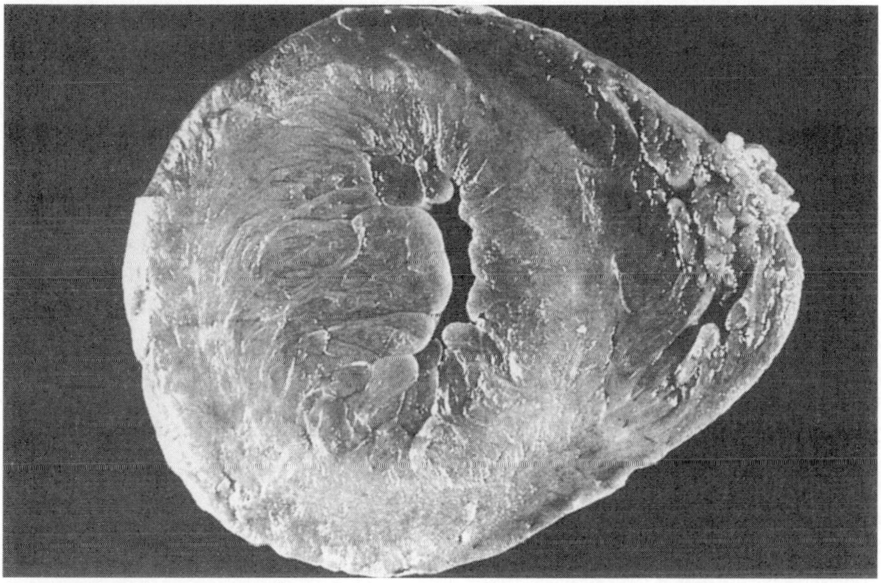

(Reprinted with permission from Golden A, Powell D, Jennings C: *Pathology: Understanding Human Disease,* 2nd ed. Baltimore, Williams & Wilkins, 1985, p 136.)

(A) Aplasia
(B) Atrophy
(C) Hyperplasia
(D) Hypertrophy
(E) Hypoplasia

2. A 16-year-old girl undergoes radiologic imaging of her abdomen and is found to have only one kidney. She had been entirely unaware of this problem. Which of the following terms is most descriptive of this finding?

(A) Agenesis
(B) Atrophy
(C) Hyperplasia
(D) Hypoplasia
(E) Metaplasia

3. An impending myocardial infarction was successfully averted by thrombolytic (clot-dissolving) therapy in a 55-year-old man. Which of the following biochemical events most likely occurred during the period of hypoxia?

(A) Decreased hydrogen ion concentration
(B) Increase in oxidative phosphorylation
(C) Loss of intracellular Na^+ and water
(D) Stimulation of ATP synthesis
(E) Stimulation of anaerobic glycolysis and glycogenolysis

4. A 45-year-old man with a long history of alcoholism presents with severe epigastric pain, nausea, vomiting, fever, and an increase in serum amylase. During a previous hospitalization for a similar episode, computed tomography scanning demonstrated calcifications in the pancreas. A diagnosis of acute pancreatitis superimposed on chronic pancreatitis was made. In this condition, which of the following types of necrosis is most characteristic?

(A) Caseous
(B) Coagulative
(C) Enzymatic
(D) Fibrinoid
(E) Liquefactive

5. A 29-year-old man hospitalized for acquired immunodeficiency syndrome (AIDS) is found to have pulmonary tuberculosis. Which type of necrosis is found in the granulomatous lesions (clusters of modified macrophages) characteristic of this increasingly frequent complication of AIDS?

(A) Caseous
(B) Coagulative
(C) Enzymatic
(D) Fibrinoid
(E) Liquefactive

6. A 45-year-old woman is investigated for hypertension and is found to have enlargement of the left kidney. The right kidney is smaller than normal. Contrast studies reveal stenosis of the right renal artery. The size change in the right kidney is an example of which of the following adaptive changes?

(A) Aplasia
(B) Atrophy
(C) Hyperplasia
(D) Hypertrophy
(E) Metaplasia

7. This figure illustrates the microscopic appearance of the heart of a 56-year-old man who died after a 24-hour hospitalization for severe "crushing" chest pain complicated by hypotension and pulmonary edema. The type of necrosis shown is best described as

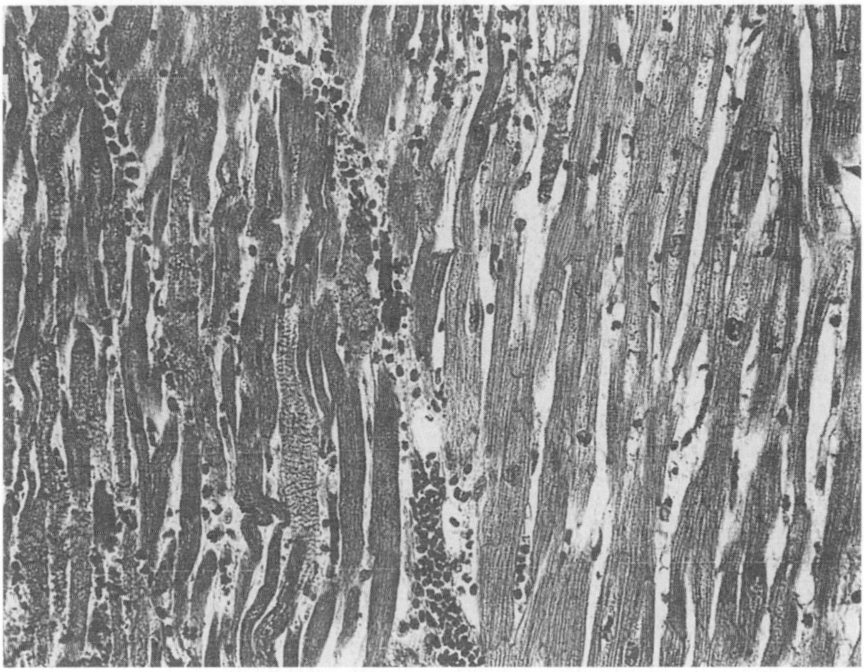

(Reprinted with permission from Golden A, Powell D, Jennings C: *Pathology: Understanding Human Disease,* 2nd ed. Baltimore, Williams & Wilkins, 1985, p 12.)

(A) Caseous
(B) Coagulative
(C) Fibrinoid
(D) Gangrenous
(E) Liquefactive

8. The illustration is from a liver biopsy of a 34-year-old woman with a long history of alcoholism. Which of the following is the best explanation for the changes shown here?

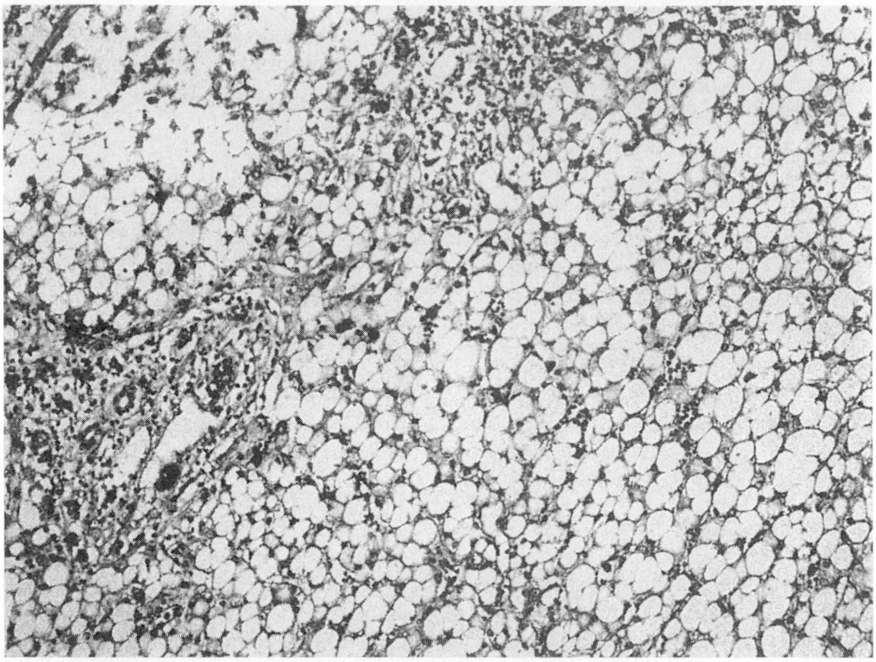

(Reprinted with permission from Golden A, Powell D, Jennings C: *Pathology: Understanding Human Disease,* 2nd ed. Baltimore, Williams & Wilkins, 1985, p 7.)

(A) Accumulation of triglycerides within hepatocytes
(B) Apoptosis with replacement of damaged cells by lipid-laden macrophages
(C) Bilirubin accumulation with mobilization of fat by bile salts
(D) Enzymatic fat necrosis with digestion of liver parenchyma by released enzymes
(E) Irreversible damage to mitochondria

9. A 56-year-old man recovered from a myocardial infarction after his myocardium was entirely "saved" by immediate thrombolytic therapy. If it had been possible to examine microscopic sections of his heart during his ischemic episode, which of the following would be the most likely cellular change to be found?

(A) Karyolysis
(B) Karyorrhexis
(C) Pyknosis
(D) Swelling of the endoplasmic reticulum

10. A 64-year-old woman presents with fever, chills, headache, neck stiffness, vomiting, and confusion. The Kernig sign (passive knee extension eliciting neck pain) and Brudzinski sign (passive neck flexion eliciting bilateral hip flexion) are both positive. Examination of the cerebrospinal fluid reveals changes consistent with bacterial meningitis, and brain imaging demonstrates a localized abscess. Which of the following types of necrosis is most characteristic of abscess formation?

(A) Caseous
(B) Coagulative
(C) Enzymatic
(D) Fibrinoid
(E) Liquefactive

11. A 20-year-old man presents with yellowing of the sclerae, skin, and oral mucosa. Which of the following accumulations underlies these findings?

(A) Bilirubin
(B) Hemosiderin
(C) Lead
(D) Melanin
(E) Silver

12. A 45-year-old man is referred because of a recent diagnosis of hereditary hemochromatosis. Which of the following is a correct statement about this disorder?

(A) Damage to organs results from abnormal deposition of lead.
(B) It can progress to liver cirrhosis, diabetes mellitus, and skin pigmentation.
(C) Most cases are due to spontaneous mutations.
(D) Skin hyperpigmentation is due to bilirubin accumulation.
(E) The total iron-binding capacity (TIBC) is characteristically increased.

13. A 60-year-old woman with breast cancer and widespread bony metastases is found to have calcification of multiple organs. The calcifications are best described as

(A) Dystrophic with decreased serum calcium
(B) Dystrophic with increased serum calcium
(C) Metastatic with decreased serum calcium
(D) Metastatic with increased serum calcium

14. A 56-year-old man dies 24 hours after the onset of substernal chest pain radiating down his left arm to the ulnar aspect of his fingertips. Which of the following morphologic myocardial findings is an indicator of irreversible injury?

(A) Cell blebs
(B) Depletion of glycogen
(C) Mitochondrial swelling
(D) Myelin figures
(E) Pyknotic nuclei

ANSWERS AND EXPLANATIONS

1-D. The illustration shows marked hypertrophy of the left ventricle. Hypertrophy of this extent, often seen in hypertensive heart disease, is caused by increased workload from increased ventricular pressure. This organ enlargement is the result of an increase in size of the individual muscle cells.

2-A. The patient has renal agenesis, absence of the kidney due to failure of organ development. The congenital lack of one kidney differs from atrophy, in which a decrease in the size of an organ results from a decrease in the mass of pre-existing cells. Unilateral renal agenesis is usually a harmless malformation, and the opposite kidney is often enlarged due to compensatory hypertrophy. Bilateral renal agenesis is incompatible with life and is of special interest since it can lead to the Potter progression (see Chapter 17).

3-E. The sequence of events in hypoxic cell damage is as follows: Hypoxia results in failure of oxidative phosphorylation, with resultant depletion of ATP and increase in AMP and ADP. Anaerobic glycolysis and glycogenolysis are stimulated (*not* inhibited) through increased phosphofructokinase and phosphorylase activities, respectively. This results in accumulation of cell lactate, with a decrease in intracellular pH and depletion of cellular glycogen stores. Decreased availability of ATP also results in failure of the Na^+K^+-ATPase pump, which then leads to increased cell Na^+ and water and decreased cell K^+.

4-C. Pancreatic enzymatic fat necrosis represents autodigestion by proteolytic and lipolytic enzymes released from damaged parenchymal cells of the pancreas. Fatty acids liberated by the digestion of fat form calcium soaps, a process referred to as saponification. The precipitated calcium in the soaps can be visualized by radiologic imaging.

5-A. Caseous necrosis occurs as part of granulomatous inflammation, typified by the lesions of tuberculosis.

6-B. The decreased size is due to restriction of the blood supply, one of the causes of atrophy. The increase in size of the opposite kidney is referred to as compensatory hypertrophy. Unilateral renal artery stenosis is a well-known cause of secondary hypertension. In this setting, increased renin excretion and stimulation of the renin-angiotensin system results in a form of hypertension that is potentially curable by surgical correction of the underlying vascular abnormality.

7-B. The figure illustrates general preservation of myocardial architecture with some fragmentation, more intense cytoplasmic staining corresponding to increased cellular eosinophilia, and loss of nuclei, all of which are characteristic of coagulative necrosis.

8-A. The figure illustrates fatty change of the liver, which is characterized by the accumulation of intracellular parenchymal triglycerides. It is seen most frequently in the liver, heart, and kidney, and commonly is secondary to alcoholism. Fatty change results from an imbalance between the uptake, utilization, and mobilization of fat from liver cells. Alcoholic fatty liver may be reversible with complete abstinence from alcohol.

9-D. If infarction is averted by immediate thrombolytic therapy, indicators of necrosis, such as karyorrhexis, pyknosis, and karyolysis, which represent irreversible changes, would not be expected. Swelling of the endoplasmic reticulum from increased cell water, one of the earliest ultrastructural changes observed in injured cells, is reversible and would be expected.

10-E. Liquefactive necrosis is characteristic of ischemic injury in the central nervous system and suppurative infections that cause abscess formation (see Chapter 2). The changes in the cerebrospinal spinal fluid characteristic of bacterial meningitis are detailed in Chapter 3.

11-A. Yellowing of the sclerae, skin, and oral mucosa are all characteristic of jaundice, the accumulation of bilirubin, the catabolic product of the heme moiety of hemoglobin. Jaundice can occur by diverse mechanisms: hemolytic (see Chapter 11), hepatocellular (see Chapter 16), or obstructive (see Chapter 16).

12-B. In advanced form, primary (hereditary) hemochromatosis is characterized by the triad of cirrhosis, diabetes, and hyperpigmentation, or so-called "bronze diabetes." The disease is most often caused by a mutation in the *Hfe* gene on chromosome 6 and is characteristically familial rather than sporadic. The manifestations of the disorder are the result of iron overload and deposition of hemosiderin in tissues such as the liver, pancreas, skin, joints, and pituitary. Laboratory abnormalities of note include increased serum iron and decreased total iron-binding capacity (TIBC). The skin hyperpigmentation is due largely to increases in melanin and to lesser accumulations of hemosiderin.

13-D. Metastatic calcification, or deposition of calcium in previously normal tissue, is caused by hypercalcemia. In this patient, tumor metastases to bone with increased osteolytic activity caused mobilization of calcium and phosphate, resulting in hypercalcemia. Metastatic calcification should be contrasted with dystrophic calcification, in which the serum calcium concentration is normal and previously damaged tissues are the sites of deposition.

14-E. Myelin figures, cell blebs, mitochondrial swelling, and glycogen depletion are all signs of reversible injury. Nuclear changes such as pyknosis, karyorrhexis, and karyolysis are signs of cell death and are, of course, irreversible.

CHAPTER 2

Inflammation

I. Introduction

- Inflammation is a vascular response to injury.

A. **Processes**
1. Exudation of fluid from vessels
2. Attraction of leukocytes to the injury. Leukocytes engulf and destroy bacteria, tissue debris, and other particulate material.
3. Activation of chemical mediators
4. Proteolytic degradation of extracellular debris
5. Restoration of injured tissue to its normal structure and function. This is limited by the extent of tissue destruction and by the regenerative capacity of the specific tissue.

B. **Cardinal signs**
1. **Rubor** (redness caused by dilation of vessels)
2. **Dolor** (pain due to increased pressure exerted by the accumulation of interstitial fluid and to mediators such as bradykinin)
3. **Calor** (heat caused by increased blood flow)
4. **Tumor** (swelling due to an extravascular accumulation of fluid)
5. **Functio laesa** (loss of function)

C. **Causes**
1. Infection
2. Trauma
3. Physical injury from thermal extremes or from ionizing radiation
4. Chemical injury
5. Immunologic injury
6. Tissue death. Inflammatory changes occur in viable tissue adjacent to necrotic areas.

II. Acute Inflammation

A. **Adhesion molecules**
1. **General considerations**
   a. Adhesion molecules play an important role in acute inflammation.
   b. They are divided into three families: selectins, immunoglobulin-family adhesion proteins, and integrins.

2. **Selectins**
   a. These molecules are induced by the cytokines interleukin-1 (IL-1) and tumor necrosis factor (TNF).
   b. **L-selectins** are expressed on neutrophils and bind to endothelial mucin-like molecules such as GlyCam-1.
   c. **E- and P-selectins** are expressed on endothelial cells and bind to oligosaccharides such as sialyl-Lewis X on the surface of leukocytes. **P-selectins,** stored in endothelial Weibel-Palade bodies and platelet alpha granules, relocate to the plasma membrane after stimulation by mediators such as histamine and thrombin.
3. **Immunoglobulin-family adhesion proteins**
   a. Intercellular adhesion molecules 1 and 2 (ICAM-1 and ICAM-2) are expressed on endothelial cells and bind to integrin molecules on leukocytes.
   b. Vascular cell adhesion molecules (VCAMs) similarly are expressed on endothelial cells and bind to integrin molecules on leukocytes.
4. **Integrins.** Examples include leukocyte LFA-1, MAC-1, and VLA-4, which bind to endothelial immunoglobulin-family adhesion proteins.

B. **Vasoactive changes**
1. These changes begin with a brief period of vasoconstriction, followed shortly by dilation of arterioles, capillaries, and postcapillary venules.
2. The resultant marked increase in blood flow to the affected area is clinically manifest by redness and increased warmth of the affected area.

C. **Increased capillary permeability**
1. This results in leakage of proteinaceous fluid, which causes edema.
2. Causes include endothelial changes that vary from contraction of endothelial cells in postcapillary venules, with widening of interendothelial gaps, to major endothelial damage involving arterioles, capillaries, and venules.

D. **Types of inflammatory cells**
1. **Neutrophils** are the most prominent inflammatory cells in foci of acute inflammation during the first 24 hours. Important causes of **neutrophilia** (increased neutrophils in the peripheral blood) include bacterial infections and other causes of acute inflammation, such as infarction. The early release of neutrophils into the peripheral blood in acute inflammation is from the bone marrow postmitotic reserve pool. There is often an increase in the proportion of less mature cells such as **band neutrophils.**
2. After 2–3 days, neutrophils are replaced mainly by **monocytes-macrophages,** which are capable of engulfing larger particles, are longer-lived, and are capable of dividing and proliferating within the inflamed tissue. Important causes of **monocytosis** (i.e., increased number of monocytes in the peripheral blood) include tuberculosis, brucellosis, typhus, and salmonella infection.
3. **Lymphocytes** are the most prominent inflammatory cells in many viral infections and, along with monocytes-macrophages and plasma cells, are the most prominent cells in chronic inflammation. **Lymphocytosis** (i.e., an increased number of lymphocytes in the peripheral blood) is most often caused by viral infections such as influenza, mumps, rubella, and infectious mononucleosis and certain bacterial infections such as whooping cough and tuberculosis.
4. **Eosinophils** are the predominant inflammatory cells in allergic reactions and parasitic infestations. The most important causes of **eosinophilia** include allergies such as asthma, hay fever, and hives and also parasitic infections. Other causes include polyarteritis nodosa and Hodgkin lymphoma.
5. **Mast cells and basophils** are sources of histamine. Important causes of **basophilia** include chronic myelogenous leukemia and other myeloproliferative diseases.

E. **Cellular response of leukocytes**

1. **Emigration** is the passage of inflammatory leukocytes between the endothelial cells into the adjacent interstitial tissue. Before emigration, circulating leukocytes from the central blood flow move toward the endothelial surface.
   a. **Margination** occurs as leukocytes localize to the outer margin of the blood flow adjacent to the vascular endothelium.
   b. **Pavementing** occurs as leukocytes line the endothelial surface.
   c. **Rolling (or tumbling)** is mediated by the action of endothelial selectins loosely binding to leukocytes, producing a characteristic "rolling" movement of the leukocytes along the endothelial surface.
   d. **Adhesion** occurs as leukocytes adhere to the endothelial surface and is mediated by the interaction of integrins on leukocytes binding to immunoglobulin-family adhesion proteins on endothelium.
   e. **Transmigration** is the movement of leukocytes across the endothelium and is mediated by platelet endothelial cell adhesion molecule-1 (PECAM-1) on both leukocytes and endothelium.
2. **Chemotaxis**
   a. This is the process by which leukocytes are attracted to and move toward an injury.
   b. Chemotaxis and other forms of cellular migration are measured in an in vitro system (Boyden chamber technique) that assesses migration of cells from an upper chamber, through a microporous membrane, to a lower chamber filled with a chemoattractant.
   c. This process is mediated by diffusible chemical agents **(Table 2-1);** movement of leukocytes occurs along a chemical gradient.
   d. **Chemotactic factors for neutrophils,** produced at the site of injury, include:
      (1) Products from bacteria
      (2) Complement components, especially C5a
      (3) Arachidonic acid metabolites, especially leukotriene B_4 (LTB_4), hydroxyeicosatetraenoic acid (HETE), and kallikrein
3. **Phagocytosis**
   a. **Definition.** Phagocytosis is the **ingestion** of particulate material (e.g., tissue debris, living or dead bacteria, other foreign cells) by phagocytic cells. **Neutrophils** and **monocytes-macrophages** are the most important phagocytic cells.

TABLE 2-1 *Chemotactic Factors*

Factor	Description	Chemotactic For
Formylated peptides	Bacterial products of *Escherichia coli*	Neutrophils
C5a	Activated complement component	Neutrophils
HETE, LTB_4	Leukotrienes	Neutrophils
Kallikrein	Product of factor XIIa-mediated conversion of prekallikrein	Neutrophils
Fibrinogen	Plasma protein	Neutrophils
PAF	AGEPC; from basophils, mast cells, and other cells	Eosinophils
PDGF	From platelets, monocytes-macrophages, smooth muscle cells, and endothelial cells	Neutrophils and macrophages
TGF-β	From platelets, neutrophils, macrophages, lymphocytes, and fibroblasts	Macrophages and fibroblasts
Fibronectin	Extracellular matrix protein	Fibroblasts and endothelial cells

PAF, platelet-activating factor; PDGF, platelet-derived growth factor; AGEPC, acetyl-glyceryl-ether phosphorylcholine; TGF-β, transforming growth factor-β.

b. **Anatomic changes**
   (1) Phagocytosis is characterized morphologically by internalization of the attached opsonized particle by pseudopodial extensions from the surface of the leukocyte, which enclose the foreign particle, forming an internalized vesicle, the **phagosome.**
   (2) Phagosomes fuse with cytoplasmic lysosomes and form **phagolysosomes.**
   (3) Phagolysosome formation is associated with leukocytic degranulation.

c. **Opsonization**
   (1) This process facilitates phagocytosis. It is the coating of particulate material by substances referred to as opsonins, which immobilize the particles on the surface of the phagocyte.
   (2) The most important opsonins are **immunoglobulin G (IgG) subtypes** and **C3b,** a complement component.
   (3) Fragments opsonized by IgG are bound to phagocytic cells by cell-surface receptors for the Fc portion of the IgG molecule.
   (4) Fragments opsonized by C3b bind to cellular receptors for C3b.

4. **Intracellular microbial killing** is mediated within phagocytic cells by oxygen-dependent and oxygen-independent mechanisms.
   a. **Oxygen-dependent microbial killing** is the most important intracellular microbicidal process.
      (1) Phagocytosis initiates activity of the hexose monophosphate shunt, causing an oxidative burst and supplying electrons to an NADPH oxidase in the phagosomal membrane.
      (2) One of the products of the NADPH oxidase reaction is superoxide anion ($O_2{\bullet}^-$), which is further converted to hydrogen peroxide (H_2O_2) by dismutation. H_2O_2 may be further converted to the activated hydroxyl radical (OH•).
      (3) In the presence of the leukocyte enzyme myeloperoxidase and a halide ion such as chloride, H_2O_2 oxidizes microbial proteins and disrupts cell walls. This entire process is referred to as the **myeloperoxidase-halide system of bacterial killing.**
   b. **Oxygen-independent microbial killing**
      (1) This process is much less effective than oxygen-dependent microbial killing.
      (2) This process is mediated by proteins, such as lysozyme, lactoferrin, major basic protein of eosinophils, and cationic proteins such as bactericidal permeability-increasing protein and defensins.

F. **Exogenous and endogenous mediators of acute inflammation**
- These mediators influence chemotaxis, vasomotor phenomena, vascular permeability, pain, and other aspects of the inflammatory process **(Table 2-2).**

1. **Exogenous mediators** are most often of microbial origin (e.g., formylated peptides of *Escherichia coli,* which are chemotactic for neutrophils).
2. **Endogenous mediators** are of host origin.
   a. **Vasoactive amines**
      (1) **Histamine** mediates the increase in capillary permeability associated with contraction of endothelial cells in postcapillary venules that occurs with mild injuries.
         (a) Histamine is liberated from **basophils, mast cells,** and **platelets.**
         (b) **Basophils and mast cells.** Histamine is liberated by degranulation triggered by the following stimuli:
            (i) Binding of specific antigen to basophil and mast cell membrane-bound **IgE** (complement is not involved)
            (ii) Binding of complement fragments C3a and C5a, **anaphylatoxins,** to specific cell-surface receptors on basophils and mast cells (specific antigen and IgE antibodies are not involved)
            (iii) Physical stimuli such as heat and cold
            (iv) Cytokine IL-1
            (v) Factors from neutrophils, monocytes, and platelets

TABLE 2-2 *Vasoactive Mediators*

Activity	Mediator
Vasoconstriction	TxA_2
	LTC_4, LTD_4, LTE_4
	PAF
Vasodilation	PGI_2
	PGD_2, PGE_2, $PGF_{2\alpha}$
	Bradykinin
	PAF
Increased vascular permeability	Histamine
	Serotonin
	PGD_2, PGE_2, $PGF_{2\alpha}$
	LTC_4, LTD_4, LTE_4
	Bradykinin
	PAF
	Nitric oxide

LTC_4, leukotriene C_4; LTD_4, leukotriene D_4; LTE_4, leukotriene E_4; TxA_2, thromboxane A_2; PAF, platelet-activating factor; PGI_2, prostacyclin (prostaglandin I_2); PGD_2, prostaglandin D_2; PGE_2, prostaglandin E_2; $PGF_{2\alpha}$, prostaglandin $F_{2\alpha}$.

(c) **Platelets.** Histamine is liberated from platelets by platelet aggregation and the release reaction, which can be triggered by endothelial injury and thrombosis or by platelet-activating factor (PAF).

(i) PAF is derived from the granules of basophils and mast cells and from endothelial cells, macrophages, neutrophils, and eosinophils. PAF is acetylglyceryl-ether phosphorylcholine, also known as AGEPC.

(ii) PAF activates and aggregates platelets, with the release of histamine and serotonin; causes vasoactive and bronchospastic effects; and activates arachidonic acid metabolism.

(2) **Serotonin (5-hydroxytryptamine)**

(a) This substance acts similarly to histamine.

(b) It is derived from platelets. It is liberated from platelets, along with histamine, during the release reaction.

b. **Arachidonic acid metabolites.** Phospholipase A_2 stimulates the release of arachidonic acid from membrane phospholipids. The metabolism of arachidonic acid proceeds along two pathways:

(1) **The cyclooxygenase (cyclic endoperoxide) pathway** is catalyzed by two enzymic isoforms, referred to as cyclooxygenase-1 (COX-1) and cyclooxygenase-2 (COX-2).

(a) This pathway is inhibited by aspirin and other anti-inflammatory drugs.

(b) It yields thromboxanes and prostaglandins: thromboxane A_2 (TxA_2) in platelets, prostacyclin (PGI_2) in endothelial cells, and other prostaglandins in other tissues.

(i) **Platelet TxA_2** is a powerful vasoconstrictor and platelet aggregant.

(ii) **Endothelial PGI_2** is a powerful vasodilator and inhibitor of platelet aggregation.

(2) **The lipoxygenase pathway** yields hydroperoxyeicosatetraenoic acid (**HPETE**) and its derivatives, **12-HPETE** in platelets and **5-HPETE** and **15-HPETE** in leukocytes.
  (a) **5-HPETE** in turn gives rise to **HETE,** a chemotactic factor for neutrophils.
  (b) **5-HPETE** also gives rise to **leukotrienes:**
    (i) LTB_4, a chemotactic factor for neutrophils
    (ii) LTC_4, LTD_4, and LTE_4, potent vasoconstrictors, bronchoconstrictors, and mediators of increased capillary permeability, which are sometimes jointly referred to as the **slow-reacting substance of anaphylaxis**
  (c) **5-HPETE** also indirectly gives rise to **lipoxins.** LXA_4 and LXB_4 inhibit polymorphonuclear neutrophils and eosinophils and also activates monocytes and macrophages. It is proposed that these lipoxins are involved in resolving inflammation and are potential anti-inflammatory mediators that may have therapeutic value.

c. **Cytokines.** These **soluble proteins** are secreted by several types of cells. They can act as effector molecules that influence the behavior of other cells.
  (1) Cytokines are mediators of immunologic response [e.g., interferon-γ (produced by T cells and natural killer cells) activates monocytes].
  (2) The cytokines **IL-1** and **TNF** are secreted by monocytes-macrophages and other cells and have several effects on inflammation.
  (3) IL-1 and TNF induce **acute phase responses,** such as
    (a) **Systemic effects** of inflammation, including fever and leukocytosis
    (b) **Hepatic synthesis** of acute phase proteins, such as C-reactive protein, serum amyloid–associated protein, complement components, fibrinogen, prothrombin, α_1-antitrypsin, α_2-macroglobulin, ferritin, and ceruloplasmin
    (c) **Synthesis of adhesion molecules**
    (d) **Neutrophil degranulation**
  (4) IL-1 and TNF reduce the thromboresistant properties of endothelium, thus promoting thrombosis.

d. **Kinin system.** The kinin system is initiated by activated Hageman factor (factor XIIa). Factor XIIa also activates the intrinsic pathway of coagulation and the plasminogen (fibrinolytic) system. Activation of this system in turn activates the complement cascade. Thus, **factor XIIa links the kinin, coagulation, plasminogen, and complement systems.**
  (1) This system converts prekallikrein to kallikrein (a chemotactic factor).
  (2) It results in the cleavage, by kallikrein, of high-molecular-weight kininogen to **bradykinin,** which is a peptide nine amino acids in length that mediates vascular permeability, arteriolar dilation, and pain.

e. **Complement system.** The complement system consists of a group of **plasma proteins** that participate in immune lysis of cells and plays a significant role in inflammation.
  (1) **C3a and C5a** (anaphylatoxins) mediate degranulation of basophils and mast cells with the release of histamine. C5a is chemotactic, mediates the release of histamine from platelet-dense granules, induces expression of leukocyte adhesion molecules, and activates the lipoxygenase pathway of arachidonic acid metabolism.
  (2) **C3b** is an opsonin.
  (3) **C5b-9,** the membrane attack complex, is a lytic agent for bacteria and other cells.

f. **Nitric oxide** (formerly known as endothelium-derived relaxing factor)
  (1) This is produced by endothelial cells.
  (2) It stimulates relaxation of smooth muscle, thus playing a role in controlling vascular tone.
  (3) It inhibits platelet aggregation, contributing to endothelial thromboresistance.

G. **Outcome of acute inflammation**

1. **Resolution of tissue structure and function** often occurs if the injurious agent is eliminated.

2. **Tissue destruction and persistent acute inflammation**
   a. **Abscess.** This is a cavity filled with pus (neutrophils, monocytes, and liquefied cellular debris).
      (1) It is often walled off by fibrous tissue and is relatively inaccessible to the circulation.
      (2) It results from tissue destruction by lysosomal products and other degradative enzymes.
      (3) It is usually caused by bacterial infections, often by staphylococci.
   b. **Ulcer**
      (1) This is the loss of surface epithelium.
      (2) This can be caused by acute inflammation of epithelial surfaces (e.g., peptic ulcer, ulcers of the skin).
   c. **Fistula.** This is an abnormal communication between two organs or between an organ and a surface.
   d. **Scar.** This is the final result of tissue destruction, with resultant distortion of structure and, in some cases, altered function.
3. **Conversion to chronic inflammation**
   a. This change is marked by the replacement of neutrophils and monocytes with lymphocytes, plasma cells, and macrophages.
   b. It often includes proliferation of fibroblasts and new vessels, with resultant scarring and distortion of architecture.

H. **Hereditary defects that impair the acute inflammatory response**

1. **Deficiency of complement components**
   a. This defect manifests clinically as increased susceptibility to infection.
   b. Notable deficiencies include C2, C3, and C5.
2. **Defects in neutrophils**
   a. **Chronic granulomatous disease of childhood**
      (1) This disease is most commonly an **X-linked** disorder characterized by **deficient activity of** one of the enzymes involved in **NADPH oxidase** activity and the oxidative burst. Autosomal recessive variants also occur.
      (2) The disease is marked by phagocytic cells that ingest but do not kill certain microorganisms.
      (3) **Catalase-positive organisms** are ingested but not killed. These organisms (e.g., *Staphylococcus aureus*) can destroy H_2O_2 generated by bacterial metabolism. Because enzyme-deficient neutrophils cannot produce H_2O_2 and bacterial H_2O_2 is destroyed by bacterial catalase, H_2O_2 is not available as a substrate for myeloperoxidase. Thus, the myeloperoxidase–halide system of bacterial killing fails.
      (4) **Catalase-negative organisms** are ingested and killed. These organisms (e.g., streptococci) produce sufficient H_2O_2 to permit oxygen-dependent microbicidal mechanisms to proceed. In effect, the substrate for myeloperoxidase is produced by the bacteria, and the bacteria in a sense kill themselves.
   b. **Myeloperoxidase deficiency**
      (1) This defect is rarely associated with recurrent bacterial infections but often has little clinical consequence.
      (2) In some instances, this defect has been associated with a marked increase in susceptibility to infections with *Candida albicans.*
   c. **Chédiak-Higashi syndrome**
      (1) This autosomal recessive disorder is characterized by neutropenia, albinism, cranial and peripheral neuropathy, and a tendency to develop repeated infections.
      (2) It is marked by the presence of abnormal white blood cells, which are characterized as follows:
         (a) **Functionally,** by abnormal microtubule formation, affecting movement, with impaired chemotaxis and migration
         (b) **Morphologically,** by large cytoplasmic granules (representing abnormal lysosomes) in granulocytes, lymphocytes, and monocytes and by large abnormal melanosomes in melanocytes, all caused by impaired membrane fusion of lysosomes

d. **Leukocyte adhesion deficiency (LAD) types 1 and 2**
  (1) **LAD type 1 deficiency** is associated with recurrent bacterial infections and is caused by deficiency of β_2-integrins.
  (2) **LAD type 2 deficiency** is also associated with recurrent bacterial infections and results from mutations in the gene that codes for fucosyltransferase, required for the synthesis of sialyl-Lewis X on neutrophils.

III. Chronic Inflammation

A. **General considerations**
1. Chronic inflammation can occur when the inciting injury is persistent or recurrent or when the inflammatory reaction is insufficient to completely degrade the agent (e.g., bacteria, tissue debris, foreign bodies) that incites the inflammatory reaction.
2. It often occurs de novo, without a preceding acute inflammatory reaction.
3. It occurs in two major patterns: chronic nonspecific inflammation and granulomatous inflammation.

B. **Chronic nonspecific inflammation**
1. A **cellular reaction** with a preponderance of **mononuclear (round) cells** (macrophages, lymphocytes, and plasma cells), often with a **proliferation of fibroblasts and new vessels. Scarring** and **distortion of tissue architecture,** is characteristic.
2. This type of inflammation is mediated by the interaction of monocytes-macrophages with lymphocytes.
3. Monocytes are recruited from the circulation by various chemotactic factors.
4. Cytokines derived from monocytes-macrophages activate lymphocytes. The activated lymphocytes, in turn, are the source of additional cytokines that activate monocytes-macrophages.
5. B lymphocyte activation by macrophage-presented antigen results in the formation of antibody-producing plasma cells.

C. **Granulomatous inflammation**
1. This type of inflammation is characterized by granulomas, which are nodular collections of specialized macrophages referred to as **epithelioid cells.** Granulomas are usually surrounded by a rim of lymphocytes.
2. Activation of macrophages by interactions with T lymphocytes is involved. Poorly digestible antigen is presented by macrophages to CD4+ lymphocytes. Interaction with the antigen-specific T-cell receptor of these cells triggers the release of cytokines (especially interferon-γ), which mediate the transformation of monocytes and macrophages to epithelioid cells and giant cells.
3. **Caseous necrosis** is often characteristic (especially in tuberculosis), resulting from the killing of mycobacteria-laden macrophages by T lymphocytes and possibly by cytokines or sensitized macrophages. **Noncaseating pulmonary granulomatous disease is caused most often by sarcoidosis.**
4. The presence of **multinucleated giant cells** derived from macrophages is also characteristic. The **Langhans giant cell** has nuclei arranged in a horseshoe-shaped pattern about the periphery of the cell and is particularly characteristic of, but not specific for, the granulomatous inflammation of tuberculosis. The **foreign body giant cell** has scattered nuclei.
5. Granulomatous inflammation is the characteristic form of inflammation associated with a number of diverse etiologic agents, including:
  a. **Infectious agents**
    (1) *Mycobacterium tuberculosis* and *M. leprae*
    (2) *Blastomyces dermatitidis, Histoplasma capsulatum, Coccidioides immitis,* and many other fungi

(3) *Treponema pallidum*
(4) The bacterium of cat-scratch disease
b. **Foreign bodies**
c. **Unknown etiology,** including sarcoidosis

IV. Tissue Repair

A. **Restoration of normal structure.** This occurs when the connective tissue infrastructure remains relatively intact. It requires that the surviving affected parenchymal cells have the capacity to regenerate.

1. **Labile cells**
   a. These cells divided actively throughout life to replace lost cells.
   b. They are capable of regeneration after injury.
   c. They include cells of the epidermis and gastrointestinal mucosa, cells lining the surface of the genitourinary tract, and hematopoietic cells of the bone marrow.
2. **Stable cells**
   a. Characteristically, these cells undergo few divisions but are capable of division when activated; that is, they can regenerate from G_0 cells when needed.
   b. They are also capable of regeneration following injury.
   c. They include hepatocytes, renal tubular cells, parenchymal cells of many glands, and numerous mesenchymal cells (e.g., smooth muscle, cartilage, connective tissue, endothelium, osteoblasts).
3. **Permanent cells**
   a. These cells have been considered to be incapable of division and regeneration (a view challenged by recent provocative new evidence involving stem cells).
   b. They include neurons and myocardial cells.
   c. They are replaced by scar tissue (typically fibrosis; gliosis in the central nervous system) after irreversible injury and cell loss.

B. **Cellular proliferation.** This process is mediated by an assemblage of growth factors.

1. **Platelet-derived growth factor (PDGF)** is a **competence factor** that promotes the proliferative response of fibroblasts and smooth muscle cells on concurrent stimulation by **progression factors** (e.g., other growth factors). Indirectly in this manner, PDGF promotes the synthesis of collagen.
   a. PDGF is synthesized by platelets and several other cells.
   b. PDGF promotes the chemotactic migration of fibroblasts and smooth muscle cells.
   c. PDGF is chemotactic for monocytes.
   d. PDGF reacts with specific cell-surface receptors. Generally, growth factor receptors are transmembrane proteins that respond to ligand interaction by conformational changes that induce tyrosine kinase activity in their intracellular domains.
2. **Epidermal growth factor (EGF)** is a progression factor that promotes the growth of endothelial cells and fibroblasts as well as epithelial cells.
3. **Fibroblast growth factors (FGFs)** promote the synthesis of extracellular matrix protein (including fibronectin) by fibroblasts, endothelial cells, monocytes, and other cells. **Fibronectin** is a glycoprotein with the following characteristics:
   a. It is chemotactic for fibroblasts and endothelial cells.
   b. It promotes angiogenesis (new vessel formation).
   c. It links other extracellular matrix components (e.g., collagen, proteoglycans) and macromolecules (e.g., fibrin, heparin) to cell-surface integrins. Integrins mediate interactions between cells and extracellular matrix.
4. **Transforming growth factors (TGFs)**
   a. **TGF-α** functions similarly to EGF.
   b. **TGF-β** is a **growth inhibitor** for many cell types and may aid in modulating the repair process; it is also a chemotactic factor for macrophages and fibroblasts.
5. **Macrophage-derived growth factors (IL-1 and TNF)** promote the proliferation of fibroblasts, smooth muscle cells, and endothelial cells.

C. **The repair process**

1. **Removal of debris** begins in the early stages of inflammation and is initiated by liquefaction and removal of dead cellular material and other debris.
2. **Formation of granulation tissue**
   a. Granulation tissue is highly vascular, newly formed connective tissue consisting of **capillaries** and **fibroblasts;** it fills defects created by liquefaction of cellular debris.
   b. Granulation tissue is not related to granulomas or granulomatous inflammation.
3. **Scarring**
   a. **Collagen** is produced by fibroblasts. As the amount of collagen in granulation tissue progressively increases, the tissue becomes gradually less vascular and less cellular.
   b. Progressive **contraction of the wound** also occurs, often resulting in deformity of the original structure.

D. **Factors that delay or impede repair**

1. Retention of debris
2. Impaired circulation
3. Persistent infection
4. Metabolic disorders, such as diabetes mellitus (associated with both susceptibility to infection and impaired circulation)
5. Dietary deficiency of ascorbic acid or protein, which are required for collagen formation

Q REVIEW TEST

***Directions:** Each of the numbered items or incomplete statements in this section is followed by answers or by completions of the statement. Select the **one** lettered answer or completion that is best in each case.*

1. A 72-year-old man presents with a 3-day history of progressively worsening productive cough, fever, chills, and signs of toxicity. Prominent physical findings include signs of consolidation and rales over the right lung base. Sputum culture is positive for *Streptococcus pneumoniae*. An intra-alveolar exudate filling the alveoli of the involved portion of the lung is present. Which of the following types of inflammatory cells is most likely a prominent feature of this exudate?

(A) Basophils
(B) Eosinophils
(C) Lymphocytes
(D) Monocytes-macrophages
(E) Neutrophils

2. A routine complete blood count performed on a 22-year-old medical student reveals an abnormality in the differential leukocyte count. She has been complaining of frequent sneezing and "watery" eyes during the past several weeks and reports that she frequently had such episodes in the spring and summer. Which of the following cell types is most likely to be increased?

(A) Basophils
(B) Eosinophils
(C) Lymphocytes
(D) Monocytes
(E) Neutrophils

3. A 16-year-old boy presents with a 24-hour history of severe abdominal pain, nausea, vomiting, and low-grade fever. The pain is initially periumbilical in location but has migrated to the right lower quadrant of the abdomen, with maximal tenderness elicited at a site one third between the crest of the ileum and the umbilicus (McBurney point). The leukocyte count is 14,000/mm^3, with 74% segmented neutrophils and 12% bands. Surgery is performed. Which of the following describes the expected findings at the affected site?

(A) Fistula (abnormal duct or passage) connecting to the abdominal wall
(B) Granulation tissue (new vessels and young fibroblasts) with a prominent infiltrate of eosinophils
(C) Granulomatous inflammation with prominent aggregates of epithelioid cells and multinucleated giant cells
(D) Massive infiltration of lymphocytes and plasma cells
(E) Prominent areas of edema, congestion, and a purulent reaction with localized areas of abscess formation

4. A 2-year-old boy presents with recurrent infections involving multiple organ systems. Extensive investigation results in a diagnosis of chronic granulomatous disease of childhood. Which of the following most closely characterizes the abnormality in this patient's phagocytic cells?

(A) Decreased killing of microorganisms because of enhanced production of hydrogen peroxide
(B) Deficiency of NADPH oxidase activity
(C) Impaired chemotaxis and migration caused by abnormal microtubule formation
(D) Inability to kill streptococci
(E) Increased myeloperoxiidase-halide-mediated killing of catalase-positive organisms as compared to catalase-negative organisms

5. A laboratory experiment is performed to evaluate the chemotactic potential of a group of potential mediators. Which of the following substances most likely has the greatest affinity for neutrophils?

(A) C5a
(B) Fucosyl transferase
(C) β_2-Integrin
(D) P-selectin
(E) Tumor necrosis factor-α

6. The accompanying figure is representative of the pulmonary pathology of a 54-year-old man who sought medical care for low-grade fever, anorexia, fatigue, night sweats, weight loss, and persistent cough with bouts of hemoptysis. A chest X-ray had revealed a right apical infiltrate with beginning cavitation, and examination of the sputum had revealed acid-fast bacilli. This condition is typified by a form of inflammation that *invariably* includes which of the following?

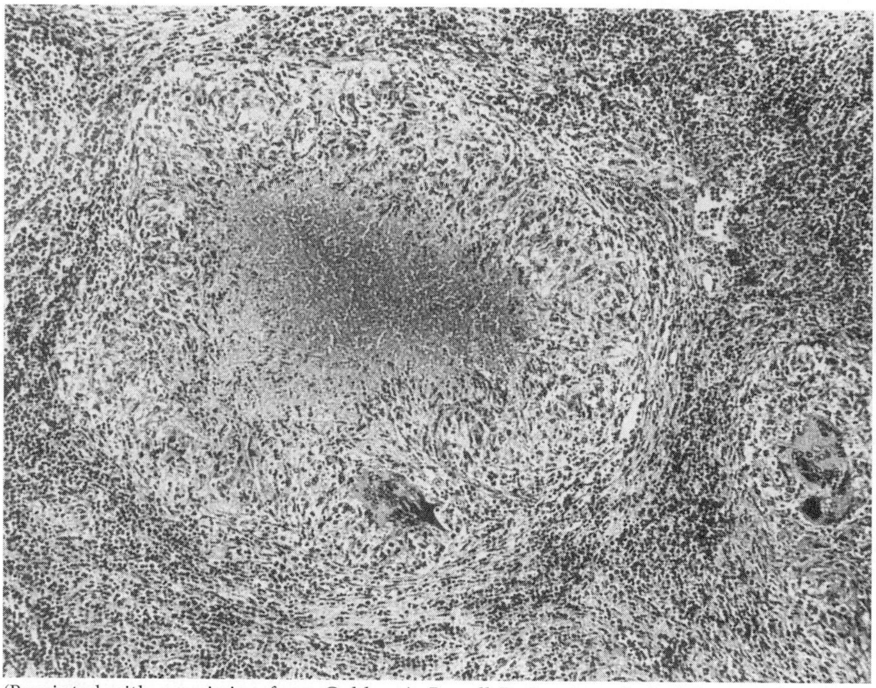

(Reprinted with permission from Golden A, Powell D, Jennings C: *Pathology: Understanding Human Disease,* 2nd ed. Baltimore, Williams & Wilkins, 1985, p 40.)

(A) A morphologically identifiable etiologic agent
(B) Caseous necrosis
(C) Clusters of epithelioid cells
(D) Multinucleated giant cells
(E) Prominent granulation tissue

7. A 26-year-old African-American woman has bilateral hilar adenopathy, and radiography reveals multiple reticular densities in both lung fields. A bronchoscopic biopsy reveals granulomatous inflammation with multiple giant cells of the Langhans type and no evidence of caseous necrosis. Which of the following is the most likely diagnosis?

(A) Aspergillosis
(B) Coccidioidomycosis
(C) Histoplasmosis
(D) Sarcoidosis
(E) Tuberculosis

8. In a laboratory exercise for medical students, an unknown compound is studied. The students are informed that the compound has been isolated from endothelial cells and that its synthesis can be inhibited by aspirin. In the laboratory, the students demonstrate that the compound is a potent vasodilator and platelet antiaggregant. Given these findings, the substance is most likely which of the following mediators?

(A) 5-Hydroperoxyeicosatetraenoic acid (5-HPETE)
(B) Leukotriene (LTC_4)
(C) Lipoxin A_4 (LXA_4)
(D) Prostacyclin (PGI_2)
(E) Thromboxane A_2 (TxA_2)

9. A 70-year-old man presents with the sudden onset of left-sided weakness, spasticity, and hyperactive and pathologic reflexes. The most serious consequences of this disorder are the result of damage to which of the following cell types?

(A) Labile cells
(B) Multipotent adult progenitor cells
(C) Permanent cells
(D) Stable cells

ANSWERS AND EXPLANATIONS

1-E. The patient has bacterial pneumonia due to *Streptococcus pneumoniae,* a classic example of severe acute inflammation. In the early stages of acute inflammation, the neutrophil is the most prominent inflammatory cell. It is noteworthy that in many instances, bacterial infections are characterized by neutrophilic infiltrates. It is also noteworthy that *S. pneumoniae* (also known as the "pneumococcus") is the most common etiologic agent of lobar pneumonia (see Chapter 14).

2-B. This type of reaction is primarily mediated by the release of histamine from tissue mast cells, and the associated cellular infiltrate and peripheral blood findings represent mobilization and increased numbers of eosinophils. The symptoms reported are those of seasonal rhinitis, better known as "hay fever," a manifestation of type I hypersensitivity (see Chapter 5).

3-E. The clinical findings are typical of acute appendicitis, another example of severe acute inflammation. Because the danger of perforation is great, early appendectomy is the treatment of choice. Suppurative or purulent inflammation is characterized by the prominent areas of edema resulting from increased vascular permeability, congestion, and a purulent (pus-containing) exudate consisting of necrotic cells and large numbers of neutrophils. In addition, other signs of acute inflammation, such as congestion, are prominent. The patient responds with the sensation of pain (induced by increased hydrostatic pressure in tissue and by chemical mediators such as bradykinin) and the acute phase reaction (in this instance, fever and neutrophilic leukocytosis with a "shift to the left").

4-B. Chronic granulomatous disease of childhood, a condition characterized by repeated infections and most commonly X-linked inheritance, is marked by failure of the myeloperoxidase-halide system of killing within phagocytic cells. It is caused by deficiency of NADPH oxidase activity. This results in a secondary deficiency of reactive oxygen metabolites, including H_2O_2, which, along with halide ions, functions as a substrate for myeloperoxidase. A hallmark of the disorder is the failure of intracellular killing of catalase-positive organisms, exemplified by staphylococci. These organisms are ingested but not killed. The impaired phagocytic cell is incapable of producing H_2O_2, and any H_2O_2 produced by the microorganism itself is inactivated by endogenous catalase. In contrast, catalase-negative microorganisms, such as streptococci, are ingested and killed. They too produce endogenous H_2O_2, which is thus available as one of the substrates for myeloperoxidase. In a sense, the microorganisms assist in their own killing.

5-A. Several substances have chemotactic potential for neutrophils (see Table 2-1). C5a is a prominent example.

6-C. The clinical description and the figure are both typical of advanced secondary tuberculosis. Although this disorder is now relatively uncommon, its incidence is increasing, especially in association with immunodeficiency. Tuberculosis is a classic cause of granulomatous inflammation, which is characterized by the presence of "granulomas," which by definition consist of clusters of modified macrophages referred to as epithelioid cells. Additional features such as caseous necrosis, giant cell formation, and identifiable etiologic agents may or may not be present and are not invariable features of this form of inflammation. Granulation tissue is a feature of early repair and is totally unrelated to granulomatous inflammation.

7-D. The histologic hallmark of sarcoidosis is the finding of noncaseating granulomatous inflammation. Although this finding is not entirely specific, a non-necrotizing granulomatous response of the lung is rarely seen in patients with tuberculosis or deep-seated fungal infections. These infections usually have a necrotizing component.

8-D. Prostacyclin (PGI_2) is a prostaglandin that is synthesized and expressed primarily in endothelial cells. It is a product of the cyclooxygenase pathway of arachidonic acid metabolism, which is inhibited by aspirin. PGI_2 is a potent vasodilator and platelet antiaggregant. These properties are often contrasted with those of thromboxane A_2 (TxA_2), which is primarily synthesized in platelets and is a vasoconstrictor and platelet aggregant. The other compounds are products of the lipoxygenase pathway of arachidonic acid metabolism, which is not inhibited by aspirin.

9-C. The clinical findings are those of "stroke," or cerebrovascular disease. This group of entities encompasses injury to the brain caused by disorders of the cerebral vasculature, such as thrombosis, embolism, and hemorrhage (see Chapter 3). The most important consequence is damage to neurons, because neurons are considered to be "permanent" cells, incapable of division and replication (however, this has been recently challenged as the result of provocative stem cell research). Permanent cells are exemplified by neurons and myocardial cells. Labile cells, such as cells of the epidermis or gastrointestinal mucosa, divide throughout the life of the individual. Stable cells, such as hepatocytes and renal tubular cells, do not divide regularly but have the capacity to divide and regenerate as needed.

CHAPTER 3

Hemodynamic Dysfunction

I. Hemorrhage

A. **General considerations**

1. Hemorrhage is the **escape of blood** from the vasculature into surrounding tissues, a hollow organ or body cavity, or to the outside.
2. Hemorrhage is most often caused by **trauma.**

B. **Hematoma.** This localized hemorrhage occurs within a tissue or organ.

C. **Hemothorax, hemopericardium, hemoperitoneum, and hemarthrosis.** Hemorrhage may occur in the pleural cavity, pericardial sac, peritoneal cavity, or a synovial space, respectively.

D. **Petechial hemorrhages, petechiae, or purpura.** These small, punctate hemorrhages occur in the skin, mucous membranes, or serosal surfaces.

E. **Ecchymosis.** This diffuse hemorrhage is usually in skin and subcutaneous tissue.

II. Hyperemia

This is a **localized increase in the volume of blood** in capillaries and small vessels.

A. **Active hyperemia.** The cause is localized arteriolar dilation (e.g., blushing, inflammation).

B. **Passive congestion (passive hyperemia).** The cause is obstructed venous return or increased back pressure from congestive heart failure (CHF).

1. **Acute passive congestion** occurs in shock, acute inflammation, or sudden right-sided heart failure.
2. **Chronic passive congestion**
   a. **Chronic passive congestion of the lung** is caused most often by **left-sided heart failure** or **mitral stenosis.**
      (1) **Congestion and distention of alveolar capillaries** lead to **capillary rupture** and passage of red cells into the alveoli.
      (2) Phagocytosis and degradation of red cells result in intra-alveolar hemosiderin-laden macrophages called **heart failure cells.**
      (3) In long-standing congestion, fibrosis of interstitium and hemosiderin deposition result in **brown induration** of the lung.

b. **Chronic passive congestion of the liver and lower extremities** is most often caused by **right-sided heart failure.**
   (1) **Nutmeg liver, a** speckled, nutmeg-like appearance on cut section, may occur.
   (2) This condition is produced by a combination of dilated, congested central veins and the surrounding brownish-yellow, often fatty, liver cells.

III. Infarction

A. **Definition. Infarction is necrosis resulting from ischemia** caused by obstruction of the blood supply; the necrotic tissue is referred to as an **infarct.**

B. **Anemic infarcts**
1. These infarts are **white or pale infarcts.**
2. They are usually caused by arterial occlusions in the **heart, spleen, and kidney.**

C. **Hemorrhagic infarcts**
1. These infarcts are **red infarcts,** in which red cells ooze into the necrotic area.
2. They occur characteristically in the **lung and gastrointestinal tract** as the result of arterial occlusion. These sites are loose, well-vascularized tissues with redundant arterial blood supplies (in the lung, from the pulmonary and bronchial systems; in the gastrointestinal tract, from multiple anastomoses between branches of the mesenteric artery), and **hemorrhage into the infarct** occurs from the nonobstructed portion of the vasculature.
3. They can also be caused by **venous occlusion.** This is an important contribution to infarcts associated with volvulus, incarcerated hernias, and postoperative adhesions.

IV. Thrombosis

A. **General considerations**
1. Thrombosis is **intravascular coagulation of blood,** often causing significant interruption of blood flow.
2. It is pathologically predisposed by many conditions, including venous stasis, usually from immobilization; CHF; polycythemia; sickle cell disease; visceral malignancies; and the use of oral contraceptives, especially in association with cigarette smoking.

B. **Thrombogenesis.** This process results from the interaction of platelets, damaged endothelial cells, and the coagulation cascade.
1. **Platelets**
   a. **Platelet functions**
      (1) Maintain the physical integrity of the vascular endothelium
      (2) Participate in endothelial repair through the contribution of platelet-derived growth factor (PDGF)
      (3) Form platelet plugs
      (4) Promote the coagulation cascade through the platelet phospholipid complex
   b. **Reactions involving platelets**
      (1) **Adhesion**
         (a) Vessel injury exposes subendothelial collagen, leading to **platelet adhesion** (adherence to the subendothelial surface).
         (b) Interaction of specific platelet-surface **glycoprotein receptors** and subendothelial collagen is mediated by **von Willebrand factor.**
      (2) **Release reaction.** Soon after adhesion, platelets release adenosine diphosphate (ADP), histamine, serotonin, PDGF, and other platelet granule constituents.

(3) **Activation of coagulation cascade.** Conformational change in the platelet membrane makes the platelet phospholipid complex available, thus contributing to the activation of the coagulation cascade, leading to the formation of thrombin.

(4) **Arachidonic acid metabolism.** Arachidonic acid, provided by activation of platelet membrane phospholipase, proceeds through the **cyclooxygenase pathway** to the production of **thromboxane A_2 (TxA_2).** Platelet TxA_2 is a potent vasoconstrictor and platelet aggregant. The inhibition of cyclooxygenase by low-dose aspirin is the basis of aspirin therapy for prevention of thrombotic disease.

(5) **Platelet aggregation**

(a) Platelets stick to each other (as contrasted to adhesion, the adherence of platelets to the underlying subendothelium).

(b) Additional platelets are recruited from the circulation to produce the initial hemostatic platelet plug.

(c) The process is mediated by the glycoprotein IIb-IIIa complex on the surface of platelets that is required for the linking of platelets by fibrinogen bridges.

(d) Agonists that promote aggregation include **ADP, thrombin,** and **TxA_2,** as well as **collagen, epinephrine,** and **platelet-activating factor,** derived from the granules of basophils and mast cells.

(6) **Stabilization of the platelet plug.** Fibrinogen bridges bind the aggregated platelets together. The platelet mass is stabilized by fibrin.

(7) **Limitation of platelet plug formation.** Prostacyclin (PGI_2), another product of the cyclooxygenase pathway, is synthesized by endothelial cells. Endothelial PGI_2 is antagonistic to platelet TxA_2 and limits further platelet aggregation. Fibrin degradation products are also inhibitors of platelet aggregation.

2. **Endothelial cells**

a. These cells are resistant to the thrombogenic influence of platelets and coagulation proteins. **Intact endothelial cells** act to modulate several aspects of **hemostasis** and oppose coagulation after injury by **thromboresistance.**

b. Some **functions of endothelial cells include:**

(1) Producing **heparin-like molecules,** endothelial proteoglycans that activate **antithrombin III,** which neutralizes thrombin and other coagulation factors, including factors IXa and Xa

(2) Secreting plasminogen activators, such as **tissue plasminogen activator (TPA)**

(3) Degrading ADP

(4) Taking up, inactivating, and clearing **thrombin**

(5) Synthesizing **thrombomodulin,** a cell-surface protein that binds thrombin and converts it to an activator of **protein C,** a vitamin K–dependent plasma protein. Activated protein C (APC) cleaves factors Va and VIIIa, thus inhibiting coagulation.

(6) Synthesizing **protein S,** a cofactor for APC

(7) Synthesizing and releasing **PGI_2**

(8) Synthesizing and releasing nitric oxide, which has actions similar to those of PGI_2

3. **Coagulation cascade.** This has been classically described as following two distinct, but interconnected, pathways **(Figure 3-1).**

a. **Extrinsic pathway of coagulation** is initiated by **tissue factor,** which activates **factor VII** and forms a **tissue factor–factor VIIa complex.** The complex initiates coagulation through the activation of **factor X to factor Xa** (and additionally factor IX to factor IXa). Factor Xa converts **prothrombin (factor II) to thrombin (factor IIa). Factor Va** is a cofactor required in the conversion of prothrombin to thrombin. Thrombin converts **fibrinogen to fibrin.**

(1) The prothrombin-mediated cleavage of fibrinogen results in a fibrin monomer, which is polymerized and stabilized by **factor XIII,** thus forming the fibrin clot.

(2) The action of the tissue factor–factor VIIa complex is limited by tissue factor pathway inhibitor.

(3) The extrinsic pathway is clinically evaluated by the **prothrombin time (PT),** which is a measure of factors II, V, VII, X, and fibrinogen.

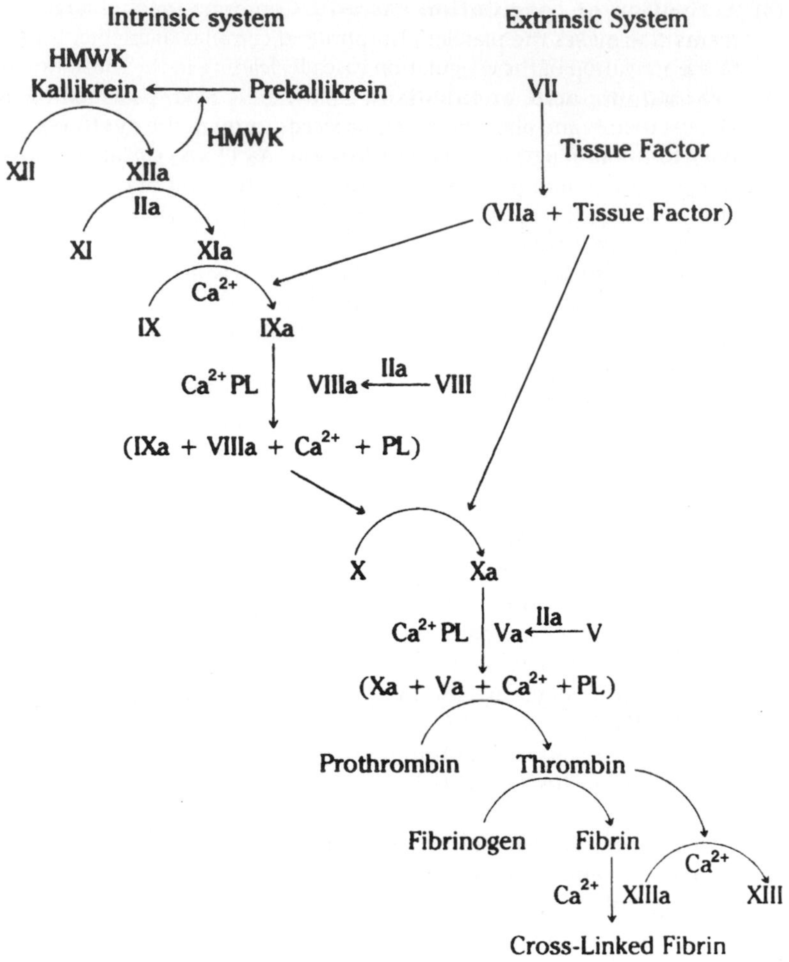

Figure 3-1 Classic representation of the coagulation cascade. This simplified conceptualization is useful for laboratory testing, but the division into extrinsic and intrinsic pathways is somewhat artificial. The role of the contact factors (factor XII, prekallikrein, and high-molecular-weight kininogen [HMWK]) in physiologic clotting has been questioned, and there are interactions between the so-called intrinsic and extrinsic pathways, the most important of which is the activation of factor IX to factor IXa by the tissue factor–factor VIIa complex. Additionally, thrombin is an activator of factor V to factor Va, factor VIII to factor VIIIa, and factor XI to factor XIa. (Modified from Kjeldsberg C, Beutler E, et al: *Practical Diagnosis of Hematologic Disorders.* Chicago, ASCP Press, 1989, p 527.)

b. **Intrinsic pathway of coagulation** involves activation of all clotting factors with the exception of factors VII and XIII.
   (1) This pathway may involve **contact activation** with interactions of the so-called contact factors: **factor XII** (Hageman factor), **prekallikrein,** and **high-molecular-weight kininogen** as well as **factor XI.** Contact activation is important in in vitro clotting in glass containers and in laboratory testing, but its physiologic role has been questioned because a deficiency of the contact factors is not associated with abnormal bleeding.
   (2) It is probably initiated by the tissue factor–factor VIIa complex (from the extrinsic pathway), activating **factor IX to factor IXa.** Factor IXa, in turn, leads to the conversion of factor X to factor Xa, catalyzed by **factor VIIIa.** It can also be activated by the **platelet phospholipid complex,** which becomes available through conformational changes in the platelet membrane.

(3) Thrombin production further stimulates the pathway by the activation of **factor XI to factor XIa** and by activation of the cofactors factor V to factor Va and factor VIII to factor VIIIa.

(4) The intrinsic pathway can be evaluated by the **partial thromboplastin time (PTT),** which is a measure of factors II, V, VIII, IX, X, XI, XII, and fibrinogen.

C. **Fibrinolysis (thrombus dissolution).** This is concurrent with thrombogenesis and modulates coagulation. It restores blood flow in vessels occluded by a thrombus and facilitates healing after inflammation and injury.

1. The proenzyme **plasminogen** is converted by proteolysis to **plasmin,** the most important fibrinolytic protease.
2. Plasmin splits fibrin.
3. It is a classic teaching that factor XII to XIIa activation links the fibrinolytic system, coagulation system, complement system, and kinin system.

D. **Thrombotic disorders**

1. **Classification**
   a. Thrombotic disorders can be **antithrombotic** (hemorrhagic), leading to pathologic bleeding states such as hemophilia, Christmas disease, and von Willebrand disease. The hemorrhagic disorders are discussed further in Chapter 13.
   b. They can also be **prothrombotic,** leading to hypercoagulability with pathologic thrombosis.
2. **Hereditary thrombophilia**
   a. **General considerations.** Hereditary thrombophilia is a prothrombotic familial syndrome occurring most often in adolescents or young women.
      (1) Characteristic features include recurrent venous thrombosis and thromboembolism.
      (2) The syndrome can be caused by deficiency of a number of antithrombotic proteins, including **antithrombin III, protein C,** and **protein S.**
   b. **Factor V Leiden**
      (1) This is the most frequent cause of hereditary thrombophilia.
      (2) This is an abnormal factor V protein with a specific mutation that alters the cleavage site targeted by APC. The mutation prevents the cleavage and inactivation of the mutant factor Va by APC, a phenomenon referred to as "hereditary resistance to activated protein C."
   c. **Prothrombin 20210A transition**
      (1) This is the second most common cause of hereditary thrombophilia (as of this writing).
      (2) This G-to-A mutation in the 3′-untranslated region of the prothrombin gene is associated with elevated plasma prothrombin levels and an increase in venous thrombosis.
   d. **Methylene tetrahydrofolate reductase mutation (MTHFR C677T)**
      (1) This results in a moderate increase in serum homocysteine, which is associated with both arterial and venous thrombosis. The increased homocysteine can be reduced by dietary supplementation with folic acid and vitamins B_6 (pyridoxine) and B_{12} (cobalamin).
      (2) This is also associated with an increased risk of neural tube defects and possibly a number of diverse neoplasms.
   e. **Increased levels of factor VIII, factor IX, factor XI, or fibrinogen** are also associated with increased venous thrombosis.
3. **Antiphospholipid antibody syndrome**
   a. This prothrombotic disorder is characterized by autoantibodies directed against a number of protein antigens complexed to phospholipids. It is further characterized by recurrent venous and arterial thromboembolism, fetal loss, thrombocytopenia, and a variety of neurologic manifestations.

b. This syndrome is most often diagnosed because of an incidental finding of a prolonged PTT. This is a paradoxical abnormality, because a prolonged PTT is usually considered to be an indicator of antithrombotic or hemorrhagic syndromes, just the reverse of the prothrombotic characteristics of the antiphospholipid antibody syndrome. The prolonged PTT is thought to be an in vitro artifact caused by interaction of the antiphospholipid antibodies with the phospholipid reagent used in the PTT test.

c. Sometimes (but not always), this syndrome is associated with systemic lupus erythematosus (SLE). For this reason, an antiphospholipid antibody that prolongs the PTT is sometimes referred to as the **lupus anticoagulant.** Another antiphospholipid antibody associated with SLE is the anticardiolipin antibody, which can cause a false-positive serologic test for syphilis.

4. **Disseminated intravascular coagulation (DIC)**
   a. DIC is both a prothrombotic and antithrombotic disorder characterized by widespread thrombosis and hemorrhage resulting from the consumption of platelets and coagulation factors.
   b. DIC is discussed further in Chapter 13.
5. **Heparin-induced thrombocytopenia (HIT) syndrome**
   a. This syndrome is characterized by heparin-induced thrombocytopenia (and thrombosis) and is a consequence of therapy with high-molecular-weight heparin.
   b. It is thought to be caused by antibodies to the complex of heparin and platelet factor 4 (PF4).

E. **Morphologic characteristics of thrombi and clots**

1. **Arterial thrombi**
   a. These thrombi are formed in areas of **active blood flow.**
   b. When mature, they demonstrate alternate dark gray layers of platelets interspersed with lighter layers of fibrin. This layering results in the **lines of Zahn.**
   c. Eventually they liquefy and disappear or are organized with fibrous tissue formation. Recanalization, new blood vessel formation within a thrombus, restores blood flow.
2. **Venous thrombi (phlebothrombosis)**
   a. These thrombi are formed in areas of **less active blood flow,** most often in the **veins of the lower extremities** and in the periprostatic or other pelvic veins.
   b. They are predisposed by **venous stasis,** with a high incidence occurring in hospitalized patients on bed rest.
   c. They are **dark red** with a higher concentration of red cells than arterial thrombi. Lines of Zahn are not prominent or are absent.
   d. They are often associated with concurrent venous inflammatory changes. Inflammation of veins with thrombus formation is referred to as **thrombophlebitis.**
3. **Postmortem clots**
   a. These clots appear soon after death and are not true thrombi. In contrast to true thrombi, they are not attached to the vessel wall.
   b. Settling of red cells results in a two-layered appearance: **currant jelly appearance** in the red cell-rich lower layer and a **chicken fat appearance** in the cell-poor upper layer.

V. Embolism

This is the passage and eventual trapping within the vasculature of any of a wide variety of mass objects.

A. **Thromboembolism.** Embolism of fragments of **thrombi** is the most frequent form of embolism.

1. **Pulmonary emboli**
   a. These emboli are an important cause of sudden death, usually occurring in **immobilized postoperative patients** and in those with **CHF.**

b. Immobilization leads to **venous thrombosis** in the lower extremities. Portions of the friable thrombus break away, travel through the venous circulation, and lodge in branches of the pulmonary artery.

c. Pulmonary emboli vary in size from **saddle emboli** obstructing the bifurcation of the pulmonary artery, which can produce sudden death, to less clinically significant small emboli. Emboli of intermediate size can cause pulmonary hypertension and acute right ventricular failure.

d. Obstruction of the pulmonary artery leads to **pulmonary infarction,** a term often used interchangeably with pulmonary embolism. **Hemorrhagic pulmonary infarcts** result. These are characteristically wedge-shaped and located just beneath the pleura.

2. **Arterial emboli**

a. **Sites of origin.** Arterial emboli usually arise from a mural thrombus, a thrombus that adheres to one wall of a heart chamber or major artery.

(1) Mural thrombi in the left atrium are associated especially with **mitral stenosis** with atrial fibrillation.

(2) Mural thrombi in the left ventricle are caused by **myocardial infarction.**

(3) Thrombi at the junction of the internal and external carotid arteries are a cause of thrombotic brain infarcts and can also be a site of origin of emboli.

b. **Sites of arrest**

(1) **Branches of the carotid artery,** most frequently the **middle cerebral artery,** leading to **cerebral infarction**

(2) **Branches of the mesenteric artery,** leading to **hemorrhagic infarction of the intestine**

(3) **Branches of the renal artery,** producing characteristic wedge-shaped **pale infarcts of the renal cortex**

3. **Paradoxical emboli** are left-sided emboli that originate in the venous circulation but gain access to the arterial circulation through a right-to-left shunt, most often a **patent foramen ovale** or an **atrial septal defect.**

B. **Other forms of embolism**

1. **Fat emboli**

a. These emboli are **particles of bone marrow and other fatty intraosseous tissue** that enter the circulation as a **result of severe (often multiple) fractures.**

b. They lodge in the lungs, brain, kidneys, and other organs.

c. They may be asymptomatic or may be manifest clinically by the potentially fatal **fat embolism syndrome,** characterized by pulmonary distress, cutaneous petechiae, and various neurologic manifestations.

2. **Air emboli**

a. These emboli result from the **introduction of air into the circulation,** most often by a penetrating chest injury or as a consequence of a clumsily performed criminal abortion.

b. They can occur as **decompression sickness,** observed in deep-sea divers who return to the surface too rapidly. Bubbles of relatively insoluble nitrogen come out of solution and obstruct the circulation, producing musculoskeletal pain (**"the bends"**) and small infarcts (**caisson disease**) in the central nervous system, bones, and other tissues. Because nitrogen has an affinity for adipose tissue, obese persons are at increased risk for this disorder.

3. **Amniotic fluid emboli**

a. These emboli are caused by escape of amniotic fluid into the maternal circulation.

b. They can activate the coagulation process, leading to **DIC.**

c. They can cause maternal death.

4. **Miscellaneous sources of emboli** include fragments of **atherosclerotic plaques,** clumps of inflamed, **infected tissue,** and **tumor fragments.**

VI. Edema

This is an abnormal accumulation of fluid in interstitial tissue spaces or body cavities.

A. **Causes of edema**
1. **Increased hydrostatic pressure** is exemplified by CHF.
   a. Right-sided heart failure results in **peripheral edema.**
   b. Left-sided heart failure results in **pulmonary edema.**
2. **Increased capillary permeability** occurs in inflammation or with injury to capillary endothelium, as may occur in burn injury.
3. **Decreased oncotic pressure** is from hypoalbuminemia caused by:
   a. Increased loss of protein, as, for example, by renal loss in the **nephrotic syndrome**
   b. Decreased production of albumin in **cirrhosis of the liver**
4. **Increased sodium retention** can occur as either a primary or secondary phenomenon.
   a. Primary sodium retention, associated with **renal disorders**
   b. Secondary sodium retention, such as occurs in **CHF**
      (1) Decreased cardiac output results in decreased renal blood flow, which activates the renin-angiotensin system.
      (2) In turn, this activates aldosterone production, with resultant retention of sodium and water.
5. **Blockage of lymphatics** results in **lymphedema.**

B. **Types of edema**
1. **Anasarca** is generalized edema.
2. **Hydrothorax** is accumulation of fluid in the pleural cavity.
3. **Hydropericardium** is abnormal accumulation of fluid in the pericardial cavity.
4. **Hydroperitoneum (ascites)** is abnormal accumulation of fluid in the peritoneal cavity.
5. **Transudate**
   a. This noninflammatory edema fluid results from **altered intravascular hydrostatic or osmotic pressure.**
   b. It has a low protein content and a specific gravity less than 1.012.
6. **Exudate**
   a. This edema fluid results from **increased vascular permeability** caused by **inflammation.**
   b. It has a high protein content, a specific gravity exceeding 1.020, and characteristically contains large numbers of **inflammatory leukocytes.** Because the metabolically active leukocytes consume glucose, the glucose content is often greatly reduced.

VII. Shock

This condition represents circulatory collapse with resultant hypoperfusion and decreased oxygenation of tissues.

A. **Causes of shock**
1. **Decreased cardiac output,** as occurs in hemorrhage or severe left ventricular failure
2. **Widespread peripheral vasodilation,** as occurs in sepsis or severe trauma, with hypotension often being a prominent feature

B. **Types of shock**
1. **Hypovolemic shock** is circulatory collapse resulting from the acute reduction in circulating blood volume caused by:
   a. Severe **hemorrhage** or massive **loss of fluid** from the skin, from extensive burns, or from severe trauma
   b. Loss of fluid from the gastrointestinal tract, through severe **vomiting** or **diarrhea**

2. **Cardiogenic shock** is circulatory collapse resulting from pump failure of the left ventricle, most often caused by massive myocardial infarction.
3. **Septic shock** is most characteristically associated with gram-negative infections, which cause **gram-negative endotoxemia;** also occurs with gram-positive and other infections.
   a. Initially, vasodilation may result in an overall increase in blood flow. However, significant peripheral pooling of blood from peripheral vasodilation results in relative **hypovolemia** and **impaired perfusion.**
   b. **Lipopolysaccharide** (endotoxin from the outer membrane of gram-negative bacteria) and other bacterial products appear to induce a cascade of cytokines (e.g., TNF, IL-1, IL-6, and IL-8), activate complement components and the kinin system, and **cause direct toxic injury to vessels.**
   c. **Endothelial injury** can lead to **activation of the coagulation pathways** and to DIC.
   d. Another group of toxic molecules, the so-called superantigens, produces septic shock-like manifestations. The release of these molecules occurs in the "toxic shock syndrome," which is most often associated with *Staphylococcus aureus* infection.
4. **Neurogenic shock** is most often associated with **severe trauma** and reactive peripheral vasodilation.

C. **Stages of shock**

1. **Nonprogressive (early) stage. Compensatory mechanisms,** including increased heart rate and increased peripheral resistance, maintain perfusion of vital organs.
2. **Progressive stage.** This stage is characterized by tissue hypoperfusion and the onset of circulatory and metabolic imbalance, including **metabolic acidosis** from lactic acidemia. Compensatory mechanisms are no longer adequate.
3. **Irreversible stage.** Organ damage and metabolic disturbances are so severe that **survival is not possible.**

D. **Morphologic manifestations**

1. A wide variety of anatomic findings are observed in shock. The most important of these is **acute tubular necrosis** of the kidney, which is potentially reversible with appropriate medical management.
2. Other anatomic findings in shock include:
   a. Areas of necrosis in the brain
   b. Centrilobular necrosis of the liver
   c. Fatty change in the heart or liver
   d. Patchy mucosal hemorrhages in the colon
   e. Depletion of lipid in the adrenal cortex
   f. Pulmonary edema

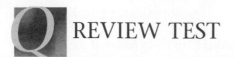

REVIEW TEST

Directions: *Each of the numbered items or incomplete statements in this section is followed by answers or by completions of the statement. Select the* ***one*** *lettered answer or completion that is best in each case.*

1. A 40-year-old woman dies after a long history of an illness characterized by dyspnea, orthopnea, hepatomegaly, distended neck veins, and peripheral edema. The cut surface of the liver as it appears at autopsy is shown in the illustration. Which of the following disorders is the most likely cause of these findings?

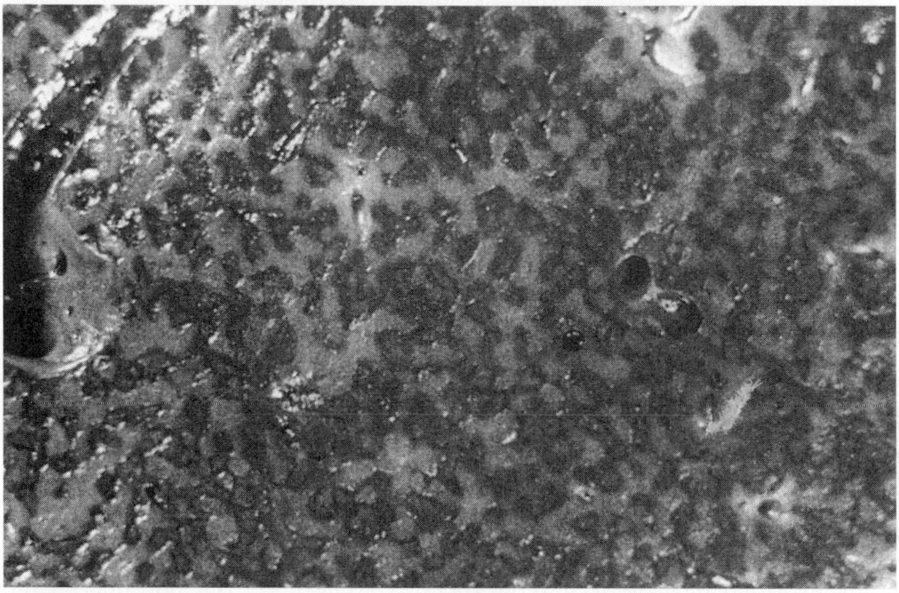

(Reprinted with permission from Golden A, Powell D, and Jennings C: *Pathology: Understanding Human Disease,* 2nd ed. Baltimore, Williams & Wilkins, 1985, p 161.)

(A) Chronic alcoholism
(B) Diabetes mellitus
(C) Niemann-Pick disease
(D) Right-sided heart failure
(E) Viral hepatitis

2. A 70-year-man seeks medical attention because of shortness of breath on minimal exertion. A posteroanterior chest radiograph reveals blunting of the right costophrenic sulcus interpreted as a right-sided pleural effusion. The aspirated fluid is straw-colored and clear. The protein concentration is low, and the specific gravity is 1.011. Microscopic examination reveals an occasional mesothelial cell. Which of the following is the most likely cause of the effusion?

(A) Decreased oncotic pressure
(B) Left ventricular heart failure
(C) Mesothelioma
(D) Pneumonia
(E) Tuberculosis

3. A 26-year-old woman dies after a short illness beginning in the late stages of labor. At autopsy, blood vessels in the lungs contained fetal debris (e.g., squamous cells, vernix, mucin), as did other vessels of multiple organs. Review of the clinical history reveals that she had become acutely ill with dyspnea, hypotension, and seizures, and a chest radiograph had demonstrated evidence of pulmonary edema. This was all followed by prolonged hemorrhage from the vagina and generalized bleeding from multiple other sites. The changes that were found within multiple blood vessels most likely are

(A) bone marrow emboli
(B) fat emboli
(C) gas emboli
(D) septic emboli
(E) widespread thrombosis

4. Two days following a cholecystectomy, a 32-year-old hospitalized woman has sudden onset of dyspnea, pleural pain, and cough productive of frothy, blood-tinged sputum. Ventilation-perfusion scintigraphy indicates a perfusion defect. If it were possible to examine a portion of the affected lung, which of the following would most likely have been found?

(A) Air embolism
(B) Anemic (white or pale) infarct
(C) Disseminated intravascular coagulation (DIC)
(D) Generalized thrombosis
(E) Hemorrhagic (red) infarct

5. A 50-year-old right-handed man with a long history of rheumatic heart disease with mitral stenosis and atrial fibrillation is brought to the emergency department after collapsing to the floor at home. He is unable to speak or walk and has right hemiplegia with a right extensor plantar response. These findings most likely result from embolism to which of the following arteries?

(A) Anterior cerebral
(B) Anterior communicating
(C) Middle cerebral
(D) Posterior communicating
(E) Superior cerebellar

6. An 86-year-old man with a history of recurrent urinary tract infection presents with fever, tachypnea, tachycardia, mental obtundation, and reduced blood pressure. Which of the following forms of shock is most likely?

(A) Anaphylactic shock
(B) Cardiogenic shock
(C) Hypovolemic shock
(D) Neurogenic shock
(E) Septic shock

7. A 60-year-old man with unstable angina (a form of acute coronary syndrome) is treated with an intravenously administered glycoprotein IIb-IIIa inhibitor. The mechanism of action of this agent is the ability to

(A) dilate coronary arteries
(B) inhibit atherogenesis
(C) inhibit platelet adhesion
(D) inhibit platelet aggregation
(E) lyse thrombi

8. A 23-year-old man undergoes surgery for fractures of the pelvis and left femur resulting from a high-speed motor vehicle accident. The following day he develops dyspnea, speech difficulties, and a petechial skin rash. Which of the following types of embolism is the likely cause of these findings?

(A) Air
(B) Amniotic fluid
(C) Fat
(D) Paradoxical
(E) Thrombotic

9. A 56-year-old man is surgically treated by a four-vessel coronary artery bypass graft procedure and placed on prophylactic daily aspirin therapy. Aspirin has been shown to prevent recurrent myocardial infarction through its ability to inhibit the synthesis of

(A) adenosine diphosphate (ADP)
(B) leukotriene B_4 (LTB_4)
(C) nitric oxide (NO)
(D) prostaglandin I_2 (PGI_2)
(E) thromboxane A_2 (TxA_2)

10. A bedridden elderly patient experiences the sudden onset of pleuritic pain and hemoptysis. The underlying lesion that led to this complication was most likely located in which of the following sites?

(A) Hepatic veins
(B) Lower extremity veins
(C) Pelvic veins
(D) Portal vein
(E) Pulmonary veins

11. Fluid is aspirated from the grossly distended abdomen of a 47-year-old chronic alcoholic man. The fluid is straw-colored and clear and is found to have a protein content (largely albumin) of 2.5 g/dL. Which of the following is a major contributor to the fluid accumulation in this patient?

(A) Blockage of lymphatics
(B) Decreased oncotic pressure
(C) Decreased sodium retention
(D) Increased capillary permeability
(E) Inflammatory exudation

12. A 36-year-old man dies during cardiac surgery. He had a history of long-standing rheumatic heart disease with mitral stenosis. At autopsy, the pathologist reports findings consistent with mitral stenosis and noted the presence of "heart failure cells." This finding results from

(A) activation of the coagulation cascade
(B) chronic passive congestion of the lungs
(C) hypoxic myocardial injury
(D) myocardial hyperemia

13. During a laboratory exercise on coagulation testing, a 23-year-old medical student is found to have a prolonged bleeding time. She has had a long history of "easy bleeding," with frequent bleeding of the gums, epistaxis, cutaneous bleeding, and menorrhagia. Further testing revealed a deficiency of von Willebrand factor. Which of the following thrombogenic processes involving platelets is most directly impaired?

(A) Adhesion
(B) Conformational change with activation of phospholipid surface
(C) Formation of fibrinogen bridges
(D) Release reaction
(E) Stabilization of platelet plug

14. A 28-year-old woman is evaluated for possible thrombophilia since she has had two episodes of deep vein thrombosis as well as two pregnancies that terminated in spontaneous abortion. The activated partial thromboplastin time is prolonged, and she has a positive VDRL screening test for syphilis. This combination of findings is most suggestive of

(A) antiphospholipid antibody syndrome
(B) disseminated intravascular coagulation
(C) factor V Leiden
(D) methylene tetrahydrofolate reductase mutation
(E) prothrombin 20210A transition

A ANSWERS AND EXPLANATIONS

1-D. The clinical findings described in the question are typical of right-sided heart failure, as is the illustration, which reveals the nutmeg-like appearance of hepatic chronic passive congestion. The gross morphologic appearance is caused by congested centrilobular areas alternating with pale portal areas.

2-B. A clear, straw-colored fluid with low protein and low specific gravity is a transudate, and the term hydrothorax refers to the accumulation of a significant volume of transudate within the pleural cavities (to be detected by chest radiograph, about 200 to 400 mL of pleural fluid must be present). The most common cause of hydrothorax is cardiac failure that may be either unilateral or bilateral (bilateral is more common). It is incumbent that the clinician distinguish pleural transudates from exudates, because the causes of each are quite different.

3-E. The history is typical of amniotic fluid embolism, one of the major obstetric causes of disseminated intravascular coagulation (DIC). Other obstetric complications associated with DIC include retained dead fetus and abruptio placentae (premature separation of the placenta). Nonobstetric causes include neoplasms or tissue damage from infection, immunologic mechanisms, or trauma. Neoplastic causes include tumors of the lung, pancreas, prostate, and stomach, and FAB M3 acute myeloblastic (promyelocytic hypergranular) leukemia. Tissue damage can result from trauma such as lung surgery, from hemolysis or hemolytic transfusion reactions, and from inflammatory causes, such as gram-negative sepsis and immune complex disease.

4-E. The history is that of pulmonary embolism and infarction, a danger of immobilization and the postoperative state. The infarct consists of an area of coagulative necrosis with superimposed hemorrhage, a combination referred to as a hemorrhagic, or red, infarct. Red infarcts are typical of tissues with a redundant arterial blood supply. Prominent examples are the lung with its double circulation from the pulmonary and bronchial arteries and the gastrointestinal tract with its multiple anastomoses between branches of the mesenteric artery. When a portion of the blood supply is obstructed, other portions remain patent, which can lead to hemorrhage into the infarcted area.

5-C. The findings are consistent with occlusion of the middle cerebral artery, the most common site of arrest of arterial emboli in branches of the carotid artery. Such emboli usually arise from a mural thrombus in the left atrium or left ventricle. Left atrial mural thrombi are especially associated with mitral stenosis with atrial fibrillation. Mural thrombi in the left ventricle are caused by myocardial infarction. Thrombi at the junction of the internal and external carotid arteries are a cause of thrombotic brain infarcts and can also be a site of origin of emboli.

6-E. The diagnosis is septic shock, most likely a result of gram-negative sepsis originating from a urinary tract infection. Gram-negative organisms contain lipopolysaccharide in the outer membrane, which triggers the release of cytokines such as tumor necrosis factor, resulting in a cascade of events culminating in increased capillary permeability and redistribution of circulatory volume into the interstitium. Anaphylactic shock is a result of a type I hypersensitivity. Cardiogenic shock often results from myocardial infarction. Hypovolemic shock is a result of blood or fluid loss. Neurogenic shock can result from spinal cord injuries.

7-D. Glycoprotein IIb-IIIa inhibitors prevent the action of the corresponding platelet surface receptor glycoprotein complex, which is required for formation of fibrinogen bridges between adjacent platelets.

8-C. The patient has the fat embolism syndrome, which is characterized by pulmonary distress, cutaneous petechiae, and various neurologic manifestations. Fat embolism is a well-known complication of fractures of long bones, such as the femur, and other bones with abundant fatty marrow. On fracture, marrow fat can enter the circulation, and small fat droplets can lodge in vessels of the skin, lung, and microvasculature of the brain, resulting in the clinical manifestations of this disorder.

9-E. Thromboxane A_2 (TxA_2) promotes platelet aggregation, as does ADP. Aspirin irreversibly inhibits the enzymes cyclooxygenase 1 and 2 and thereby the synthesis of TxA_2, thus inhibiting platelet aggregation, which is thought to be an important early step in atherogenesis. A negative but apparently unimportant consequence of aspirin prophylaxis is the parallel inhibition of synthesis of the antiaggregant endothelial PGI_2, also a product of the cyclooxgenase pathway.

10-B. The clinical description is characteristic of pulmonary infarction, which in turn most often results from thromboembolism originating from thrombosis in the lower extremity veins. Because venous thrombosis is associated with impaired blood flow, this condition is particularly characteristic of immobilization, which is often seen in elderly, debilitated, or chronically bedridden persons.

11-B. The patient has cirrhosis of the liver secondary to chronic alcoholism. A prominent manifestation of this disorder is decreased hepatic synthesis of albumin, the most significant contributor to plasma oncotic pressure. In addition, ascites is associated with increased sodium and water retention because of stimulation of the renin-angiotensin system. Also, hydrostatic forces (because of intrahepatic scarring and partial obstruction of the portal venous return) result in fluid transudation and increased secretion of hepatic lymph.

12-B. "Heart failure cells" are intra-alveolar hemosiderin-laden macrophages and are indicative of marked chronic passive congestion of the lung. Red cells leak from congested alveolar capillaries into the alveoli, where they are engulfed and degraded by macrophages.

13-A. Von Willibrand factor is required for platelet adhesion to the subendothelium of damaged blood vessels. See further discussion of von Willebrand disease in Chapter 13.

14-A. The combination of a prolonged activated partial thromboplastin time (APTT), a positive VDRL test for syphilis, recurrent thromboses (arterial or venous), and spontaneous abortion is highly suggestive of the antiphospholipid antibody syndrome. As the name implies, antibodies directed at phospholipids are a characteristic finding. Because of the prolonged APTT and frequent association with systemic lupus erythematosus (SLE), the antibody has been referred to as the "lupus anticoagulant," a misleading term because affected subjects have a thrombotic rather than hemorrhagic diathesis and not all subjects have SLE. The term primary antiphospholipid antibody syndrome is used when there is no evident underlying disease. It should be contrasted to secondary antiphospholipid antibody syndrome, in which the patient has a well-defined autoimmune disorder such as SLE.

CHAPTER

4

Genetic Disorders

I. Chromosomal Disorders

A. **Changes in chromosome number or structure.** Normal cells are **diploid,** containing 46 chromosomes, 22 pairs of autosomes and 1 pair of sex chromosomes, XX in females or XY in males.

1. **Aneuploidy** is a chromosome number that is not a multiple of 23, the normal **haploid** number. It is caused most often by an addition or loss of one or two chromosomes; this change may result from nondisjunction or anaphase lag.
   a. **Nondisjunction**
      (1) Nondisjunction is failure of chromosomes to separate during meiosis or mitosis. **Meiotic nondisjunction** is the most common cause of aneuploidy.
      (2) This process is responsible for disorders such as trisomy 21, the most common form of **Down syndrome.**
   b. **Anaphase lag**
      (1) Anaphase lag results in the **loss of a chromosome** during meiotic or mitotic division.
      (2) In early embryonic life, this can result in **mosaicism,** in which an individual develops two lines of cells, one with a normal chromosome complement and another with **monosomy,** a single residual chromosome, for the affected chromosome pair.
2. **Polyploidy** is a chromosome number that is a multiple greater than two of the haploid number.
   a. Triploidy is three times the haploid number; tetraploidy is four times the haploid number.
   b. Polyploidy is rarely compatible with life and usually results in **spontaneous abortion.**
3. **Deletion**
   a. Deletion is most often absence of a portion of a chromosome, although it can be loss of an entire chromosome.
   b. This change is denoted by a minus sign following the number of the chromosome and the sign for the chromosomal arm involved, *p* for the short arm and *q* for the long arm. For example, **cri du chat syndrome,** characterized by partial loss of the short arm of chromosome 5, is designated as 46,XY,5p− in males or 46,XX,5p− in females.
4. **Inversion.** This is **reunion** of a chromosome broken at two points, in which the internal fragment is reinserted in an **inverted position.**
5. **Translocation**
   a. This is an **exchange** of chromosomal segments between nonhomologous chromosomes. It is denoted by a *t* followed by the involved chromosomes in numeric order. For example, the translocation form of Down syndrome is designated as t(14q;21q).

b. **Reciprocal or balanced translocation** is a break in two chromosomes leading to an exchange of chromosomal material. Because no genetic material is lost, balanced translocation is often **clinically silent.**

c. **Robertsonian translocation** is a variant in which the long arms of two **acrocentric chromosomes,** chromosomes in which the short arm is very short, are joined with a common centromere, and the short arms are lost. One important example leads to a hereditable form of Down syndrome. Chromosome 21 is joined to a second acrocentic chromosome, commonly chromosome 14 or 22. The union of a gamete with this translocation with a gamete from an unaffected person can result in trisomy 21 (1 in 3 theoretic chance).

6. **Isochromosome formation.** This is the result of **transverse** rather than longitudinal division of a chromosome, forming two new chromosomes, each consisting of either two long arms or two short arms. One of the two isochromosomes, usually the short-arm isochromosome, often is lost.

B. **Sex chromosomes: X inactivation and Barr body formation**

- **Extreme karyotype deviations** in the sex chromosomes are compatible with life; this is believed to be due to X inactivation **(lyonization)** and the relatively scanty genetic information carried by the Y chromosome.

1. **Barr bodies.** Also known as **sex chromatin,** these are clumps of chromatin in the interphase nuclei of all somatic cells in females.
   a. According to the Lyon hypothesis, each Barr body represents one **inactivated X chromosome.** Thus, normal female cells (XX) have one Barr body; normal male cells (XY) have no Barr bodies; and XXXY cells have two Barr bodies. The number of Barr bodies is always one less than the number of X chromosomes.
   b. Assessment of the presence or absence of Barr bodies and their number was once an important diagnostic tool, but it has now been supplanted by more definitive and sophisticated analytic procedures.
2. **X inactivation**
   a. This is the process by which all X chromosomes except one are **randomly inactivated** at an early stage of embryonic development. It results in all normal females being **mosaics,** with two distinct cell lines, one with an active maternal X, another with an active paternal X.
   b. It can be demonstrated if the female is heterozygous for an **X-linked gene;** if individuals demonstrate inheritable differences that distinguish the protein products of one X chromosome from the other, members of the two cell lines can be identified.
   c. The X-inactive-specific transcript (XIST) is a large untranslated RNA molecule that is associated with "coating" and inactivation of one of the two X chromosomes. All except a single remaining X chromosome are inactivated.
   d. The phenotypic differences between XO, XX, and multiple X genotypes are thought to be caused by residual genes on the X chromosome that escape inactivation.

C. **Abnormalities of autosomal chromosomes**

1. **Down syndrome** is the most frequently occurring chromosomal disorder.
   a. **Causes of Down syndrome**
      (1) **Trisomy 21**
         (a) The vast majority of cases (95%) are caused by trisomy 21, and the **incidence increases with maternal age.**
         (b) **Maternal meiotic nondisjunction** is the usual cause. When the cause is paternal nondisjunction, there is no relation to paternal age.
      (2) **Translocation**
         (a) Translocation leads to a **familial form** of Down syndrome, with significant risk of the syndrome in subsequent children.
         (b) From 3% to 5% of cases result from translocation, and there is **no relation to maternal age.**

(c) The cause is parental meiotic translocation between chromosome 21 and another chromosome. The fertilized ovum has three chromosomes bearing the chromosome 21 material, the functional equivalent of trisomy 21.

b. **Characteristics of Down syndrome**

(1) Severe **mental retardation** is marked.

(2) Changes in appearance include:

(a) Large forehead, broad nasal bridge, wide-spaced eyes, **epicanthal folds,** large protruding tongue, and small low-set ears

(b) **Brushfield spots,** small white spots on the periphery of the iris

(c) Short, broad hands with curvature of the fifth finger; **simian crease,** a single palmar crease; and an unusually wide space between the first and second toes

c. **Complications of Down syndrome**

(1) **Congenital heart disease,** especially defects of the endocardial cushion, including atrioventricular valve malformations and atrial and ventricular septal defects

(2) Acute **leukemia** (20-fold increase), most often lymphoblastic

(3) Increased **susceptibility to infection**

(4) In patients surviving into middle age, morphologic **changes in the brain similar to those of Alzheimer disease**

d. **Maternal screening for Down syndrome**

(1) α-Fetoprotein—low

(2) Human chorionic gonadotropin (hCG)—high

(3) Unconjugated estriol—low

2. **Cri du chat (5p−, cry of the cat) syndrome**

a. The cause is the **deletion** of the short arm of chromosome 5.

b. Characteristics are **severe mental retardation, microcephaly,** and an **unusual catlike cry.** Additional manifestations include low birth weight, round face, **hypertelorism** (wide-set eyes), low-set ears, and epicanthal folds.

3. **DiGeorge/velocardiofacial syndrome (microdeletion of 22q11, CATCH 22 syndrome)**

a. This syndrome leads to a spectrum of clinical abnormalities formerly thought to be at least two separate and distinct disorders.

b. Characteristics include a set of findings summed up in the acronym **CATCH 22,** which denotes **c**ardiac abnormalities, **a**bnormal facies, **T**-cell deficit because of thymic hypoplasia, **c**left palate, **h**ypocalcemia because of hypoparathyroidism, and microdeletion 22q11. In about 30% of cases, this syndrome is also associated with behavior disorders and psychosis (bipolar disorder and schizophrenia) that develop during adolescence.

4. **Edwards syndrome (trisomy 18)**

a. Most frequently, trisomy 18 results from **nondisjunction.**

b. Characteristics include mental retardation, prominent occiput, **micrognathia** (small lower jaw), low-set ears, **rocker-bottom feet,** flexion deformities of the fingers (index overlapping third and fourth), and **congenital heart disease.**

5. **Patau syndrome (trisomy 13).** Characteristics include mental retardation, microcephaly, **microphthalmia,** brain abnormalities, cleft lip and palate, polydactyly, rocker-bottom feet, and congenital heart disease.

D. **Abnormalities of sex chromosomes**

1. **Klinefelter syndrome**

a. Klinefelter syndrome occurs when there are **at least two X chromosomes and one or more Y chromosomes.** The most striking clinical changes are male **hypogonadism** and its secondary effects. Most often, the **karyotype 47,XXY** is characteristic. Variants include additional X chromosomes (e.g., XXXY) and rare mosaic forms.

b. The disorder is always manifested by a male phenotype with testes. Affected individuals have **atrophic testes; tall stature,** because fusion of the epiphyses is delayed; and a eunuchoid appearance with **gynecomastia.** In addition, they have **decreased testosterone production** and **increased pituitary gonadotropins** from loss of feedback inhibition.

c. The disorder is a frequent cause of male infertility.
d. **Usually,** there is **no association with mental retardation.** If present, mental retardation is usually mild, and the extent of retardation increases with increased number of X chromosomes.
e. Most often, the cause is **maternal meiotic nondisjunction,** and incidence increases with maternal age.
f. Usually, Klinefelter syndrome is undiagnosed before puberty.

2. **XYY syndrome**
a. XYY syndrome occurs with increased frequency among criminals demonstrating **violent behavior;** the significance of this association is unknown, because only about 2% of XYY individuals display such behavioral abnormalities.
b. Characteristics include tallness, **severe acne,** and **only rarely mild mental retardation.**

3. **Turner syndrome**
a. Turner syndrome is a disorder that occurs when there is complete or partial monosomy of the X chromosome.
b. An **XO karyotype** (45,X) is characteristic.
c. The most striking clinical changes are **female hypogonadism** and its secondary effects. **Turner syndrome is also often associated with autoantibody-mediated hypothyroidism.**
d. Other characteristics of Turner syndrome include the following:
(1) Replacement of the ovaries by **fibrous streaks**
(2) Decreased estrogen production and increased pituitary gonadotropins from loss of feedback inhibition
(3) **Infantile genitalia** and poor breast development
(4) **Short stature, webbed neck,** shield-like chest with widely spaced nipples, and wide carrying angle of the arms
(5) Lymphedema of the extremities and neck
(6) Coarctation of the aorta and other congenital malformations
e. Turner syndrome, the most common cause of **primary amenorrhea, is generally considered not to be a cause of mental retardation.**

4. **XXX syndrome (47,XXX) and other multi-X chromosome anomalies.** These syndromes are usually unaccompanied by any clinical abnormalities, although they may be marked by menstrual irregularities. Additional X chromosomes beyond XXX are marked by progressively increasing mental deficiency, depending on the number of additional X chromosomes.

E. **Abnormalities due to increased numbers of trinucleotide repeats**

1. **General considerations.** Several disorders have been found to be associated with the **expansion of the number of tandem trinucleotide repeats** in certain critical genes.
a. The number of repeats often increases from generation to generation and is associated with earlier onset and **more severe manifestations in successive generations.** This phenomenon is referred to as **anticipation.**
b. Prominent examples of trinucleotide repeat disorders include fragile X syndrome, Huntington disease, and myotonic dystrophy. Because fragile X syndrome can be detected as a karyotypic abnormality, it is discussed here. Huntington disease is discussed in Chapter 23, and myotonic dystrophy is discussed in Chapter 22.

2. **Fragile X syndrome**
a. Fragile X syndrome is an important cause of hereditary **mental retardation second in frequency only to Down syndrome.**
b. The cause is a **cytogenetically demonstrable defect** on the long arm of the X chromosome that leads to chromosome breakage in vitro. Fragile X syndrome is considered to be an X-linked disorder; however, the pattern of inheritance has a number of unusual features.
(1) Both males and females can be asymptomatic carriers. Such carriers have an **increased number of CGG tandem repeats** in the 5′ untranslated region of the familial mental retardation (*FMR*-1) gene. This increased number of repeats is referred to as a premutation. In carrier females (but not carrier males), premutations

can expand in the germline to even greater increases in the number of tandem repeats. These increased numbers are referred to as full mutations.

(2) Carrier males (transmitting males) can transmit premutations through their daughters, who remain clinically unaffected but who can become carriers of X chromosomes with full mutations due to germline expansion of the repeats.

(3) Carrier females can transmit the affected X chromosome to both sons and daughters.

(a) Sons with full mutations exhibit mental retardation and often bilateral **macro-orchidism** (enlarged testes). The genetic defect can be further transmitted to all of their daughters.

(b) Daughters with full mutations may or may not (~50%) exhibit mental retardation. This unexplained phenomenon is possibly due to selective X inactivation, in which affected females have a greater number of somatic cells with full mutations than do unaffected females.

F. **Disorders associated with genomic imprinting.** In these hereditary disorders, different phenotypes occur depending on whether an abnormal gene is of maternal or paternal origin.

1. It is thought that epigenetic changes occurring during gametogenesis mark at least some genes as of either maternal or paternal origin and can modify the later expression of these genes when they are passed to the next generation. Such marking is referred to as **genomic imprinting.** The most likely explanation for this phenomenon is differing levels of DNA methylation in the female and male gonads, making certain genes nonactive (i.e., not able to be transcribed).
2. This phenomenon is illustrated by two rare syndromes in which the same cytogenetic deletion, del(15)(q11q13), results in differing phenotypes in progeny depending on whether the deletions were transmitted by the mother or the father.
   a. **Paternal transmission** results in the **Prader-Willi syndrome,** characterized by hypogonadism, hypotonia, mental retardation, behavior problems, and uncontrolled appetite leading to obesity and diabetes.
   b. **Maternal transmission** results in the **Angelman syndrome,** sometimes referred to as the "happy puppet" syndrome, which is also characterized by mental retardation but is additionally characterized by ataxia, seizures, and inappropriate laughter. In some instances, this condition is associated with alterations in a gene involved in the ubiquitin-proteosome system.

II. Modes of Inheritance of Monogenic Disorders (Figure 4-1)

A. **Autosomal dominant inheritance**

1. One heterozygous parent carries a gene associated with phenotypic expression of a disorder and the other parent is normal, by far the most likely case in nonconsanguineous matings.
2. One half of the children are expected to inherit the gene and are themselves heterozygotes who phenotypically manifest the gene.
3. Distribution of the phenotype is the same in both sexes.

B. **Autosomal recessive inheritance**

1. Both parents are heterozygotes who do not phenotypically manifest the disorder.
2. One in four of their children will be homozygous for the trait and, in the case of disease states, will phenotypically manifest the disorder. Similarly, one in four of the children will not inherit the trait. Two of the children will be heterozygotes.
3. Distribution of the disordered phenotype is the same in both sexes.

C. **X-linked recessive inheritance**

1. In the most frequent disease setting, the **female parent is a heterozygous carrier,** and the male parent is genotypically and phenotypically unaffected.

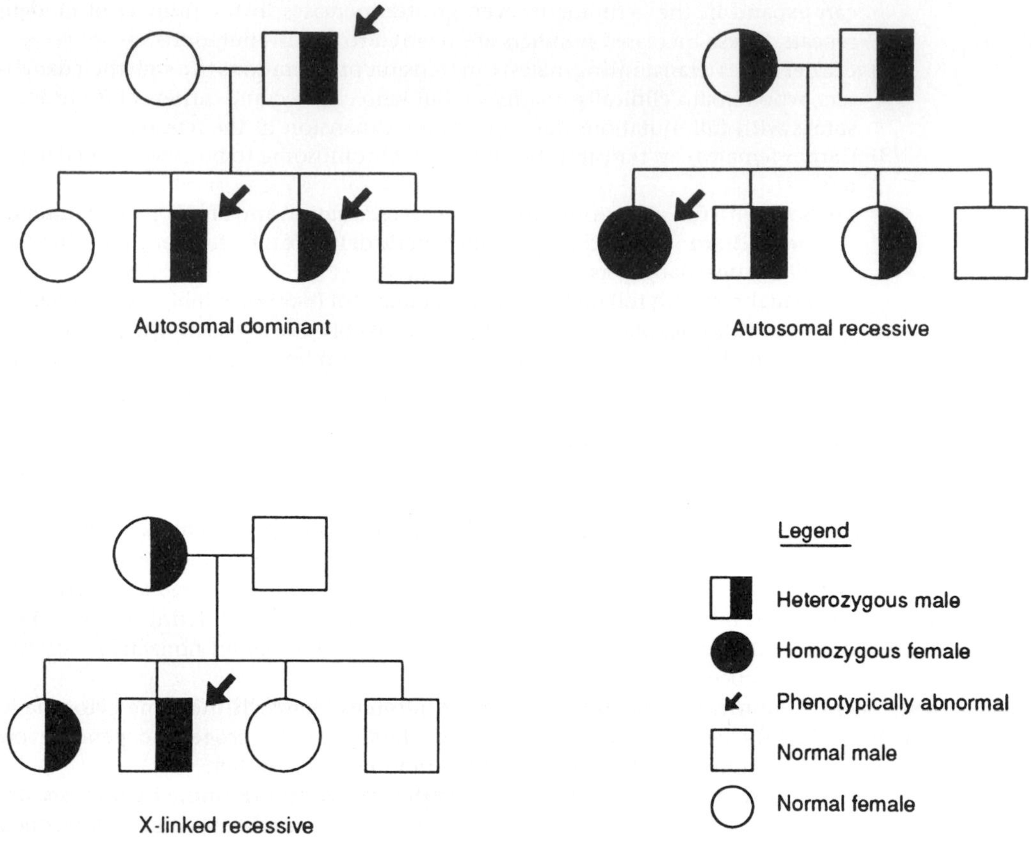

Figure 4-1 Modes of inheritance.

2. The affected X chromosome will be inherited by one in two children; **male children who inherit the affected X chromosome phenotypically manifest the disorder;** heterozygous female children are carriers.
3. In a variant setting, the male parent carries the affected gene on the X chromosome and the female parent is unaffected. All female children inherit the paternal X chromosome and become carriers; all male children are genotypically and phenotypically unaffected.

D. **Other modes of inheritance**
   1. **X-linked dominant inheritance** is a rare variant of X-linked inheritance. Heterozygous females as well as hemizygous males phenotypically manifest the disorder.
   2. **Mitochondrial inheritance** is mediated by cytoplasmic (mitochondrial) genes, which are **inherited exclusively by maternal transmission.**

III. Mendelian Disorders

A. **Autosomal dominant disorders**
   1. **Adult polycystic kidney disease** is the most frequently occurring hereditary renal disorder.
      a. Characteristics include **numerous bilateral cysts** that replace and ultimately destroy the renal parenchyma.

b. The disease becomes clinically manifest between 20 and 40 years of age even though the genetic defect is present at birth; death usually occurs at about 50 years of age. (Similarly, Huntington disease, a condition associated with multiple trinucleotide repeats, does not become manifest until adult life.)

2. **Familial hypercholesterolemia** is a genetic defect characterized by anomalies of receptors for low-density lipoprotein (LDL) receptors.
   a. The disease results in decreased transport of LDL cholesterol into cells, which causes hypercholesterolemia and a striking increase in incidence and in earlier onset of **atherosclerosis** and its complications.
   b. Additional manifestations include **xanthomas,** raised yellow lesions filled with lipid-laden macrophages, in the skin and tendons.
3. **Hereditary hemorrhagic telangiectasia (Osler-Weber-Rendu syndrome)** is a rare disorder seen with increased frequency in certain populations, such as in Mormon families of Utah. Characteristics include localized **telangiectases of the skin and mucous membranes** and by recurrent **hemorrhage** from these lesions.
4. **Hereditary spherocytosis**
   a. The cause is a variety of inherited defects of erythrocyte membrane-associated skeletal proteins.
   b. Characteristics include **spheroidal erythrocytes** that are sequestered and destroyed in the spleen, producing **hemolytic anemia.**
5. **Marfan syndrome** is a **defect of connective tissue** characterized by faulty scaffolding.
   a. The apparent cause is a deficiency of fibrillin, a glycoprotein constituent of microfibrils.
   b. Characteristics include defects in skeletal, visual, and cardiovascular structures.
      (1) Patients are tall and thin with abnormally long legs and arms, spider-like fingers **(arachnodactyly)**, and hyperextensible joints.
      (2) Dislocation of the ocular lens (**ectopia lentis**) is frequent.
      (3) Cystic medial necrosis can lead to aortic dilation with resultant **aneurysm of the proximal aorta,** aortic valvular insufficiency, and **dissecting aneurysm of the aorta.** Loss of connective tissue support may lead to **mitral valve prolapse.**
6. **Neurofibromatosis (von Recklinghausen disease)**
   a. Distinguishing features include **multiple neurofibromas** in skin and other locations, schwannomas of the VIIIth nerve, **café au lait spots**, and pigmented iris hamartomas (**Lisch nodules**). The benign neurofibromas can become malignant.
   b. **Skeletal disorders,** such as scoliosis and bone cysts, and **increased incidence of other tumors,** especially pheochromocytoma and malignancies such as Wilms tumor, rhabdomyosarcoma, and leukemia, also occur.
   c. The cause is mutations in the *NF1* gene, a tumor suppressor gene that normally codes for a GTPase-activating protein (GAP) that facilitates the conversion of active ras-GTP to inactive ras-GDP.
7. **Tuberous sclerosis**
   a. Characteristics include the presence of **glial nodules** and **distorted neurons** in the cerebral cortex. **Seizures, mental retardation,** and adenoma sebaceum (a facial skin lesion consisting of malformed blood vessels and connective tissue) also occur.
   b. Associated symptoms include rhabdomyomas of the heart and with **renal angiomyolipomas,** lesions consisting of malformed blood vessels, smooth muscle, and fat cells.
8. **von Hippel-Lindau disease**
   a. Characteristics include **hemangioblastoma** or **cavernous hemangioma** of the cerebellum, brain stem, or retina; **adenomas;** and **cysts** of the liver, kidney, pancreas, and other organs.
   b. A remarkably increased incidence of **renal cell carcinoma** is associated with von Hippel-Lindau disease. The gene for von Hippel-Lindau disease has been localized to the short arm of chromosome 3, deletion of which has been noted in many cases of sporadic renal cell carcinoma.

TABLE 4-1 *Some Autosomal Recessive Disorders*

Disorder	Enzyme Deficiency	Accumulation
Tay-Sachs disease	Hexosaminidase A	GM_2 ganglioside
Gaucher disease	Glucocerebrosidase	Glucocerebroside
Niemann-Pick disease	Sphingomyelinase	Sphingomyelin
Hurler syndrome	α-L-Iduronidase	Heparan sulfate, dermatan sulfate
Von Gierke disease (type I glycogenosis)	Glucose-6-phosphatase	Glycogen
Pompe disease (type II glycogenosis)	α-1,4-glucosidase	Glycogen
Cori disease (type III glycogenosis)	Amylo-1,6-glucosidase	Glycogen
McArdle syndrome (type V glycogenosis)	Muscle phosphorylase	Glycogen
Galactosemia	Galactose-1-phosphate uridyl transferase	Galactose-1-phosphate
Phenylketonuria	Phenylalanine hydroxylase	Phenylalanine and its degradation products
Alkaptonuria	Homogentisic oxidase	Homogentisic acid

B. **Autosomal recessive disorders.** These include most **inborn errors of metabolism** (Table 4-1).

1. **Lysosomal storage diseases** are a group of disorders characterized by **deficiency of a specific single lysosomal enzyme,** resulting in an accumulation of abnormal metabolic products.
   a. **Tay-Sachs disease (amaurotic familial idiocy)** is the most common form of gangliosidosis and occurs primarily in those of Ashkenazi (central European origin) Jewish descent.
      (1) The cause is a deficiency of **hexosaminidase A,** with consequent accumulation of **GM_2 ganglioside,** especially in neurons.
      (2) Characteristics include **central nervous system (CNS) degeneration,** severe mental and motor deterioration, **blindness** (amaurosis), a characteristic **cherry-red spot** in the macula, and death before 4 years of age.
   b. **Gaucher disease** is a disorder of lipid metabolism caused by a deficiency of **glucocerebrosidase,** which results in an accumulation of **glucocerebroside** in cells of the mononuclear phagocyte system.
      (1) This disorder can be identified by the presence of **Gaucher cells,** enlarged histiocytes with a distinctive "wrinkled tissue paper" cytoplasmic appearance.
      (2) There are three major variants:
         (a) **Type I,** or adult Gaucher disease, which accounts for about 80% of cases, is characterized by **hepatosplenomegaly, erosion of the femoral head and of the long bones,** and **mild anemia.** Gaucher cells are seen in the liver, spleen, lymph nodes, and bone marrow. A normal lifespan is possible.
         (b) **Type II,** or infantile Gaucher disease, is marked by **severe CNS involvement** and results in **death before 1 year of age.** There is no detectable glucocerebrosidase in the tissues.
         (c) **Type III,** or juvenile Gaucher disease, involves both the brain and the viscera but is **less severe than type II.** Onset is usually in early childhood.

c. **Niemann-Pick disease**
   (1) Often, the cause is a deficiency of **sphingomyelinase,** with consequent **sphingomyelin** accumulation in phagocytes (types A and B Niemann-Pick disease). More commonly, the cause is a defect in a gene involved in cholesterol transport with cholesterol accumulation within phagocytes (type C Niemann-Pick disease).
   (2) Characteristics include **"foamy histiocytes,"** containing sphingomyelin, which proliferate in the liver, spleen, lymph nodes, and skin, as well as **hepatosplenomegaly,** anemia, fever, and, in some variants, neurologic deterioration. About half of the patients have a cherry-red spot in the macula similar to that of Tay-Sachs disease. Death occurs by 3 years of age.

d. **Hurler syndrome**
   (1) This mucopolysaccharidosis is caused by deficiency of **α-L-iduronidase,** with consequent accumulations of the mucopolysaccharides **heparan sulfate** and **dermatan sulfate** in the heart, brain, liver, and other organs.
   (2) Characteristics include progressive deterioration, hepatosplenomegaly, dwarfism, gargoyle-like facies, stubby fingers, corneal clouding, progressive mental retardation, and death by 10 years of age.
   (3) The syndrome is clinically similar to, but should not be confused with, Hunter syndrome, which is an X-linked recessive disorder.

2. **Glycogen storage diseases** are a group of disorders caused by defects in the synthesis or degradation of glycogen.
   a. **von Gierke disease** is glycogen storage disease type I, or hepatorenal glycogenosis.
      (1) The cause is a deficiency of **glucose-6-phosphatase,** with consequent accumulation of glycogen, primarily in the liver and kidney.
      (2) Characteristics include **hepatomegaly** and sometimes intractable **hypoglycemia.**
   b. **Pompe disease** is glycogen storage disease type II but can also be classified as a lysosomal storage disease.
      (1) The cause is a deficiency of **α-1,4-glucosidase** (a lysosomal enzyme), with consequent accumulation of glycogen, especially in the liver, heart, and skeletal muscle.
      (2) Characteristics include cardiomegaly, muscle hypotonia, and splenomegaly; death occurs from cardiorespiratory failure before 3 years of age.
      (3) The disease can also be characterized by intractable hypoglycemia.
   c. **Cori disease** is glycogen storage disease type III.
      (1) The cause is a deficiency of the **debranching enzyme, amylo-1,6-glucosidase,** leading to variable accumulation of glycogen in the liver, heart, or skeletal muscle.
      (2) Characteristics include stunted growth, hepatomegaly, and hypoglycemia.
   d. **McArdle syndrome** is glycogen storage disease type V.
      (1) The cause is deficiency of **muscle phosphorylase,** with consequent glycogen accumulation in skeletal muscle.
      (2) This disease produces painful muscle cramps and muscle weakness following exercise.

3. **Disorders of carbohydrate metabolism: galactosemia**
   a. **Classic galactosemia**
      (1) The cause is deficiency of **galactose-1-phosphate uridyl transferase,** with resultant accumulation of **galactose-1-phosphate** in many tissues.
      (2) Characteristics include **failure to thrive, infantile cataracts, mental retardation,** and progressive hepatic failure leading to **cirrhosis** and death. Most of these changes can be prevented by **early removal of galactose from the diet.**
   b. **Galactokinase-deficiency galactosemia** is much less frequent than classic galactosemia. The disorder is often marked only by infantile cataracts.

4. **Disorders of amino acid metabolism**
   a. **Phenylketonuria (PKU)**
      (1) In most cases, PKU is caused by mutation of the **phenylalanine hydroxylase** gene. Phenylalanine hydroxylase deficiency results in failure of conversion of phenylalanine to tyrosine in the liver.

(2) PKU results in high serum concentrations of **phenylalanine,** which are neurotoxic and cause progressive cerebral demyelination. Minor pathways of phenylalanine catabolism come into play, and metabolites such as **phenylpyruvic acid** ("phenylketone") and phenylacetic acid accumulate. These are found in large amounts in the urine of children with PKU.

(3) Characteristics include progressive **mental deterioration,** usually pronounced by 1 year of age. Other manifestations include seizures, hyperactivity, and other neurologic abnormalities; decreased pigmentation of hair, eyes, and skin (children are characteristically **blond and blue-eyed**); and **mousy or musty body odor** from phenylacetic acid in urine and sweat.

(4) Successful treatment is a phenylalanine-free diet. Screening tests for serum phenylalanine or urinary catabolites are usually performed on the third or fourth day of life. Earlier screening may result in false-negative results.

(5) Even though a phenylalanine-free diet is usually abandoned in adult patients, there is special danger of maternal PKU during pregnancy. If PKU is not controlled by reinstitution of a phenylalanine-deficient diet in the affected mother, the infant (who does not have PKU) is at risk of congenital heart disease, growth retardation, microcephaly, and mental retardation.

b. **Alkaptonuria**

(1) The cause is incomplete metabolism of phenylalanine and tyrosine due to deficiency of **homogentisic oxidase,** leading to accumulation and urinary excretion of **homogentisic acid.**

(2) Characteristics include urine that turns dark and finally black on standing; **ochronosis,** dark pigmentation of fibrous tissues and cartilage; and incapacitating ochronotic arthritis. Cardiac valves may also be involved.

c. **Maple syrup urine disease**

(1) This rare inborn error of metabolism can be caused by any of a number of defects in the proteins that make up the branched-chain α-keto acid dehydrogenase (keto acid decarboxylase) complex.

(2) Characteristics include mental and physical retardation, feeding problems, and a maple syrup odor to the urine, as well as high urinary levels of the keto acids of leucine, isoleucine, and valine.

(3) If untreated, maple syrup urine disease results in mental and physical disabilities and often leads to neonatal death. This disease can be detected by newborn screening programs and can be minimized in severity when treated with protein-modified diets.

5. **Cystic fibrosis (mucoviscidosis, fibrocystic disease of the pancreas)** is one of the most common lethal genetic diseases among whites.

a. The cause is mutations in the **cystic fibrosis transmembrane conductance regulator (CFTR) gene,** which has been localized to the midsection of the long arm of **chromosome 7.** This gene codes for a membrane protein that facilitates the movement of chloride and other ions across membranes. In 70% of cases, the cause involves deletion of the three base pairs that code for phenylalanine at position 508 (ΔF508 mutation), an important example of deletion of an entire codon.

b. Characteristics include **malfunction of exocrine glands,** resulting in **increased viscosity of mucus** and **increased chloride concentration in sweat** and tears. Clinical manifestations include:

(1) **Chronic pulmonary disease** is caused by retention of viscid mucus, which leads to secondary infection; recurrent bouts of pneumonia, severe chronic bronchitis, bronchiectasis, and lung abscess are common. Infection with *Pseudomonas aeruginosa* is a common cause of death in cystic fibrosis.

(2) **Pancreatic insufficiency** is a deficiency of pancreatic enzymes that leads to malabsorption and steatorrhea.

(3) **Meconium ileus** is small-bowel obstruction in the newborn caused by thick, viscous meconium.

c. The **sweat test** is an important diagnostic procedure. Secretion by sweat glands of chloride and sodium is normal, but their reabsorption by sweat ducts is impaired.

Table 4-2 *Examples of X-linked Disorders*

Disorder	Enzyme Deficiency	Accumulation
Hunter syndrome	L-Iduronosulfate sulfatase	Heparan sulfate, dermatan sulfate
Fabry disease	α-Galactosidase A	Ceramide trihexoside
G6PD deficiency	G6PD	—
Classic hemophilia (hemophilia A)	Factor VIII	—
Lesch-Nyhan syndrome	HGPRT	Uric acid
Duchenne muscular dystrophy	Dystrophin	—

G6PD = glucose-6-phosphate dehydrogenase; HGPRT = hypoxanthine-guanine phosphoribosyltransferase.

C. **X-linked recessive disorders** (Table 4-2)
1. **Hunter syndrome** is a lysosomal storage disease, a form of mucopolysaccharidosis clinically similar to, but less severe than, Hurler syndrome.
   a. This disorder is caused by deficiency of **L-iduronosulfate sulfatase,** resulting in accumulations of **heparan sulfate** and **dermatan sulfate.**
   b. Characteristics include hepatosplenomegaly, micrognathia, retinal degeneration, joint stiffness, mild mental retardation, and cardiac lesions.
2. **Fabry disease (angiokeratoma corporis diffusum universale)** is a lysosomal storage disease caused by deficiency of **α-galactosidase A,** with resultant accumulation of **ceramide trihexoside** in body tissues.
   a. Characteristics include **skin lesions (angiokeratomas)** over the lower trunk, febrile episodes, severe burning pain in the extremities, and cardiovascular and cerebrovascular involvement.
   b. Death results in early adult life from **renal failure.**
3. **Classic hemophilia (hemophilia A)** is a relatively common X-linked disorder caused by mutations affecting the **factor VIII gene,** which has been localized to the tip of the long arm of the X chromosome. The disease is manifest as a deficiency of coagulation factor VIII.
   a. Symptoms and signs include **hemorrhage** from minor wounds and trauma, bleeding from oral mucosa, hematuria, and hemarthroses.
   b. Recurrent hemarthroses can lead to progressive crippling deformities.
4. **Lesch-Nyhan syndrome**
   a. The cause is a deficiency of **hypoxanthine-guanine phosphoribosyltransferase (HGPRT),** with resultant impaired purine metabolism and excess production of uric acid.
   b. Characteristics include **gout,** mental retardation, choreoathetosis, spasticity, **self-mutilation,** and aggressive behavior.

IV. Balanced Polymorphism

A. **General considerations**
1. Balanced polymorphism refers to the increased incidence of deleterious (usually in homozygotes) alleles among certain populations in environments in which the same allele is associated with a potential survival advantage (usually in heterozygotes).
2. This condition has been observed in both autosomal and X-linked disorders.

B. **Hemoglobin S.** Heterozygotes are thought to be relatively resistant to *Plasmodium falciparum* malaria, and homozygotes have sickle cell anemia.

C. **Glucose-6-phosphate dehydrogenase (G6PD) deficiency.** In this X-linked disorder, hemizygotes manifest drug-related (classically primaquine, an antimalarial) or oxidant-related hemolytic anemia and are also resistant to malaria. In this instance, selection working both positively and negatively clearly represents a manifestation of the balance implied by the term balanced polymorphism.

D. **Phenylketonuria**. Unaffected heterozygotes have a lower incidence of spontaneous abortion. It is thought that modestly increased concentrations of phenylalanine exert a protective effect on pregnancy. This should not be confused with maternal PKU, which is discussed elsewhere in this chapter

E. **Tay-Sachs disease,** in which there may be a protective effect against tuberculosis.

F. **Cystic fibrosis,** in which there is an apparent protective effect against cholera. It is thought that the enterotoxin of cholera facilitates the egress of chloride and water from intestinal mucosa by enhanced activity of chloride channels. Both heterozygous carriers and homozygous affected subjects with cystic fibrosis are relatively resistant to this effect, because insufficient chloride channels are available.

V. Polygenic and Multifactorial Disorders

A. These disorders are more common than monogenic disorders.

B. The causes are abnormalities of complex processes that are regulated by the protein products of two or more genes. Environmental factors also play an important role in the modulation of the genetic defects.

C. Common polygenic disorders include ischemic heart disease, diabetes mellitus, hypertension, gout, schizophrenia, bipolar disorder, and neural tube defects.

VI. Disorders of Sexual Differentiation

These occur when genetic sex, gonadal sex, or genital sex of an individual are discordant.

A. **Definitions**

1. **Genetic sex** is determined by the **presence or absence of a Y chromosome.** At least one Y chromosome is necessary for male gender to be manifest.
2. **Gonadal sex** is determined by the **presence of ovaries or testes.** The gene responsible for development of the testes, the sex-determining region Y gene (SRY gene), is localized to the Y chromosome.
3. **Genital sex** is based on the **appearance of the external genitalia.**

B. **True hermaphrodite**

1. This rare condition is characterized by both ovarian and testicular tissue, with ambiguous external genitalia and both X and Y chromosomes.
2. One possible mechanism is the parthenogenetic division of a haploid ova into two haploid ova, followed by double fertilization and then fusion of the two zygotes in early embryonic development.

C. **Pseudohermaphrodite.** This organism has gonads of only one sex, but the appearance of the external genitalia does not correspond to the gonads present.

1. **Male pseudohermaphrodite**. The gonads are testes, but the external genitalia are not clearly male. The cause may be tissue resistance to androgens (testicular feminization), defects in testosterone synthesis, or hormones administered to the mother during preg-

nancy. The condition has also been linked to **chromosomal anomalies,** such as 46,XY/45,X mosaicism.

2. **Female pseudohermaphrodite.** The gonads are ovaries, but the external genitalia are not clearly female. The condition is most often caused by increased androgenic hormones from congenital adrenal hyperplasia, an androgen-secreting adrenal or ovarian tumor in the mother, or hormones administered to the mother during pregnancy.

REVIEW TEST

Directions: *Each of the numbered items or incomplete statements in this section is followed by answers or by completions of the statement. Select the* ***one*** *lettered answer or completion that is best in each case.*

1. A 19-year-old college sophomore is referred by his ophthalmologist because of the finding of ectopia lentis (dislocation of the lens), which has resulted in visual difficulties that have interfered with his performance on the varsity basketball team. The patient is very tall, with long limbs and long, slender, spiderlike fingers. His chest has a "caved-in" appearance, and he also has a modest degree of scoliosis. A midsystolic "click" is heard, and an echocardiogram reveals mitral valve prolapse. The most likely diagnosis is

(A) Ehlers-Danlos syndrome
(B) Fabry disease
(C) Hurler syndrome
(D) Marfan syndrome
(E) Pompe disease

2. A 20-year-old woman has a robertsonian translocation involving chromosome 21 and a second acrocentric chromosome. What is the theoretic likelihood of a functional trisomy trisomy 21 if one of her ova is fertilized by a normal sperm?

(A) 1 in 1
(B) 1 in 2
(C) 1 in 3
(D) 1 in 4
(E) 1 in 1500

3. A 1-year-old female infant is hospitalized for pneumonia. Bacterial cultures of the sputum have grown *Pseudomonas aeruginosa*. She has had two prior hospitalizations for severe respiratory infections. Her mother has noted that when she kisses her child, the child tastes "salty." The child has had weight loss that the mother attributes to frequent vomiting and diarrhea with bulky, foul-smelling fatty stools. The child is small for her age. Which of the following critical proteins is altered in this condition?

(A) Cystic fibrosis transmembrane conductance regulator
(B) Dystrophin
(C) α-1,4-Glucosidase
(D) α-L-Iduronidase
(E) Lysyl hydroxylase

4. A newly described neurologic disorder is found to affect multiple family members in three generations that were available for study. In the first generation, two sisters and one brother were affected. In the second generation, all of the children of the first generation sisters were affected, but none of the descendants of the first generation son. In the third generation, all of the children of the affected second-generation women were affected, but none of the descendants of the second-generation men. The mode of inheritance exemplified here is

(A) autosomal dominant
(B) autosomal recessive
(C) mitochondrial
(D) X-linked dominant
(E) X-linked recessive

5. As part of a fourth-year elective, a medical student rotating through a medical genetics service is assigned to counsel a patient who is concerned about a family history of hypertension. To be properly prepared for the counseling session, the student reviews course notes on modes of inheritance of various disorders. Knowledge of which of the following modes of inheritance is most pertinent to the upcoming discussion with the patient?

(A) Autosomal dominant
(B) Autosomal recessive
(C) Multifactorial
(D) X-linked dominant
(E) X-linked recessive

6. A 2-year-old child has been followed for mental retardation and slow development as well as multiple birth defects. The child has a high-pitched catlike cry. On examination, microcephaly, hypertelorism, micrognathia, epicanthal folds, low-set ears, and hypotonia are noted. Karyotypic analysis would be expected to show

(A) 5p−
(B) 22q11−
(C) 45,XO
(D) 46,XY
(E) 47,XXY

7. The parents of a 17-year-old boy with Down syndrome seek counseling because they are concerned that their son may develop a life-threatening disorder known to be associated with his chromosomal abnormality. The physician should be prepared to discuss which of the following disorders in terms of its association with Down syndrome?

(A) Berry aneurysm of the circle of Willis
(B) Creutzfeldt-Jakob disease
(C) Lymphoblastic leukemia
(D) Medullary carcinoma of the thyroid
(E) Osteosarcoma

8. A 14-year-old girl with amenorrhea is concerned because of the delayed onset of menses. She has shortened stature and a wide, webbed neck; broad chest; and secondary sexual characteristics consistent with those of a much younger girl. Which of the following chromosomal changes is most consistent with these findings?

(A) 5p
(B) 22q11 −
(C) 45,XO
(D) 46,XY
(E) 47,XXY

9. A 50-year-old woman of Eastern European Jewish ancestry has a history of recurrent fractures and easy bruising and is found to have hepatosplenomegaly and mild anemia. Serum assays reveal elevations of chitotriosidase and angiotensin-converting enzyme. Assay of cultured leukocytes most likely reveals marked deficiency of which of the following enzymes?

(A) Glucocerebrosidase
(B) α-1,4-Glucosidase
(C) Hexosaminidase A
(D) α-L-Iduronidase
(E) Sphingomyelinase

10. During a routine physical examination, a 41-year-old woman is noted to have blue-black pigmented patches in the sclerae and gray-blue discoloration of the ear cartilages. The extensor tendons of the hands exhibit similar discoloration when she is asked to "make a fist." On questioning, the patient vaguely remembers hearing her mother say that the patient had dark discoloration on her diapers when she was an infant. Her only current complaint is slowly increasing pain and stiffness of the lower back, hips, and knees. A urine sample darkens on standing. These findings are characteristic of a deficiency of which of the following enzymes?

(A) Homogentisic oxidase
(B) Hypoxanthine guanine phosphoribosyltransferase
(C) L-Iduronosulfate sulfatase
(D) Ketoacid decarboxylase
(E) Phenylalanine hydroxylase

11. A screening test for phenylketonuria (PKU) is performed on umbilical cord blood from a fair-skinned blond, blue-eyed infant born to dark-complexioned parents. The test is reported as negative, and no dietary restrictions are imposed. At 1 year of age, the child is seen again, this time with obvious signs of severe mental retardation, and a diagnosis of PKU is made. The diagnosis was missed at birth because

(A) cord blood is not a good source of fetal blood
(B) the screening (Guthrie) test has low sensitivity
(C) the test should have been performed on maternal blood
(D) the test should have been performed on urine rather than blood
(E) the test was performed too early

12. A 56-year-old man dies of a 15-year progressive illness characterized by athetoid movements and deterioration leading to hypertonicity, fecal and urine incontinence, anorexia and weight loss, and eventually dementia and death. The disease is known to have an autosomal dominant mode of inheritance and to be due to an abnormality in a gene on chromosome 4 that is altered by increased numbers of intragenic trinucleotide repeats. In addition, this disorder has an earlier onset and is more debilitating in successive generations, a phenomenon that might be due to

(A) a shift from trinucleotide repeats to pentanucleotide repeats
(B) an increase in the number of trinucleotide repeats in successive generations
(C) defects in membrane receptors and transport systems
(D) imprinting variability in successive generations
(E) increased medical awareness of the condition

A ANSWERS AND EXPLANATIONS

1-D. Marfan syndrome, an autosomal dominant disorder caused by mutations of the fibrillin gene on chromosome 15, is a frequent cause of ectopia lentis. Other cardinal features include skeletal and cardiovascular abnormalities. Patients are tall and thin, with notably long limbs and digits. An anterior chest deformity known as pectus excavatum is sometimes seen, and vertebral abnormalities include scoliosis and lordosis. In addition, a highly arched palate and crowding of the teeth may occur. Cardiovascular complications include mitral valve prolapse and mitral regurgitation. Cystic medial necrosis can lead to dilation of the aortic root and aortic regurgitation. Life-threatening complications are aortic aneurysm and aortic dissection.

2-C. Theoretically, a person who carries a robertsonian translocation with chromosome 21 and a second acrocentric chromosome has a 1 in 3 chance of having a child with trisomy 21. However, the risk of a live birth of a child with Down syndrome is actually much less, presumably because of a high incidence of spontaneous abortion of such fetuses. The important point is that a robertsonian translocation predisposes to a hereditable form of Down syndrome. The risk is not related to maternal age and is much higher than the risk in the general population, which is 1 in 1500 for women 20 years of age and younger, increasing to 1 in 25 in women older than 45 years of age.

3-A. The diagnosis is cystic fibrosis, the most common lethal genetic disease in Caucasian populations. The disorder is due to a defect in the cystic fibrosis transmembrane conductance regulator protein, and about 70% of cases have a deletion of phenylalanine in position 508 (ΔF508 mutation). Affected patients often have multiple pulmonary infections and pancreatic insufficiency with steatorrhea and failure to thrive. Death is often due to respiratory failure secondary to repeated pulmonary infections, facilitated by the buildup of thick, tenacious mucus in the airways. Increased concentration of chloride in sweat and tears is characteristic, and the sweat test is an important diagnostic adjunct.

4-C. In mitochondrial inheritance, inheritance is entirely maternal in transmission. Affected males do not transmit the trait to any of their children, and affected females transmit the trait to all of their children. Abnormalities of mitochondrial inheritance typically involve genes that code for enzymes of oxidative phosphorylation.

5-C. Multifactorial disorders are among the most common familial abnormalities and are much more common than monogenic disorders. They include a number of common entities, such as ischemic heart disease, diabetes mellitus, hypertension, gout, schizophrenia, bipolar disorder, and neural tube defects.

6-A. The clinical presentation is that of the cri du chat (or 5p−) syndrome.

7-C. Patients with Down syndrome are at increased risk of lymphoblastic leukemia. In addition, there is common occurrence of congenital heart disease, especially defects of the endocardial cushion (atrioventricular valve malformations and atrial and ventricular septal defects), and increased susceptibility to infection. Many patients with Down syndrome who are older than 35 years of age show clinical signs, symptoms, and pathologic findings of Alzheimer-type dementia, with an incidence much higher than in the general population.

8-C. Although most patients with Turner syndrome have a 45,XO karyotype, the syndrome is thought to be caused by the absence of one set of genes from the short arm of one X chromosome, and a variety of chromosome abnormalities may be found. Many patients are mosaics (e.g., 45,XO/46,XX or 45,XO/47,XXX), and the phenotype is highly variable. A deletion of the *SHOX* gene can cause an identical phenotype and may be considered to be a variant of Turner syndrome.

9-A. The clinical findings are those of type I Gaucher disease, which is a manifestation of glucocerebrosidase deficiency. The disorder is most often seen in persons of European (Ashkenazic) Jewish lineage. Prominent findings include bone pain and fractures, easy bruising, hepatosplenomegaly, anemia, and thrombocytopenia. Bone marrow aspiration reveals numerous typical Gaucher cells, but specific enzyme assay is required to confirm the diagnosis. This lysosomal storage disease is relatively mild compared to a number of other such entities, such as Tay-Sachs disease and Niemann-Pick disease, which are rarely seen in adults. The disease is highly variable in its clinical manifestations, and assays of chitotriosidase and angiotensin-converting enzyme, markers of macrophage proliferation, are useful measures of the extent of disease and of its control.

10-A. The patient has homogentisic oxidase deficiency, a rare inborn error of metabolism (actually the first such disorder described by Garrod in 1902), clinically manifest by alkaptonuria and ochronosis. The term alkaptonuria refers to urinary excretion of unmetabolized homogentisic acid imparting a dark color to urine on standing. The term ochronosis refers to pigment deposition in multiple tissues, most prominently in cartilage and connective tissue. Most symptoms result from joint involvement, which can lead to disabling arthritis as patients age. Other affected structures include the eyes, larynx and bronchi, heart and vessels, prostate, and sweat glands.

11-E. The concentration of phenylalanine in affected infants is usually normal at birth and increases rapidly during the first days of life. False-negative results are common immediately after birth but are rare on the second and third days of life. Consequently, the blood sample for phenylketonuria is usually taken from the infant's heel within 2 to 3 days after birth. If the test is performed too early, the diagnosis could be missed.

12-B. The phenomenon of earlier and more severe manifestations of a disorder in successive generations (anticipation) is a characteristic of many trinucleotide repeat disorders, the best known examples of which are fragile X syndrome (discussed in this chapter) and Huntington disease (described in this clinical scenario and further discussed in Chapter 23). The degree of expansion is closely related to the gender of the parent with the genetic abnormality. In the fragile X syndrome, expansion occurs during oogenesis. In Huntington disease, expansion occurs during spermatogenesis. Even though trinucleotide repeats almost always involve guanine and cytosine (G and C), the third nucleotide is different in the two conditions: CGG in fragile X syndrome and CAG in Huntington disease.

CHAPTER 5

Immune Dysfunction

I. Cells of the Immune System

A. **Lymphocytes. These** include B cells, T cells, and natural killer (NK) cells. They are identified by cell-surface glycoproteins specific for both cell type and stage of differentiation.

1. **B cells** originate from stem cells in the bone marrow. They continue their differentiation within the bone marrow and peripherally, where they cluster in the **germinal centers of lymph nodes** and in the **lymphoid follicles of the spleen.**
   a. The presence of **surface immunoglobulin** is characteristic.
   b. Approximately 15% of circulating peripheral blood lymphocytes are B cells.
2. **T cells** originate from stem cells in the bone marrow and differentiate in the **thymus.** They populate the **paracortical and deep medullary areas of lymph nodes** and **periarteriolar sheaths of the spleen.**
   a. Approximately 70% of circulating peripheral blood lymphocytes are T cells.
   b. T cells are subclassified by surface markers as follows:
      (1) **CD4+ T cells** (T4+ T cells), which account for approximately 60% of circulating T cells
      (2) **CD8+ T cells** (T8+ T cells), which account for approximately 30% of circulating T cells. The normal 2:1 ratio of CD4+ to CD8+ T cells is dramatically altered in some disease states. For example, in AIDS, the ratio is often 0.5:1 or less.
3. **NK cells** are also called **large granular lymphocytes (LGLs)** because of their distinctive large size, pale cytoplasm, and prominent granulation.
   a. NK cells kill tumor cells, fungi, and cells altered by viral infection. Neither specific sensitization nor antibody is involved in this type of cell killing. NK cells can also lyse cells by **antibody-dependent cell-mediated cytotoxicity (ADCC).**
   b. Approximately 15% of circulating lymphocytes are NK cells.

B. **Macrophages.** These derivatives of peripheral blood monocytes are members of the mononuclear phagocyte system of cells.

1. Macrophages secrete a variety of cytokines, including **interleukin-1 (IL-1),** as well as other products, such as acid hydrolases, neutral proteases, and prostaglandins. In addition, they process and present antigen [along with human leukocyte antigen (HLA) class II antigens] to CD4+ T cells.
2. Macrophages also participate in **delayed hypersensitivity reactions.** They may be capable of directly killing tumor cells.

C. **Dendritic cells of lymphoid tissue** are characterized by **dendritic cytoplasmic processes.**

1. Dendritic cells express large quantities of **cell surface HLA class II antigens.**
2. In contrast to macrophages, dendritic cells are poorly phagocytic. However, like macrophages, dendritic cells are antigen-presenting cells.

D. **Langerhans cells of the skin**
1. Ultrastructural characteristics include the presence of **Birbeck granules,** tennis racket-shaped cytoplasmic structures.
2. Like dendritic cells of lymphoid tissue, Langerhans cells of the skin express HLA class II antigens and are antigen-presenting cells.

II. Cytokines

These soluble proteins are secreted by lymphocytes (lymphokines), monocytes—macrophages (monokines), and NK cells, as well as other cell types. They act as effector molecules influencing the behavior of B cells, T cells, NK cells, monocytes, macrophages, hematopoietic cells, and many other cell types (Table 5-1).

III. Complement System

This system consists of about 20 plasma proteins and their products, which can be activated by way of the classic or alternate pathway to form a final product—the membrane attack complex—that lyses targeted cells.

A. **Classic pathway. This pathway** is initiated by reaction with **antigen-antibody complexes.** The final lytic form of activated complement is the result of a series of **enzymatic cleavages** and recombinations of cleavage products.

TABLE 5-1 *Cytokine Functions*

Cytokine	Source	Major Functions
Interleukin-1 (IL-1)	Monocytes, macrophages, and other cells	Stimulates T cell proliferation and IL-2 production
Interleukin-2 (IL-2)	Macrophages, T cells, and NK cells	Stimulates proliferation of T cells, B cells, and NK cells; activates monocytes
Interleukin-3 (IL-3)	T cells	Acts as growth factor for tissue mast cells and hematopoietic stem cells
Interleukin-4 (IL-4)	T cells	Promotes growth of B and T cells; enhances expression of HLA class II antigens
Interleukin-5 (IL-5)	T cells	Promotes end-stage maturation of B cells into plasma cells
Interleukin-6 (IL-6)	T cells, monocytes, and other cells	Promotes maturation of B and T cells; inhibits growth of fibroblasts
Interferon-α (IFN-α)	B cells and macrophages	Has antiviral activity
Interferon-β (IFN-β)	Fibroblasts	Has antiviral activity
Interferon-γ (IFN-γ)	T cells and NK cells	Has antiviral activity; activates macrophages; enhances expression of HLA class II antigens
Tumor necrosis factor-α (TNF-α, cachectin)	Macrophages, T cells, and NK cells	Stimulates T cell proliferation and IL-2 production: cytotoxic to some tumor cells
Tumor necrosis factor-β (TNF-β)	T cells	Stimulates T cell proliferation and IL-2 production; cytotoxic to some tumor cells

HLA = human leukocyte antigen; NK = natural killer.

B. **Alternate pathway. This pathway** is initiated directly by **nonimmunologic stimuli,** such as invading microorganisms, and, like the classic pathway, leads to cleavage products that cause cell lysis. It bypasses the initial stages of the classic pathway.

IV. Human Leukocyte Antigen System

The HLA system consists of a group of related proteins referred to as **HLA antigens.** The genes that code for HLA antigens are called **histocompatibility genes** and are localized to a region on the short arm of chromosome 6, known as the **major histocompatibility complex.** The HLA system is important in **organ transplantation,** where HLA typing and matching of donor and recipient are now widely used to predict tissue compatibility.

A. **HLA antigens.** The two major classes are separated on the basis of structure and tissue distribution.

1. **Class I antigens** include the HLA-A, HLA-B, and HLA-C antigens, which are found on almost all human cells.
   a. Class I antigens are the principal antigens involved in **tissue graft rejection.** Serologic testing for HLA-A and HLA-B antigens is used to predict the likelihood of long-term graft survival.
   b. Standard serologic techniques are used for identification.
2. **Class II antigens** are chiefly found on immunocompetent cells, including macrophages, dendritic cells, Langerhans cells, B cells, and some T cells.
   a. The HLA-DP, HLA-DQ, and HLA-DR antigens are identifiable by standard serologic techniques or by mixed lymphocyte reactions.
   b. The HLA-D antigens are identifiable only by mixed lymphocyte reactions.

B. **Association of HLA antigens with disease.** There is a significant association of certain HLA antigens with a number of specific diseases. Many HLA-associated disorders involve immunologic abnormalities, but the mechanisms for these observed associations await full explanation.

1. **HLA-B27 antigen** is associated with almost 90% of cases of **ankylosing spondylitis.**
2. Specific HLA antigens are also associated with insulin-dependent diabetes mellitus, rheumatoid arthritis, uveitis, and Reiter syndrome (urethritis, conjunctivitis, and arthritis), as well as with many other entities.

V. Mechanisms of Immune Injury

Adverse reactions caused by immune mechanisms are termed **hypersensitivity reactions.** The classification of Gell and Coombs divides hypersensitivity reactions into four types (Table 5-2). Types I, II, and III require the active production of antibody by plasma cells (terminally differentiated B cells). Type IV is mediated by the interaction of T cells and macrophages.

A. **Type I (immediate or anaphylactic) hypersensitivity**

1. **Steps in the reaction**
   a. **Immunoglobulin E (IgE)** antibody production by IgE B cells is stimulated by antigen. The IgE antibody is then bound to the Fc receptors of **basophils** and **tissue mast cells.**
   b. On **subsequent exposure,** antigen (allergen) reacts with bound IgE antibody (complement is not involved), resulting in cytolysis and degranulation of basophils or tissue mast cells. This reaction requires bridging (cross-linking) of adjacent IgE molecules on the mast cell surface.
   c. **Degranulation** results in **histamine** release, which increases vascular permeability. Various other substances are produced, many of which are vasoactive or smooth muscle spasm-inducing.

TABLE 5-2 *Mechanisms of Immune Injury (Modified Gell and Coombs Classification)*

Type of Hypersensitivity	Mechanism	Examples
Type I (immediate or anaphylactic)	Antigen reacts with IgE bound to surface of basophils or tissue mast cells, causing degranulation with release of histamine and other substances, many of which are vasoactive, smooth muscle spasm-inducing, or chemotactic	Hay fever; allergic asthma; hives; anaphylactic shock
Type II (antibody-mediated or cytotoxic)	Antibodies react with antigens that are intrinsic components of cell membrane or other structures, such as basement membranes, resulting in direct damage, complement-mediated increased susceptibility to phagocytosis, or antibody-dependent cell-mediated cytotoxicity; also may be caused by inactivation of cell-surface receptors by anti-receptor antibodies	Warm antibody autoimmune hemolytic anemia; hemolytic disease of the newborn; Goodpasture syndrome; Graves disease
Type III (immune complex)	Insoluble complement-bound aggregates of antigen-antibody complexes are deposited in vessel walls or on serosal surfaces or other extravascular sites; neutrophils are chemotactically attracted and release lysosomal enzymes, prostaglandins, kinins, and free radicals, resulting in tissue damage	Serum sickness; Arthus reaction; polyarteritis nodosa; SLE; immune complex-mediated glomerular diseases
Type IV (cell-mediated)	Delayed hypersensitivity; proliferation of antigen-specific CD4+ memory T cells, with secretion of IL-2 and other cytokines, which in turn recruit and stimulate phagocytic macrophages; may also involve cytotoxic CD8+ T lymphocyte killing of specific target cells	Tuberculin reaction; contact dermatitis; tumor cell killing; virally infected cell killing

d. Chemotactic substances recruit eosinophils, resulting in tissue and peripheral blood **eosinophilia.**

2. **Clinical examples**

a. **Allergic** or **atopic** reactions, such as **seasonal rhinitis** (hay fever), allergic **asthma,** or **urticaria** (hives)

b. **Systemic anaphylaxis (anaphylactic shock),** which is a potentially fatal reaction. Rapid onset of urticaria, bronchospasm, laryngeal edema, and shock after exposure to an offending antigen is characteristic.

c. **Angioedema,** which is acute edema of cutaneous or mucosal structures, most commonly involving the lips and eyelids. Laryngeal edema can occur and be life threatening. Hereditary angioedema is caused by deficiency of C1 esterase inhibiter and is not a manifestation of type I hypersensitivity. Serum C4 is low and other complement components such as C3 are consumed.

B. **Type II (antibody-mediated or cytotoxic) hypersensitivity**

1. **Complement-fixing antibodies** react directly with antigens that are integral components of the target cell. The interaction of complement with the cell surface results in cell lysis and destruction. Serum complement is characteristically decreased.
   a. The antigens involved are usually localized to tissue basement membranes or blood cell membranes.
   b. Clinical examples include **warm antibody autoimmune hemolytic anemia, hemolytic transfusion reactions,** and **hemolytic disease of the newborn** (erythroblastosis fetalis), in which the antigens are components of red blood cell membranes; and **Goodpasture syndrome** (antiglomerular basement membrane antibody disease), in which the pulmonary alveolar and glomerular basement membranes are affected.
2. **Antibody-dependent cell-mediated cytotoxicity (ADCC)**
   a. Antibody reacts directly with integral surface antigens of targeted cells.
   b. The free Fc portion of the antibody molecule reacts with the Fc receptor of a variety of cytotoxic leukocytes, most importantly **NK cells.** Other leukocytes, including monocytes, neutrophils, and eosinophils, also bear Fc receptors and can participate in ADCC.
   c. The target cells are killed by the Fc receptor-bound cytotoxic leukocytes. Complement is not involved.
3. **Reaction of anti-receptor antibodies with cell-surface receptor protein**
   a. This variant, sometimes classified separately as type V hypersensitivity, is exemplified by the reaction of **thyroid-stimulating immunoglobulin** with the thyroid-stimulating hormone (TSH) receptor of thyroid follicular cells in **Graves disease.**
   b. In this disorder, the antigen-antibody reaction mimics the effect of TSH on the follicular cells and results in glandular hyperplasia and hyperproduction of thyroid hormone with clinical hyperthyroidism.

C. **Type III (immune complex) hypersensitivity**

1. Exogenous antibody produced in response to exposure to antigen combines with antigen, resulting in circulating **antigen-antibody complexes.** In contrast to type II hypersensitivity, the **antigen is not an intrinsic component of the target cells.**
2. Immune complexes are most often removed by cells of the mononuclear phagocyte system without adverse effect. In other cases, insoluble aggregates of immune complex are deposited in vessel walls or on serosal surfaces or other extravascular sites. This involves smaller immune complexes that are less easily removed by the mononuclear phagocyte system.
3. The immune complexes bind **complement,** which is highly chemotactic for neutrophils. The neutrophils release lysosomal enzymes, resulting in tissue damage, which can also result from other substances released by neutrophils, including prostaglandins, kinins, and free radicals. Serum complement is decreased.
4. **Hageman factor (factor XII)** is also activated, with further activation of the intrinsic pathway of coagulation, resulting in thrombosis in nearby small vessels, and activation of the kinin system, resulting in vasodilation and edema.
5. **Platelet aggregation** causes microthrombus formation and leads to the release of vasoactive amines from platelet dense granules.
6. **Clinical examples**
   a. **Serum sickness** is a systemic deposition of antigen-antibody complexes in multiple sites, especially the heart, joints, and kidneys. In the past, antibody-containing foreign serum (most often horse serum) was administered therapeutically for passive immunization against microorganisms or their toxic products. Because of the danger of serum sickness, this mode of therapy is no longer employed.
   b. **Systemic lupus erythematosus** is also an example of a multisystem immune complex disease.
   c. **Arthus reaction** is a localized immune complex reaction that occurs when exogenous antigen is introduced, either by injection or by organ transplant, in the presence of an excess of preformed antibodies.

d. **Polyarteritis nodosa** is a generalized immune complex disease especially involving small- and medium-sized arteries.

e. **Immune complex-mediated glomerular diseases** include poststreptococcal glomerulonephritis, membranous glomerulonephritis, and lupus nephropathy.

D. **Type IV (cell-mediated) hypersensitivity**

1. **Delayed hypersensitivity**

a. The T-cell receptor of **CD4+ lymphocytes** interacts with antigen, presented by **macrophages,** and with **HLA class II antigens** on macrophages, resulting in stimulation of antigen-specific CD4+ memory T cells.

(1) On subsequent contact with antigen, the CD4+ memory T cells proliferate and secrete cytokines.

(2) IL-2 and other cytokines secreted by the CD4+ T cells recruit and stimulate the phagocytic activity of macrophages.

b. **Examples**

(1) The **tuberculin reaction** is a localized inflammatory reaction initiated by the intracutaneous injection of tuberculin and marked by proliferation of lymphocytes, monocytes, and small numbers of neutrophils, with a tendency toward cellular accumulations about small vessels (perivascular cuffing). Induration (hardening) results from fibrin formation.

(2) **Contact dermatitis** may result from either delayed hypersensitivity or direct chemical injury to the skin.

2. **Cytotoxic T lymphocyte–mediated cytotoxicity** is direct **CD8+ T cell–mediated killing** of target cells (typically tumor cells or virus-infected cells).

a. Specific target cell antigen is recognized by the T-cell receptor of CD8+ lymphocytes.

b. Target cell **HLA class I antigens** recognized as self-antigens are also required.

c. Cytokines are not involved.

VI. Transplantation Immunology

A. **General considerations**

1. For a successful graft, donor and recipient must be matched for ABO blood groups and, ideally, for as many HLA antigens as possible.

2. Adverse immune responses can be suppressed by immunosuppressant drugs, radiation, or recipient T-cell depletion. However, these processes can result in clinically significant immunodeficiency.

B. **Types of transplant rejection.** Three basic patterns of graft rejection are well illustrated by rejection following kidney transplantation.

1. **Hyperacute rejection**

a. Rejection is primarily **antibody-mediated** and occurs in the presence of preexisting antibody to donor antigens.

b. Rejection most often **occurs within minutes** of transplantation.

c. Rejection is a **localized Arthus reaction** marked by acute inflammation, fibrinoid necrosis of small vessels, and extensive thrombosis.

2. **Acute rejection**

a. Rejection is primarily **T cell-mediated.**

b. Rejection generally occurs **days to weeks after transplantation.**

c. Rejection is characterized by infiltration of lymphocytes and macrophages. When antibody-mediated mechanisms are prominent, it may show evidence of arteritis with thrombosis and cortical necrosis.

3. **Chronic rejection**

a. Rejection is primarily caused by **antibody-mediated vascular damage.**

b. Rejection may occur **months to years after an otherwise successful transplantation.**

c. Rejection is characterized histologically by marked vascular fibrointimal proliferation, often resulting in a small, scarred kidney. It is becoming more common with the success of immunosuppression in overcoming acute rejection.

C. **Graft-versus-host disease.** This is a significant problem in **bone marrow transplantation** because immunocompetent cells are transplanted in this procedure. It can also be caused by **whole blood transfusion in patients with severe combined immunodeficiency (SCID).**

1. The rejection of "foreign" host cells by engrafted T and B cells is characteristic.
   a. CD8+ T cells from graft directly damage host cells.
   b. Cytokines from graft CD4+ T cells recruit macrophages, which damage host cells.
   c. Clinical features include fever, rash, hepatosplenomegaly, and jaundice.
   d. Principal target organs are **liver, skin,** and **gastrointestinal mucosa.**

VII. Immunodeficiency Diseases

A. **X-linked agammaglobulinemia of Bruton.** This disorder occurs in male infants but is usually not manifest clinically until **after 6 months of age** because of the persistence of maternal antibodies.

1. **Immune system defects**
   a. Failure of antibody synthesis caused by a block in maturation of pre-B cells to B cells due to a mutation in the B cell tyrosine kinase (*Btk*) gene. Cell-mediated immunity is unaffected.
   b. **Absence of plasma cells** in tissue results in virtual **absence of serum immunoglobulins.**
   c. **Absent or poorly defined germinal centers** in lymphoid tissue occur.
2. **Effects**
   a. A propensity to **recurrent bacterial infections** with organisms such as pneumococci, streptococci, staphylococci, and *Haemophilus influenzae* may occur.
   b. Resistance to viral and fungal infections or phagocytosis and killing of bacteria by neutrophils is not affected.

B. **Isolated IgA deficiency**

1. The most common inherited B cell defect, isolated IgA deficiency occurs in approximately 1 in 700 persons.
2. It results from the inability of IgA B cells to mature to plasma cells. Other immunoglobulins are normal.
3. Most often, the disorder is asymptomatic, but it may be characterized by occasional anaphylactic reactions to transfused blood. It may also be associated with infections, especially those involving mucosal surfaces, and manifest as recurrent upper respiratory tract infections and frequent episodes of diarrhea.

C. **Common variable immunodeficiency.** This diverse group of disorders is caused by **failure of terminal B-cell maturation,** resulting in diminution in the number of plasma cells and thus **hypogammaglobulinemia.** It is manifest clinically by **recurrent bacterial infection.**

D. **DiGeorge syndrome (thymic hypoplasia)**

1. This **congenital T-cell deficiency** results from aberrant embryonic development of the third and fourth branchial arches, leading to hypoplasia of the thymus and parathyroid glands as well as abnormalities of the mandible, ear, and aortic arch.
2. Failure of T-cell maturation resulting in **lymphopenia** is characteristic. B cells remain unimpaired.
3. Clinical manifestations include **recurrent viral and fungal infections** and **tetany** from hypoparathyroidism with hypocalcemia.

4. DiGeorge syndrome can be summed up by the popular acronym **CATCH 22,** which denotes **C**ardiac defects, **A**bnormal facies, **T**hymic hypoplasia, **C**left palate, **H**ypocalcemia, and microdeletion of chromosome ***22***.

E. **Severe combined immunodeficiency disease (SCID).** This disorder is also known as **Swiss-type agammaglobulinemia.**

1. Marked deficiency of **both B and T cells** manifest as profound lymphopenia and severe defects in both humoral and cell-mediated immunity.
2. SCID, which can be caused by a wide variety of genetic defects, occurs in both autosomal recessive and X-linked forms. Approximately 50% of autosomal recessive cases are caused by adenosine deaminase **(ADA) deficiency,** which leads to an accumulation of deoxyadenosine and deoxy-ATP, substances that are toxic to lymphocytes.
3. **Clinical manifestations**
   a. **Severe infections** (bacterial, viral, and fungal)
   b. High incidence of **malignancy**
   c. **Failure to thrive,** usually with fatal outcome in infancy
   d. **Graft-versus-host disease** as a result of blood transfusions
4. **Anatomic manifestations**
   a. Thymic hypoplasia with absent or greatly reduced thymic lymphoid component
   b. Hypoplasia of lymph nodes, tonsils, and other lymphoid tissues
5. **Treatments**
   a. Bone marrow or stem cell transplantation
   b. ADA gene transplantation (presently on hold)

F. **Immunodeficiency with thrombocytopenia and eczema (Wiskott-Aldrich syndrome)**

1. This syndrome is an **X-linked** disorder.
2. Characteristics include **eczema, thrombocytopenia, recurrent infections,** and poor antibody response to polysaccharide antigens. Total immunoglobulins most often are normal.

G. **Acquired immunodeficiency syndrome (AIDS)**

1. **Cause.** AIDS is caused by **human immunodeficiency virus (HIV)** infection and has become a worldwide epidemic since the first clinical description in 1981. The vast majority of AIDS cases in the U.S. and Europe are caused by infection with the retrovirus **HIV-1.**
2. **Mechanisms of HIV infection**
   a. The HIV virion expresses a cell surface protein, **gp120,** with binding sites for the CD4 molecule on the surface of **CD4+ T cells**. The interaction of viral gp120 with cellular CD4 explains the affinity of HIV for CD4+ T cells. In addition, two recognition sites on gp120 for the coreceptors CCR5 and CXCR4 are involved in the entry of HIV into the cell. Of considerable interest is the finding that **individuals homozygous for mutated CCR5 receptor are highly resistant to some strains of HIV.**
   b. **Other CD4+ cell types** that are targets for HIV infection include monocytes, macrophages, dendritic cells, Langerhans cells, and microglial cells of the central nervous system (CNS).
      (1) **Monocytes and macrophages** may function as reservoirs for HIV and possibly as vehicles for viral entry into the CNS.
      (2) HIV may infect **neural cells** directly by way of CD4 receptors or may compete (through the gp120 protein) for neural receptor sites for neuroleukin, a neural tissue growth factor.
   c. After cellular binding of gp120 to CD4 and internalization of HIV into the cell, proviral DNA is synthesized by reverse transcription from genomic viral RNA.
   d. **Proviral DNA** is integrated into the host genome.
      (1) In its proviral form, HIV may remain latent for an extended period until activation, possibly by infection with other viruses, such as cytomegalovirus or Epstein-Barr virus (EBV).

(2) Low-level virion production, with resultant infectivity, occurs even during the latent period.

e. The HIV virus is found in blood, semen, vaginal secretions, breast milk, and saliva.

f. Diagnosis by the ELISA test is presumptive; follow-up tests include Western blot and direct assessment of viral RNA.

3. **High-risk populations: AIDS**

a. **Homosexual or bisexual men** (75% of cases)

(1) The risk is apparently greater with anal receptive intercourse.

(2) In Central Africa, the incidence in both sexes is about equal and is no higher in homosexual or bisexual men than in the general population.

b. **Intravenous drug abusers** (15% of cases). The virus is spread by sharing needles used by infected drug users.

c. **Heterosexual partners of persons in high-risk groups** (4% of cases). Sexual transmission from intravenous drug abusers is the major mode of entry of HIV into the heterosexual population.

d. **Patients receiving multiple blood transfusions** (2% of cases). Risk has been greatly diminished by screening donor blood for anti-HIV antibodies, HIV p24 antigen and HIV-1 RNA.

e. **Hemophiliacs** (1% of cases). Most likely, the entire cohort of hemophiliacs who received factor VIII concentrates between 1981 and 1985 became infected with HIV. Since 1985, HIV screening and heat inactivation of HIV in factor VIII concentrates have become universal.

f. **Infants of high-risk parents.** Infection can be transplacental or can occur at the time of delivery.

4. **Pathogenesis of AIDS**

a. Infection with HIV results in the **depletion of CD4+ T cells.** The number of circulating lymphocytes is greatly decreased, and this decrease is accounted for by a loss of CD4+ T cells. The CD4+:CD8+ ratio is also greatly reduced, often to less than 1.0.

b. The loss of CD4+ (helper) T cells causes **failure in humoral and cell-mediated hypersensitivity reactions.**

c. Despite the inability to produce specific antibodies, patients with AIDS paradoxically demonstrate **hypergammaglobulinemia** from polyclonal B cell activation.

5. **Clinical characteristics of AIDS**

a. Severe immunodeficiency manifested by **opportunistic infection** with organisms such as ***Pneumocystis carinii*, cytomegalovirus, *Mucor* species,** and **typical and atypical mycobacteria such as *Mycobacterium avium-intracellulare*;** other opportunistic infections often found include *Candida, Cryptosporidium, Coccidioides, Cryptococcus, Toxoplasma, Histoplasma,* and *Giardia* infections.

b. Increased incidence of malignancy, particularly multifocal **Kaposi sarcoma,** an otherwise rare lesion that in AIDS is almost entirely confined to the homosexual male population, and B-cell **non-Hodgkin lymphoma;** an increased incidence of Hodgkin disease and hepatocellular carcinoma also occurs.

c. **Central and peripheral nervous system manifestations** occur due to opportunistic infections, CNS tumors, or direct neural infection with HIV.

6. **Stages of HIV infection.** HIV disease may be asymptomatic for many years. Before fully developed AIDS occurs, there is acute illness resembling infectious mononucleosis; a long latent phase followed by generalized lymphadenopathy; and a stage marked by chronic fever, weight loss, and diarrhea.

a. **HIV seropositivity** begins soon after initial HIV infection. Antibodies to the proteins coded by the genes of retroviral *gag, env,* and *pol* regions can be demonstrated, especially antibodies to the gp120 and p24 proteins. HIV infection can also be demonstrated by amplification of viral genetic sequences by polymerase chain reaction or by viral culture.

b. The last stage, defined as **AIDS,** is marked by HIV infection complicated by specified secondary opportunistic infection or malignant neoplasms.

VIII. Autoimmunity

A. **General considerations**

1. Autoimmunity results in disease caused by immune reactions directed toward tissues of the host, with apparent inability to distinguish self from nonself. Examples include a number of autoimmune disorders, including **autoimmune hemolytic anemia, Hashimoto thyroiditis, idiopathic adrenal atrophy,** and a group of disorders referred to as **connective tissue diseases.**
2. One or more of the following associations are often characteristic: the presence of autoantibodies (incidence increases with age); comorbidity with other autoimmune diseases; morphologic changes such as lymphoid follicle formation, as prominently exemplified by Hashimoto thyroiditis; and association with specific HLA haplotypes.
3. A number of possible mechanisms may mediate autoimmunity.

B. **Antigens**

1. Host antigens may be recognized as nonself if modified by infection, inflammation, or complexing with a drug.
2. Antigens usually isolated from the immune system may be exposed by trauma or inflammation and become recognized as foreign. Examples include thyroglobulin, lens protein, and spermatozoa.
3. A foreign antigen may share a common structure with a host antigen.

C. **Antibodies**

1. Many autoimmune disorders are characterized by the presence of **specific autoantibodies,** antibodies directed against host tissue.
2. The demonstration of autoantibodies is presumptive (but not entirely conclusive) evidence of the autoimmune nature of a disorder.

D. **Disordered immunoregulation**

1. **Increase in helper T-cell function** or **decrease in suppressor T-cell function**
2. **Nonspecific B-cell activation** by EBV may trigger polyclonal antibody formation
3. **Thymic defects or B-cell defects**

E. **Genetic factors**

1. **Genetic predisposition** is suggested because several autoimmune disorders, including Hashimoto thyroiditis, pernicious anemia, type 1 diabetes mellitus (also known as insulin-dependent diabetes mellitus, or IDDM), and Sjögren syndrome, are associated with an increased incidence of other autoimmune disorders.
2. Some **HLA antigens** are associated with increased incidence of certain autoimmune disorders. For example, incidence of Hashimoto thyroiditis is increased in HLA-DR5- and HLA-B5-positive individuals, and incidence of type 2 diabetes is increased in HLA-DR3- and HLA-DR4-positive individuals.

F. **Environmental factors**

1. Infection (particularly viral) or other environmental agents may initiate autoimmune reactions in genetically susceptible individuals.
2. Some viruses apparently trigger autoimmune islet cell inflammation and resultant type 1 diabetes.

IX. Connective Tissue (Collagen) Diseases

These encompass a group of loosely related conditions, most of which feature **fibrinoid change** in connective tissue. They may be of autoimmune origin; **antinuclear antibodies (ANAs)** and various other autoantibodies are often present.

A. **Systemic lupus erythematosus (SLE)**
   1. SLE, the prototype connective tissue disease, most often affects **women** (80% of patients), usually those of childbearing age.
   2. SLE is marked by the presence of a spectrum of ANAs and by **extensive immune complex-mediated inflammatory lesions** involving multiple organ systems, especially the joints, skin, serous membranes, lungs, and kidneys. The lesions of greatest clinical importance in SLE are those in the **kidney.**
   3. **Clinical manifestations**
      a. **Fever, malaise, lymphadenopathy, and weight loss**
      b. **Joint symptoms,** including arthralgia and arthritis
      c. Skin rashes, including a **characteristic butterfly rash** over the base of the nose and malar eminences, often with associated photosensitivity
      d. **Raynaud phenomenon,** manifested by vasospasm of small vessels, most often of the fingers
      e. **Serosal inflammation,** especially pericarditis and pleuritis
      f. **Diffuse interstitial pulmonary fibrosis,** manifest as interstitial pneumonitis or diffuse fibrosing alveolitis
      g. **Endocarditis** of the characteristic atypical nonbacterial verrucous (Libman-Sacks) form, in which vegetations are seen on both sides of the mitral valve leaflet. The tricuspid valve is less frequently involved.
      h. **Immune complex vasculitis** in vessels of almost any organ. In the spleen, perivascular fibrosis with concentric rings of collagen around splenic arterioles results in a characteristic onion-skin appearance.
      i. **Glomerular changes** varying from minimal involvement to severe diffuse proliferative disease with marked subendothelial and mesangial immune complex deposition, endothelial proliferation, and thickening of basement membranes; can be indistinguishable from idiopathic membranous glomerulonephritis.
         (1) Subendothelial immune complex deposition in the glomeruli has considerable diagnostic significance. This change results in the wire-loop appearance seen by light microscopy.
         (2) Thickening of basement membranes can result in changes indistinguishable from those of membranous glomerulonephritis.
      j. **Neurologic and psychiatric manifestations**
      k. **Eye changes,** with yellowish, cotton wool-like fundal lesions (cytoid bodies)
   4. **Laboratory findings**
      a. **LE test** is based on the LE phenomenon, which occurs in vitro.
         (1) In this procedure, morphologically characteristic LE cells are formed in a mixture of mechanically damaged neutrophils and autoantibody-containing patient serum.
         (2) The LE test is positive in only about 70% of cases and has now been largely replaced by more sensitive determinations.
      b. **A positive test result for ANA** is seen in almost all patients with SLE. ANAs are also found in patients with other connective tissue diseases.
         (1) The ANA test becomes almost specific for SLE when the antinuclear antibodies react with **double-stranded DNA.** When this reaction is assessed by microscopic examination of cells using immunofluorescent techniques, a characteristic peripheral nuclear staining, or **"rim" pattern,** is seen.
         (2) ANAs that react with **Sm (Smith) antigen,** a ribonucleoprotein, are also highly specific for SLE.
      c. **Serum complement is often greatly decreased,** especially in association with active renal involvement.
      d. **Immune complexes at dermal-epidermal junction** are demonstrable in skin biopsies.
      e. **Biologic false-positive tests for syphilis** (due to anticardiolipins, a form of antiphospholipid antibody) occur in approximately 15% of patients. This may be the earliest laboratory abnormality in some cases of SLE.

B. **Progressive systemic sclerosis (PSS, scleroderma)**
1. PSS involves **widespread fibrosis and degenerative changes** that affect the skin, gastrointestinal tract (especially the esophagus), heart, muscle, and other organs such as the lung and kidney. The disease occurs most frequently in young women.
2. PSS is marked by the presence of the ANA **anti-Scl-70** in one third of patients. ANA with anticentromere activity is characteristic of a PSS variant, the **CREST syndrome** (**C**alcinosis, **R**aynaud phenomenon, **E**sophageal dysfunction, **S**clerodactyly, and **T**elangiectasia).
3. The initial presentation usually includes skin changes, polyarthralgias, and esophageal symptoms.
4. Characteristics include:
   a. **Hypertrophy of collagen fibers of the subcutaneous tissue,** leading to tightening of the facial skin and a characteristic **fixed facial appearance**
   b. **Sclerodactyly** (claw-like appearance of the hand)
   c. **Raynaud phenomenon** in approximately 75% of patients
   d. **Visceral organ involvement,** especially of the esophagus, gastrointestinal tract, kidneys, lungs, and heart
      (1) The **esophagus** is frequently affected, and dysphagia is common.
      (2) **Interstitial pulmonary fibrosis** is a serious complication.
      (3) **Hypertension** often occurs.

C. **Sjögren syndrome.** This disease **most often affects women in late middle age.**
1. **Clinical manifestations**
   a. **Triad** of **xerostomia** (dry mouth), **keratoconjunctivitis sicca** (dry eyes), and **one of several connective tissue or other autoimmune diseases,** most often rheumatoid arthritis
      (1) Other associated disorders may include SLE, PSS, polymyositis, or Hashimoto thyroiditis.
      (2) **Sicca syndrome** is a variant characterized by xerostomia and keratoconjunctivitis alone.
   b. **Involvement of salivary glands,** often with bilaterally enlarged parotids diffusely infiltrated by lymphocytes and plasma cells. This cellular infiltration can partly or completely obscure the parenchyma of the parotid gland and can mimic, or in some cases lead to, malignant lymphoma.
   c. **Involvement of lacrimal glands**
2. **Laboratory findings**
   a. Significant polyclonal **hypergammaglobulinemia** (a broad-based elevation of serum gamma globulins demonstrable by electrophoresis)
   b. ANAs, including the highly specific **anti-SS-B** and somewhat less specific anti-SS-A

D. **Polymyositis.** This **chronic inflammatory process** especially involves the proximal muscles of the extremities. When the skin is also involved, with a characteristic reddish-purple rash over exposed areas of the face and neck, the condition is called **dermatomyositis.** It occurs mainly in women and is often associated with malignancy.
1. **Increased serum creatine kinase** and frequent presence of ANAs are characteristic.
2. The condition can be confirmed by muscle biopsy, which demonstrates necrotic muscle cells and a lymphocytic infiltrate.

E. **Mixed connective tissue disease (MCTD).** This occurs mainly in women (80% of patients), with a peak incidence at 35 to 40 years of age.
1. MCTD shares clinical features with other connective tissue disorders, but in MCTD, renal involvement is uncommon. It is often manifest clinically by arthralgias, Raynaud phenomenon, esophageal hypomotility, and myositis.
2. Most uniquely, MCTD is characterized by **specific ANAs** (high-titer anti-nRNP and an immunofluorescent speckled nuclear appearance on morphologic ANA analysis).

F. **Polyarteritis nodosa**

1. This **immune complex vasculitis** is characterized by segmental fibrinoid necrosis in the walls of **small and medium arteries** of almost any organ. This form of vasculitis occurs predominantly in **men** (in contrast to the other connective tissue diseases).
2. The **antigen** is usually unknown but may be:
   a. **Hepatitis B** antigen is implicated in 30% of cases.
   b. **Drugs,** such as sulfonamides and penicillin, may form immunogenic hapten-protein complexes.
3. **Clinical manifestations**
   a. Symptoms and signs may include abdominal pain, hypertension, uremia, polyneuritis, allergic asthma, urticaria or rash, splenomegaly, fever, leukocytosis, and proteinuria.
   b. The lung may be involved, resulting in chest pain, cough, dyspnea, and hemoptysis. Severe dyspnea and eosinophilia occur in 20% of patients.

X. Amyloidosis

This group of disorders is characterized by the deposition of amyloid, a proteinaceous material with certain physicochemical features.

A. **Amyloid**

1. **Structure**
   a. Amyloid is not a single substance but a group of substances that share a common physical structure that can be formed by a number of different proteins (Table 5-3).
   b. It always has a **β-pleated sheet configuration** (demonstrable by x-ray diffraction).
2. **Morphologic features**
   a. Amyloid is characteristically **extracellular** in distribution, most often appearing as accumulations proximate to basement membranes.
   b. It has an amorphous eosinophilic appearance in routine hematoxylin and eosin sections.
   c. It is characteristically stained by **Congo red** dye, demonstrating apple green **birefringence** when viewed under polarized light and confirming the suspected presence of amyloid. It can also be demonstrated by a variety of other methods, including immunochemical, fluorescent, and metachromatic techniques.

TABLE 5-3 *Associations of Various Amyloid Proteins*

Type of Amyloidosis	
Systemic amyloidosis	**Amyloid Protein**
Primary (immunocytic dyscrasia)	AL protein derived from immunoglobulin light chains
Secondary (reactive systemic)	AA protein derived from precursor serum protein
Other amyloid-associated conditions	
Portuguese type of polyneuropathy	Transthyretin
Alzheimer disease	A4 amyloid (or Aβ-protein)
Familial Mediterranean fever	AA amyloid
Medullary carcinoma of the thyroid	Amyloid protein derived from calcitonin
Insulin-resistant diabetes mellitus	Amylin (islet amyloid polypeptide, IAPP)
Senile amyloidosis	Transthyretin

AL = amyloid light chain; AA = amyloid-associated.

B. **Clinical patterns of amyloidosis**

1. **Primary amyloidosis (immunocytic dyscrasia amyloidosis)**
   a. The cause is deposition of amyloid fibrils derived from **immunoglobulin light chains,** referred to as **AL (amyloid light chain) protein.**
   b. Amyloid deposition in tissues of mesodermal origin, such as **heart, muscle,** and **tongue** is characteristic. It **may involve the kidney,** with amyloid deposits in the glomerular mesangium as well as in the interstitial tissue between tubules.
   c. Primary amyloidosis is the form frequently associated with **plasma cell disorders** such as multiple myeloma, Waldenström macroglobulinemia, and other less defined disorders.
2. **Secondary amyloidosis (reactive systemic amyloidosis)**
   a. Deposition of fibrils consisting of the amyloid protein called **AA protein,** which is formed from a precursor, serum amyloid-associated protein (SAA) is characteristic. Chronic tissue destruction leads to increased SAA.
   b. Usually, involvement of parenchymatous organs, especially the **kidney** (nephrotic syndrome is very common), **liver, adrenals, pancreas, lymph nodes,** and **spleen** is seen. Perifollicular involvement in the spleen results in "sago spleen," an appearance reminiscent of tapioca-like granules.
   c. Secondary amyloidosis characteristically is a complication of **chronic inflammatory disease** such as rheumatoid arthritis, tuberculosis, osteomyelitis, syphilis, or leprosy. It also may complicate noninflammatory disorders such as renal cell carcinoma and Hodgkin disease.
3. **Other forms of amyloidosis**
   a. **Portuguese type of polyneuropathy** is associated with amyloid derived from a protein known as **transthyretin** (a serum protein that **trans**ports **thy**roxine and **retin**ol). It is characterized by severe peripheral nerve involvement caused by amyloid deposits.
   b. **Alzheimer disease** is characterized by deposits of an amyloid protein referred to as **A4 amyloid,** or **amyloid β-protein,** which differs from AL, AA, and transthyretin-derived amyloid. The gene that codes for the protein precursors of A4 amyloid has been localized to **chromosome 21.**
   c. **Familial Mediterranean fever** is an autosomal recessive disorder occurring in persons of Eastern Mediterranean origin. It is is characterized by episodic fever and polyserositis. The distribution and type of amyloid are similar to that of **secondary amyloidosis** (AA amyloid).
   d. **Medullary carcinoma of the thyroid** is characterized by prominent **amyloid deposits** within the tumor, apparently derived from calcitonin.
   e. **Diabetes mellitus** in the insulin-resistant adult-onset form (type 2) is characterized by **deposits of amyloid in islet cells.** This amyloid is thought to be derived from either insulin or glucagon and is referred to as **amylin** or, alternatively, **islet amyloid polypeptide.** It is postulated that amylin interferes with insulin sensing by beta cells.
   f. **Senile amyloidosis** is characterized by minor deposits of amyloid found at autopsy in the very elderly. This condition may involve the heart, brain, and other organs. When senile amyloidosis occurs in the heart, the amyloid protein is derived from **transthyretin.**
   g. **Dialysis-associated amyloidosis** is characterized by amyloid deposits in the joints of patients who have undergone hemodialysis for several years. The amyloid is derived from β-microglobulin, a protein not readily filtered by the dialysis membrane.

REVIEW TEST

Directions: *Each of the numbered items or incomplete statements in this section is followed by answers or by completions of the statement. Select the* ***one*** *lettered answer or completion that is best in each case.*

1. A 28-year-old woman is found to have pulmonary sarcoidosis. Flow cytometric analysis of T cells isolated from the alveoli and lung interstitium reveals the presence of large numbers of T helper (T_H1) cells. These cells are known to secrete which of the following substances?

(A) Complement component C5A
(B) Elastase and lysyl-hydroxylase
(C) Interleukin-2 (IL-2) and interferon-γ
(D) IL-8 and transforming growth factor-β
(E) Leukotrienes C_4 and C_5

2. A pathologist examines a renal biopsy from a 45-year-old man with the nephrotic syndrome and requests a Congo red stain to confirm the nature of an amorphous acidophilic extracellular hyaline substance localized within the mesangial matrix of the glomeruli. A positive test confirms the presence of

(A) α_1-antitrypsin
(B) amyloid
(C) copper
(D) glycogen
(E) hemosiderin

3. Within minutes of a bee sting, a 23-year-old woman develops generalized pruritus and hyperemia of the skin, followed shortly by swelling of the face and eyelids, dyspnea, and laryngeal edema. This reaction is mediated by

(A) antigen-antibody complexes
(B) cytotoxic T cells
(C) IgA antibodies
(D) IgE antibodies
(E) IgG antibodies

4. A 25-year-old woman with membranous glomerulonephritis receives a kidney transplant. The donor is her HLA-matched sister. She does well initially, but after several weeks, there is a progressive increase in serum creatinine. Assuming that this represents acute cellular rejection, an infiltrate with which of the following types of inflammatory cells is most likely to be a prominent finding on renal biopsy?

(A) Eosinophils
(B) Lymphocytes
(C) Mast cells
(D) Monocytes-macrophages
(E) Neutrophils

5. A 12-month-old boy has had repeated pyogenic infections with streptococci, staphylococci, and *Haemophilus* for the past 6 months. Tests for T-cell function, granulocyte function, and complement activity have all been unaffected. Serum IgG is 50 mg/dL (normal 500 mg/dL). Flow cytometry revealed absent expression of heavy-chain μ on blood lymphocytes. T lymphocytes were slightly increased in number, with a normal CD4+ . CD8+ ratio. Expected findings on examination of a lymph node biopsy from this patient include which of the following?

(A) Absent germinal centers
(B) Follicular hyperplasia with exuberant proliferation of immature B cells
(C) Massive T_H1 cell infiltration into lymphoid follicles
(D) Normal lymphoid tissue development
(E) Plasma cell hyperplasia

6. A 20-year-old woman presents with malar rash, arthralgias, low-grade fever, and high titer antibodies to double-stranded DNA and to the Sm (Smith) antigen. Which of the following forms of hypersensitivity is the primary mechanism of the abnormalities found in this disorder?

(A) Type I (immediate or anaphylactic) hypersensitivity
(B) Type II (antibody-mediated or cytotoxic) hypersensitivity
(C) Type III (immune complex-mediated disorders) hypersensitivity
(D) Type IV (cell-mediated) hypersensitivity

7. An HIV–positive intravenous drug user is suspected of having active tuberculosis, and a tuberculin (Mantoux) intradermal skin test is performed. After 48 hours, 10 cm of induration is observed. Which of the following are involved in this form of hypersensitivity reaction?

(A) B cells and antibodies
(B) Basophils and IgE
(C) Immune complexes and complement
(D) Plasma cells and IgM
(E) T cells and macrophages

8. A 1-year-old girl with an inborn error of metabolism resulting in a lysosomal storage disease receives a hematopoietic stem cell transplant intended to replace her macrophage population. The gene of interest has a "marker" small nucleotide polymorphism within a noncoding intron of the affected gene in which an A (patient gene) is substituted for a G (donor gene). She does quite well for the first 3 weeks. She tests positive for the missing enzyme, her previously abnormally enlarged organs begin to diminish in size, and assay of peripheral blood lymphocytes reveals increasing numbers of cells with the G polymorphism. However, the attending physicians are now concerned because repeated genetic testing reveals a progressive increase in lymphocytes with the A polymorphism. Which of the following is the best explanation for this finding?

(A) Generalized immune complex formation
(B) Graft-versus-host disease
(C) Immune paralysis
(D) Immune tolerance
(E) Rejection of the stem cell transplant

9. A 24-year-old woman who had previously been uneventfully transfused receives a blood transfusion during surgery and shortly thereafter develops itching, generalized urticaria, laryngeal edema, and dyspnea with wheezing respiration. She has a past history of recurrent upper respiratory tract infections and frequent episodes of diarrhea. Laboratory studies are most likely to reveal decreased concentrations of which of the following immunoglobulins?

(A) IgA
(B) IgD
(C) IgE
(D) IgG
(E) IgM

10. A 22-year-old woman with acute myeloblastic leukemia receives an allogeneic bone marrow transplant with apparent successful engraftment. Three weeks later, early jaundice, as well as a generalized maculopapular rash is noted. Profuse diarrhea follows. A skin biopsy reveals vacuolar changes, necrotic epidermal cells, and a lymphocytic infiltrate. These findings are most likely caused by

(A) antibody-dependent cellular cytotoxicity
(B) attack on host epithelial cells by donor CD8+ T cells
(C) contamination of the donor transplant cells with hepatitis C virus
(D) IgE and mast cell-mediated anaphylactic hypersensitivity
(E) secretion of interleukin-2 and interferon-γ by T_H1 cells.

11. A 19-year-old intravenous drug user has regularly sought human immunodeficiency virus (HIV) testing, always with negative results. He admits to carelessly sharing needles on multiple occasions with individuals later found to be HIV-positive. He has heard that there is an inherited genetic basis for some people to be relatively "immune" to HIV infection. The genetic change that he is referring to is a mutation in a gene coding for which of the following proteins?

(A) CCR5
(B) CD4
(C) gp120
(D) gp41
(E) Reverse transcriptase

12. A 2-year-old boy has eczema and thrombocytopenia. There is also a history of recurrent infection. His brother has similar abnormalities, but none of his three sisters are affected. Patients with this disorder are known to have impaired antibody response to which of the following types of antigen?

(A) Deoxyribonucleic acid
(B) Phospholipid
(C) Polysaccharide
(D) Ribonucleic acid
(E) Steroid

13. A 45-year-old woman is seen because of varied complaints. She has been troubled by small painful lumps under the skin of her fingers, some of which have ruptured and leaked a chalky white substance. She also complains of painful episodes in her fingers and toes, which blanch and turn blue on exposure to cold. In addition, questioning reveals increasing "heartburn" and difficulty swallowing. Examination reveals thickening of the skin of the fingers and toes, resulting in a claw-like appearance. Telangiectatic clusters of vessels, appearing as small focal red lesions, are observed in the skin of the face, upper trunk, and hands, and on the mucosal surface of the lips. Antibodies to which of the following are most characteristic of the findings presented by this patient?

(A) Centromeric proteins
(B) Histidyl-t-RNA synthetase (Jo-1)
(C) Histones
(D) Mitochondria
(E) Native DNA

14. A 7-month-old boy has had multiple bouts of otitis media, sinusitis, bronchitis, oral candidiasis, and multiple viral infections. Cessation of the recurrent infections follows successful engraftment of a bone marrow transplant. The basis of the clinical improvement is

(A) direct transfusion of antibody-producing B cells
(B) direct transfusion of donor CD4+ and CD8+ lymphocytes
(C) donor suppression of recipient cytotoxic T cells
(D) infusion of donor-derived cytokines
(E) maturation of donor lymphoid progenitor cells

ANSWERS AND EXPLANATIONS

1-C. T helper (T_H1) cells secrete interleukin-2 and interferon-γ, which in turn facilitate T-cell expansion and macrophage activation.

2-B. A positive Congo red test confirms the presence of amyloid. Apple green birefringence is observed under polarized light.

3-D. The clinical description is characteristic of systemic anaphylaxis, an IgE-mediated type I hypersensitivity reaction. In type I hypersensitivity, reaction of antigen with preformed IgE antibodies fixed by Fc receptors to the surface of basophils or tissue mast cells results in cytolysis and degranulation of these cells, with release of histamine and other mediators.

4-B. Acute cellular rejection is characterized by an infiltrate of both CD4+ and CD8+ lymphocytes. Acute rejection occurs over a variable time period, ordinarily days to weeks to months after transplant.

5-A. The diagnosis is X-linked agammaglobulinemia of Bruton. Failure of maturation of pre-B cells is associated with absence of mature B lymphocytes and plasma cells; failure of antibody synthesis; marked serum hypogammaglobulinemia; and recurrent bacterial infections, especially sinopulmonary infections. Histologic examination of lymphoid tissue reveals marked underdevelopment of germinal centers. T cells are unaffected, as are T-cell functions such as cell-mediated immunity and resistance to most viral infections. The disease is X-linked and is due to mutations in the B cell tyrosine kinase (*Btk*) gene.

6-C. The diagnosis is systemic lupus erythematosus, and the most characteristic lesions are mediated by immune complex deposition (type III hypersensitivity). In this form of hypersensitivity, antibody combines with antigen, resulting in antigen-antibody complexes. Insoluble aggregates of immune complex are deposited in vessel walls, serosal surfaces, and other extravascular sites, and complement is bound. The antigen-antibody-complement complexes are highly chemotactic for neutrophils, which release lysosomal enzymes and other mediators of tissue damage (prostaglandins, kinins, and free radicals).

7-E. The tuberculin test is a classic example of delayed hypersensitivity, a form of cell-mediated hypersensitivity involving CD4+ T cells and macrophages. Native CD4+ T cells are converted to T_H1 cells that secrete cytokines, especially interferon-γ, which is a central mediator of delayed hypersensitivity. Among the many actions of interferon-γ, the most important is activation of macrophages.

8-E. Rejection of the stem cell transplant is occurring, as evidenced by reappearance of the marker for the patient's original gene. Small nucleotide polymorphisms are the most frequent form of DNA variation. As the name implies, they are typically small in size, often a single nucleotide. They may occur in any portion of the gene, even in intergenic regions of the genome, and are of increasing importance as genetic markers, as illustrated by the example presented here.

9-A. Isolated IgA deficiency is most often asymptomatic but can be characterized by anaphylactic reactions to transfused blood. It also can be associated with frequent episodes of diarrhea and recurrent infections, especially those involving mucosal surfaces. This inherited B-cell defect is due to inability of IgA B cells to mature into IgA-producing plasma cells. Interestingly, the defect leading to systemic anaphylaxis involves both IgA and IgE antibody formation. Patients lacking IgA can develop IgE antibodies against the IgA antibodies present in transfused blood. This sensitization can result in susceptibility to anaphylaxis on subsequent transfusion.

10-B. Graft-versus-host disease is most often manifest by clinical findings related to the three principal target organs: the skin, liver, and gastrointestinal tract. The skin manifestations are often initiated by a pruritic rash. Elevation of bilirubin and liver enzymes signals the hepatic involvement. Effects on the ileum and colon present as diarrhea and abdominal pain. The lesions are caused by donor lymphocytes, with targeting of host epithelial cells by CD8+ T cells.

11-A. Either of two coreceptors, CCR5 or CXCR4, is involved in the initial binding of the virus to the cell surface molecule gp120 on CD4+ cells. It is of considerable interest that certain mutations in the CCR5 gene are associated with what appears to be total resistance to infection with some common strains of HIV. Homozygotes are totally resistant, and heterozygotes develop a more slowly progressive disease.

12-C. Wiskott-Aldrich syndrome is an X-linked disorder characterized by eczema, thrombocytopenia, recurrent infections, and poor antibody response to polysaccharide antigens. Bloody diarrhea is also common. Death before 6 years of age occurs frequently and is most often due to bleeding, infection, or malignancy (most often lymphoma).

13-A. The patient exhibits the cardinal findings of the CREST syndrome, a less severe variant of systemic sclerosis (scleroderma) characterized by ***C***alcinosis, ***R***aynaud phenomenon, ***E***sophogeal dysfunction, ***S***clerodactyly, and ***T***elangiectasia. Although a number of antinuclear antibodies can be found in this disorder, the most characteristic is directed at centromeric proteins (the antibody is often referred to as anticentromere).

14-E. Severe combined immunodeficiency disease is characterized by failure to thrive and increased susceptibility to bacterial, fungal, and viral infections. Laboratory studies reveal decreased numbers of both B cells and T cells and deficiency of immunoglobulins. The treatment of choice is bone marrow (or other sources of hematopoietic stem cells) transplantation and is based on maturation of donor lymphoid progenitor cells.

CHAPTER

6

Neoplasia

I. General Considerations

Neoplasia is the uncontrolled, disorderly proliferation of cells, resulting in a benign or malignant tumor, or neoplasm.

A. **Dysplasia**

1. This **reversible** change often precedes malignancy.
2. Morphologic manifestations include disorderly maturation and spatial arrangement of cells; marked variability in nuclear size and shape (pleomorphism); and increased, often abnormal, mitosis.
3. Examples include dysplasia occuring in squamous epithelium of the cervix. This change is often a precursor of malignancy.

B. **Neoplasms**

1. If the resemblance to tissue of origin is close, the neoplasm is termed **well differentiated;** if little resemblance to the tissue of origin is seen, it is **poorly differentiated.**
2. Neoplasms grow at the expense of function and vitality of normal tissue without benefit to the host and are largely independent of host control mechanisms.

II. Classification and Nomenclature of Tumors

Neoplasms are classified as either **malignant** or **benign,** based on their behavior. They are also described by terms derived from the **appearance** of the neoplasm, **tissue of origin,** or degree of **differentiation.**

A. **Malignant tumors (cancer)**

1. **General considerations**
    a. **Invasion** (spread of the neoplasm into adjacent structures) and **metastasis** (implantation of the neoplasm into noncontiguous sites) are characteristic. Metastasis is the most important **defining characteristic of malignancy,** although there are some malignant tumors, such as basal cell carcinoma of the skin, that rarely metastasize.
    b. Malignant tumors are usually less differentiated than benign tumors.
    c. **Anaplasia,** in which tumor cells are very poorly differentiated and exhibit **pleomorphism, hyperchromatism** (dark-staining nuclei), an **increased nuclear-cytoplasmic ratio,** abnormal mitoses, cellular dyspolarity, and often **prominent nucleoli** is a common feature. In general, highly anaplastic tumors are very aggressive, and well-differentiated tumors are less aggressive. Paradoxically, the most aggressive

tumors often respond well to chemotherapy and radiotherapy, because these modalities are most effective with rapidly dividing cells.

2. **Carcinoma** is a malignant tumor of **epithelial** origin and can be seen in the following variations:
   a. **Squamous cell carcinoma**
      (1) Squamous cell carcinoma originates from stratified squamous epithelium of, for example, the skin, mouth, esophagus, and vagina, as well as from areas of squamous metaplasia, as in the bronchi or the squamocolumnar junction of the uterine cervix.
      (2) It is marked by the production of keratin.
   b. **Transitional cell carcinoma** arises from the transitional cell epithelium of the urinary tract.
   c. **Adenocarcinoma** is carcinoma of **glandular epithelium** and includes malignant tumors of the gastrointestinal mucosa, endometrium, and pancreas. It is often associated with **desmoplasia,** tumor-induced proliferation of non-neoplastic fibrous connective tissue, particularly in adenocarcinoma of the **breast, pancreas,** and **prostate.**
3. **Sarcoma** is a malignant tumor of **mesenchymal origin.** It is often used with a prefix that denotes the tissue of origin of the tumor, as in **osteosarcoma** (bone), **rhabdomyosarcoma** (skeletal muscle), **leiomyosarcoma** (smooth muscle), and **liposarcoma** (fatty tissue).
4. **Eponymically named tumors** include Burkitt lymphoma, Hodgkin disease, and Wilms tumor.
5. **Teratoma** is a neoplasm derived from all **three germ cell layers,** which may contain structures such as skin, bone, cartilage, teeth, and intestinal epithelium. It may be either malignant or benign and usually arises in the ovaries or testes.

B. **Benign tumors**
1. **General considerations**
   a. Benign tumors are usually **well differentiated** and closely resemble the tissue of origin.
   b. They grow slowly and do not metastasize. If their growth compresses adjacent tissues, they can be harmful. For example, benign intracranial tumors can be more lethal than some malignant skin tumors.
   c. They tend to become **encapsulated.**
   d. They are denoted by the suffix -oma, as in lipoma and fibroma. However, this suffix is also applied to some malignant neoplasms, such as hepatoma, melanoma, lymphoma, and mesothelioma, as well as several non-neoplastic swellings, including granuloma and hematoma.
2. **Papilloma.** This benign neoplasm most often arises from **surface epithelium** such as squamous epithelium of the skin, larynx, or tongue. It may also develop from **transitional epithelium** of the urinary bladder, ureter, or renal pelvis. The tumor consists of delicate **finger-like epithelial processes** overlying a core of connective tissue stroma that contains blood vessels.
3. **Adenoma.** This benign neoplasm of **glandular epithelium** occurs in several variants:
   a. **Papillary cystadenoma** is characterized by adenomatous papillary processes that extend into cystic spaces, as in cystadenoma of the ovary.
   b. **Fibroadenoma** is marked by proliferation of connective tissue surrounding glandular epithelium; for example, fibroadenoma of the breast. In this instance, either the connective tissue or the stroma may be neoplastic.
4. **Benign tumors of mesenchymal origin** are most often named by the tissue of origin (e.g., leiomyoma, rhabdomyoma, lipoma, fibroma, chondroma). They include the most common neoplasm of women, the uterine leiomyoma, or fibroid tumor.
5. **Choristoma.** This is a small non-neoplastic area of **normal tissue misplaced within another organ,** such as pancreatic tissue within the wall of the stomach.
6. **Hamartoma.** This is a non-neoplastic, disorganized, tumor-like overgrowth of cell types regularly found within an affected organ; **hemangioma,** an irregular accumulation of blood vessels, is an example.

III. Properties of Neoplasms

A. **Monoclonality.** This denotes origin from a single precursor cell.

1. **Most neoplasms are monoclonal;** in contrast, **polyclonal proliferations are almost always non-neoplastic.**
2. Monoclonality is assessed by a variety of approaches using isoenzyme patterns or other markers in individuals who are heterozygous for the measured trait.
   a. **Monoclonal tumors** express only one of the isoenzymes or other markers of clonality.
   b. **Polyclonal cellular proliferations** exhibit both isoenzymes or markers.
3. **Glucose-6-phosphate dehydrogenase (G6PD) isoenzymes and other X-linked markers**
   a. These are the first described and classic indicators of monoclonality in tumors.
   b. Because of X inactivation in early embryonic life, tissues of females heterozygous for G6PD isoenzymes consist of a mosaic of cell types, with random cells expressing one or the other of the two isoenzymes. However, in the case of G6PD, one of the two polymorphic forms of these isoenzymes occurs with significant frequency only in women of African lineage, limiting the application of this technique.
   c. Other polymorphic X-linked markers such as iduronate-2-sulfatase and phosphoglycerate kinase can be used in a broader spectrum of patients.
4. **Human androgen receptor gene (*HUMARA*)**
   a. This gene has now become the most common marker used to determine clonality.
   b. This method involves study of methylation patterns adjacent to high-frequency polymorphisms in multiple populations.
5. **Specific translocations.** If present, genes such as the 8;14 translocation can also be used to assess clonality in certain neoplasms (e.g., in Burkitt lymphoma).
6. **Monoclonality of cells of lymphoid origin**
   a. **Indicators of monoclonality in malignancies of B-cell origin**
      (1) **Immunoglobulins** are produced by B-cell malignant tumors and are demonstrable as cytoplasmic or surface immunoglobulin or, in the case of multiple myeloma, are secreted and are demonstrable in the serum.
         (a) If monoclonal, the resultant mixture of immunoglobulin molecules exhibits **either kappa or lambda chain specificity,** but not both, a characteristic finding in neoplastic B-cell proliferations.
         (b) If B-cell or plasma cell proliferations are polyclonal, they result in the production of heterogeneous immunoglobulin molecules, some of which express kappa specificity and others that express lambda specificity.
      (2) **Immunoglobulin gene rearrangement** is a characteristic of B-cell maturation. The number of possible combinations achieved by rearrangement is almost countless; it can be assumed that each normal B cell is marked by a unique rearrangement pattern. **Neoplastic proliferation** results in large numbers of cells, all demonstrating the same pattern of immunoglobulin gene rearrangement denoting their common origin from a single cell.
         (a) Assessment is by molecular diagnostic techniques.
         (b) Because immunoglobulin heavy chain rearrangement is limited to B cells, this approach also demonstrates the B-cell origin of a tumor.
   b. **Indicators of monoclonality in malignancies of T-cell origin**
      (1) **Surface antigens (markers)** are demonstrable as T cells mature; they may be characteristic of either the stage of maturation or functional subclass. **Cellular proliferations** in which large numbers of T cells share surface markers in common are suggestive of monoclonality. In addition to many others, these markers include the CD4 antigen marking helper T cells and the CD8 antigen marking suppressor T and cytotoxic T cells.

(2) **T-cell receptor gene arrangement** is analogous to immunoglobulin gene rearrangement and is used in a similar manner to demonstrate both the T-cell origin of a tumor and its monoclonality.

B. **Invasion and metastasis**

1. **Invasion** is aggressive infiltration of adjacent tissues by a malignant tumor.
   a. It often extends into lymphatics and blood vessels, with the formation of tumor emboli that may be carried to distal sites.
   b. Not all tumor emboli result in metastatic tumor implants, and the presence of tumor cells within blood vessels or lymphatics indicates only the penetration of basement membranes and is not synonymous with metastasis.
2. **Metastasis** is implantation in distal sites.
   a. **Multistep process of metastasis**
      (1) **Growth and vascularization** of the primary tumor
      (2) **Invasiveness** and penetration of basement membranes into lymphatics or blood vessels
      (3) **Transport and survival** of tumor cells in the circulation
      (4) **Arrest of tumor emboli** in the target tissue and passage again across basement membranes
      (5) **Overcoming of target tissue defense mechanisms**
      (6) Development of **successful metastatic implants**
   b. **Preferential routes of metastasis** vary with specific neoplasms.
      (1) **Carcinomas** tend to metastasize via lymphatic spread.
      (2) **Sarcomas** tend to invade blood vessels early, resulting in widespread blood-borne (hematogenous) dissemination.
      (3) Notable exceptions include renal cell and hepatocellular carcinoma, which are marked by early venous invasion and hematogenous dissemination.
   c. **Target organs** are most commonly the liver, lungs, brain, adrenal glands, lymph nodes, and bone marrow. They rarely include skeletal muscle or the spleen.
   d. **Tumor progression** is characterized by the accumulation of successive cytogenetic or molecular abnormalities.
      (1) It is exemplified by the progression of changes from normal colonic epithelium to adenoma to carcinoma to metastasis, with parallel changes in the *APC, K-ras, DCC, p53,* and possibly other genes.
      (2) Individual neoplastic cells within a tumor may have varying metastatic potential.

C. **Other clinical manifestations of malignancy.** These are mediated by mechanisms other than invasion and metastasis.

1. **Cachexia and wasting.** The origin is complex; it is characterized by weakness, weight loss, anorexia, anemia, infection, and hypermetabolism. This process may be mediated in part by **cachectin** (tumor necrosis factor-α, TNF-α), a product of macrophages that promotes catabolism of fatty tissue.
2. **Endocrine abnormalities** are caused by tumors of endocrine gland origin, which may actively elaborate hormones, leading to a variety of syndromes.
   a. **Pituitary abnormalities**
      (1) **Prolactinoma,** leading to amenorrhea, infertility, and sometimes galactorrhea
      (2) **Somatotropic (acidophilic) adenoma,** leading to gigantism in children and acromegaly in adults
      (3) **Corticotropic (most often basophilic) adenoma,** leading to Cushing disease (adrenal hypercorticism of pituitary origin)
   b. **Adrenocortical abnormalities** include adrenogenital syndrome, Conn syndrome, and Cushing syndrome of adrenal origin, resulting from adrenal cortical tumors.
   c. **Ovarian abnormalities**
      (1) **Granulosa-theca cell tumor,** leading to hyperestrinism
      (2) **Sertoli-Leydig cell tumor,** leading to excess androgen production

d. **Trophoblastic tissue abnormalities** include hyperproduction of human chorionic gonadotropin from hydatidiform mole or choriocarcinoma.

3. **Paraneoplastic syndromes**
   a. **Endocrinopathies** are caused by ectopic production of hormones or chemically unrelated substances inducing effects similar to those of a given hormone. They include the following:
      (1) **Cushing syndrome** is caused by production of ACTH-like substances by small cell (oat cell) carcinoma of the lung.
      (2) **Inappropriate secretion of antidiuretic hormone** may be caused by a variety of tumors, most commonly small cell carcinoma of the lung.
      (3) **Hypercalcemia** is caused by metastatic disease in bone, secretion of a substance similar to parathormone by squamous cell bronchogenic carcinoma, or secretion of a substance similar to osteoclast-activating factor by the malignant plasma cells of multiple myeloma.
      (4) **Hypoglycemia** is caused by secretion of insulin-like substances by hepatocellular carcinomas, mesotheliomas, and some sarcomas.
      (5) **Polycythemia** is caused by elaboration of erythropoietin by renal tumors and other neoplasms.
      (6) **Hyperthyroidism** is caused by production of substances such as thyroid-stimulating hormone by hydatidiform moles, choriocarcinomas, and some lung tumors.
   b. **Neurologic abnormalities** may occur in the absence of metastatic disease. They include degenerative cerebral changes with dementia, cerebellar changes with resultant gait dysfunction, and peripheral neuropathies.
   c. **Skin lesions** may be associated with visceral malignancies. They include acanthosis nigricans and dermatomyositis.
   d. **Coagulation abnormalities** include migratory thrombophlebitis associated with carcinoma of the pancreas and other visceral malignancies (Trousseau phenomenon), and disseminated intravascular coagulation associated with various neoplasms.
4. **Oncofetal antigens**
   a. These are proteins normally expressed only in fetal or embryonic life; their expression by neoplastic cells is considered a manifestation of dedifferentiation (i.e., the undifferentiated neoplastic cells tend to resemble their embryonic counterparts).
   b. They include **carcinoembryonic antigen (CEA),** which is associated with colon cancer and other cancers and preneoplastic processes, and **α-fetoprotein (AFP),** which is associated with hepatocellular carcinoma and many germ cell tumors. AFP is also increased in fetal anencephaly and other neural tube defects.

IV. Carcinogenesis and Etiology

The transformation of normal to neoplastic cells is caused by both endogenous and exogenous factors, including chemical and physical agents, viruses, activation of cancer-promoting genes, and inhibition of cancer-suppressing genes.

A. **Chemical carcinogenesis**
1. **Association between chemicals and cancer** (Table 6-1)
2. **Types of carcinogens**
   a. **Direct-reacting carcinogens** do not need to be chemically altered to act.
   b. **Indirect-reacting carcinogens** require metabolic conversion from **procarcinogens** to active **ultimate carcinogens.** For example, a mucosal glucuronidase in the urinary bladder converts β-naphthylamine glucuronide to the carcinogen β-naphthylamine.
3. **Stages of chemical carcinogenesis**
   a. **Initiation** is the first critical carcinogenic event, and it is usually a reaction between a carcinogen and DNA. Two or more agents (e.g., chemicals, viruses, radiation) may act together as **cocarcinogens.**

TABLE 6-1 *Some Environmental Factors, Drugs, and Chemicals Associated with Human Cancer*

Factor	Type of Malignancy
Cigarette smoking	Carcinoma of lung; carcinoma of larynx
Excess sun exposure	Squamous cell carcinoma and basal cell carcinoma of skin; melanoma
Alkylating agents	Acute leukemia
Asbestos	Carcinoma of lung; pleural and peritoneal mesothelioma; gastrointestinal tract cancers
Smoked foods rich in nitrosamines	Adenocarcinoma of stomach
Alcohol	Carcinoma of mouth and esophagus (especially in association with cigarette smoking)
	Hepatocellular carcinoma (in association with cirrhosis of liver; all forms of cirrhosis predispose to hepatocellular carcinoma)
Arsenic	Squamous cell and basal cell carcinoma of skin
Low-fiber diet	Adenocarcinoma of colon
High-fat diet	Breast carcinoma
Aniline dyes, aromatic amines, β-naphthylamine	Transitional cell carcinoma of bladder (caused by action of bladder mucosal glucuronidase on detoxified glucuronides of these compounds)
Aflatoxin B_1	Hepatocellular carcinoma
Benzene	Acute leukemia
Polyvinyl chloride	Hepatic hemangiosarcoma (angiosarcoma)
Thorotrast	Hepatic hemangiosarcoma (angiosarcoma)
Diethylstilbestrol (DES)	Clear-cell adenocarcinoma of vagina (occurs in daughters of patients who received DES during pregnancy)
Nickel	Carcinoma of lung
Chromium	Carcinoma of lung
Uranium	Carcinoma of lung

b. **Promotion** is induced by a stimulator of cell proliferation and enhances the carcinogenic process. A promoter, not carcinogenic in itself, enhances other agents' carcinogenicity. For example, phorbol esters react with membrane receptors, stimulating cell replication. This may enhance clonal selection, resulting in cells with increasingly deleterious DNA changes.

B. **Radiation carcinogenesis**

1. **Exposure to ultraviolet radiation** in the form of sunlight is clearly related to the frequency of skin cancers such as squamous cell and basal cell carcinomas and melanomas.
   a. The process is thought to act by inducing dimer formation between neighboring thymine pairs in DNA. In most cases, such dimers are successfully repaired by enzymatically mediated mechanisms.
   b. That skin cancer may be induced by such dimer formation is suggested by the greatly increased incidence of skin tumors seen in **xeroderma pigmentosum,** an autosomal recessive disorder characterized by failure of DNA excision repair mechanisms.
2. **Ionizing radiation** is a classic cause of cancer, exemplified by the increased incidence of cancers in those exposed to radiation. There are several historic examples:

TABLE 6-2 ***Viruses and Other Infectious Agents Associated with Human Malignancy***

Infectious Agent	Neoplasm	Etiologic Role
HTLV-1	Adult T cell leukemia/lymphoma	Definite
HPV	Genital tract neoplasms, especially premalignant lesions and cancers of the cervix and vulva; laryngeal papillomas	Almost certain
EBV	Nasopharyngeal carcinoma Burkitt lymphoma	Almost certain Stimulates proliferation of B cells; increases opportunity for translocation and oncogene activation
HBV	Hepatocellular carcinoma	Almost certain
HHV-8	Kaposi sarcoma	Definite
Helicobacter pylori	Adenocarcinoma and B-cell lymphomas (MALTomas) of stomach	High suspect

HTLV-1 = human T lymphotrophic virus type 1; HPV = human papillomavirus; EBV = Epstein-Barr virus; HBV = hepatitis B virus; HHV-8 = human herpes virus-8 (also known as Kaposi sarcoma-associated herpesvirus)

a. Skin cancer and myeloid leukemias in radiologists
b. Lung cancer in uranium miners
c. Thyroid cancer in patients who have received head and neck radiation therapy
d. Acute and chronic myeloid (but not lymphoid) leukemias in survivors of atomic blasts
e. Osteosarcoma in radium watch-dial workers

C. **Viral carcinogenesis** (Table 6-2)

1. **Virus types**
   a. **DNA viruses**
      (1) These viruses integrate viral DNA into host genomes, perhaps resulting in host cell expression of viral mRNA coding for specific proteins.
      (2) Examples include human papillomavirus, Epstein-Barr virus, and hepatitis B virus as prominent suspects that play a role in human carcinogenesis.
   b. **Retroviruses** are marked by transcription of viral genomic RNA sequences into DNA by action of viral reverse transcriptase. In the case of retroviruses that are tumorigenic in experimental animals, retroviruses are frequently characterized by substitutions of genomic sequences known as viral oncogenes.
2. **Viral oncogenes (v-oncs)** are named with a three-letter abbreviation, preceded by ***v*** **for viral** (Table 6-3). They exhibit homology for DNA sequences of man and other eukaryotic species; these eukaryotic DNA sequences are called **proto-oncogenes,** or **cellular oncogenes (c-oncs),** and are identified with the same three-letter abbreviations preceded by ***c*** **for cellular.**

D. **Oncogenes and cancer.** The protein products of proto-oncogenes play essential roles in DNA replication and transcription.

1. **Mechanisms of action of oncogene protein products**
   a. **Activation by binding of guanosine triphosphate (GTP).** ***Ras*** **oncogenes** code for proteins known as p21 proteins, which are functionally similar to G proteins, membrane-signaling proteins activated by GTP binding, which mediate signal transduction from the cell surface.
      (1) **Characteristics—*Ras* proteins and G proteins** are located at the plasma membrane and have GTP binding and GTPase activities.

TABLE 6-3 *Examples of Retroviral Oncogenes*

Oncogene	Source
v-*src*	Rous sarcoma virus of chickens
v-*abl*	Abelson murine leukemia virus
v-*sis*	Simian sarcoma virus
v-*myc*	MC29 viral isolate from chickens
v-H-*ras*	Harvey rat sarcoma virus
v-K-*ras*	Kirsten rat sarcoma virus
v-*erb*	Erythroblastosis virus of chickens
v-*fms*	Feline McDonough sarcoma virus
v-*fos*	FBJ osteosarcoma virus of mice
v-*ros*	UR2 avian sarcoma virus
v-*myb*	Avian myeloblastosis virus

(a) GTPase hydrolytically converts active ras-GTP to inactive ras-GDP. These proteins are inactivated by ras-GTPase mediated by GTPase-activating protein (GAP).

(b) GTP activation of ras can stimulate or depress adenylate cyclase activity, altering intracellular cAMP levels, thus affecting cellular behavior.

(2) **Mutation of the *ras* gene** usually occurs at codon 12, resulting in an aberrant p21 protein product with intact GTP binding but with a loss of GTPase activity.

(a) Mutant ras proteins can be activated by GTP binding but cannot be inactivated by GTPase activity.

(b) The *ras* gene is mutated in 25%–30% of malignancies.

b. **Protein tyrosine kinase activity** is exhibited by the following:

(1) The oncogene product of the Rous sarcoma virus (designated as $pp60^{src}$)

(2) Other oncogene products, usually oncogenic analogs of transmembrane receptor proteins

c. **Growth factor or growth factor receptor activity.** Alterations in expression or structural changes in oncogene products may result in inappropriate activation of receptor proteins or their oncogenic analogs, thus mimicking the actions of growth factors.

(1) On stimulation with the appropriate growth factor, receptor proteins often demonstrate tyrosine kinase activity of their cytoplasmic domains.

(2) Significant homologies occur between several oncogenes and the genes for cellular growth factors and their receptors. For example:

(a) v-*sis* and the gene for the β chain of platelet-derived growth factor

(b) v-*erb* and the gene for the epidermal growth factor (EGF) receptor

(c) v-*fms* and the gene for the colony-stimulating factor-1 receptor

(d) c-*neu* and the gene for the EGF receptor

d. **Nuclear proteins.** Some oncogene products, including the protein products of *myc, fos,* and *myb,* are confined to the cell nucleus.

2. **Oncogenes and human cancer.** Mechanisms by which c-oncs become tumorigenic include the following:

a. **Promoter insertion (insertional mutagenesis)**

(1) Insertion of retroviral promoter or enhancer sequences into the host genome can lead to increased expression of a nearby oncogene.

(2) This mechanism is similar to the promoter-induced hyperexpression associated with translocations characteristic of several human leukemias and lymphomas.

b. **Point mutations.** These are exemplified by single nucleotide changes in codon 12 of the *ras* family of genes that are associated with a number of human tumors.

c. **Chromosomal translocation.** Frequent association with malignancy seen in these genetic rearrangements has been clarified by demonstrating that important genes are situated at the sites of chromosomal breaks. For example:

(1) **8;14 translocation and Burkitt lymphoma.** The c-*myc* proto-oncogene on chromosome 8 is translocated to a site adjacent to the immunoglobulin heavy chain locus on chromosome 14. Major regulatory sequences within the immunoglobulin gene are thought to increase the expression of c-*myc*.

(2) **14;18 translocation and follicular lymphoma.** The immunoglobulin heavy chain locus on chromosome 14 is transposed to a site adjacent to *bcl*-2, an oncogene on chromosome 18. This results in enhanced expression of *bcl*-2, thus inhibiting apoptosis.

(3) **9;22 translocation and chronic myeloid leukemia (CML).** The c-*abl* proto-oncogene on chromosome 9 is transposed to a site adjacent to *bcr* (breakpoint cluster region), an oncogene on chromosome 22.

(a) The union of *bcr* and *abl* results in a **hybrid,** or chimeric, ***bcr-abl*** fusion gene that codes for a protein with increased tyrosine kinase activity.

(b) The altered chromosome carrying this hybrid gene, the **Philadelphia chromosome,** can be demonstrated by cytogenetic techniques in hematopoietic cells of patients with CML.

(4) **15;17 translocation and acute promyelocytic leukemia (FAB M3 AML).** The translocation involves the *PML* gene on chromosome 15 and the retinoic acid receptor-α (*RAR*-α) gene on chromosome 17. Therapy with the retinoic acid analogue all-*trans* retinoic acid can result in maturation of these leukemic cells and clinical remission.

d. **Gene amplification**

(1) This reduplication of the gene, with multiple resultant genomic DNA copies, can sometimes result in a thousand or more copies of the amplified gene.

(2) Extensive amplification can result in small free chromosome-like bodies called **double minute chromosomes** or in band-like structures within chromosomes called **homogeneously staining regions,** which are both demonstrable cytogenetically.

(3) Several human neoplasms involve gene amplification.

(a) **Neuroblastoma** is an aggressive childhood tumor characterized by marked N-*myc* amplification that correlates inversely with the degree of differentiation of the neuroblastoma cells.

(b) **Some breast cancers** are marked by amplification of the *HER-2/neu* oncogene (c-*erb*B2). Such amplification is correlated with a poor prognosis.

3. **Cancer suppressor genes (anti-oncogenes).** In contrast to the preceding mechanisms, cancer suppressor genes promote cellular proliferation when the gene is inactivated (most often by deletion). A single residual copy of the anti-oncogene suppresses tumor formation, but homozygous inactivation (i.e., loss of function of both copies) promotes the expression of the neoplastic phenotype.

a. The prototype is **retinoblastoma,** an intraocular childhood tumor caused by inactivation of the *Rb* gene. The **"two-hit" hypothesis of Knudson** holds that two mutagenic events are required to induce alterations on both chromosomes.

(1) In the familial forms of retinoblastoma, the gene on one chromosome in the germline is inactivated or deleted, and the gene on the other chromosome is affected by a somatic mutation.

(2) In sporadic nonfamilial cases of retinoblastoma, both deletions occur as somatic mutations.

b. Inactivation of the *Rb* gene is also a factor in the genesis of other tumors, especially **osteosarcoma,** which often occurs following successful surgical cure of familial retinoblastoma.

c. There are several other important cancer suppressor genes:

(1) ***p53***

(a) This gene, which has been called the "guardian of the genome," is mutated in more than 50% of all malignant tumors.

(b) In the setting of DNA damage, the *p53* gene causes cell cycle arrest in G_1, providing time for DNA repair. If repair is successful, cells re-enter the cell cycle. If repair is not successful, p53 product causes cell death by apoptosis (events involve transcription of p21, inhibition of the formation of cyclin-CDK complexes, and inhibition of Rb phosphorylation, and also the transcription of *bax*, an apoptosis-promoting gene).

(c) Familial loss causes the Li-Fraumeni syndrome, which is characterized by a wide variety of tumors: breast tumors, soft tissue sarcomas, brain tumors, and leukemias.

(2) ***WT*-1 and *WT*-2**. Inactivation or deletion of either of these genes, which are located on chromosome 11, is associated with Wilms tumor, the most common renal neoplasm of children.

(3) ***APC*.** Inactivation is common in familial polyposis coli and adenocarcinoma of the colon as well as a few other tumors (e.g., gastric and esophageal cancers).

(4) ***BRCA*-1.** Inactivation is associated with familial propensity to breast and ovarian carcinomas. (*BRCA*-2 inactivation is associated with breast cancer alone.)

E. **Epidemiology.** Important epidemiologic factors include geographic and racial differences, heredity, age, sex and hormonal differences, dietary factors, environmental toxins, and infection (see Table 6-1).

V. Other Neoplastic Disorders with Known DNA Defects

A. von Recklinghausen neurofibromatosis type 1 and *NF*-1

1. Characteristics include multiple benign neurofibromas, café au lait spots, iris hamartomas, and an increased risk of developing fibrosarcomas (see Chapter 4).
2. The cause of the disorder is mutations in the *NF*-1 tumor suppressor gene (which functions as a GAP protein that inactivates ras).

B. Multiple endocrine neoplasia type IIa (MEN IIa) and *ret* (see Chapter 20 for descriptions of MEN I and MEN IIb)

1. MEN is the familial occurrence of the combination of medullary thyroid carcinoma, bilateral pheochromocytomas, and hyperparathyroidism due to hyperplasia or tumor.
2. The cause is mutations of the *ret* proto-oncogene that are transmitted in the germline. Thus, demonstration of a *ret* mutation in a patient with medullary thyroid carcinoma would indicate the need for surveillance for the development of pheochromocytoma or hyperparathyroidism.

C. Hereditary nonpolyposis colon cancer (HNPCC, or Lynch syndrome)

1. The cause of HNPCC is an inherited mutation in certain DNA repair genes, resulting in genomic instability. The mutation, referred to as the replication error phenotype, is involved in mismatch repair and is detected as instability in microsatellite repeat sequences. HNPCC predisposes to mutations in other genes more directly related to transformation.
2. Characteristics include familial right-sided colorectal carcinomas and increased risk of other carcinomas.

D. **Xeroderma pigmentosum**

1. This autosomal recessive disorder is manifest by an increased incidence of skin cancers (basal cell carcinoma, squamous cell carcinoma, malignant melanoma) caused by hypersensitivity to ultraviolet light.
2. It involves defects in genes that function in nucleotide excision repair, which is required for repair of ultraviolet-induced pyrimidine (often thymine) dimers (cross-linked pyrimidine residues).

VI. Grading and Staging

These clinical measures are used for prognostic evaluation and planning of clinical management.

A. **Grading.** This histopathologic evaluation of the lesion is based on the **degree of cellular differentiation.**

B. **Staging.** This is clinical assessment of the **degree of localization** or spread of the tumor.

1. Staging generally correlates better with prognosis than does histopathologic grading. However, both approaches are useful.
2. It is exemplified by the generalized **TNM system,** which evaluates the size and the extent of the tumor (**T**), lymph node involvement (**N**), and metastasis (**M**).
3. It is sometimes oriented toward specific tumors, as exemplified by the **Dukes system** for colorectal carcinoma and the **Ann Arbor system** for Hodgkin disease and non-Hodgkin lymphomas.

REVIEW TEST

***Directions:** Each of the numbered items or incomplete statements in this section is followed by answers or by completions of the statement. Select the **one** lettered answer or completion that is best in each case.*

1. A 54-year-old woman who has been diagnosed with early stage breast cancer undergoes surgery for a lumpectomy to remove a small tumor detected by mammography. The pathology report confirms the early stage of the cancer and further comments on the fact that there is significant desmoplasia in the surrounding tissue. The term desmoplasia refers to

(A) an irregular accumulation of blood vessels
(B) maturation and spatial arrangement of cells
(C) metastatic involvement of surrounding tissue
(D) normal tissue misplaced within another organ
(E) proliferation of non-neoplastic fibrous connective tissue

2. A 24-year-old woman with a history of heavy and painful menstrual periods has been having difficulty conceiving despite months of trying to become pregnant. Further workup includes a bimanual pelvic examination and an ultrasound, which demonstrates a mass in the uterus that is presumed to be a leiomyoma. This mass is a

(A) benign tumor of mesenchymal tissue
(B) benign tumor of surface epithelium
(C) malignant tumor of epithelial tissue
(D) malignant tumor of glandular epithelium
(E) malignant tumor of mesenchymal tissue

3. A 68-year-old man has a long history of prostate cancer that was metastatic at the time of diagnosis. Over the past 2 months, he has had significant weight loss, loss of appetite, and loss of energy. His current spectrum of conditions can be attributed to which of the following?

(B) Fibroblast growth factor
(C) Interleukin-2
(A) Platelet-derived growth factor
(D) Tumor necrosis factor-α
(E) Vascular endothelial growth factor

4. A 58-year-old man with a 700-pack-per-year smoking history presents to the emergency department with shortness of breath and hemoptysis. Portable chest radiography demonstrates a large mass centrally located within the left lung field. The serum calcium is 13.0 mg/dL (normal 8.5 to 10.2). The metabolic abnormality described here is likely due to elaboration of which substance?

(A) Adrenocorticotropic hormone–like substance
(B) Antidiuretic hormone
(C) Carcinoembryonic antigen
(D) Erythropoietin
(E) Parathyroid-related hormone

5. An 8-year-old boy is referred to the dermatologist for numerous "suspicious" pigmented lesions on the face and neck. Further history reveals that the patient has had difficulty seeing out of his right eye; he is referred to the ophthalmologist, who diagnoses an ocular melanoma. Based on the patient's symptoms, the diagnosis of xeroderma pigmentosum is considered. This condition results from

(A) aberrant expression of a receptor tyrosine kinase
(B) an inborn defect in DNA repair
(C) chemical carcinogenesis
(D) DNA viral infection
(E) retroviral infection

6. A 46-year-old woman with prominent splenomegaly presents with a 3-month history of malaise, easy fatigability, weakness, weight loss, and anorexia. A complete blood count and differential demonstrates a white blood cell count of $250,000/mm^3$ (normal $3000–10,000/mm^3$) with a predominance of myelocytes, metamyelocytes, band cells, and segmented neutrophils. Cytogenetic analysis is most likely to reveal which of the following translocations?

(A) t(8;14)
(B) t(9;22)
(C) t(11;22)
(D) t(14;18)
(E) t(15;17)

7. A 63-year-old woman discovers a lump in her right breast. Mammography confirms the presence of a suspicious "lump," and a needle core biopsy is performed to determine whether the mass is malignant. The pathology report confirms that the mass is indeed cancerous and that the tissue demonstrates amplification of the *Her-2/neu* oncogene. The gene product of *Her-2/neu* is what kind of protein?

(A) GTPase
(B) GTPase-activating protein
(C) Nuclear transcription factor
(D) Receptor tyrosine kinase
(E) A retinoic acid receptor protein

8. A 27-year-old woman has recently been diagnosed with a glioma (a malignant brain tumor). Further family history reveals that her 4-year-old son has been diagnosed with leukemia and has been undergoing chemotherapy. In addition, the patient's mother died at 36 years of age due to metastatic breast cancer. Li-Fraumeni syndrome is suspected, given the familial clustering of this group of malignancies. The gene mutated in Li-Fraumeni syndrome normally functions in what capacity?

(A) Activates the GTPase activity of the gene product of the *Ras* oncogene
(B) Excises ultraviolet light–induced thymidine dimers
(C) Functions as a cytoplasmic tyrosine kinase
(D) Functions as a transmembrane tyrosine kinase
(E) Halts the cell cycle if DNA damage is detected

9. An 8-year-old child is evaluated by the pediatrician, who notes what appears to be ten small café-au-lait spots on the child's torso. In addition, on close inspection of the eyes, the presence of Lisch nodules is noted. The patient is diagnosed with von Recklinghausen neurofibromatosis type 1. The protein that is mutated in this disorder normally

(A) activates the GTPase activity of Ras
(B) cleaves cellular proteins during apoptosis
(C) functions as a regulator of the cell cycle
(D) promotes angiogenesis in the growing tumor mass
(E) promotes the cell to undergo apoptosis

10. A 78-year-old Navy veteran with a 600-pack per-year history of cigarette smoking presents with cancer. During his military career, he was involved in fireproofing naval combat ships with asbestos insulation. Given his environmental exposure to both tobacco and asbestos, to which cancer do both of these carcinogens contribute?

(A) Bladder cancer
(B) Bronchogenic cancer
(C) Cancer of the throat
(D) Esophageal cancer
(E) Mesothelioma

ANSWERS AND EXPLANATIONS

1-E. Desmoplasia refers to proliferation of non-neoplastic fibrous connective tissue within a tumor and is quite common in cases of breast cancer. An irregular accumulation of blood vessels is known as a hemangioma. An area of tissue misplaced within another organ is known as a choristoma.

2-A. A leiomyoma (fibroid) is a benign tumor of the smooth muscle of the uterus and is thus is an example of a benign tumor of mesenchymal origin. Profuse, painful menses and infertility are major complications of this most common tumor of the female genital tract. A leiomyosarcoma is the malignant counterpart. Malignant tumors of epithelial cells are carcinomas, and these are known as adenocarcinomas if they involve glandular epithelium. Benign tumors of surface epithelium are termed papillomas.

3-D. Cachexia, or wasting due to cancer, manifests with weakness, weight loss, anorexia, anemia, and infection. The principal cytokine responsible for such changes is tumor necrosis factor-α (TNF-α). Both platelet-derived growth factor and fibroblast growth factor are involved in wound healing. Interleukin-2 (IL-2) is an immunostimulating cytokine produced by activated T cells. Vascular endothelial growth factor is important in the proliferation of blood vessels in a growing tumor.

4-E. The man is likely to have a lung tumor, given his clinical presentation and the radiographic results. The patient's hypercalcemia is likely due to a paraneoplastic syndrome, such as that due to the elaboration of parathyroid-related hormone (PTrH). PTrH is produced by squamous cell carcinoma, whereas adrenocorticotropic-like substance and antidiuretic hormone are produced by yet another form of lung cancer, small cell carcinoma of the lung. Carcinoembryonic antigen is an oncofetal antigen produced by colon cancer cells. Erythropoietin causes secondary polycythemia and is related to renal cell carcinoma.

5-B. Xeroderma pigmentosum is a hereditary DNA defect with a deficiency in the ability to repair ultraviolet (sunlight)-induced thymidine dimers. Faulty repair leads to increased sun sensitivity, with a predilection to develop skin lesions and skin cancers on exposed skin as well as ocular melanomas. Aberrant expression of the gene for a receptor tyrosine kinase such as the Her-2/neu gene product can cause breast cancer. A retrovirus is responsible for the development of T-cell leukemia/lymphoma. The DNA virus human papillomavirus can cause cervical cancer.

6-B. The translocation t(9;22) is the characteristic translocation associated with chronic myelogenous leukemia, forming the so-called "Philadelphia chromosome." The resultant fusion protein, p210, has increased tyrosine kinase activity that contributes to the uncontrolled proliferation in this form of leukemia. The translocation t(14;18) is seen in follicular lymphoma; t(8;14) in Burkitt's lymphoma; t(15;17) in the M3 variant of acute promyelocytic leukemia (AML); and t(11;22) in Ewing sarcoma, a relatively uncommon tumor of bone.

7-D. Her-2/neu, also known as (c-erbB2), is a receptor tyrosine kinase related to epidermal growth factor receptor and is amplified at the DNA level and overexpressed at the protein level in some breast cancers. Ras is a GTPase that is mutated in a number of cancers. NF-1 is a GTPase-activating protein (GAP) aberrantly expressed in neurofibromatosis. An aberrant version of a retinoic acid receptor is expressed in M3 AML.

8-E. Li-Fraumeni syndrome is a hereditary syndrome characterized by sarcomas, breast cancer, leukemia, and brain tumors. Xeroderma pigmentosum results from a defect in repair of UV damage. Numerous transmembrane tyrosine kinases, such as Her-2/neu, are implicated in numerous cancers. C-*abl* codes for a cytoplasmic tyrosine kinase that forms a fusion protein with bcr in chronic myelogenous leukemia. NF-1, mutated in neurofibromatosis, normally activates the GTPase activity of the gene product of the *Ras* oncogene. The gene *p53*, the "guardian of the genome," arrests the cell cycle in G_1 in the event that DNA damage is detected.

9-A. The normal function of NF-1 is to promote the intrinsic GTPase function of the *Ras* oncogene. When the Ras protein is bound to GTP, the growth-promoting function of the molecule is "ON." On hydrolysis of the GTP to GDP, Ras is converted to an inactive state. GTPase-activating proteins (GAPs) such as NF-1 suppress cell growth by stimulating GTP hydrolysis. Patients with a mutation in NF-1 are susceptible to fibrosarcomas as a result of loss of function of this GAP. The molecule Bax is pro-apoptotic and antagonizes Bcl-2. Vascular endothelial growth factor promotes tumor angiogenesis. The protein p53 regulates the cell cycle if DNA damage is detected. Lastly, caspases function to cleave cellular proteins once apoptosis is triggered.

10-B. Tobacco contributes to the development of many cancers, including those of the bladder, lung, throat, and esophagus. Asbestos exposure carries a risk of lung cancer as well as mesothelioma, a cancer of the pleura. Tobacco and asbestos function as cocarcinogens in the pathogenesis of lung cancer, with an approximately 50-fold greater risk of developing bronchogenic cancer of the lung than in those without such exposure.

CHAPTER 7

Environmental Pathology

I. Physical Injury

A. Mechanical injury. Causes are various and include blunt force, sharp objects, or bullets. Mechanical injury can produce damage by cutting, tearing, or crushing of tissues; by severe blood loss; or by interruption of blood or air supply.

1. **Terminology**
   a. An **abrasion or scrape** is a superficial tearing away of epidermal cells.
   b. A **laceration** is a jagged tear, often with stretching of the underlying tissue.
   c. An **incision** is a clean cut by a sharp object.
   d. A **puncture** is a deep tubular wound produced by a sharp, thin object.
   e. A **contusion** is a bruise caused by disruption of underlying small blood vessels; commonly the skin is affected, but internal organs may also be involved.
2. **Causes of death**
   a. **Hemorrhage** into body cavities
   b. **Fat embolism** from bone fractures
   c. **Ruptured viscera**
   d. **Secondary infection**
   e. **Renal shutdown** caused by acute tubular necrosis, especially when associated with myoglobin casts arising from crush injury of skeletal muscle
3. **Blunt force injuries**
   a. **Head injury**
      (1) **Brain damage,** with possible skull fracture, can be the direct result of cerebral trauma or caused by intracranial hemorrhage.
      (2) **Brain laceration** can be caused by fracture with penetrating injury by skull fragments.
      (3) **Brain contusion** may occur at the point of impact (**coup injury**) or on the opposite side of the brain (**contrecoup injury**).
   b. **Abdominal injury** may result in the following conditions:
      (1) **Contusion**
      (2) **Rupture of the spleen or liver,** sometimes with severe hemorrhage
      (3) **Rupture of the intestine,** which can result in **peritonitis**
   c. **Thoracic injury** may result in the following conditions:
      (1) **Rib fracture,** possibly with penetration into pulmonary parenchyma or thoracic wall vessels
      (2) **Hemothorax,** or hemorrhage in the pleural cavity
      (3) **Pneumothorax,** or air in the pleural cavity
4. **Knife and stab wounds** can be incisions or puncture wounds and result in highly variable consequences, depending on the site of the injury.
5. **Gunshot wounds**

a. The entrance wound is usually smaller and rounder than the exit wound (and in some cases even smaller than the bullet because the skin is elastic).
b. Exit wounds may be significantly larger than the bullet due to tumbling of the bullet (and tissue and bone fragments accompanying the bullet) and are usually irregular or stellate rather than round.
c. In contact wounds, there may be burning around the margins of the wound (abrasion ring).
d. Contact wounds over the skull and other areas with skin closely overlying bone may demonstrate a stellate (star-shaped) appearance due to gases from the gun undermining the skin margins.
e. Close-range wounds (20 inches or less) demonstrate unburned powder particles in the skin (tattooing or stippling) and deposits of soot on the skin.
f. Long-range wounds are usually round or oval, demonstrating clean margins without evidence of stippling or fouling.

B. **Thermal injury**
1. **Burns**
a. **Classification**
(1) **First-degree burns (partial-thickness burns)** are characterized by hyperemia without significant epidermal damage; they generally heal without intervention.
(2) **Second-degree burns (partial-thickness burns)** are characterized by blistering and destruction of the epidermis with slight damage to the underlying dermis; they generally heal without intervention.
(3) **Third-degree burns (full-thickness burns)** are characterized by damage to the epidermis, dermis, and dermal appendages; skin and underlying tissue are often charred and blackened; these burns often require skin grafting.
b. **Complications**
(1) **Inhalation of smoke or toxic fumes** result in pulmonary or systemic damage.
(2) **Hypovolemia** results from fluid and electrolyte loss.
(3) **Curling ulcer** (acute gastric ulcer associated with severe burns)
(4) **Infection** is the most common cause of late fatalities. The most frequent organism is *Pseudomonas aeruginosa.*
2. **Freezing**
a. Tissue damage may be generalized, resulting in **death.**
b. Tissue damage may be localized, resulting in **frostbite;** exposed areas such as fingers, toes, earlobes, or nose are usually affected.
c. Severe, prolonged frostbite may result in **intracellular ice crystals, intravascular thrombosis,** and sometimes local **gangrene.**

C. **Electrical injury.** When electric current passes through an individual, thus completing an electric circuit, electrical injury occurs.
1. Fatal electrical injury is usually caused by current passing through the brain or heart. It may cause **respiratory or cardiac arrest** or **cardiac arrhythmias.**
2. Electrical injury may result in small **cutaneous burns** with blister formation at the point of entry or exit of the electric current. At times, burns may be severe.

D. **Radiation injury**
1. **Ultraviolet light (sunlight)**
a. Ultraviolet radiation causes **sunburn,** which is characterized by erythema, often with superficial desquamation and, in severe cases, blister formation.
b. It is associated with premalignant cutaneous lesions **(actinic keratosis)** and malignant cutaneous lesions such as **squamous and basal cell carcinomas and melanoma.**
2. **Ionizing radiation**
a. Ionizing radiation is from x-ray, radioactive waste, nuclear disasters, and other exposures.

TABLE 7-1 *Radiosensitivity of Specialized Cells*

Degree of Sensitivity	Types	Characteristics
Radiosensitive	Lymphoid, hematopoietic, germ, gastrointestinal mucosal, rapidly dividing tumor cells	Regularly actively divide, especially those cells undergoing mitosis
Intermediate radiosensitivity	Fibroblasts; cells of endothelium, elastic tissue, salivary glands, eye	...
Radioresistant	Cells of bone, cartilage, muscle, central nervous system, kidney, liver, and most endocrine glands	Cease division shortly after fetal development is complete

b. Cell damage results from the formation of toxic free radicals, affecting vital cell components such as DNA and intracellular membranes.

c. **Localized radiation** results in the following conditions:

(1) **Skin changes** include dermatitis, ulceration, and skin malignancies.

(2) **Pulmonary changes** include acute changes similar to those of adult respiratory distress syndrome; and chronic changes, such as septal fibrosis, bronchiolar metaplasia, and hyaline thickening of blood vessel walls

(3) **Gastrointestinal inflammation and ulceration**

(4) **Hematopoietic alterations,** including bone marrow depression or leukemia

(5) **Neoplasia includes** myeloid (but not lymphoid) leukemias and cancers of bone, skin, thyroid, lung, or breast.

d. **Severe and generalized radiation** occurs in whole body irradiation such as that seen in nuclear disasters.

(1) **Severe central nervous system (CNS) injury** primarily caused by capillary damage

(2) **Gastrointestinal mucosal denudation**

(3) **Acute bone marrow failure**

3. **Radiosensitivity of specialized cells (Table 7-1)**

a. Lymphocytes are the earliest blood cells to be affected.

b. The most sensitive cells are lymphoid, hematopoietic, germ, gastrointestinal mucosal, and those from rapidly dividing tumors.

II. Chemical Abuse

A. **Alcohol abuse.** This is an important cause of death and disability from several causes ranging from automobile accidents to homicides. A constellation of changes that are collectively grouped as **chronic alcoholism** is characteristic, and common pathologic findings include:

1. **Alcoholic hepatitis and cirrhosis**
2. **Acute and chronic pancreatitis**
3. **Gastritis**
4. **Oral, pharyngeal, laryngeal, esophageal, and gastric carcinoma** (especially in association with combined abuse of alcohol and tobacco)
5. **Alcoholic (dilated) cardiomyopathy**
6. **Aspiration pneumonia**
7. **Myopathy**
8. **Peripheral neuropathy**
9. **Cerebral dysfunction,** such as thiamine deficiency-mediated **Wernicke-Korsakoff syndrome,** sometimes referred to as alcoholic encephalopathy

a. The cause is a combination of alcoholism and thiamine deficiency.
b. The syndrome is often associated with hemorrhagic necrosis of mamillary bodies.
c. Wernicke syndrome is a combination of ataxia, confusion, ophthalmoplegia, and often nystagmus.
d. Korsakoff syndrome is manifest by memory loss and confabulation.

10. **Fetal alcohol syndrome,** which involves microcephaly, mental retardation, facial and cardiac defects

B. **Tobacco abuse.** Associated conditions include:

1. Squamous cell carcinoma of the larynx, squamous cell and small cell bronchogenic carcinoma, and transitional cell carcinoma of the urinary bladder
2. Chronic obstructive pulmonary disease
3. Atherosclerosis and other vascular occlusive diseases, such as Buerger disease

C. **Drug abuse**

1. **Cocaine** can result in the following effects and complications:
   a. **Mood elevation,** sometimes followed by irritability, anxiety, and depression, which may lead to suicide
   b. **Increased myocardial irritability,** which can lead to fatal arrhythmias
   c. **Hypertension,** which can predispose to cerebral hemorrhage
   d. **Nasal congestion, ulceration, or septal perforation,** from intranasal use
   e. **Burn injury,** due to volatile inflammable substances used in cocaine free-base preparation
   f. **Viral** [human immunodeficiency virus (HIV) or hepatitis B] or **bacterial** (infective endocarditis) **infection** (from intravenous use). Infective endocarditis due to intravenous drug abuse often involves the valves of the right side of the heart.
   g. Epileptic seizures, respiratory arrest, myocardial infarction, and, in newborns of addicted mothers, multiple small cerebral infarcts
2. **Heroin** is usually administered intravenously and can result in the following effects and complications:
   a. **Physical dependence,** with severe withdrawal symptoms
   b. **Infections,** such as HIV, hepatitis B, and infective endocarditis
   c. **Adult respiratory distress syndrome**
   d. **Death** from respiratory or cardiac arrest or from pulmonary edema

III. Environmental Chemical Injuries (Table 7-2)

A. **Methyl alcohol (methanol)**

1. This chemical is converted to the cellular toxins formaldehyde and formic acid, resulting in transient metabolic acidosis.
2. It damages the cells of the retina, optic nerve, and CNS, resulting in **blindness.**

B. **Carbon monoxide (CO)**

1. This gas inhibits the capacity of hemoglobin to function as an oxygen carrier because hemoglobin has an affinity for CO that is 200 times greater than its affinity for oxygen.
2. It can result in irreversible **hypoxic injury,** often leading to death; neurons of the brain are most vulnerable. Foci of neuronal necrosis in the basal ganglia, lenticular nuclei, and cortical gray areas are characteristic. When fatal, it causes a **cherry-red color of the skin, blood, viscera, and muscles.**

C. **Carbon tetrachloride (CCl_4).** This chemical induces **centrilobular necrosis and fatty change** in the liver.

D. **Cyanide**

1. This chemical **inhibits intracellular cytochrome oxidase** by binding with ferric iron, thus preventing cellular oxidation. **Death** occurs within minutes.
2. Generalized petechial hemorrhages and a scent of bitter almonds are noted at autopsy.

TABLE 7-2 *Some Environmental Toxins and Their Effects*

Toxin	Predominant Adverse Effects
Methyl alcohol	Blindness
Carbon monoxide	Severe hypoxic injury caused by displacement of oxyhemoglobin by carboxyhemoglobin
Carbon tetrachloride	Hepatic centrilobular necrosis and fatty change
Cyanide	Cessation of intracellular oxidation because of cytochrome oxidase inhibition
Lead	Anemia; basophilic stippling of erythrocytes; encephalopathy; neuropathy; lead line; Fanconi syndrome
Mercuric chloride	Gastrointestinal ulcerations; calcification and necrosis of renal convoluted tubules

E. **Lead.** This chemical may be **ingested,** particularly from lead in paint, or may be **inspired,** particularly from automotive emissions. When ingested or inhaled in toxic amounts, is manifested clinically by:

1. **Red blood cell changes**
   a. **Basophilic stippling**
   b. **Hypochromic microcytic anemia**
      (1) The cause is deficient heme synthesis mediated by the inhibition of **δ-aminolevulinic acid (ALA) dehydratase** and by decreased incorporation of iron into heme.
      (2) Defects result in accumulation of both ALA and erythrocyte protoporphyrin, leading to protoporphyrinemia, porphyrinuria, and aminolevulinic aciduria.
2. **Encephalopathy,** characterized by irritability and sometimes by seizures and coma
3. **Neuropathy,** characterized by wristdrop and footdrop
4. **Fanconi syndrome,** characterized by impaired proximal renal tubular reabsorption of phosphate, glucose, and amino acids
5. **Lead line,** characterized by mucosal deposits of lead sulfide at the junction of the teeth and gums
6. **Increased radiodensity of the epiphyses of the long bones**

F. **Mercuric chloride.** Ingestion results in **focal gastrointestinal ulceration and severe renal damage** with widespread necrosis and calcification of the proximal convoluted tubules. Proximal convoluted tubular necrosis is characteristic of injury from a number of nephrotoxins.

G. **Vinyl chloride.** This chemical can lead to hemangiosarcoma (angiosarcoma) of liver.

H. **β-Naphthylamine and aniline dyes.** These chemicals can lead to transitional cell carcinoma of the urinary bladder.

I. **Ethylene glycol.** This chemical can cause acute tubular necrosis as well as tubular precipitation of calcium oxalate crystals, which can be visualized with polarized light.

J. **Polychlorinated biphenyls (PCBs)**

1. These nonbiodegradable **environmental pollutants** were used to manufacture a variety of products, such as adhesives and plasticizers. Because of their toxicity, their production is now outlawed.
2. Exposure produces a syndrome of chloracne, impotence, and visual changes.

IV. Adverse Effects of Therapeutic Drugs

These effects can be manifest by a wide variety of clinically significant abnormalities. For example:

A. **Antibiotics**
   1. **Development of drug-resistant organisms** is often mediated by plasmids carrying specific drug-resistant genes.
   2. **Fatal aplastic anemia** can occur as a result of an idiosyncratic reaction to chloramphenicol.

B. **Sulfonamides**
   1. **Immune complex disease,** such as polyarteritis nodosa, can develop when sulfonamides, acting as haptens, stimulate antibody production.
   2. **Crystallization of sulfonamides within the renal collecting system,** cause calculi with obstruction, infection, or both.
   3. **Bone marrow failure**
   4. **Acute, self-limited hemolytic anemia** may be induced in individuals with erythrocyte glucose-6-phosphate dehydrogenase (G6PD) deficiency.

C. **Analgesics**
   1. **Aspirin**
      a. **Gastroduodenal bleeding** may be caused by aspirin-induced gastritis or peptic ulcer or by inhibition of platelet cyclooxygenase with resultant thromboxane A_2 deficiency and impaired platelet plug formation.
      b. **Reye syndrome** occurs in children following an acute febrile viral illness, almost always in association with aspirin intake. It is characterized by microvesicular fatty change in the liver and encephalopathy.
      c. **Allergic reactions** include urticaria, asthma, nasal polyps, and angioneurotic edema.
   2. **Phenacetin**
      a. **Chronic analgesic nephritis and renal papillary necrosis** (the drug has been withdrawn from the U.S. market)
      b. **Urothelial neoplasms,** especially transitional cell carcinoma of the renal pelvis
      c. **Acute hemolysis** in G6PD-deficient individuals

D. **Cancer chemotherapeutic drugs**
   1. **Toxic effects,** including hair loss, gastrointestinal erosions and ulcerations, and, most significantly, bone marrow failure
   2. **Acute leukemia or other malignancies**

REVIEW TEST

Directions: *Each of the numbered items or incomplete statements in this section is followed by answers or by completions of the statement. Select the* ***one*** *lettered answer or completion that is best in each case.*

1. A 32-year-old man is involved in a high-speed motor vehicle accident and brought by ambulance to a Level I trauma center because of the severity of his injuries. On arrival, it is determined that he is bleeding internally, and he is taken immediately to surgery, where the surgeons find that the source of his bleeding is a severe liver laceration. A laceration is a

(A) bruise caused by disruption of underlying blood vessels
(B) clean cut by a sharp object
(C) deep tubular wound produced by a sharp, thin object
(D) jagged tear, often with stretching of the underlying tissue
(E) superficial tearing away of epidermal cells

2. A forensic pathologist is asked to evaluate a fatal gunshot wound involving the left thorax of a 27-year-old man, a known drug dealer. Even though a gun and suicide note were found next to the body, the pathologist has concluded that the wound was probably not self-inflicted. Which of the following findings is most supportive of that conclusion?

(A) The entrance wound is smaller than the exit wound.
(B) The entrance wound is stellate-shaped.
(C) The exit wound is irregularly shaped.
(D) There is no stippling of the skin, and the wound is oval with clean margins.
(E) There is stippling of the skin from unburned gunpowder.

3. A 4-year-old girl is brought by her mother to the emergency department after the girl was "placed in a hot bath." The patient appears to have extensive blistering of the thighs and buttocks, with slight damage to the underlying dermis. Her burns are best described as

(A) first-degree burns
(B) fourth-degree burns
(C) full-thickness burns
(D) second-degree burns
(E) third-degree burns

4. A 38-year-old woman is receiving radiation therapy to her abdomen as adjuvant therapy for the treatment of cervical cancer. The radiosensitivity of organs or tissues within the treatment field is a limiting factor in determining the dose of radiation that can be administered? Which of the following is most susceptible to radiation damage?

(A) Bone
(B) Gastrointestinal mucosa
(C) Peripheral nervous tissue
(D) Renal parenchyma
(E) Skeletal musculature of the abdomen

5. A 50-year-old chronic alcoholic is seen in the emergency department with ataxic gait, confusion, confabulation, and nystagmus. This constellation of findings is the classic presentation of

(A) Fetal alcohol syndrome
(B) Li-Fraumeni syndrome
(C) Lynch syndrome
(D) Wernicke-Korsakoff syndrome
(E) Wiskott-Aldrich syndrome

6. A 50-year-old man who works for a chemical company is being held on charges of murdering his wife. When the police found the woman's body, they noted no signs of physical injury but detected a scent of bitter almonds. A small sample of cyanide was recently reported missing from the husband's workplace. Based on these investigational findings, a justifiable working hypothesis for the forensic pathologist is that the death resulted from

(A) acute tubular necrosis
(B) induction of direct DNA damage
(C) inhibition of intracellular oxidative phosphorylation
(D) inhibition of the oxygen-carrying capacity of hemoglobin
(E) rhabdomyolysis

7. A 78-year-old man is found in his closed room unresponsive in bed after the first cold day of winter. There is a kerosene heater still on from the previous night. On attempts to arouse him, officers note the cherry hue of his lips, cheeks, and mucous membranes. The likely mechanism of his death was

(A) accidental ingestion of ethylene glycol
(B) binding of carbon monoxide to hemoglobin
(C) hepatic necrosis with fatty change
(D) inhibition of hemoglobin production
(E) inhibition of incorporation of iron into hemoglobin

8. A 3-year-old child is brought to the emergency department because of a week-long history of abdominal discomfort, irritability, and weakness. A complete blood count and blood smear demonstrate microcytic hypochromic anemia with basophilic stippling of the red blood cells. Further history reveals that the family lives in an old apartment complex. The most likely cause of the hematologic findings is

(A) binding of carbon monoxide to hemoglobin
(B) inhibition of cytochrome oxidase
(C) inhibition of hemoglobin production
(D) iron deficiency
(E) iron intoxication

9. A 27-year-old man who was badly burned in an industrial accident requires multiple skin grafting. While in the intensive care unit, he is found to have blood in his stools, and endoscopy confirms the presence of many small ulcers in his stomach. This complication is referred to as

(A) aplastic anemia
(B) Curling ulcer
(C) Cushing ulcer
(D) Reye syndrome
(E) Stevens-Johnson syndrome

10. Following his return home from a party, a 22-year-old man develops crushing chest pain and is brought to the emergency department by ambulance. Questioning reveals no cardiac risk factors. Electrocardiographic and serum enzyme findings are consistent with acute myocardial infarction. It is suspected that the cardiac damage is related to toxicity of a drug of abuse. Which of the following drugs is most likely?

(A) Cocaine
(B) Ethyl alcohol
(C) Heroin
(D) Methyl alcohol
(E) Phenacetin

ANSWERS AND EXPLANATIONS

1-D. A laceration, especially of internal organs, is common in cases of blunt trauma, as in a motor vehicle accident. By definition, a laceration is a jagged tear, often with stretching of the underlying tissue. An incision is a clean cut by a sharp object, as in a clean cut by a surgeon. A contusion is a bruise caused by disruption of underlying blood vessels. A puncture is a deep tubular wound produced by a sharp, thin object. An abrasion is a superficial tearing away of epidermal cells.

2-D. Lack of stippling is a characteristic of gunshot wounds inflicted from long distances. In addition, the wounds are often oval with clean margins. Such evidence is more consistent with a homicide than a "staged" suicide. In general, entrance wounds are smaller than exit wounds, which are often irregularly shaped. Stellate-shaped wounds are associated with wounds over bony areas. Wounds from close range, as in a suicide, would be expected to have stippling and tattooing of skin caused by unburned gunpowder.

3-D. First-and second-degree burns are both partial-thickness burns. Because the findings in this patient reveal both epithelial and dermal involvement, the burns are, by definition, second-degree in type. Both third- and fourth-degree burns are classified as full-thickness burns; they entail total destruction of dermis and epidermis along with underlying skin appendages that normally serve as a source of cells for regeneration. As such, these wounds require skin grafting.

4-B. Gastrointestinal mucosal cells are examples of labile cells, and thus are among the most radiosensitive of the tissues or organs listed in the question. The symptoms associated with damage to these cells (nausea, diarrhea, and malabsorption) are likely to limit the total dose of radiation the patient can receive. The other tissues listed are relatively radioresistant and are unlikely to limit the amount of radiation a patient can receive.

5-D. Wernicke-Korsakoff syndrome presents with the classic triad of ataxia, confabulation, and ophthalmoplegia and is seen in alcoholics secondary to a deficiency of the vitamin thiamine. Fetal alcohol syndrome occurs in infants born to mothers who consume alcohol during pregnancy and results in microcephaly, mental retardation, and facial and cardiac defects. Li-Fraumeni syndrome and the Lynch syndrome are both familial defects in DNA repair that lead to a propensity to develop particular cancers. Wiskott-Aldrich syndrome is an inborn immune defect presenting with eczema, thrombocytopenia, and recurrent infections.

6-C. Cyanide is an inhibitor of the electron transport chain (ETC) within the mitochondria. Inhibition of the ETC results in the inhibition of intracellular oxidative phosphorylation, with depletion of cellular energy stores and, ultimately, death. Acute tubular necrosis can occur under many circumstances, as in cases of rhabdomyolysis secondary to crush injury. Inhibition of the oxygen-carrying capacity of hemoglobin can result from carbon monoxide poisoning. Induction of direct DNA damage can result from radiation exposure.

7-B. Carbon monoxide (CO) binds to hemoglobin with approximately 200 times greater affinity than oxygen, preventing delivery of oxygen to tissues. In addition, CO is an inhibitor of cytochrome oxidase, impairing cellular respiration. Ethylene glycol (antifreeze) is associated with kidney damage and the formation of birefringent calcium oxalate crystals in the urinary tract. Hepatic necrosis and fatty change result from carbon tetrachloride poisoning. Lead inhibits a key enzyme in hemoglobin synthesis as well as iron incorporation in hemoglobin.

8-C. This is a typical presentation of lead poisoning. Lead inhibits hemoglobin synthesis by inhibiting both aminolevulinic acid dehydratase and ferroketolase. This inhibits not only the synthesis of hemoglobin but also the incorporation of iron into the molecule. Cyanide and carbon monoxide (CO) inhibit cytochrome oxidase. CO also binds to hemoglobin, preventing adequate oxygen transport. Iron deficiency can lead to similar hematologic findings.

9-B. Punctate ulcers associated with extensive burn injuries are known as Curling ulcers. A similar phenomenon occurs in patients with head trauma, in which the lesions are known as Cushing ulcers. Aplastic anemia can result from an idiosyncratic reaction in patients taking the antibiotic chloramphenicol. Likewise, sulfonamides can cause a necrotizing eruption around mucous membranes in some individuals. Reye syndrome is associated with extensive microvesicular fatty change of the liver in children taking aspirin during an acute viral illness. The Stevens-Johnson syndrome is characterized by erosions and crusts of the lips and oral mucosa as a component of an extensive form of erythema multiforme, a maculopapular, vesiculobullous eruption often related to drugs (such as sulfonamides), neoplasia, or connective tissue disorders.

10-A. Cocaine is associated with increased myocardial irritability and sometimes with myocardial infarction, hypertension, and cerebral vascular accident. Both ethyl alcohol and tobacco are long-term contributors to heart disease but are unlikely to cause an acute event in a young patient. Methyl alcohol can lead to blindness as well as kidney damage. Phenacetin, an analgesic related to acetaminophen, can lead to kidney damage and is no longer used in this country.

CHAPTER

8

Nutritional Disorders

I. Malnutrition

A. **In affluent countries,** malnutrition is found in children living below the poverty level, the elderly, alcoholics, persons on fad diets and with eating disorders such as anorexia nervosa, and patients with severe wasting diseases.

B. **In developing countries, protein-calorie malnutrition** occurs in two forms—marasmus and kwashiorkor.

1. **Marasmus** is caused by widespread **deficiency of almost all nutrients,** notably protein and calories.
   a. It often coexists with vitamin deficiencies.
   b. It typically occurs in children younger than 1 year of age who are not breast-fed and do not have an adequate intake of substitute nutrients.
   c. Clinical characteristics include retarded growth and loss of muscle and other protein-containing tissue, as well as subcutaneous fat ("wasting away").
2. **Kwashiorkor** is caused by **protein deficiency** but with adequate caloric intake.
   a. It usually affects children older than 1 year of age who are no longer breast-fed and receive a starch-rich, protein-poor diet.
   b. Clinical characteristics include retarded growth and muscle wasting, caused by inadequate protein intake, but with preservation of subcutaneous fat.
   c. Kwashiokor is distinguished from marasmus by the presence of the following abnormalities:
      (1) Fatty liver
      (2) **Severe edema** due to protein deficiency and decreased oncotic pressure
      (3) Anemia
      (4) Malabsorption due to atrophy of the small intestinal villi
      (5) **Depigmented bands** with pale streaking in the hair or skin

II. Vitamins

A. **Water-soluble vitamins** (Table 8-1)

1. **General considerations.** Water-soluble vitamins include the **B complex vitamins:** B_1 (thiamine), B_2 (riboflavin), B_3 (niacin), B_6 (pyridoxine), and B_{12} (cobalamin); folic acid; and vitamin C (ascorbic acid).
   a. Because these vitamins are not stored in the body, regular intake is essential, except for vitamin B_{12}. Vitamin B_{12} is stored in the liver in quantities sufficiently large so that deprivation for months or years is necessary for deficiency to develop.
   b. Toxicity from excessive intake is rare, because excess vitamin is excreted in the urine.

TABLE 8-1 *Water-Soluble Vitamins*

	Metabolic Functions	Clinical Manifestations of Deficiency
Vitamin B_1 (thiamine)	Coenzyme thiamine pyrophosphate plays a key role in carbohydrate and amino acid intermediary metabolism	Wet beriberi; dry beriberi; Wernicke-Korsakoff syndrome
Vitamin B_2 (riboflavin)	Component of FAD and FMN and is essential in a variety of oxidation-reduction processes	Cheilosis; corneal vascularization; glossitis; dermatitis
Vitamin B_3 (niacin, nicotinic acid)	Component of NAD and NADP, essential to glycolysis, the citric acid cycle, and to a variety of oxidations (can be synthesized from tryptophan); deficiency requires diet lacking both niacin and tryptophan	Pellagra
Vitamin B_6 (pyridoxine)	Required for transamination, porphyrin synthesis, synthesis of niacin from tryptophan	Cheilosis; glossitis; anemia; convulsions in infants; neurologic dysfunction
Vitamin B_{12} (cobalamin)	1-Carbon transfers required for folate synthesis and activation of FH_4; $N^{5,10}$-methylene FH_4 is required for conversion of dUMP to dTMP in DNA synthesis	Megaloblastic anemia; neurologic dysfunction
Folic acid	1-Carbon transfers in a number of metabolic reactions; $N^{5,10}$-methylene FH_4 required for DNA synthesis	Megaloblastic anemia; neurologic dysfunction is not a feature (as it is in vitamin B_{12} deficiency)
Vitamin C (ascorbic acid)	Required for hydroxylation of proline and lysine, which are essential for collagen synthesis; hydroxylation of dopamine in synthesis of norepinephrine; enhances maintenance of reduced state of other metabolically active agents, such as iron and FH_4	Scurvy, defective formation of mesenchymal tissue and osteoid matrix; defective wound healing; hemorrhagic phenomena

FAD = flavin adenine dinucleotide; FMN = flavin mononucleotide; NAD = nicotinamide adenine dinucleotide; NADP = nicotinamide adenine dinucleotide phosphate; FH_4 = tetrahydrofolate; $N^{5,10}$-methylene FH_4 = activated tetrahydrofolate.

2. **Dietary sources**
   a. **B complex vitamins** (except vitamin B_{12}): whole grain cereals, green leafy vegetables, fish, meat, and dairy foods
   b. **Vitamin B_{12}:** foods of animal origin only (vitamin B_{12} is synthesized by intestinal bacteria in animals)
   c. **Folic acid:** leafy vegetables, cereals, fruits, and a number of animal products
   d. **Vitamin C:** fruits (especially citrus fruits and tomatoes), vegetables, various meats, and milk
3. **Deficiencies.** Clinical manifestions are often shared. The most striking clinical manifestations are in tissues with active metabolism, because these vitamins are involved in the release and storage of energy. In B complex vitamins, deficiencies are often marked by glossitis, dermatitis, and diarrhea.
   a. **Vitamin B_1 (thiamine) deficiency** is most often associated with severe malnutrition. (In Western countries, it is usually associated with alcoholism and fad diets.) It results in three distinct syndromes:

(1) **Dry beriberi** is characterized by **peripheral neuropathy** with resultant atrophy of the muscles of the extremities.
(2) **Wet beriberi**
(a) This condition is marked by **high-output cardiac failure,** often with dilated cardiomyopathy.
(b) It results from peripheral dilation of arterioles and capillaries, leading to increased arteriovenous shunting, hypervolemia, and cardiac dilation.
(3) **Wernicke-Korsakoff syndrome** most often occurs in a setting of thiamine deficiency and alcoholism.
(a) This condition is manifest by degenerative changes in the brain stem and diencephalon, with **hemorrhagic lesions** of cortical and bilateral paramedian masses of gray matter and the **mamillary bodies.**
(b) It is characterized by **confusion, ataxia,** and **ophthalmoplegia** (Wernicke triad) and also by marked **memory loss and confabulation.**

b. **Vitamin B_2 (riboflavin) deficiency** is rare in the United States because riboflavin is almost always added to commercially prepared bread and cereals.
(1) This condition occurs in chronic alcoholics, fad dieters, the elderly, and in persons with chronic debilitating diseases.
(2) It manifests clinically by **cheilosis** (skin fissures at the angles of the mouth), **glossitis, corneal vascularization,** and **seborrheic dermatitis** of the face, scrotum, or vulva.

c. **Vitamin B_3 (niacin) deficiency**
(1) This condition develops only when the diet lacks both niacin and tryptophan (niacin can be synthesized from the essential amino acid tryptophan). Niacin is a component of the nicotinamide adenine dinucleotides (NAD and NADP) and as such is essential to glycolysis, the citric acid cycle, and other metabolic processes.
(2) It is manifest clinically as **pellagra,** which is characterized by the "three Ds": **dementia, dermatitis,** and **diarrhea.** Dermatitis affects exposed areas, such as the face and neck and the dorsa of the hands and feet.

d. **Vitamin B_6 (pyridoxine) deficiency** may cause convulsions in infants, due to decreased activity of pyridoxal-dependent glutamate decarboxylase, which leads to deficient production of γ-aminobutyric acid (GABA), a neurotransmitter. It results in clinical manifestations similar to those of vitamin B_2 (riboflavin) deficiency. Although pyroxidine deficiency is uncommon, it occurs in the following conditions:
(1) Chronic alcoholism
(2) Association with therapeutic drugs, such as isonicotinic acid hydrazide (INH, an antituberculous agent), which react as competitive inhibitors for pyridoxine binding sites
(3) A variety of syndromes characterized by an increased need for pyridoxine, including:
(a) **Homocystinuria,** an inborn error of metabolism
(b) **Pyridoxine-responsive anemia,** a microcytic anemia characterized by reduced heme synthesis

e. **Vitamin B_{12} (cobalamin) deficiency** results in a marked reduction in DNA replication and cell division.
(1) This condition is manifest clinically by **megaloblastic anemia** with **prominent neurologic dysfunction.**
(2) The cause is almost always malabsorption but may occur in rare cases on a dietary basis in strict vegetarians. Cobalamin deficiency is not found in other settings of malnutrition such as alcoholism.
(a) The most common malabsorption disease is **pernicious anemia,** in which there is a lack of gastric intrinsic factor, a carrier protein essential to vitamin B_{12} absorption in the terminal small bowel.
(b) Less commonly, malabsorption can result from a number of diverse causes, including Crohn disease (which often affects the terminal ileum), blind loop syndrome, and *Diphyllobothrium latum* (giant fish tapeworm) infestation.

f. **Folic acid deficiency**
   (1) This condition is most commonly of dietary origin and often occurs in alcoholics and fad dieters. It can be secondary to intestinal malabsorption or it can occur, without gross dietary deprivation, as a relative deficiency because of increased demand for folate (e.g., in pregnancy and in hemolytic anemia, which is due to shortening of the life span of the red blood cell). Sometimes it is secondary to cancer chemotherapy containing folic acid antagonists.
   (2) The result is **megaloblastic anemia.**
   (3) Folic acid deficiency **does not cause neurologic changes** (in contrast to vitamin B_{12} deficiency).

g. **Vitamin C (ascorbic acid) deficiency**
   (1) Characteristics include **defective formation of mesenchymal tissue and osteoid matrix** due to **impaired synthesis of hydroxyproline and hydroxylysine,** for which vitamin C is a cofactor. **Defective collagen fibrillogenesis** contributes to **impaired wound healing.** Defective connective tissue also leads to fragile capillaries, resulting in **abnormal bleeding.**
   (2) Ascorbic acid deficiency results in **scurvy,** which is characterized by muscle, joint, and bone pain; swollen, bleeding gums; subperiosteal hemorrhage; and perifollicular petechial hemorrhages. **Bone changes** in scurvy are secondary to **defective osteoid matrix formation.**

B. **Fat-soluble vitamins (vitamins A, D, E,** and **K;** Table 8-2)
   1. **General considerations**
      a. Deficiency may result from malnutrition and intestinal **malabsorption syndromes, pancreatic exocrine insufficiency,** or **biliary obstruction,** all of which are associated with poor absorption of fats.

TABLE 8-2 *Fat-Soluble Vitamins*

	Metabolic Functions	Clinical Manifestations of Deficiency
Vitamin A	Precursor in rhodopsin synthesis; important in glycoprotein synthesis; regulator of epithelial differentiation	Night blindness; squamous metaplasia in many tissues, most importantly in eyes, where blindness may result
Vitamin D (calciferol)	Active form 1α, 25-dihydroxycholecalciferol (1,25-$(OH)_2D_3$, calcitriol) promotes intestinal calcium and phosphorus absorption and stimulates parathyroid hormone–mediated renal tubular reabsorption of calcium; thus maintains physiologic concentration of serum calcium; enhances calcification of bone	Rickets in children; osteomalacia in adults
Vitamin E (α-tocopherol)	Antioxidant; maintenance of cell membranes, probably by modulation of lipid peroxidation	Possible neurologic dysfunction
Vitamin K	Glutamyl carboxylation required for synthesis of γ-carboxyglutamyl residues of active serine proteases (e.g., clotting factors II, VII, IX, and X)	Hemorrhagic diatheses such as hemorrhagic disease of the newborn

b. Excess intake (i.e., **hypervitaminosis**), with resultant toxicity, may occur, especially with vitamins A and D.

2. **Vitamin A** is a term for a group of compounds (retinoids) with similar activities that are provided by animal products, such as liver, egg yolk, and butter. Also, a variety of vegetables (e.g., carrots and green leafy vegetables) supply β-carotene, a vitamin A precursor. Vitamin A is essential to the maintenance of mucus-secreting epithelium. A derivative, retinol, is a component of the visual pigment rhodopsin.
   a. **Vitamin A deficiency** can be caused by dietary deficiency or fat malabsorption. Clinical manifestations include:
      (1) **Night blindness,** due to insufficient retinal rhodopsin
      (2) **Squamous metaplasia** of the trachea, bronchi, renal pelvis (often associated with renal calculi), conjunctivae, and tear ducts. Ocular abnormalities can result in **xerophthalmia** (dry eyes) and **blindness** or in **keratomalacia** (corneal softening).
   b. **Hypervitaminosis A** is most often caused by excessive intake of vitamin A preparations. It is manifest by **alopecia, hepatocellular damage,** and **bone changes.**
3. **Vitamin D** is synthesized in the skin by ultraviolet light from the precursor 7-dehydrocholesterol; exposure to sunlight is required for this biosynthesis. Other sources include foods such as milk, butter, and eggs.
   a. Vitamin D promotes intestinal calcium absorption mediated by a specific calcium-binding intestinal transport protein as well as intestinal phosphorus absorption. In addition, vitamin D enhances bone calcification, apparently through its role in intestinal calcium absorption.
   b. **Vitamin D deficiency** manifests clinically as **rickets in children** and as **osteomalacia in adults,** both due to **deficient calcification of osteoid matrix.** It can be caused by the following factors:
      (1) **Malnutrition**
      (2) **Intestinal malabsorption**
      (3) **Inadequate exposure to sunlight**
      (4) **Liver disease,** with impaired hepatic conversion of vitamin D to the 25-hydroxyl form, a precursor of active vitamin D, 1α,25-dihydroxycholecalciferol (1,25-$(OH)_2D_3$, calcitriol)
      (5) **Renal disease,** with incomplete synthesis of active vitamin D
      (6) **Vitamin D-resistant rickets** due to hereditary renal 1α-hydroxylase deficiency which causes impaired synthesis of active vitamin D, impaired calcium absorption, and increased parathyroid hormone activity.
   c. **Hypervitaminosis D** is manifest in children by **growth retardation** and is manifest in adults by **hypercalciuria, nephrocalcinosis,** and **renal calculi.**
4. **Vitamin E deficiency** is rare but is thought to result in neurologic dysfunction.
5. **Vitamin K**
   a. This vitamin is essential for carboxylation of glutamyl residues in the synthesis of the γ-carboxyglutamyl forms (active forms) of **clotting factors II, VII, IX,** and **X,** and of **protein C.**
   b. It is provided by green and yellow vegetables and by dairy products.
   c. It is synthesized by intestinal microorganisms.
   d. **Vitamin K deficiency** results from fat malabsorption or alterations in the intestinal flora caused by antibiotics.
      (1) This condition is characterized by a **hemorrhagic diathesis** (abnormal bleeding) marked by prolongation of the prothrombin and activated partial thromboplastin times.
      (2) It is the cause of **hemorrhagic disease of the newborn,** which may result from a variety of causes, including deficient intake combined with inadequate intestinal bacterial colonization.
   e. There are no known clinical manifestations of excess vitamin K.

III. Obesity

A. Obesity is associated with increased risk of type 2 (non-insulin-dependent) diabetes mellitus, hypertension, gallstones, and osteoarthritis.

B. When central in distribution (fat deposits principally surrounding abdominal viscera and subcutaneous areas of the trunk), it may be associated with an increased incidence of coronary artery disease.

C. It may, as is suggested by animal studies, be partly related to secretion of leptin, an antiobesity hormone produced by adipocytes, and neuropeptide Y, a pro-obesity polypeptide secreted by the hypothalamus in response to leptin deficiency.

Q REVIEW TEST

Directions: *Each of the numbered items or incomplete statements in this section is followed by answers or by completions of the statement. Select the* ***one*** *lettered answer or completion that is best in each case.*

1. While working with an international group of physicians to administer polio vaccine, a medical student sees several children with abdominal distention and pale streaks in the hair and skin. Cursory physical examination reveals significant hepatomegaly. The children likely suffer from

(A) anorexia
(B) beriberi
(C) bulimia
(D) kwashiorkor
(E) marasmus

2. A 57-year-old man is admitted to the hospital for treatment of chronic pancreatitis. In patients with chronic pancreatitis, deficiency of which of the following vitamins is most likely?

(A) Folic acid
(B) Vitamin B_2 (riboflavin)
(C) Vitamin B_6 (pyridoxine)
(D) Vitamin B_{12} (cobalamin)
(E) Vitamin D

3. A 54-year-old Native American living on a reservation in southwest Arizona presents to a clinic with impaired memory, diarrhea, and a rash on the face, neck, and dorsum of the hands. It is likely that this patient has a deficiency of which of the following nutrients?

(A) Ascorbic acid
(B) Folic acid
(C) Homocysteine
(D) Niacin
(E) α-Tocopherol (vitamin E)

4. A 52-year-old recent Asian immigrant is brought to the emergency department after experiencing several convulsions. Further history reveals that she has been diagnosed with tuberculosis and has recently been started on a multidrug regimen that includes isoniazid. Which of the following is the likely cause of her convulsions?

(A) Vitamin B_1 (thiamine) deficiency
(B) Vitamin B_2 (riboflavin) deficiency
(C) Vitamin B_3 (niacin) deficiency
(D) Vitamin B_6 (pyridoxine) deficiency
(E) Vitamin C (ascorbic acid) deficiency

5. A 64-year-old man undergoes a total gastric resection for adenocarcinoma of the stomach. He has done well for 4 years but now presents with profound anemia, fatigue, and vague neurologic complaints. Position and vibration sensation are markedly diminished, and hyperreflexia is pronounced. Laboratory studies, including examination of the bone marrow, reveal pancytopenia and other findings compatible with a megaloblastic anemia. He is likely suffering a deficiency of which essential vitamin?

(A) Folate
(B) Vitamin B_{12}
(C) Vitamin C
(D) Vitamin D
(E) Vitamin K

6. A 62-year-old woman with a long history of rheumatoid arthritis was recently placed on therapy with methotrexate (a folic acid antagonist). The physician should be on the alert for which of the following side effects of this newly added medication?

(A) Defective osteoid matrix production
(B) Hemorrhagic lesions of the mamillary bodies
(C) High-output heart failure
(D) Impaired wound healing
(E) Megaloblastic anemia

7. A woman from a rural Appalachian community who had recently given birth to a newborn boy at home with the aid of a midwife now brings to her infant to the hospital because of continued bleeding and oozing from the umbilical stump. It is likely that the bleeding problem is secondary to a deficiency of which of the following vitamins?

(A) Folic acid
(B) Vitamin A
(C) Vitamin D
(D) Vitamin E
(E) Vitamin K

8. A 4-year-old Eskimo child is brought to the pediatrician because of concern about progressive bowing of the legs and enlargement of the costochondral junctions (rachitic rosary). The underlying defect in this disorder is a defect in

(A) calcification of osteoid matrix
(B) fibrillin
(C) formation of osteoid matrix
(D) hydroxylation of proline residues in collagen
(E) type I collagen

9. An abused child is found living in the basement of his parents' home after they are arrested on drug charges. In addition to being severely malnourished, the child is found to have bleeding gums and easy bruisability, along with numerous poorly healing skin ulcerations. Assuming that these findings resulted from vitamin C deficiency, what is the likely mechanism of these findings?

(A) Defective DNA synthesis
(B) Defective production of γ-aminobutyric acid
(C) Impaired carboxylation of coagulation factors II, VII, IX, and X
(D) Impaired hydroxyproline and hydroxylysine production
(E) Impaired renal 1α-hydroxylase

10. An 18-year-old young man with known cystic fibrosis presents to the physician with his third episode of kidney stones in the past year. In addition, he has begun to complain of difficulty seeing at night. Such changes can be attributed to a deficiency of which vitamin?

(A) Pyridoxine
(B) Vitamin A
(C) Vitamin B_1
(D) Vitamin B_{12}
(E) Vitamin D

ANSWERS AND EXPLANATIONS

1-D. These children suffer from kwashiorkor, a form of protein-calorie malnutrition that is associated with a protein-poor diet. Kwashiorkor should be distinguished from the relative deficiency of all calories, known as marasmus. Anorexia and bulimia are psychiatric eating disorders that are significantly more prevalent in developed countries. Beriberi is due to deficiency of thiamine.

2-E. Deficiency of fat-soluble vitamins (vitamins A, D, E, and K) can occur in chronic pancreatitis due to loss of exocrine pancreas function. Vitamin B_{12} (cobalamin), folic acid, vitamin B_2 (riboflavin), and vitamin B_6 (pyridoxine) are all water-soluble vitamins. It should be noted that most patients with chronic pancreatitis also are alcoholics and that alcoholics often have multiple nutritional deficiencies, including lack of water-soluble vitamins.

3-D. The clinical scenario depicts the classic findings of pellagra, or niacin deficiency, with diarrhea, dementia, and dermatitis. Niacin is synthesized from the essential amino acid tryptophan, which is particularly deficient in corn-based diets. Vitamin C deficiency results in scurvy. Folic acid deficiency often manifests with anemia. Decreased levels of homocysteine, an amino acid, have been associated with cardiovascular disease. Vitamin E deficiency is rare and can result in neurologic abnormalities.

4-D. Isoniazid is a competitive inhibitor of pyridoxine (vitamin B_6), which is required for the synthesis of the inhibitory neurotransmitter γ-aminobutyric acid. Riboflavin deficiency is rare and can result in cheilosis, glossitis, and other epithelial changes. Niacin deficiency results in pellagra. Pyridoxine deficiency can be manifest by convulsions. Vitamin C deficiency results in defects in collagen synthesis. Thiamine deficiency results in neuropathy, cardiomyopathy, and mental status changes.

5-B. Both folate and vitamin B_{12} deficiency lead to megaloblastic anemia, secondary to impaired DNA replication. In marked contrast to folate deficiency, vitamin B_{12} deficiency causes neurologic dysfunction associated with damage to the lateral and dorsal spinal columns. The history of gastric resection is consistent with a deficiency of intrinsic factor, which is required for absorption of vitamin B_{12} in the terminal ileum.

6-E. Folate is required for DNA replication in rapidly dividing cells such as red blood cells, and a deficiency results in megaloblastic anemia. Hemorrhagic lesions of the mamillary bodies and high-output heart failure occur with thiamine deficiency. Impaired wound healing and defective osteoid matrix production result from vitamin C deficiency.

7-E. Deficiency of vitamin K results in abnormal bleeding, based on the requirement of the vitamin for γ-carboxylation of clotting factors II, VII, IX, and X. Because newborns have inadequate intestinal flora, the primary source of vitamin K, vitamin K deficiency is relatively common and is estimated to occur in approximately 3% of neonates. The resultant bleeding disorder is termed hemorrhagic disease of the newborn. Folic acid deficiency during early embryogenesis can result in neural tube defects. Vitamin A deficiency results in changes in vision and defects in epithelial cell function. Vitamin D deficiency in children results in rickets.

8-A. Vitamin D is required for calcification of osteoid matrix, and defective calcification leads to bowing of the legs and the abnormalities in the costochondral junctions known as the rachitic rosary. Mutations in genes involved in the synthesis of type I collagen lead to osteogenesis imperfecta, and defects in fibrillin lead to Marfan syndrome. Defects in hydroxylation of proline residues occur both in the Ehlers-Danlos syndrome and in vitamin C deficiency, leading to defects in the synthesis of osteoid matrix.

9-D. Because vitamin C is a required cofactor for the synthesis of hydroxyproline and hydroxylysine, which are both required for collagen synthesis, vitamin C deficiency can lead to impaired capillary formation, with consequent bleeding, as well as to impaired wound healing. Both vitamin B_{12} and folic acid are required for DNA synthesis. Pyridoxine is required for γ-aminobutyric acid synthesis. Vitamin K is required for carboxylation of clotting factors. Patients with vitamin D-resistant rickets have a deficiency of renal 1α-hydroxylase.

10-B. Patients with cystic fibrosis often have impaired exocrine pancreas function, resulting in a deficiency of fat-soluble vitamins. Of the fat-soluble vitamins, vitamin A deficiency results in night blindness, xerophthalmia, keratomalacia, and squamous metaplasia of the urinary tract, contributing to the formation of recurrent renal calculi.

CHAPTER 9

Vascular System

I. Arterial Disorders

A. **Arteriosclerosis.** This is a general term for three types of vascular disease, all characterized by rigidity (sclerosis), and often thickening, of blood vessels.

1. **Mönckeberg arteriosclerosis (medial calcific sclerosis)** involves the **media** of medium-sized muscular arteries, most typically the **radial and ulnar arteries,** and usually affects persons older than 50 years of age. It **does not obstruct arterial flow** because the intima is not involved.
   a. **Ring-like calcifications** in the media of the arteries are characteristic.
   b. Stiff, calcific **"pipestem" arteries** result.
   c. This form of arteriosclerosis may coexist with atherosclerosis but is distinct from and unrelated to it.
2. **Arteriolosclerosis** is characterized by hyaline thickening or proliferative changes of **small arteries and arterioles,** especially in the kidneys, and is usually associated with **hypertension** or **diabetes mellitus.** It occurs in two variants.
   a. **Hyaline arteriolosclerosis** is characterized by **hyaline thickening** of arteriolar walls. In the kidneys, this is called **benign nephrosclerosis** and is associated with hypertension.
   b. **Hyperplastic arteriolosclerosis** is marked by **concentric, laminated, "onion-skin" thickening of the arteriolar walls.** It may be accompanied by **necrotizing arteriolitis,** intramural deposition of fibrinoid material in arterioles with vascular necrosis and inflammation. In the kidneys, it is called **malignant nephrosclerosis** and is associated with malignant hypertension.
3. **Atherosclerosis** is the most frequent cause of significant morbidity caused by vascular disease. It is seen worldwide, but the highest incidence occurs in Finland, Great Britain, other northern European countries, the United States, and Canada. The incidence is more than 10-fold greater in Finland than in Japan.
   a. **Characteristics of atherosclerosis.** Fibrous plaques, or **atheromas,** occur within the intima of arteries, most frequently the proximal portions of the coronary arteries, the larger branches of the carotid arteries, the circle of Willis, the large vessels of the lower extremities, and the renal and mesenteric arteries.
      (1) The plaques have a **central core** of cholesterol and cholesterol esters; lipid-laden macrophages, or foam cells; calcium; and necrotic debris.
      (2) The core is covered by a subendothelial **fibrous cap,** which is made up of smooth muscle cells, foam cells, fibrin and other coagulation proteins, as well as extracellular matrix material, such as collagen, elastin, glycosaminoglycans, and proteoglycans.
      (3) The plaques may be complicated by:
         (a) **Ulceration, hemorrhage** into the plaque, or **calcification of the plaque**

(b) **Thrombus formation** at the site of the plaque, producing obstructive disease
(c) **Embolization** of an overlying thrombus or of plaque material itself

(4) The atheromas can develop from the **fatty streak,** a lesion that is characterized by focal accumulations in the intima of lipid-laden foam cells that may appear as early as the first year of life and that is present in the aorta of most older children.

b. **Consequences of atherosclerosis**

(1) The most significant consequence is **ischemic heart disease and myocardial infarction,** the most common cause of death in the United States.
(2) Other significant complications include **stroke** from cerebral ischemia and infarction, **ischemic bowel disease, peripheral vascular occlusive disease** with findings varying from claudication to ischemic necrosis and gangrene, and **renal arterial ischemia** with secondary hypertension.
(3) Weakening of the vessel wall may lead to **aneurysm** formation.

c. **Risk factors for atherosclerosis**

(1) Incidence increases with **age.**
(2) **Gender** plays a role. Atherosclerosis is **more common in men** in all age groups, although the incidence increases in **postmenopausal women.**
(3) Considerable evidence links **hypercholesterolemia** with atherosclerosis.

(a) Serum cholesterol may be of **dietary,** or exogenous, origin or of **biosynthetic, endogenous** origin. Cholesterol and dietary fats associate with apolipoprotein molecules and circulate as **lipoproteins.** Figure 9-1 briefly summarizes lipoprotein transport and metabolism.

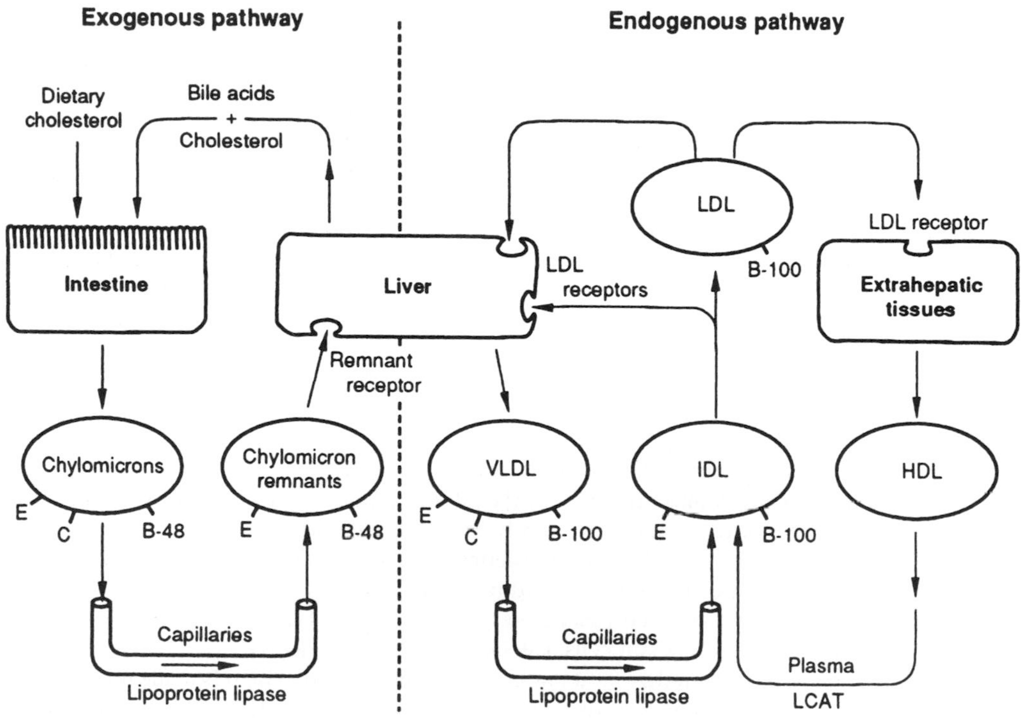

Figure 9-1 Lipoprotein transport and metabolism. HDL = high-density lipoprotein; LCAT = lecithin:cholesterol acetyltransferase; LDL = low-density lipoprotein; IDL = intermediate-density lipoprotein; VLDL = very low density lipoprotein. (Reprinted with permission from Goldstein J, Kita T, Brown M: Defective lipoprotein receptors and atherosclerosis. N Engl J Med 309:288, 1983.)

(b) Relative concentrations of lipoprotein fractions are used as **clinical predictors of atherogenesis;** ideally, the ratio between low-density lipoprotein (LDL) and high-density lipoprotein (HDL) cholesterol should be 4:1.

(c) Serum concentrations of **LDL,** also known as "bad" cholesterol, are directly related to the risk of atherosclerosis, as is the total cholesterol concentration.

(d) An inverse relationship exists between the HDL concentration and the risk of atherosclerosis. **HDL,** also known as "good" cholesterol, appears to exert its protective effect by **removing cholesterol** from tissues and from atherosclerotic plaques.

(4) **Hypertension** is a major risk factor for, and is associated with, premature atherosclerosis.

(5) **Diabetes mellitus** is associated with premature atherosclerosis. Atherosclerotic **peripheral vascular occlusive disease,** often leading to gangrene of the lower extremities, is common in diabetic patients.

(6) **Cigarette smoking** is also a well-established risk factor.

(7) Less firmly established are **obesity, physical inactivity, "type A" personality** with stress factors in life-style, **hyperuricemia,** hyperhomocysteinemia, methylene tetrahydrofolate reductase mutations, lipoprotein A, infection with *Chlamydia pneumoniae,* and use of **oral contraceptive drugs,** especially in association with cigarette smoking.

d. **Pathogenesis of atherosclerosis**

(1) **Older concepts**

(a) **Insudation hypothesis** proposed that the **infiltration of the intima with lipid and protein** is the primary atherogenic event, a process accelerated by hypercholesterolemia.

(b) **Encrustation or thrombogenic hypothesis** proposed that **organization of repeated mural thrombi on the intimal surface** leads to buildup of plaques filled with lipid derived from the breakdown of platelets and leukocytes.

(c) **Monoclonal hypothesis** proposed that **smooth muscle migration and proliferation** is analogous to tumor growth and is a primary rather than a secondary event. Smooth muscle proliferations within atheromas are often monoclonal—that is, like neoplasms, they are derived from single cell precursors. This hypothesis held that stimuli such as **hyperlipidemia may incite the proliferation.**

(2) **Current concept: reaction to injury formulation**

(a) Overall, this view considers the primary event as **injury to (or dysfunction of) arterial endothelium,** which may be produced by hypercholesterolemia, mechanical injury, hypertension, immune mechanisms, toxins, or viruses or other infectious agents. **Hyperlipidemia** may initiate endothelial injury, promote foam cell formation, act as a chemotactic factor for monocytes, inhibit macrophage motility, or injure smooth muscle cells.

(b) It leads to the following:

(i) **Entry of monocytes and lipid into subendothelium occurs, sometimes with platelet adhesion and aggregation** at the injury site.

(ii) **Mitogenic factors** (platelet-derived growth factor and possibly fibroblast growth factor, epidermal growth factor, and transforming growth factor-α) **are released** from platelets and perhaps also from monocytes.

(iii) These growth factors induce proliferation and migration of smooth muscle cells into the intima, with the production of connective tissue matrix proteins (collagen, elastin, glycosaminoglycans, and proteoglycans).

(iv) Monocytes and smooth muscle cells engulf lipid and contribute to the deposition of lipid into lesions. Monocyte conversion to **lipid-laden foam cells** is mediated by specific monocyte receptors, the β-VLDL receptor, and the scavenger receptor, which recognizes modified LDL.

B. **Aneurysms.** These localized **abnormal dilations** of either arteries or veins can erode adjacent structures or **rupture.** They may be of several different types.

1. **Atherosclerotic aneurysms** most frequently occur in the **descending, especially the abdominal, aorta.**
2. **Aneurysms due to cystic medial necrosis** are the most frequent aneurysms of the aortic root.
3. **Berry aneurysms** are small, saccular lesions most often seen in the smaller arteries of the brain, especially in the **circle of Willis.** They are unrelated to atherosclerosis.
   a. Berry aneurysms are not present at birth but develop at sites of congenital medial weakness at **bifurcations of cerebral arteries.** These aneurysms are the **most frequent cause of subarachnoid hemorrhage.**
   b. Often, there is an association with adult polycystic kidney disease.
4. **Syphilitic (luetic) aneurysm**
   a. This aneurysm is a manifestation of **tertiary syphilis,** which has become rare with better treatment and control of the disease. It is caused by **syphilitic aortitis,** which is characterized by obliterative endarteritis of the vasa vasorum and necrosis of the media. Grossly, these changes result in a "tree-bark" appearance.
   b. Unlike atherosclerotic aneurysms, syphilitic aneurysms characteristically involve the **ascending aorta.** Dilation of the ascending aorta may widen the aortic commissures, leading to **aortic valve insufficiency.**
5. **Dissecting aneurysm (dissecting hematoma)**
   a. This aneurysm is a **longitudinal intraluminal tear,** usually in the wall of the ascending aorta, forming a second arterial lumen within the media. It is typically associated with **hypertension** or with **cystic medial necrosis** (can be a component of Marfan syndrome), which is characterized by degenerative changes in the media with destruction of elastic and muscular tissue. It has no relation to atherosclerosis.
   b. Severe, tearing chest pain, often radiating through to the back, is clinically dominant. A radiograph may reveal widening of the aortic shadow.
   c. Dissecting aneurysms may be clinically confused with acute myocardial infarction, but the electrocardiogram, serum troponin I, and serum myocardial enzymes are normal.
   d. The characteristic result is **aortic rupture,** most often into the pericardial sac, causing hemopericardium and fatal cardiac tamponade.
6. **Arteriovenous fistula (aneurysm)**
   a. This aneurysm is an **abnormal communication between an artery and a vein.**
   b. It can be **secondary to trauma** or other pathologic processes that mechanically penetrate the walls of both vessels.
   c. Resulting changes may include **ischemic changes** from the diversion of blood, ballooning and **aneurysm formation** from increased venous pressure, and **high-output cardiac failure** from hypervolemia.

II. Venous Disorders

A. **Venous thrombosis (phlebothrombosis)**

1. Venous thrombosis arises most often in the **deep veins of the lower extremities.** It is often associated with inflammation and is then termed **thrombophlebitis.**
2. Predisposing factors include **venous circulatory stasis** or partially obstructed venous return such as occurs with cardiac failure, pregnancy, prolonged bed rest, or varicose veins.
3. **Embolism** with resultant pulmonary infarction may develop. Pulmonary infarcts are characteristically hemorrhagic, subpleural, and wedge-shaped.

B. **Varicose veins.** These abnormally **dilated and tortuous veins** occur most often in superficial veins of the lower extremities. Predisposing factors include **increased venous pressure** such as occurs with pregnancy, obesity, or thrombophlebitis, and in persons whose occupations require prolonged standing.

III. Tumors of Blood Vessels

A. **Benign vascular tumors.** These are usually not true neoplasms but are better characterized as malformations or hamartomas and include:

1. **Spider telangiectasia** is a dilated small vessel surrounded by radiating fine channels. It is associated with **hyperestrinism,** as seen in chronic liver disease or pregnancy.
2. **Hereditary hemorrhagic telangiectasia (Osler-Weber-Rendu syndrome)** is an autosomal dominant condition characterized by localized dilation and convolution of venules and capillaries of the skin and mucous membranes. It is often complicated by epistaxis or gastrointestinal bleeding.
3. **Hemangioma (angioma)** is a malformation of a larger vessel composed of masses of channels filled with blood. It is the most common tumor of infancy and is responsible for **port-wine stain birthmarks.** It includes the following types:
   a. **Capillary hemangioma** consists of a tangle of closely packed capillary-like channels that may occur in the skin, subcutaneous tissues, lips, liver, spleen, or kidneys.
   b. **Cavernous hemangioma** consists of large cavernous vascular spaces in the skin and mucosal surfaces and in internal organs such as the liver, pancreas, spleen, and brain. It can occur in **von Hippel-Lindau (VHL) disease,** an autosomal dominant disorder that is also marked by hemangioblastomas of the cerebellum, brain stem, and retina and is also characterized by adenomas and cysts of the liver, kidneys, pancreas, and other organs, and by an increased incidence of renal cell carcinoma.
4. **Glomangioma (glomus tumor)** is a small, purplish, painful subungual nodule in a finger or toe.
5. **Cystic hygroma** is a cavernous **lymphangioma** that occurs most often in the neck or axilla.

B. **Malignant vascular tumors.** These uncommon tumors include the following:

1. **Hemangioendothelioma** is intermediate in behavior between a benign and a malignant tumor.
2. **Hemangiopericytoma** arises from **pericytes** and varies in behavior from benign to malignant.
3. **Hemangiosarcoma (angiosarcoma)**
   a. This rare, malignant, vascular tumor occurs in the skin, musculoskeletal system, breast, or liver.
   b. It is associated with toxic exposures to **arsenic** or the **radioactive diagnostic agent thorium dioxide (Thorotrast). Polyvinyl chloride** is specifically associated with angiosarcoma of the liver.
4. **Kaposi sarcoma (KS)** is a malignant vascular tumor that occurs in several forms.
   a. Classic KS most often affects older men of Ashkenazi Jewish or Mediterranean origin.
   b. Endemic (or African) KS tends to affect young African men and children and accounts for as many as 10% of all cancers in Africa.
   c. Epidemic KS occurs as a component of **acquired immunodeficiency syndrome (AIDS),** especially in the homosexual male risk group and is caused by a virus that has been termed *KS herpesvirus*. KS is a feature of immunosuppression associated with causes other than AIDS.

IV. Vasculitis Syndromes (Vasculitides)

- These **inflammatory and often necrotizing vascular lesions** occur in almost any organ and are usually mediated by immune mechanisms, most often immune complex depositions. Frequent antigens in immune complexes include DNA, hepatitis B surface antigen, and hepatitis C RNA.

A. **Polyarteritis nodosa**

1. This condition is characterized by **necrotizing immune complex inflammation** of small- and medium-sized arteries. It is marked by destruction of arterial media and internal elastic lamella, resulting in **aneurysmal nodules.**
2. There is an association with **hepatitis B viral infection** in 30% of patients.
3. Clinical manifestations often include fever, weight loss, malaise, abdominal pain, headache, myalgia, and hypertension. Polyarteritis nodosa is seen in the following sites:
   a. Kidneys, with immune complex **vasculitis in the arterioles and glomeruli;** renal lesions and hypertension cause most deaths from polyarteritis nodosa.
   b. Coronary arteries, resulting in **ischemic heart disease**
   c. Musculoskeletal system, resulting in **myalgia, arthralgia,** or **arthritis**
   d. Gastrointestinal tract, manifesting as nausea, vomiting, or **abdominal pain**
   e. Central nervous system (CNS) or peripheral nervous system, the eye, or skin
4. Laboratory studies often show serum antibodies to neutrophilic myeloperoxidase. These antibodies are referred to as perinuclear antineutrophil cytoplasmic antibodies (**P-ANCAs**).

B. **Churg-Strauss syndrome (allergic granulomatous angiitis).** This is a necrotizing vasculitis considered by some to be a variant of polyarteritis nodosa. It is characterized by prominent involvement of the pulmonary vasculature, marked peripheral eosinophilia, and clinical manifestations of asthma.

C. **Hypersensitivity (leukocytoclastic) vasculitis**

1. This is a group of **immune complex-mediated vasculitides** characterized by acute inflammation of small blood vessels (arterioles, capillaries, venules); the multiple lesions tend to be of the same age. These are in contrast to the findings in polyarteritis nodosa.
2. It is manifest by **palpable purpura** when the skin is involved but can involve any site, including the glomeruli or the gastrointestinal tract.
3. It may be precipitated by **exogenous antigens** such as drugs, foods, or infectious organisms; may also occur as a **complication of systemic illnesses** such as connective tissue disorders or malignancies.
4. It presents clinically in distinctive syndromes, including:
   a. **Henoch-Schönlein purpura** is most common in young children.
      (1) Characteristics include **hemorrhagic urticaria** of extensor surfaces of the arms, legs, and buttocks, with fever, arthralgias, and gastrointestinal and renal involvement (often similar to IgA nephropathy; see Chapter 17).
      (2) This disorder can sometimes be poststreptococcal in origin. It is associated with antecedent **upper respiratory infections,** suggesting that infectious agents may be the inciting antigens; other antigens may include drugs or foods.
   b. **Serum sickness**
      (1) This syndrome is seen in the experimental model in which rabbits, after serial injections of bovine serum albumin, develop **generalized deposition of antigen-antibody complexes** in the heart, joints, and kidneys.
      (2) Serum sickness is now rare in humans, but in the past, it was caused by therapeutic administration of various antitoxins (foreign serum containing specialized antibodies prepared by immunization of animals such as horses).

D. **Wegener granulomatosis.** This disease of unknown etiology is characterized by **necrotizing granulomatous vasculitis** of the small- to medium-sized vessels of the **respiratory tract, kidneys,** and other organs.

1. Wegener granulomatosis is dominated clinically by **respiratory tract signs and symptoms,** especially of the **paranasal sinuses** and lungs, and **necrotizing glomeru-**

lonephritis (sometimes with immune complex deposition). Manifestations include **fibrinoid necrosis** of small arteries and veins, **early infiltration by neutrophils,** subsequent mononuclear cell infiltration, and fibrosis. **Granuloma formation** with giant cells is prominent.

2. In most cases, Wegener granulomatosis is associated with circulating antineutrophil cytoplasmic antibodies with a cytoplasmic staining pattern (**C-ANCAs**).

E. **Giant cell arteritides** are seen in medium- to large-sized arteries and are characterized by granuloma formation with giant cells as well as by infiltrates of mononuclear cells, neutrophils, and eosinophils. They include two distinct clinical syndromes:

1. **Temporal arteritis** is the most frequently occurring form of vasculitis.
   a. This **systemic vasculitis** occurs most often in **elderly persons.** It usually affects **branches of the carotid artery,** particularly the temporal artery.
   b. Clinical manifestations include:
      (1) Malaise and fatigue
      (2) **Headache** or claudication of the jaw
      (3) **Tenderness,** absent pulse, and **palpable nodules along the course of the involved artery**
      (4) **Visual impairment,** especially with involvement of the ophthalmic artery
      (5) **Polymyalgia rheumatica,** a complex of symptoms including proximal muscle pain, periarticular pain, and morning stiffness
      (6) Markedly elevated erythrocyte sedimentation rate
2. **Takayasu arteritis (pulseless disease)** is characterized by inflammation and stenosis of medium- and large-sized arteries with frequent involvement of the aortic arch and its branches, producing **aortic arch syndrome.** Clinical manifestations include:
   a. **Absent pulses** in carotid, radial, or ulnar arteries
   b. Nonspecific findings such as fever, night sweats, malaise, myalgia, arthritis and arthralgia, eye problems, and painful skin nodules

F. **Mucocutaneous lymph node syndrome (Kawasaki disease)** is an acute, self-limited illness of **infants and young children** characterized by **acute necrotizing vasculitis** of small- and medium-sized vessels.

1. This syndrome is manifest clinically by fever; hemorrhagic edema of conjunctivae, lips, and oral mucosa; and cervical lymphadenopathy.
2. It can be a cause of coronary artery vasculitis with aneurysm formation.

G. **Thromboangiitis obliterans (Buerger disease)** is an **acute inflammation** involving **small- to medium-sized arteries** of the extremities, extending to adjacent veins and nerves. It occurs with greater frequency in Jewish populations and is most common in **young men.**

1. This disease results in **painful ischemic disease,** often leading to gangrene.
2. It is clearly exacerbated by heavy **cigarette smoking.**

H. **Lymphomatoid granulomatosis** is a rare granulomatous vasculitis characterized by **infiltration by atypical lymphocytoid and plasmacytoid cells.** It may progress from a chronic inflammatory condition to a fully developed lymphoproliferative neoplasm, most often a **T-cell non-Hodgkin lymphoma.**

V. Functional Vascular Disorders

A. **Raynaud disease** is manifest by **recurrent vasospasm** of small arteries and arterioles, with resultant pallor or cyanosis, most often in the fingers and toes. This disease most commonly occurs in young, healthy women. It is most often precipitated by **chilling.**

B. **Raynaud phenomenon** is clinically similar to Raynaud disease but is always secondary to an underlying disorder, most characteristically systemic lupus erythematosus or progressive systemic sclerosis (scleroderma).

VI. Hypertension (Table 9-1)

A. **Essential hypertension** is hypertension of unknown etiology, accounting for the majority of cases. It represents an interaction of predisposing determinants with a number of exogenous factors.

1. **Determinants of essential hypertension**
   a. **Genetic factors**
      (1) **Family history** of hypertensive disease is seen in three of four patients with the disorder.
      (2) It is more common and usually more severe in persons of **African lineage.**
   b. **Environmental factors**
      (1) Evidence linking levels of **dietary sodium intake** with hypertension prevalence in population groups is impressive, although not everyone with excessive salt intake develops hypertension.
      (2) **Stress,** probably mediated by neurogenic vasoconstriction, is a factor in the development of hypertension.
      (3) Other factors include **obesity, cigarette smoking,** and **physical inactivity.**

TABLE 9-1 *Types of Hypertension*

Type or Cause	Comments
Primary (essential) hypertension	Unknown etiology; accounts for 90% –95% of cases
Secondary hypertension	
Renal parenchymal diseases, such as postinfectious glomerulonephritis, diabetic nephropathy, adult polycystic disease	Stimulation of renin–angiotensin system
Renovascular disease	Stimulation of renin–angiotensin system
Hyperparathyroidism	...
Cushing syndrome, of pituitary or adrenal origin	Excessive production of cortisol
Primary aldosteronism	Increased aldosterone secretion; sodium and water retention, often with hypokalemic alkalosis
Congenital adrenal hyperplasia	Occurs in several forms; hypervolemia mediated by increased production of mineralocorticoids in 17-hydroxylase deficiency and 11-hydroxylase deficiency
Pheochromocytoma	Secretion of epinephrine and norepinephrine, resulting in sustained or paroxysmal hypertension, which may be cured by resection of the tumor
Oral contraceptive use	Hypertension an infrequent effect
Coarctation of aorta	Upper extremity hypertension only, with increased collateral circulation in the intercostal arteries, resulting in notching of ribs
Toxemia of pregnancy	Hypertension usually ceases after delivery
Increased intracranial pressure	From brain tumors or other expanding intracranial lesions
Toxic hypertension	Poisoning by lead, cadmium, and other agents

2. **Results of essential hypertension**
   a. If untreated, essential hypertension can lead eventually to retinal changes, left ventricular hypertrophy and cardiac failure, and benign nephrosclerosis.
   b. It can predispose to **ischemic heart disease** or stroke.

B. **Secondary hypertension** is secondary to known causes, including:
1. **Renal disease** is by far the most common cause of secondary hypertension.
   a. **Causes of renal hypertension**
      (1) **Disorders of the renal parenchyma**
      (2) **Unilateral renal artery stenosis** can be caused by atherosclerosis or unilateral fibromuscular dysplasia. It is marked by atrophy of the affected kidney and may be corrected surgically.
   b. **Mechanism of renal hypertension** occurs through **stimulation of the renin-angiotensin system.**
      (1) Juxtaglomerular cells respond to decreased vascular tone by secreting **renin,** which facilitates the conversion of angiotensinogen to angiotensin I, which is further converted to angiotensin II.
      (2) **Angiotensin II** promotes hypertension by acting both as a vasoconstrictor and as an activator of aldosterone secretion.
      (3) **Aldosterone** promotes sodium and water retention.
2. **Endocrine disorders**
   a. **Primary aldosteronism, or Conn syndrome,** which is usually associated with an adrenocortical adenoma or bilateral adrenal hyperplasia. In addition to hypertension, it is marked by increased serum sodium and reduced serum potassium.
   b. **Acromegaly, Cushing syndrome** of pituitary or adrenocortical origin, **pheochromocytoma,** and **hyperthyroidism**
   c. **Diabetes mellitus** (when complicated by diabetic glomerulosclerosis; see Chapter 17)
3. **Other causes** include **coarctation of the aorta** (which causes hypertension limited to the upper body) and other congenital anomalies; **toxemia** of pregnancy; **CNS disorders,** especially brain tumors; and **drugs and chemicals,** notably amphetamines and steroids.

C. **Malignant hypertension** can be a complication of either essential (primary) or secondary hypertension. It follows an **accelerated** clinical course.
1. Malignant hypertension occurs in less than 5% of patients with elevated blood pressure, most often in **young African-American males.**
2. Characteristic features include a marked increase in diastolic blood pressure, focal retinal hemorrhages and **papilledema,** left ventricular hypertrophy, and left ventricular failure.
3. It most often results in **early death** from congestive heart failure, cerebrovascular accident, or renal failure.
4. It produces the renal changes of **malignant nephrosclerosis:** arterioles or glomerular capillaries rupture, resulting in "**flea-bitten**" **kidney,** multiple pinpoint petechial hemorrhages on the kidney surface; large, swollen kidneys; necrotizing arteriolitis and glomerulitis with fibrinoid necrosis; and hyperplastic arteriolosclerosis, affecting both the glomeruli and arterioles.

REVIEW TEST

***Directions:** Each of the numbered items or incomplete statements in this section is followed by answers or by completions of the statement. Select the **one** lettered answer or completion that is best in each case.*

1. A 45-year-old man presents with abdominal pain and hypertension. On physical examination, he is found to have an abdominal mass. Further workup confirms the diagnosis of adult polycystic kidney disease. Which of the following vascular complication is associated with this condition?

(A) Arteriovenous fistula
(B) Atherosclerotic aneurysm
(C) Berry aneurysm
(D) Dissecting aneurysm
(E) Luetic aneurysm

2. A 65-year-old man who has a long history of hypertension presents to the emergency department with tearing chest pain that radiates to the back. An electrocardiogram is normal, as are cardiac enzymes. A "stat" chest radiograph demonstrates widening of the mediastinum. Which of the following is the most likely?

(A) Arteriovenous fistula
(B) Atherosclerotic aneurysm
(C) Berry aneurysm
(D) Dissecting aneurysm
(E) Syphilitic aneurysm

3. The arterial lesion shown in the figure is observed at autopsy in a 56-year-old man who dies suddenly on rising in the morning. Which of the following abnormalities is considered a major risk factor for the development of this lesion?

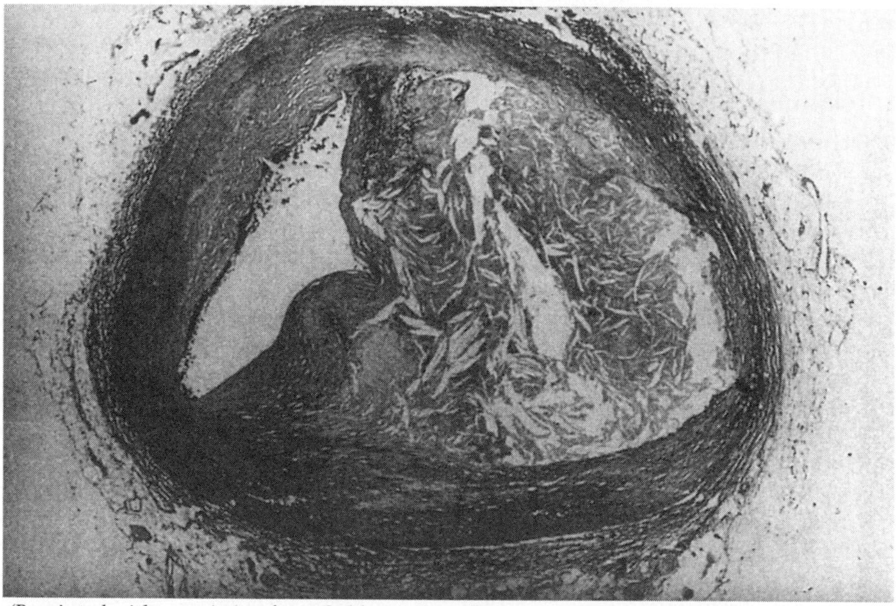

(Reprinted with permission from Golden A, Powell D, and Jennings C: *Pathology: Understanding Human Disease,* 2nd ed. Baltimore, Williams & Wilkins, 1985, p 189.)

(A) Congenital vascular muscle weakness
(B) Cystic medial necrosis
(C) Hypercholesterolemia
(D) Medial calcification
(E) Syphilis

4. A 14-year-old boy is brought by his family to your clinic in Utah with a long history of recurrent epistaxis. His father also reports such a history. Of the following, which is the most likely condition consistent with these findings?

(A) Cavernous hemangioma
(B) Glomangioma
(C) Hemangioendothelioma
(D) Osler-Weber-Rendu syndrome
(E) Varicose veins

5. A 23-year-old man known to have acquired immunodeficiency syndrome (AIDS) is seen by his primary care physician. The patient is concerned by the development of multiple red-to-purple skin plaques that have become nearly confluent on his arms and legs. The skin disorder is most likely

(A) angioedema
(B) angiosarcoma
(C) erythema multiforme
(D) Kaposi sarcoma
(E) multiple telangiectasias of Osler-Weber-Rendu syndrome

6. A 23-year-old man presents with fever, weight loss, malaise, abdominal pain, and myalgias. Workup reveals that the patient has polyarteritis nodosa. Which of the following is associated with this form of vasculitis?

(A) Arsenic
(B) Chlamydia pneumonia
(C) Hepatitis B virus
(D) Herpesvirus 8
(E) Human immunodeficiency virus

7. A 19-year-old young woman who emigrated from Taiwan 8 years ago presents with fever, malaise, myalgias, and arthritis and "coldness" in her upper extremities. She has a weak radial pulse bilaterally, and a magnetic resonance angiogram demonstrates nearly 75% stenosis of the main arteries originating from the aorta. She likely has which of the following rheumatologic conditions?

(A) Buerger disease
(B) Kawasaki disease
(C) Raynaud disease
(D) Takayasu arteritis
(E) Temporal arteritis

8. A 74-year-old woman presents to her primary care physician with malaise, proximal muscle pain, morning stiffness, and claudication of the jaw, along with occasional visual impairment. On examination, palpation along the lateral aspect of the head elicits tenderness. This is likely a result of

(A) giant cell arteritis
(B) hypersensitivity vasculitis
(C) Kawasaki disease
(D) Takayasu arteritis
(E) Wegener granulomatosis

9. A 3-year-old boy is brought by his parents to the emergency department because they are concerned that he has had a high fever for several days. On examination, the boy has conjunctival and oral erythema. He has palpable cervical lymphadenopathy and erythema of his palms and soles. What is a potential life-threatening complication of this disorder?

(A) Aneurysm of the abdominal aorta
(B) Aneurysm of the coronary arteries
(C) Dissection of the thoracic aorta
(D) Ischemia and gangrene of the extremities
(E) Rupture of a berry aneurysm

10. A 35-year-old African-American man is transported to the emergency department because of unrelenting, severe, excruciating headache. His blood pressure is 245/150 mm Hg, and bilateral papilledema is evident on ophthalmoscopic examination of the retina. Despite all interventions, including administration of nitroprusside, the patient dies. At autopsy, which of the following is a likely finding?

(A) Immune complex vasculitis of the glomeruli
(B) Longitudinal intraluminal tears of the ascending aorta
(C) Multiple punctuate hemorrhages on the surface of both kidneys ("flea-bitten kidneys")
(D) "Tree-bark" appearance of the ascending aorta
(E) Unilateral renal artery stenosis

11. A 32-year-old woman returns to her physician for follow-up of hypertension that has been poorly controlled in spite of numerous antihypertensive medications. It is decided to evaluate the patient for possible "secondary" hypertension. Which of the following is a well-known cause of secondary hypertension?

(A) Ethnicity
(B) Obesity
(C) Renal artery stenosis
(D) Smoking
(E) Stress

A ANSWERS AND EXPLANATIONS

1-C. Berry aneurysms, which occur in 10-15% of patients with adult polycystic kidney disease, are small saccular lesions that develop at the site of congenital weakness of cerebral arteries, especially those of the circle of Willis. Rupture of these aneurysms is the most common cause of subarachnoid hemorrhage. Arteriovenous fistulas are often secondary to trauma. Dissecting aneurysm is associated with hypertension or with diseases affecting the vascular media, most notably Marfan syndrome. Syphilitic (luetic) aneurysm is associated with tertiary syphilis.

2-D. The clinical presentation of a dissecting aortic aneurysm mimics that of a myocardial infarction. However, electrocardiographic changes and increased concentration of cardiac enzymes are notably absent. The mediastinum is often widened by radiographic examination. Although there is an association with hypertension and disorders of connective tissue (e.g., Marfan syndrome and Ehlers-Danlos syndrome), there is no association with atherosclerosis. The presentation exemplified by this scenario is a true surgical emergency!

3-C. The figure shows a large atheromatous plaque narrowing the lumen of an artery. The plaque consists of a mixture of fibrous tissue and cleft-like spaces indicating the presence of cholesterol crystals.The incidence of atherosclerosis is strongly associated with hypercholesterolemia. Renal disease is the most frequent cause of secondary hypertension. Endocrine disorders, such as pheochromocytoma, Conn syndrome, and acromegaly, represent the next most common cause. Coarctation of the aorta is a frequent cause of hypertension limited to the upper extremities.

4-D. The hemorrhagic phenomena in this patient likely represent recurrent rupture of the convolutions of venules and capillaries in the mucous membranes of the nose, as occurs in the Osler-Weber-Rendu syndrome (hereditary hemorrhagic telangiectasia). This disorder is inherited as an autosomal dominant condition and also affects the vessels of the gastrointestinal tract. Characteristic lesions can often be seen on the lips, conjunctivae, and mucous membranes of the nose or mouth. Cavernous hemangioma is a common lesion. On occasion, it can be seen as a component of the von Hippel Lindau syndrome. A glomangioma is a benign tumor of blood vessels on the fingers or toes. A hemangioendothelioma is a rare malignant tumor of blood vessels. Varicose veins are a manifestation of incompetency of the valves in the superficial veins of the legs of older patients.

5-D. Kaposi sarcoma is a malignant vascular tumor that occurs in men infected with the Kaposi sarcoma-associated herpesvirus (KSHV), often as a complication of AIDS. Angiosarcoma is a malignant tumor of blood vessels associated with thorium dioxide (Thorotrast); arsenic; or in the case of angiosarcoma of the liver, polyvinyl chloride. Polyarteritis nodosa is a vasculitis sometimes associated with hepatitis B infection. Serum sickness is due to deposition of antigen-antibody complexes.

6-C. Although the significance remains unclear, 30% of patients with polyarteritis nodosa have serum antibodies to hepatitis B virus. Arsenic is associated with the development of angiosarcoma. Chlamydia pneumonia has been implicated in the development of atherosclerosis. Kaposi sarcoma herpesvirus, herpesvirus 8, causes Kaposi sarcoma in individuals infected with human immunodeficiency virus.

7-D. Inflammation and stenosis of branches of the aortic arch is known as Takayasu arteritis, or "pulseless disease." It most commonly occurs in young Asian females. Buerger disease usually affects young Jewish males and involves the arteries of the extremities. The disease is exacerbated by smoking and can lead to gangrene of the extremities. Kawasaki disease affects the branches of the coronary arteries. Raynaud disease is due to vasospasm of small vessels of the fingers and toes, leading to cyanosis and pallor of the affected tissues. Temporal arteritis is usually encountered in older patients and affects the branches of the carotid artery, most commonly the temporal artery.

8-A. This is the typical presentation of temporal, or giant cell, arteritis. Along with involvement of the branches of the carotid artery, such as the temporal or ophthalmic arteries, there is a close association with a complex of symptoms of proximal muscles termed polymyalgia rheumatica. Hypersensitivity vasculitis manifests with palpable purpura and is associated with drugs, food, or infectious agents. Takayasu arteritis involves the vessels of the aortic arch, whereas Kawasaki disease involves the coronary arteries. Wegener granulomatosis involves vessels of the respiratory tract and kidney.

9-B. The patient presents with mucocutaneous lymph node syndrome, or Kawasaki disease. It is often a self-limiting condition, although as many as 20% of patients develop an aneurysm of the coronary vessels. Dissection of the thoracic aorta is associated with hypertension. Rupture of a berry aneurysm can result in a subarachnoid hemorrhage. Aneurysm of the abdominal aorta is associated with atherosclerosis. Ischemia and gangrene can be a result of Buerger disease.

10-C. This is a typical presentation for a patient with malignant hypertension. The kidneys appear "flea-bitten" because of multiple petechial hemorrhages on the surface. Microscopically, the glomeruli display fibrinoid necrosis and hyperplastic arteriolosclerosis. Immune complex vasculitis of the glomeruli is typical of polyarteritis nodosa. Longitudinal intraluminal tears of the ascending aorta occur with dissecting aneurysm. A "tree-bark" appearance of the ascending aorta results from tertiary syphilis. Unilateral renal artery stenosis can result from fibromuscular dysplasia.

11-C. The great majority of cases of hypertension are classified as essential hypertension. Essential hypertension results from the interactions of predisposing determinants and exogenous factors, including family history, ethnicity, stress, obesity, sodium intake, smoking, and physical activity. A small minority of cases of hypertension are due to secondary causes. Unilateral renal artery stenosis is a secondary cause that is typically correctable by surgery.

CHAPTER

10

The Heart

I. Ischemic Heart Disease (IHD)

A. **General considerations**

1. Causes include partial or complete interruption of arterial blood flow to the myocardium. In most cases, the cause is **atherosclerotic narrowing of the coronary arteries,** sometimes acutely aggravated by superimposed thrombosis or vasospasm.
2. The ischemia may be clinically silent or manifest as angina pectoris, myocardial infarction, or chronic IHD.
3. Frequency is increased in patients who manifest the **metabolic syndrome,** a group of risk factors including central obesity, atherogenic lipid patterns, hypertension, insulin resistance (sometimes overt diabetes), and evidence of a proinflammatory state such as elevated C-reactive protein. Obesity and physical inactivity, and probably genetic factors, predispose to the metabolic syndrome.

B. **Angina pectoris** is episodic chest pain caused by inadequate oxygenation of the myocardium.

1. **Stable angina** is the most common form of angina.
   a. It is **pain that is precipitated by exertion** and is relieved by rest or by vasodilators, such as nitroglycerin.
   b. It results from severe narrowing of atherosclerotic coronary vessels, which are thus unable to supply sufficient oxygenated blood to support the increased myocardial demands of exertion.
2. **Unstable angina** is **prolonged or recurrent pain at rest.**
   a. It is often indicative of imminent myocardial infarction.
   b. It is generally caused by disruption of an atherosclerotic plaque with superimposed thrombosis. It can also be caused by embolization or vasospasm.
3. **Prinzmetal angina** is **intermittent chest pain at rest.** It is generally considered to be caused by vasospasm.

C. **Myocardial infarction**

1. **General considerations**
   a. Myocardial infarction is the most important cause of morbidity from IHD and is one of the leading causes of death in the Western world.
   b. Myocardial coagulative necrosis caused by coronary artery occlusion is characteristic.
   c. Myocardial infarction is marked by a series of progressive changes involving gross and microscopic appearance of the heart (Table 10-1). It is also marked by release of myocardial enzymes and other proteins (Table 10-2) into the bloodstream, a process caused by altered membrane permeability of necrotic myocardial cells.
   d. The cells involved in the evolution of a myocardial infarct include neutrophils, macrophages, and fibroblasts. (Lymphocytes and plasma cells are not involved.)

Table 10-1 *Progressive Morphologic Changes in Acute Myocardial Infarction*

Stage	Gross Changes	Microscopic Changes	Clinical Correlations
0–6 hours	None	No morphologic changes at first; vascular congestion at perimeter of lesion after the first few hours	Arrhythmia most common cause of death in early hours
After 12 hours	None	First appearance of neutrophils in viable tissue adjacent to the lesion	
12–24 hours	Slight swelling and change of color	Cytoplasm displays increasing affinity for acidophilic dyes, and striations are lost; nuclei disappear; neutrophils infiltrate the lesion	
By 24 hours	Pale or reddish brown infarct with surrounding hyperemia	Well-developed changes of coagulative necrosis; progressive infiltration by neutrophils	
By third day	Increasingly yellow color of infarct	Replacement of neutrophils by macrophages; phagocytosis of debris begins	
From 7 days	Yellow infarcted area surrounded by congested red border	Beginning of growth of young fibroblasts and newly formed vessels into the lesion; replacement of neutrophils by macrophages and phagocytosis of debris continue	Risk for myocardial rupture greatest within first 4–7 days
From 10 days	Red, newly formed vascular connective tissue encircles and gradually replaces yellow necrotic tissue	Growth of fibrovascular tissue continues; replacement of neutrophils by macrophages and phagocytosis of debris are almost complete	
Between second and fourth week		Progressive synthesis of collagen and other intracellular matrix proteins	
From fifth week	Increasing pallor of infarct because of progressive fibrosis	Progressive fibrosis	
Within 3–6 months	Well-developed gray-white scar	Mature fibrous tissue replaces area of infarction	Ventricular aneurysm may occur in scarred area

TABLE 10-2 ***Progressive Changes of Serum Enzymes and Other Proteins in Acute Myocardial Infarction***

	CK-MB	Troponin I	LDH
6 hours	Weakly positive	Weakly positive	
12–16 hours	Strongly positive	Strongly positive	
24 hours	Peaks	Peaks	
2 days	Persists	Persists	
3 days	Negative	Persists	Peaks
4–7 days		Persists	Persists

CK-MB = creatine kinase - MB fraction; LDH = lactate dehydrogenase.
Note: Troponin I and CK-MB elevations are highly characteristic of myocardial infarction. Total LDH and total CK are nonspecific indicators that are passing into disuse in the diagnosis of myocardial infarction.

e. There are two distinct patterns of myocardial ischemic necrosis.
   (1) **Transmural infarction** traverses the entire ventricular wall from the endocardium to the epicardium.
   (2) **Subendocardial infarction** is limited to the interior one third of the wall of the left ventricle.

2. **Complications**
   a. **Arrhythmia** is the most common cause of death in the first several hours following infarction.
   b. **Myocardial (pump) failure** can lead to congestive heart failure and/or shock. The likelihood and severity are determined by the size and location of the lesion.
   c. **Myocardial rupture** is a catastrophic complication that usually occurs within the first 4–7 days and may result in death from **cardiac tamponade,** compression of the heart by hemorrhage into the pericardial space.
   d. **Ruptured papillary muscle**
   e. **Mural thrombosis** is thrombus formation on the endocardium overlying the infarct; may lead to left-sided embolism.
   f. **Ventricular aneurysm**

II. Rheumatic Fever

A. **Definition.** Rheumatic fever is a multisystem inflammatory disorder **with major cardiac manifestations and sequelae, most often affecting children between 5 and 15 years of age.**
   1. It is also characterized by transient mild migratory polyarthritis.
   2. It usually occurs 1–4 weeks after an episode of tonsillitis or other infection caused by **group A β-hemolytic streptococci.** An elevated titer of antistreptolysin O (ASO) is evidence of a recent streptococcal infection.

B. **Etiology**
   1. Rheumatic fever is apparently of **immunologic origin** rather than a result of direct bacterial involvement; however, the precise nature of the immune mechanisms of injury remains unclear. It is postulated to occur as a result of **streptococcal antigens** that elicit an antibody response reactive to streptococcal organisms as well as to human antigens in the heart and other tissues.
   2. The incidence has been remarkably reduced in the Western world in recent years.

C. **Aschoff body**
1. This is the classic lesion of rheumatic fever.
2. This is an area of **focal interstitial myocardial inflammation** that is characterized by fragmented collagen and fibrinoid material, by large cells (Anitschkow myocytes), and by occasional multinucleated giant cells (Aschoff cells).

D. **Other anatomic changes**
- Characteristics include **pancarditis,** inflammation of the pericardium, myocardium, and endocardium.
1. **Pericarditis** may result in pericardial, pleural, or other serous effusions.
2. **Myocarditis** may lead to cardiac failure and is the cause of most deaths occurring during the early stages of acute rheumatic fever.
3. **Endocarditis** leads to valvular damage.
   a. **Rheumatic endocarditis** usually occurs in areas subject to greatest hemodynamic stress, such as the points of valve closure and the posterior wall of the left atrium, resulting in the formation of the so-called MacCallum plaque. The mitral and aortic valves, which are subjected to much greater pressure and turbulence, are more likely to be affected than are the tricuspid and pulmonary valves.
   b. In the early stage, the valve leaflets are red and swollen, and tiny, warty, bead-like, rubbery vegetations (verrucae) form along the lines of closure of the valve leaflet. The small, firm verrucae of acute rheumatic fever are nonfriable and are not a source of peripheral emboli.
   c. As a consequence of fibrotic healing, the valves become thickened, fibrotic, and deformed, often with fusion of valve cusps as well as thickening of the chordae tendineae. Calcification is often prominent. These late sequelae, which often occur many years after the episode of rheumatic fever, are grouped under the term **rheumatic heart disease.**
      (1) The **mitral valve** is the valve that is most frequently involved in rheumatic heart disease.
         (a) It is the only valve affected in almost 50% of cases.
         (b) It can be affected by stenosis with fish-mouth buttonhole deformity, insufficiency, or a combination of both.
         (c) Mitral stenosis is marked by diastolic pressure higher in the left atrium than in the left ventricle.
      (2) The **aortic valve** is affected most often along with the mitral valve. It can be affected by stenosis or insufficiency.
      (3) The **tricuspid valve** is affected along with the mitral valve and aortic valves (trivalvular involvement) in approximately 5% of cases of rheumatic heart disease.
      (4) The **pulmonary valve** is rarely involved.

E. **Noncardiac manifestations of acute rheumatic fever**
1. **Fever, malaise, and increased erythrocyte sedimentation rate**
2. **Joint involvement**
   a. **Arthralgia**—joint pain without clinically evident inflammation
   b. **Arthritis**—overt joint inflammation presenting as painful, red, swollen, hot joints, usually involving larger joints, especially the knees, ankles, wrists, and elbows
   c. **Migratory polyarthritis**—sequential involvement of multiple joints
3. **Skin lesions,** including **subcutaneous nodules,** small painless swellings usually over bony prominences, and **erythema marginatum,** a distinctive skin rash characteristic of rheumatic fever, often involving the trunk and extremities
4. **Central nervous system involvement,** including **Sydenham chorea,** characterized by involuntary, purposeless muscular movements, and bizarre grimaces, as well as emotional lability

III. Other Forms of Endocarditis

A. **Infective endocarditis. This bacterial, or sometimes fungal, infection of the endocardium,** is marked by prominent involvement of the valvular surfaces.

1. **General considerations**
   a. Characteristics include large, soft, friable, easily detached **vegetations** consisting of fibrin and intermeshed inflammatory cells and bacteria.
   b. Complications may include **ulceration,** often with perforation, of the valve cusps or **rupture** of one of the chordae tendineae.
2. **Classification**
   a. **Acute endocarditis** is caused by pathogens such as *Staphylococcus aureus* (50% of cases). This type of endocarditis is often secondary to infection occurring elsewhere in the body.
   b. **Subacute (bacterial) endocarditis** is caused by less virulent organisms such as *Streptococcus viridans* (more than 50% of cases). This type of endocarditis tends to occur in patients with congenital heart disease or preexisting valvular heart disease, often of rheumatic origin.
3. **Clinical features**
   a. **Valvular involvement**
      (1) The **mitral valve** is most frequently involved.
      (2) The **mitral valve along with the aortic valve** is involved in about 40% of cases.
      (3) The **tricuspid valve** is involved in more than 50% of cases of endocarditis of intravenous drug users, in whom endocarditis is most often caused by staphylococcal infection.
   b. **Complications**
      (1) **Distal embolization** occurs when vegetations fragment.
      (2) Embolization can occur almost anywhere in the body and can result in **septic infarcts** in the brain or in other organs.
      (3) The **renal glomeruli** may be the site of focal glomerulonephritis (focal necrotizing glomerulitis) caused by immune complex disease or by septic emboli.

B. **Nonbacterial thrombotic endocarditis (marantic endocarditis)**

1. This form of endocarditis is associated with debilitating disorders, such as metastatic cancer and other wasting conditions.
2. Characteristics include small, sterile fibrin deposits randomly arranged along the line of closure of the valve leaflets.
3. The disease can result in **peripheral embolization** but, unlike infective endocarditis, the **emboli are sterile.**

C. **Libman-Sacks endocarditis** occurs in **systemic lupus erythematosus (SLE). It** is characterized by **small vegetations on either or both surfaces of the valve leaflets.**

D. **Endocarditis of the carcinoid syndrome**

1. The cause is **secretory products of carcinoid tumors** (vasoactive peptides and amines, especially serotonin [5-hydroxytryptamine]).
2. The valves on the left side of the heart are rarely involved, because serotonin and other carcinoid secretory products are detoxified in the lung.
3. This form of endocarditis results in thickened **endocardial plaques** characteristically involving the mural endocardium or the valvular cusps of the right side of the heart.

IV. Valvular Heart Disease

A. **General considerations**

1. Valvular heart disease occurs often as a late result of **rheumatic fever.** It may be secondary to various other inflammatory processes.

2. This disease may be congenital.
3. In addition, valvular heart disease can occur even with prosthetic cardiac valves, which are subject to physical deterioration or can be the site of thrombus formation or infectious endocarditis. They can also cause mechanical disruption of red blood cells, resulting in hemolytic anemia with schistocyte formation.

B. **Mitral valve**

1. **Prolapse** is the **most frequent valvular lesion,** occurring in approximately 7% of the population, most often in young women.
   a. Characteristics include myxoid degeneration of the ground substance of the valve (it can be a component of Marfan syndrome).
   b. Results include stretching of the posterior mitral valve leaflet, producing a "floppy" cusp (parachute deformity) with prolapse into the atrium during systole. These changes produce a characteristic **systolic murmur with a midsystolic click.**
   c. The lesion is usually benign and asymptomatic but can result in **mitral insufficiency.** It is often associated with a variety of **arrhythmias** and predisposes to **infective endocarditis.**
2. **Stenosis** is almost always due to rheumatic heart disease.
3. **Insufficiency** is usually a result of rheumatic heart disease. It can also result from **mitral valve prolapse, infective endocarditis,** or **damage to a papillary muscle from myocardial infarction.** It can be secondary to left ventricular dilation, with stretching of the mitral valve ring.

C. **Aortic valve.** This valve, along with the mitral valve, is frequently involved in rheumatic heart disease and in infective endocarditis.

1. **Stenosis** often presents as **calcific aortic stenosis** caused by calcification of:
   a. An otherwise normal aortic valve as an age-related degenerative change. This condition, called **degenerative calcific aortic stenosis,** is the most common cause of calcific aortic stenosis in persons older than 60 years of age. This designation is used when the stenotic valve has three cusps.
   b. **A congenital bicuspid aortic valve**
   c. **A valve affected by rheumatic heart disease.** In this case, scarring may be evidenced by fusion of the valve commissures.
2. **Insufficiency** can be caused by:
   a. **Nondissecting aortic aneurysm** resulting from cystic medial necrosis
   b. **Rheumatic heart disease,** usually in association with mitral valve disease
   c. **Syphilitic (luetic) aortitis** (now rare) with dilation of the aortic valve ring

D. **Tricuspid valve.** This valve is rarely involved alone in rheumatic heart disease but may be involved together with the mitral and aortic valves. This trivalvular involvement accounts for approximately 5% of cases of rheumatic heart disease. The tricuspid valve may be involved in the **carcinoid syndrome.**

E. **Pulmonary valve.** This valve is most commonly affected by **congenital malformations,** occurring either alone or along with other congenital defects, such as in the tetralogy of Fallot. It is rarely involved in rheumatic heart disease, although it may be involved in the carcinoid syndrome.

V. Congenital Heart Disease (Table 10-3)

A. **Causes and associations**

1. The etiology is usually undetermined.
2. Chromosomal abnormalities, such as Down syndrome, some of the other trisomies, and Turner syndrome are often complicated by congenital heart disease.

TABLE 10-3 ***Frequently Occurring Forms of Congenital Heart Disease***

Disorder	Anatomic Changes	Comments
Atrial septal defects	Patent foramen ovale, usually clinically insignificant Septum primum, affects lower part of septum; if large, may be associated with deformities of atrioventricular valves Septum secundum, defect in the fossa ovalis Sinus venosus, affects the upper part of the septum near the entrance of the superior vena cava	Clinical manifestations often delayed until adult life; pulmonary hypertension and reversal of flow with resultant cyanosis are late complications; can lead to paradoxic embolism
	Lutembacher syndrome, atrial septal defect with mitral stenosis	Mitral stenosis is often of rheumatic origin
Ventricular septal defects	Vary greatly in size	Small defects may close spontaneously; larger defects may lead to pulmonary hypertension and eventual right-sided heart failure; reversal of flow and late cyanosis also occur
Tetralogy of Fallot	Pulmonary infundibular or valvular stenosis; ventricular septal defect; overriding aorta; right ventricular hypertrophy	Cyanosis from birth; tendency of patients to assume a squatting position, presumably because of lessening of right-to-left shunting
Patent ductus arteriosus	Failure of closure of the fetal ductus arteriosus	Patency maintained during fetal life by combined effects of low oxygen tension and prostaglandin synthesis; can be closed surgically or pharmacologically treated with indomethacin; if not closed, leads eventually to pulmonary hypertension, right ventricular hypertrophy, reversal of blood flow, and late cyanosis
Coarctation of aorta	Narrowing of the aorta, usually distal to the origin of the subclavian arteries; extensive development of collateral circulation with dilation of intercostal arteries	Hypertension limited to the upper extremities and cerebral vessels; notching of the ribs seen on x-ray
Transposition of the great vessels	Aorta arises from the right ventricle, and the pulmonary artery arises from the left ventricle	Compensatory anomaly such as patent ductus arteriosus necessary for survival

a. The association of Turner syndrome with coarctation of the aorta is notable.

b. Endocardial cushion defects, which result in atrial and ventricular septal defects and atrioventricular valve deformities, are frequent associations of Down syndrome (trisomy 21).

3. There is an apparent increase in the incidence of **patent ductus arteriosus** in patients living at high altitudes, suggesting an association with fetal oxygen deprivation.
4. **Rubella (German measles) infection** is a prominent cause of congenital heart disease.

a. There is strong evidence of a link between maternal rubella during the first trimester of pregnancy and a constellation of fetal defects, known as the **congenital rubella syndrome,** which includes cardiovascular defects, microcephaly with mental retardation, deafness, cataracts, and growth retardation.

b. **Cardiac malformations** are especially frequent and commonly include **patent ductus arteriosus,** aortic stenosis, ventricular septal defect, and pulmonary infundibular or valvular stenosis, sometimes occurring as part of the tetralogy of Fallot.

c. Before or during pregnancy, it is often important to determine the mother's immune status to rubella. Demonstration of antirubella **antibodies** of the **IgM class indicates recent primary infection,** whereas demonstration of **IgG antibodies** indicates either recent primary infection, past infection, or reinfection.

5. **Genetic predisposition.** Tetralogy of Fallot can cluster in families, probably because of multifactorial inheritance.

B. **Functional abnormalities of congenital heart disease.** These can be classified according to the presence or absence of **cyanosis.**

1. **Noncyanotic diseases** include those with no shunt (e.g., aortic stenosis, coarctation of the aorta) and those with a left-to-right shunt (e.g., patent ductus arteriosus, atrial or ventricular septal defect). In atrial septal defects, both pressure and oxygen saturation may be equalized between the two atria.
2. **Cyanotic diseases** include transposition of the great vessels (survival depends on the presence of a shunt between the left and right ventricles), malformations with a right-to-left shunt (e.g., the tetralogy of Fallot), and disorders in which a left-to-right shunt reverses to right-to-left because of increased pulmonary arterial pressure (e.g., late cyanosis, tardive cyanosis).

VI. Diseases of the Myocardium

A. **Cardiomyopathy**

1. This term refers to diseases of the heart muscle that are noninflammatory and are not associated with hypertension, congenital heart disease, valvular disease, or coronary artery disease.
2. Usually, these diseases are characterized by otherwise unexplained **ventricular dysfunction** (heart failure unresponsive to digitalis, ventricular enlargement, ventricular arrhythmias). It occurs in several forms:

a. **Congestive or dilated cardiomyopathy** is the **most common form** of cardiomyopathy.

(1) Characteristics include four-chamber hypertrophy and dilation and both right- and left-sided intractable heart failure.

(2) Etiology is most often unknown. In some cases, the cardiomyopathy is related to **alcoholism** (alcohol cardiomyopathy), **thiamine deficiency** (beriberi heart), or prior myocarditis.

b. **Restrictive cardiomyopathy**

(1) The cause is infiltrative processes within the myocardium that result in stiffening of the heart muscle, which interferes with pumping action.

(2) This cardiomyopathy is exemplified by **cardiac amyloidosis,** which may result in both right- and left-sided heart failure.

c. **Hypertrophic cardiomyopathy** is often inherited as an **autosomal dominant characteristic.**

(1) Gross characteristics include **hypertrophy of all chamber walls, especially the ventricular septum** (asymmetric septal hypertrophy).

(2) Microscopic characteristics include **disoriented, tangled, and hypertrophied myocardial fibers.**

(3) The cardiomyopathy may result in **left ventricular outflow obstruction,** placing the patient in danger of syncope and even sudden death, which often occurs unexpectedly in young athletes.

B. Myocarditis

1. This myocardial disease most often presents as biventricular heart failure in young persons who do not have valvular, rheumatic, or congenital heart disease.
2. Morphologic characteristics include diffuse myocardial degeneration and necrosis with an inflammatory infiltrate.
3. Myocarditis is most often viral, and coxsackievirus is frequently the cause.
4. In parts of South America, myocarditis may be a component of Chagas disease, which is caused by the protozoan *Trypanosoma cruzi.*

VII. Diseases of the Pericardium

A. Noninflammatory conditions

1. **Hydropericardium** is an accumulation of **serous transudate in the pericardial space.** It may result from any condition causing systemic edema. It is most often caused by congestive heart failure or by edematous conditions due to hypoproteinemia, such as the nephrotic syndrome or chronic liver disease.
2. **Hemopericardium** is an **accumulation of blood in the pericardial sac.** It is usually caused by traumatic perforation of the heart or aorta or by myocardial rupture associated with acute myocardial infarction.

B. Acute pericarditis

1. **Serous pericarditis** is associated with **systemic lupus erythematosus, rheumatic fever,** and a variety of **viral infections.** It is characterized by production of a clear, straw-colored, **protein-rich exudate** containing small numbers of inflammatory cells.
2. **Fibrinous or serofibrinous pericarditis** is characterized by a **fibrin-rich exudate.** It may be caused by **uremia, myocardial infarction, or acute rheumatic fever.**
3. **Purulent or suppurative pericarditis** is characterized by a grossly cloudy or frankly purulent **inflammatory exudate.** It is almost always caused by **bacterial infection.**
4. **Hemorrhagic pericarditis** is characterized by a **bloody inflammatory exudate.** It usually results from **tumor invasion of the pericardium** but can also result from **tuberculosis or other bacterial infection.**

C. Chronic (constrictive) pericarditis. This disease is usually of **tuberculous or pyogenic staphylococcal etiology.**

1. Characteristics include **thickening and scarring of the pericardium** with resultant loss of elasticity. This prevents the pericardium from stretching and thus interferes with cardiac action and venous return, **often mimicking the signs and symptoms of right-sided heart failure.**
2. **Proliferation of fibrous tissue** with occasional small foci of calcification is marked.

VIII. Tumors of the Heart

A. Primary tumors

1. **Myxoma of the left atrium** is the most frequently occurring cardiac tumor and is found most often in adults.
2. **Rhabdomyoma** is most common in infants and young children and is notable for its association with tuberous sclerosis.

B. Metastatic tumors are more frequent than primary tumors.

IX. Congestive Heart Failure

A. **General considerations**

1. Congestive heart failure may be failure of the left ventricle, right ventricle, or both.
2. This condition often presents with dyspnea and/or edema. Assay of B-type natriuretic peptide, which is elevated in heart failure, can aid in the distinction of heart failure from a number of other conditions such as asthma, acute coronary syndrome, chronic obstructive pulmonary disease, or pulmonary embolism, which can also present with dyspnea or edema.

B. **Left-sided heart failure**

1. **Causes**
   a. **Ischemic heart disease,** especially myocardial infarction
   b. **Hypertension**
   c. **Aortic and mitral valvular disease**
   d. **Myocardial diseases,** such as cardiomyopathies and myocarditis
2. **Clinical manifestations**
   a. **Dyspnea and orthopnea** caused by pulmonary congestion and edema regularly occurs.
   b. **Pleural effusion with hydrothorax** often results.
   c. **Reduction in renal perfusion,** causing activation of the renin-angiotensin-aldosterone system and leading to retention of salt and water, is less frequent.
   d. **Cerebral anoxia** is less frequent.

C. **Right-sided heart failure**

1. **Causes**
   a. **Left-sided heart failure** is the most common cause of right-sided heart failure.
   b. **Left-sided lesions** such as mitral stenosis
   c. **Pulmonary hypertension** often caused by chronic lung disease (cor pulmonale)
   d. **Various types of cardiomyopathy and diffuse myocarditis**
   e. **Tricuspid or pulmonary valvular disease**
2. **Clinical manifestations**
   a. **Renal hypoxia,** leading to greater **fluid retention and peripheral edema** than seen in left-sided failure. Edema occurs first in dependent areas and often manifests early as so-called pitting edema of the ankles. Other manifestations of fluid retention include pleural effusion and sometimes ascites. Hydrothorax can be a manifestation of either left-sided or right-sided heart failure.
   b. **Enlarged and congested liver and spleen.** Chronic passive congestion of the centrilobular veins of the liver surrounded by relatively pale, sometimes fatty, peripheral regions leads to a "nutmeg" pattern.
   c. **Distention of the neck veins**

X. Hypertrophy of the Heart

A. **Hypertrophy of the left ventricle** is most commonly caused by **hypertension and aortic or mitral valvular disease.**

B. **Hypertrophy of the right ventricle**

1. **Causes**
   a. **Left ventricular failure**
   b. **Chronic lung disease**
   c. **Mitral valve disease**
   d. **Congenital heart disease** with left-to-right shunt

2. **Cor pulmonale**
   a. Cor pulmonale is defined as right ventricular hypertrophy and/or dilation secondary to lung disease or primary disease of the pulmonary vasculature, such as primary pulmonary hypertension. Emphysema is a frequent cause.
   b. Characteristics include pulmonary arterial hypertension, the common characteristic among the entities that lead to cor pulmonale.

REVIEW TEST

Directions: *Each of the numbered items or incomplete statements in this section is followed by answers or by completions of the statement. Select the one lettered answer or completion that is best in each case.*

1. A 55-year-old woman presents with complaints of chest pain. She states that the chest pain predictably occurs when she climbs four flights of stairs to reach her apartment or when she has been jogging for more than 10 minutes. She is particularly concerned because her mother died of a myocardial infarction at 50 years of age. Which of the following best describes this patient's state?

(A) Arrhythmia
(B) Myocardial infarction
(C) Prinzmetal angina
(D) Stable angina pectoris
(E) Unstable angina pectoris

2. Yesterday, a 60-year-old man presented to the emergency department with dyspnea, diaphoresis, and crushing substernal chest pain that radiated to his neck and left arm. When asked to describe the pain, he put his fist to the center of his chest and stated that it felt "as if someone is squeezing my heart." An electrocardiogram demonstrated changes consistent with myocardial infarction, and serum troponin I levels were elevated. If the patient unexpectedly dies today, which of the following would almost certainly be found on histologic examination of the affected myocardium?

(A) Coagulative necrosis with neutrophil infiltration
(B) Fibrotic tissue replacing infarcted tissue
(C) No histologic changes
(D) Slight swelling of tissue and change of color
(E) Young fibroblasts and new vessels growing into the infarcted tissue

3. A 60-year-old-man is discharged after being observed in the hospital for 4 days following a myocardial infarction. He returns to his normal activities, which include sedentary work only. This point of time following a myocardial infarct is noteworthy for the special danger of which of the following?

(A) Arrhythmia
(B) Mural thrombosis
(C) Myocardial (pump) failure
(D) Myocardial rupture
(E) Ventricular aneurysm

4. A 10-year-old boy presents with migratory polyarthritis involving several large joints, fever, and malaise. Physical examination reveals a new heart murmur and friction rub on auscultation, and a painless nodule is detected on the extensor surface of the elbow. He had a severe sore throat approximately 2 weeks ago, apparently recovering without antibiotic therapy. The anti-streptolysin O (ASO) titer is elevated. Which of the following describes the most likely outcome for this patient?

(A) Development of mitral valve stenosis over many months to years
(B) Development of mitral valve stenosis over the next few months
(D) Increasing severity of the current symptoms and findings over the next few decades
(D) Persistence of the current symptoms and signs over the patient's lifetime
(E) Total recovery after 1–2 months with no further complications or sequelae

5. A 9-year-old girl is diagnosed with acute rheumatic fever. Instead of recovering as expected, her condition worsens, and she dies. Which of the following is the most likely cause of death?

(A) Central nervous system involvement
(B) Endocarditis
(C) Myocarditis
(D) Pericarditis
(E) Streptococcal sepsis

6. A 70-year-old woman has a long history of metastatic colon cancer, and she donates her body for use in medical school anatomy courses. At death, the body is emaciated and cachectic, and gross dissection reveals small fibrin deposits arranged around the line of closure of the leaflets of the mitral valve. The valvular lesions most likely represent

(A) bacterial endocarditis
(B) endocarditis of the carcinoid syndrome
(C) Libman-Sacks endocarditis
(D) nonbacterial thrombotic (marantic) endocarditis
(E) rheumatic endocarditis

7. The myocardial lesions shown in the figure were observed at autopsy examination of a pediatric patient who died after a short illness. During life, which of the following manifestations of his illness was most likely?

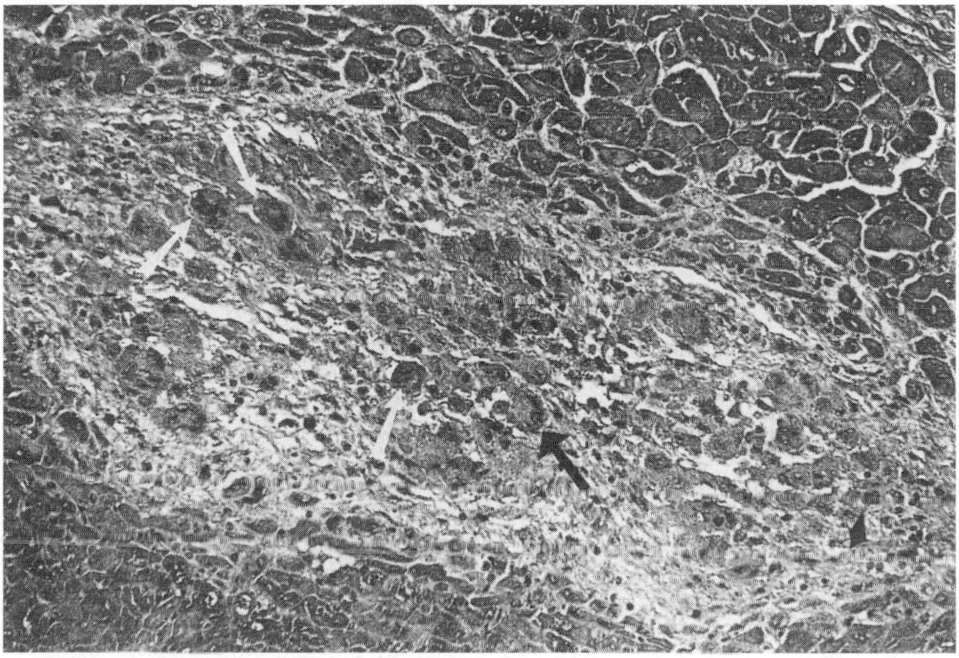

(Reprinted with permission from Golden A, Powell D, and Jennings C: *Pathology: Understanding Human Disease,* 2nd ed. Baltimore, Williams & Wilkins, 1985, p 171.)

(A) Chorea
(B) Systemic embolization
(C) Systemic lupus erythematosus
(D) Unstable angina
(E) Wasting diseases

8. A 60-year-old man presents with angina. He has no past medical history of heart disease. On questioning, the patient reveals that he had repeated sexually transmitted diseases in the past, including a painless chancre (a hard, round sore) on his penis, for which he never sought medical attention. Rapid plasma reagin (RPR), Venereal Disease Research Laboratory (VDRL) slide test, and fluorescent treponemal antibody (FTA) serologic tests (indicative of syphilis infection) are positive. Echocardiography and computed tomography of the heart are performed. The history of untreated syphilis suggests that these tests will most likely detect which of the following abnormalities?

(A) Aortic valvular insufficiency and linear calcification along the ascending aorta
(B) Bicuspid aortic valve with aortic stenosis
(C) Large valvular vegetations from bacterial endocarditis
(D) Right-sided heart failure from the carcinoid syndrome
(E) Small fibrin deposits on the mitral valve from nonbacterial thrombotic (marantic) endocarditis

9. A 50-year-old man presents with sudden weakness in his left leg. He has felt well lately and has no past medical history of coronary artery disease, hyperlipidemia, or hypertension, and no family history of myocardial infarction or stroke. Physical examination reveals motor weakness in the left leg, with no other neurologic deficits, and no cardiac murmur. Magnetic resonance imaging of the brain demonstrates a small ischemic infarct in the arterial distribution of the brain correlating with motor control of the left leg. Angiography and echocardiography reveal normal coronary arteries, normal valves with no vegetations, and a small right-to-left shunt. Which of the following is most likely associated with this scenario?

(A) Atrial septal defect
(B) Bacterial endocarditis
(C) Nonbacterial thrombotic (marantic) endocarditis
(D) Tetralogy of Fallot
(E) Ventricular septal defect

10. A 3-year-old boy presents with cyanosis and shortness of breath that develops when he plays with friends. According to his mother, the boy was born cyanotic. The boy is very small and short for his age, and he squats on the floor next to his mother. Chest radiography reveals a boot-shaped heart, normal heart size, and a right aortic arch. Echocardiography reveals a large ventricular septal defect with an overriding aorta, pulmonary stenosis, and right ventricular hypertrophy. Which of the following is the most likely diagnosis?

(A) Coarctation of the aorta
(B) Patent ductus arteriosus
(C) Rheumatic heart disease
(D) Tetralogy of Fallot
(E) Transposition of the great vessels

11. A 53-year-old woman presents with dyspnea on exertion, orthopnea, paroxysmal nocturnal dyspnea, edema in the legs and feet, and fatigue. She has no history of angina, other signs of coronary artery disease, hypertension, or valvular disease. Echocardiography reveals cardiomegaly, with four-chamber hypertrophy and dilation. Which of the following is the most likely diagnosis?

(A) Congestive or dilated cardiomyopathy
(B) Hypertrophic cardiomyopathy
(C) Myocarditis
(D) Restrictive cardiomyopathy

12. A 56-year-old woman presents with dyspnea on exertion, orthopnea, paroxysmal nocturnal dyspnea, and pulmonary edema. She also presents with severe dizziness and syncope, fatigue, weight loss, and arthralgias. After undergoing several tests, she is diagnosed with a primary heart tumor that is causing a "ball-valve obstruction" of her mitral valve. Which of the following is the most likely tumor?

(A) Fibroma
(B) Leiomyoma
(C) Lipoma
(D) Myxoma
(E) Rhabdomyoma

13. A 64-year-old woman presents with dependent peripheral edema in her ankles and feet. She has long-standing chronic obstructive lung disease and a long history of cigarette smoking. Further investigation reveals that she has cor pulmonale with right-sided heart failure. Which of the following is the most likely cause of the right-sided heart failure in this patient?

(A) Constrictive pericarditis
(B) Disease of the lungs or pulmonary vessels
(C) Left-sided heart failure
(D) Pulmonary infundibular or valvular stenosis
(E) Systemic hypertension

14. A 42-year-old man is seen because of a long history of slowly developing congestive heart failure. His blood pressure is normal. Coronary artery angiography reveals no vascular disease. No heart murmurs are heard. The white blood cell count, differential, and erythrocyte sedimentation rate are normal. The most likely diagnosis is

(A) carcinoid heart disease
(B) cardiomyopathy
(C) coarctation of the aorta
(D) constrictive pericarditis
(E) myocardial infarction

ANSWERS AND EXPLANATIONS

1-D. This is a classic case of stable angina, which is chest pain that is precipitated by exertion but relieved by rest. Stable angina is due to atherosclerosis of the coronary arteries. This patient has risk factors for ischemic heart disease, or IHD (e.g., cigarette smoking, hypertension, hyperlipidemia, diabetes, family history of IHD/coronary artery disease). Prinzmetal angina is intermittent chest pain at rest, and unstable angina is prolonged chest pain at rest.

2-A. By 24 hours, well-developed microscopic changes of coagulative necrosis can be detected in infarcted tissue. There is loss of nuclei in cells and infiltration of neutrophils into tissue.

3-D. Rupture of the left ventricle, a catastrophic complication of acute myocardial infarction, usually occurs when the necrotic area has the least tensile strength, about 4–7 days after an infarction, when repair is just beginning. The anterior wall of the heart is the most frequent site of rupture, usually leading to fatal cardiac tamponade. Internal rupture of the interventricular septum or of a papillary muscle may also occur. The risk of arrhythmia is greatest within the first 6 hours after myocardial infarct. Arrhythmias are the most important early complication of acute myocardial infarction, accounting for almost 50% of deaths shortly after myocardial infarction. Myocardial, or pump, failure and mural thrombosis are other complications that may develop as a result of permanent damage to the heart after infarct. Ventricular aneurysms may develop in the fibrotic scar within 3–6 months after myocardial infarct.

4-E. This is a case of acute rheumatic fever. Acute rheumatic fever manifests most commonly in patients 5–15 years of age with migratory polyarthritis, pancarditis, subcutaneous nodules, erythema marginatum, and Sydenham chorea. Decades later, severe valvular disease, often manifest as mitral stenosis, may develop as a feature of rheumatic heart disease. In this chronic stage of rheumatic disease, fibrotic valves may become stenotic, insufficient, or both, but much more commonly, progression to cardiac valve complication does not occur.

5-C. The most common cause of death that occurs during acute rheumatic fever is cardiac failure secondary to myocarditis.

6-D. Nonbacterial thrombotic endocarditis, or marantic endocarditis, has been associated with a variety of wasting diseases and is observed most often in patients with cancer.

7-A. The figure illustrates an Aschoff body, the characteristic lesion of rheumatic fever. This myocardial lesion is most often oval in shape and characterized by swollen, fragmented collagen and fibrinoid material and by characteristic large mesenchymal cells (Anitschkow myocytes) and multinucleated cells (Aschoff cells). Sydenham chorea is a major manifestation of rheumatic fever.

8-A. This is a case of syphilitic (luetic) aortitis. In syphilitic aortitis, the elastica of the aorta undergoes calcification and is replaced by fibrous tissue, resulting in dilation of the ascending aorta and separation of the aortic valve commissures, with resultant aortic insufficiency. Thus, echocardiography and computed tomography of the heart reveal calcification in a linear pattern along the ascending aorta, calcification in the coronary arteries (leading to anginal symptoms), and aortic valvular insufficiency.

9-A. This is a case of paradoxical embolism, which denotes the passage of an embolus of venous origin into the arterial circulation, by way of a right-to-left shunt (e.g., atrial septal defect or patent foramen ovale). Ordinarily, atrial septal defects result in a left-to-right shunt across the atrial septum, but over time may develop into a right-to-left shunt. The likelihood of right-to-left passage of an embolus is often enhanced by pulmonary hypertension, sometimes secondary to pulmonary thromboembolism.

10-D. In the tetralogy of Fallot, the characteristic lesions include ventricular septal defect, overriding aorta, pulmonary valve stenosis, and right ventricular hypertrophy. The pulmonary stenosis and overriding aorta cause increased right ventricular pressure and lead to right-to-left shunting. Cyanosis, which occurs when the arterial concentration of reduced hemoglobin exceeds 5 mg/mL, is seen with a right-to-left shunt, in which venous blood gains direct access to the arterial circulation. In contrast, patent ductus arteriosus, atrial septal defect, and ventricular septal defect are associated with left-to-right blood flow.

11-A. Congestive or dilated cardiomyopathy is the most common form of cardiomyopathy. It is characterized by four-chamber hypertrophy and dilation as well as right- and left-sided severe heart failure. In some cases, congestive (dilated) cardiomyopathy may be associated with alcoholism, thiamine deficiency, or prior myocarditis.

12-D. Myxoma of the heart, although rare, is the most common primary cardiac tumor. Because of the jelly-like appearance and myxoid histology similar to that of some organized thrombi, the neoplastic nature of this lesion was debated for many years. However, it is now generally believed that myxoma is a true neoplasm. The most common location of myxoma is in the left atrium. Due to its location, complications may develop due to physical obstruction of blood flow through the mitral valve, resulting in symptoms of congestive heart failure.

13-B. The term *cor pulmonale* refers to right ventricular hypertrophy caused by pulmonary hypertension secondary to disorders of the lungs or pulmonary vessels. Other causes of right ventricular hypertrophy and failure, such as valvular disease, congenital defects, and left-sided heart failure, are precluded by this definition. Therefore, although in general, the most common cause of right-sided heart failure is left-sided heart failure, cor pulmonale with right-sided heart failure is due to an intrinsic disease originating in the lungs. Constrictive pericarditis can clinically mimic right sided heart failure but is entirely unrelated to cor pulmonale.

14-B. Cardiomyopathies are noninflammatory myocardial disorders that are not associated with coronary artery obstruction, hypertension, valvular disease, congenital heart disease, or infectious disease. They are most often characterized by otherwise unexplained ventricular dysfunction, such as cardiac failure, ventricular enlargement, or ventricular arrhythmias.

CHAPTER 11

Anemia

I. General Concepts

A. **Definitions**

1. Anemia is a decrease in whole body red cell mass, a definition that precludes relative decreases in red blood cell count, hemoglobin, or hematocrit, which occur when the plasma volume is increased.
2. Anemia of pregnancy is not anemia but is rather a manifestation of increased plasma volume.
3. A practical working definition of anemia is a decrease in red blood cell count, hemoglobin, or hematocrit, commonly measured red cell parameters.

B. **Causes of anemia** (Table 11-1). Anemia may be caused by two major mechanisms:

1. **Decreased red cell production** resulting from:
   a. **Hematopoietic cell damage** from infection, drugs, radiation, and other similar agents
   b. **Deficiency of factors** necessary for heme synthesis (iron) or DNA synthesis (vitamin B_{12} or folate)
2. **Increased red cell loss** due to:
   a. **External blood loss**
   b. **Red cell destruction** (hemolytic anemia)

II. Acute Posthemorrhagic Anemia

A. Within the first few hours of acute blood loss, prior to hemodilution (compensatory increase in plasma volume), there may be no decrease in the hemoglobin, hematocrit, and red blood cell count because of a parallel loss of both red cells and plasma. There is often a marked reactive increase in platelet count.

B. Significant clinical findings are related to **hypovolemia.**

III. Iron Deficiency Anemia (see Table 11-1)

A. **Causes**

1. Chronic blood loss
   a. Such blood loss is the major cause of iron deficiency anemia in adults.

TABLE 11-1 *Examples of Anemia Resulting from Decreased Red Cell Production*

Type	Mechanisms	Diagnostic Features	Major Etiologic Factors
Iron deficiency anemia	Impaired heme synthesis	Hypochromia and microcytosis; decreased serum iron and increased total iron-binding capacity; decreased serum ferritin	Dietary deficiency in infants and preadolescents; excess menstrual bleeding; chronic blood loss from the gastrointestinal tract
Pernicious anemia	Autoimmune gastritis leading to lack of gastric intrinsic factor and failure of vitamin B_{12} absorption; vitamin B_{12} deficiency causes delayed DNA replication	Pancytopenia, oval macrocytes, and hypersegmented neutrophils; megaloblastic hyperplasia; achlorhydria; anti-intrinsic factor antibodies; hyperreflexia, absent position and vibration sensations; impaired vitamin B_{12} absorption corrected by intrinsic factor (abnormal Schilling test)	Autoimmunity
Folate deficiency	Delayed DNA replication	Pancytopenia, oval macrocytes, and hypersegmented neutrophils; megaloblastic hyperplasia	Dietary deficiency; malabsorption syndromes
Aplastic anemia	Greatly diminished hematopoiesis	Pancytopenia, reticulocytopenia, marked hypocellularity of bone marrow	Toxic drugs and chemicals; often idiopathic
Anemia of chronic disease	Diverse mechanisms	Anemia most often normochromic and normocytic or macrocytic; may be hypochromic and microcytic with decreased serum iron and decreased serum iron-binding capacity	Various chronic diseases, especially rheumatoid arthritis, renal disease, and chronic infection
Myelophthisic	Bone marrow replacement, usually by malignant tumor	Severe anemia; small numbers of nucleated red cells and immature granulocytes in the peripheral blood; tumor cells in the bone marrow	

b. Most often causes are **menorrhagia** or **bleeding gastrointestinal lesions,** such as carcinoma of the colon in the United States or hookworm disease in less developed countries.

2. **Dietary deficiency** is rare except in infants; because human milk is low in iron, newborn storage iron is depleted within the first 6 months unless it is replaced by dietary supplementation. Premature infants are at special risk. Dietary deficiency of iron may rarely occur in elderly persons.
3. **Increased iron requirement** may occur during **pregnancy;** iron demands of the fetus can deplete maternal iron stores. It may also occur in **infants and preadolescents** who may outgrow borderline iron stores.

B. **Clinical manifestations**

1. Signs and symptoms may include **pallor, fatigue,** or **dyspnea on exertion.** Sometimes angina pectoris may occur in persons with coronary artery narrowing caused by atherosclerotic disease.
2. When extreme, associated features may include glossitis; gastritis; koilonychia (spooning of the nails); or Plummer-Vinson syndrome, in which iron deficiency is associated with a partially obstructing upper esophageal web.

C. **Laboratory findings**

1. Decreased hemoglobin, hematocrit, and red blood cell count
2. Hypochromic microcytic erythrocytes on peripheral smear
3. Decreased serum iron and increased total iron-binding capacity (TIBC)
4. Decreased body iron stores, measured by bone marrow examination for stainable hemosiderin or by decreased serum ferritin

D. **Differential diagnosis**

1. Iron deficiency anemia must be distinguished from other causes of hypochromic microcytic anemia, such as the anemia of chronic disease and β-thalassemia minor.
2. In anemia of chronic disease, the serum iron is low (as in iron deficiency), but the TIBC is also low.
3. In β-thalassemia minor, the A_2 hemoglobin is increased.

IV. Megaloblastic Anemias

A. **General considerations**

1. Megaloblastic anemias are defined by large, abnormal-appearing **erythroid precursor cells** (megaloblasts) in the bone marrow.
2. These anemias are caused by **deficiency of vitamin B_{12} or folate.**
3. These anemias are characterized by decreased DNA synthesis, with a consequent delay in DNA replication and nuclear division, and by relatively unimpeded cytoplasmic maturation. Morphologically, they manifest as **nuclear-cytoplasmic asynchrony** of large erythroid precursor cells with an open, loose-appearing chromatin pattern.
4. Results include anemia caused by impaired red cell production; to a lesser degree, red cell destruction occurs within the bone marrow prior to release of mature erythrocytes into the peripheral blood **(ineffective erythropoiesis).**

B. **Laboratory abnormalities**

1. **Peripheral blood and bone marrow** findings are identical in all forms of megaloblastic anemias.
   a. **Peripheral blood**
      (1) **Pancytopenia** (decreased red cells, white cells, and platelets)
      (2) **Oval macrocytosis.** Mean corpuscular volume (MCV) is often greater than 110 fl (normal about 87 fl).
      (3) **Hypersegmented neutrophils** (more than five lobes)
   b. **Bone marrow: megaloblastic hyperplasia**
2. **Vitamin B_{12} and folate levels** further define the specific type of megaloblastic anemia.

C. **Types of megaloblastic anemia**

1. **Vitamin B_{12} deficiency**
   a. **Pernicious anemia**
      (1) Pernicious anemia is the most common form of vitamin B_{12} deficiency megaloblastic anemia. It is considered to be an **autoimmune disorder;** other autoimmune diseases (especially thyroid diseases) occur with increased frequency in persons with pernicious anemia.

(2) Causes include **autoimmune gastritis** (previously referred to as fundal or type A gastritis), which is associated with **failure of production of intrinsic factor,** essential for vitamin B_{12} absorption. The chronic gastritis is also associated with:
   (a) **Achlorhydria** (absent gastric free hydrochloric acid)
   (b) **Anti-intrinsic factor and antiparietal cell antibodies**
   (c) **Increased incidence of gastric carcinoma**

(3) **Clinical findings**
   (a) **Insidious onset** with extreme reduction of red blood cell count; in older persons may be preceded by a lengthy subclinical period in which clinical manifestations are minimal.
   (b) Characteristic **lemon-yellow skin color**
   (c) **Stomatitis and glossitis**
   (d) **Subacute combined degeneration of the spinal cord** (combined systems disease, posterolateral degeneration)
      (i) Morphologic characteristics include demyelination of the posterior and lateral columns.
      (ii) Clinical manifestations include ataxic gait, hyperreflexia with extensor plantar reflexes, and impaired position and vibration sensation. (Neurologic abnormalities are associated with vitamin B_{12} deficiency but not with folate deficiency.)

(4) **Laboratory findings**
   (a) **Pancytopenia, hypersegmented neutrophils, and megaloblastic hyperplasia** of the bone marrow (findings characteristic of all megaloblastic anemias)
   (b) **Anti-intrinsic factor antibodies,** which are rarely found in other conditions; antiparietal cell antibodies may be seen in other conditions but are most frequent in pernicious anemia.
   (c) **Abnormal Schilling test,** characterized by impaired absorption of vitamin B_{12} correctable by intrinsic factor
      (i) Impaired absorption not corrected by intrinsic factor is characteristic of intestinal malabsorption such as may occur in Crohn disease, blind-loop syndrome, and giant tapeworm infestation.
      (ii) Normal absorption is characteristic of vitamin B_{12} deficiency due to dietary deprivation, which may occur in absolute vegetarians.

b. **Other forms of vitamin B_{12} deficiency megaloblastic anemia.** These pernicious anemia–like illnesses can be caused by a number of other mechanisms that result in vitamin B_{12} deficiency.
   (1) **Total gastric resection;** because intrinsic factor is produced in the gastric fundus, the clinical picture is the same as in pernicious anemia.
   (2) **Disorders of the distal ileum;** intrinsic factor–vitamin B_{12} complex is absorbed in the distal ileum.
   (3) **Strict vegetarian diet;** vitamin B_{12} is found only in foods of animal origin.
   (4) **Intestinal malabsorption syndromes**
   (5) **Blind-loop syndrome;** bacterial overgrowth in a surgically induced intestinal blind loop results in depletion of vitamin B_{12}.
   (6) **Broad-spectrum antibiotic therapy;** can result in intestinal bacterial overgrowth with vitamin B_{12} depletion.
   (7) ***Diphyllobothrium latum*** infestation; the giant fish tapeworm of man, acquired by ingestion of freshwater fish, inhabits the intestine and causes vitamin B_{12} depletion.

2. **Folate deficiency**
   a. No neurologic abnormalities (in contrast to vitamin B_{12} deficiency) occur.
   b. Folate deficiency megaloblastic anemia can be caused by a number of diverse mechanisms:
      (1) **Severe dietary deprivation** (most often occurs in chronic alcoholics or fad dieters)

(2) **Pregnancy** (combination of additional demands of the fetus and borderline maternal diet)
(3) **Dilantin (phenytoin),** which interferes with the absorption of folate, or **oral contraceptive therapy**
(4) **Folic acid antagonist chemotherapy** for cancer
(5) **Relative folate deficiency** (increased demand because of compensatory accelerated erythropoiesis in hemolytic anemia)
(6) **Intestinal malabsorption** caused by:
(a) **Sprue**
(b) ***Giardia lamblia*** infection

V. Anemia of Chronic Disease.

This common form of anemia is second in incidence to iron deficiency anemia.

A. Anemia of chronic disease can be **secondary to a wide variety of primary disorders,** including rheumatoid arthritis, renal disease, or chronic infection.

B. It is often **normochromic and normocytic.** When associated with renal disease, it may be moderately macrocytic.

C. When associated with **chronic inflammatory states** (e.g., rheumatoid arthritis), it may be accompanied by **decreased serum iron** and hypochromia and microcytosis, mimicking iron deficiency anemia; however, in contrast to iron deficiency anemia, **TIBC is characteristically decreased.**

VI. Aplastic Anemia

A. **General considerations**

1. Characteristics include a markedly **hypocellular bone marrow** with almost total loss of hematopoietic cells, including erythroid and myeloid precursor cells and megakaryocytes, and **peripheral pancytopenia** (anemia, leukopenia, and thrombocytopenia) and reticulocytopenia.
2. Aplastic anemia is most often **secondary to toxic exposure;** it may also occur without evident cause. In addition, it can be caused by autoimmune dysfunction of **cytotoxic T cells,** and it can also be induced by **several other etiologic agents:**
   a. **Radiation** exposure
   b. **Chemicals,** such as **benzene** and related organic compounds
   c. **Therapeutic drugs,** such as **chloramphenicol,** sulfonamides, gold salts, chlorpromazine, various anti-inflammatory and antimalarial drugs, and **alkylating agents** used in the treatment of neoplastic diseases
   (1) In some persons who have been given chloramphenicol, there is a predictable, dose-related, usually reversible marrow response.
   (2) In other persons, there is an idiosyncratic, severe, frequently irreversible effect.
   d. **Viral infection,** such as **human parvovirus** or **hepatitis C virus**

VII. Myelophthisic Anemia.

This form of bone marrow failure is caused by replacement of the marrow, most often by a malignant neoplasm.

A. Less commonly it is due to bone marrow destruction from non-neoplastic causes such as marrow fibrosis.

B. It may be signaled by leukoerythroblastosis, in which small numbers of nucleated red cells and immature granulocytic precursors are seen in the peripheral blood smear.

VIII. Hemolytic Anemias (Table 11-2).

These anemias are due to shortening of red cell life span (increased red cell destruction).

A. **General considerations**

1. **Increased red cell destruction** with liberation of hemoglobin or its degradation products is manifested by:
   a. **Increased unconjugated (indirect reacting) bilirubin,** resulting in **acholuric jaundice,** which is jaundice not accompanied by bilirubinuria. Hyperbilirubinemia may lead to **pigment-containing gallstones** as a late complication.
   b. **Increased urine urobilinogen**
   c. **Hemoglobinemia and hemoglobinuria,** which, along with methemalbuminemia and hemosiderinuria, occur if red cell destruction is very rapid and within the circulation (intravascular hemolysis).
   d. **Disappearance of serum haptoglobins,** a group of hemoglobin-binding proteins, which combine with liberated hemoglobin and are no longer demonstrable. In instances of intravascular hemolysis, such as hemolytic transfusion reactions, elevation of serum hemoglobin does not occur until serum haptoglobins are no longer detectable.
   e. **Hemosiderosis,** systemic iron deposition
2. **Increased erythropoiesis,** compensating in part for the shortened red cell survival, is manifested by:
   a. **Normoblastic erythroid hyperplasia** in bone marrow
   b. **Reticulocytosis** (increased number of circulating newly formed red cells identified by residual stainable RNA). Because reticulocytes are larger than other red cells, the MCV may be modestly increased (up to about 105 fl).
   c. **Polychromatophilia** (increased number of somewhat larger red cells that stain with a bluish cast, roughly equivalent to increased reticulocyte count)

B. **Terminology**

1. **Intracorpuscular hemolytic anemia** is marked by defects, most often **genetically determined,** in the red cell itself.
2. **Extracorpuscular hemolytic anemia** is marked by defects, most often **acquired,** of the extraerythrocytic environment, such as circulating antibodies or an enlarged spleen.

C. **Immune hemolytic anemias** are clinically suggested by hemolytic anemia of recent onset.

1. **Warm antibody autoimmune hemolytic anemia** is the **most common form** of immune hemolytic anemia.
   a. This anemia is mediated by **IgG autoantibodies** that react with red cell surface antigens. These antibodies are optimally active at 37°C (thus their designation as "warm" antibodies). The anemia is often secondary to underlying disease states such as systemic lupus erythematosus, Hodgkin disease, or non-Hodgkin lymphomas.
   b. Clinical characteristics include the following:
      (1) **General features of hemolytic anemia**
      (2) **Spherocytosis** due to progressive loss of membrane protein by serial passage of antibody-coated red cells through the spleen
      (3) **Positive direct Coombs test** reflecting the binding of IgG autoantibody to the red cell surface
2. **Cold agglutinin disease** is mediated by **IgM antibodies** optimally active at temperatures below 30°C (cold antibodies, cold agglutinins).
   a. **Acute cold agglutinin disease** is often mediated by antibodies with specificity for the **I blood group antigen.** It is often a complication of infectious mononucleosis

or *Mycoplasma pneumoniae* infection. Diagnosis of mycoplasma pneumonia is facilitated by the demonstration of cold agglutinins.

3. **Chronic cold agglutinin disease** is often associated with **lymphoid neoplasms.** It is often mediated by **anti-i antibodies.** Characterized clinically by agglutination and hemolysis in tissue sites exposed to the cold, it may be associated with Raynaud phenomenon. These cases are marked by chronic hemolytic anemia exacerbated by cold weather, punctuated by episodes of jaundice, sometimes with hemoglobinemia and hemoglobinuria.
4. **Hemolytic disease of the newborn (erythroblastosis fetalis)** occurs when maternal antibodies cross the placenta and react with fetal red cells, resulting in **fetal hemolytic anemia.**
   a. Causes include **maternal alloimmunization** to fetal red cell antigens, classically the D antigen of the **Rh blood group system.** In the most frequently occurring form of Rh-mediated hemolytic disease of the newborn, the mother is typed as d and the fetus as D.
   b. Causes also include **ABO incompatibility.** In most instances of ABO incompatibility, the mother is blood group O and the child is blood group A or group B. Other incompatible combinations include: mother A, child B or AB; mother B, child A or AB.
   c. This disease can result in **kernicterus,** staining of the basal ganglia and other central nervous system structures by unconjugated bilirubin. Kernicterus with resultant neurologic damage is the most significant long-term consequence of hemolytic disease of the newborn. In addition, consequences include stillbirth or in **hydrops fetalis,** fetal heart failure with massive generalized edema.
   d. The incidence has been markedly reduced by preventive measures. Routine administration of anti-D IgG antiserum to D-negative mothers at the time of delivery (or at the time of termination of pregnancy) of a D-positive child results in the antibody-mediated removal of fetal red cells from the maternal circulation, preventing maternal alloimmunization.

D. **Paroxysmal nocturnal hemoglobinuria** is an uncommon acquired **intracorpuscular defect.**

1. Characteristics include increased sensitivity to complement-induced red cell lysis, resulting in intravascular hemolytic anemia, pancytopenia, and an increased incidence of venous thrombosis. The condition is often marked by the passage of hemoglobin-containing urine on awakening.
2. This defect arises from a somatic mutation in a gene known as *PIG*-A. The mutation causes impaired synthesis of the glycosylphosphatidylinositol (GPI) anchor that is required for the fixation of a number of diverse proteins to cellular surfaces. Among these proteins are CD55, CD59, and C8 binding proteins, which are required for the protection of red cells, granulocytes, and platelets from complement-mediated lysis.
3. Diagnosis now involves flow cytometry demonstrating a population of **CD59-negative erythrocytes**; the defect was formerly diagnosed by the now archaic Ham (acid serum) test, which demonstrated in vitro complement-induced hemolysis in acidified serum.

E. **Hemolytic anemias caused by membrane skeletal protein abnormalities**

1. **Hereditary spherocytosis** is an autosomal dominant hemolytic anemia. It is the most common intracorpuscular inherited hemolytic anemia observed in whites.
   a. This anemia is characterized by **spherocytes** (sphere-shaped erythrocytes) that are selectively trapped or sequestered in the spleen. **Splenomegaly** is often prominent.
   b. An increased **erythrocyte osmotic fragility** to hypotonic saline is characteristic.
   c. An **increase** in the mean corpuscular hemoglobin concentration (MCHC), an abnormality seldom observed in other forms of anemia, is also characteristic.
   d. The cause is a variety of molecular defects in the genes coding for spectrin, ankyrin, protein 4.1, and other erythrocyte membrane skeletal proteins. These defects are usually manifest as a deficiency of spectrin.

2. **Hereditary elliptocytosis (ovalocytosis)** is an autosomal dominant disorder characterized by elongated, oval red cells. It may be marked by hemolytic anemia and splenomegaly. It often does not cause anemia.

F. **Enzyme deficiency hemolytic anemias**

1. **Glucose-6-phosphate dehydrogenase (G6PD) deficiency** is the most common form of enzyme deficiency hemolytic anemia.
   a. This **X-linked** disorder occurs in approximately 10% of African Americans and also in persons of Mediterranean origin.
   b. G6PD deficiency is manifest by acute self-limited intravascular hemolytic anemia with hemoglobinemia and hemoglobinuria caused by oxidative stress induced by infection, by a wide variety of therapeutic drugs such as primaquine (an anti-malarial agent), sulfonamides, and many other oxidant drugs, or, in some persons of Mediterranean origin, by fava beans.
   c. G6PD deficiency may be suggested by the finding of "bite cells" (erythrocytes that appear as if a piece were munched out) on the peripheral blood smear.
2. **Pyruvate kinase deficiency** is the second most common enzyme deficiency hemolytic anemia.
   a. This autosomal recessive disorder is characterized by hereditary nonspherocytic hemolytic anemia.
   b. In contrast to the most common form of G6PD deficiency, in which the anemia is episodic and self-limited, the anemia is chronic and sustained.

G. **Hemoglobinopathies.** These are hemolytic anemias caused by genetically determined **abnormalities of hemoglobin structure.** In the United States, they are most importantly represented by disorders involving hemoglobin S; to a lesser extent, hemoglobin C; and in some urban centers, hemoglobin E.

1. **Hemoglobin S disorders**
   a. **General considerations**
      (1) Approximately 7% of African Americans carry the hemoglobin S gene. In some parts of Africa, more than one third of the population is affected; it is thought that the hemoglobin S gene confers resistance to falciparum malarial infection.
      (2) Similar resistance may be conferred by erythrocyte G6PD deficiency or by the absence of Duffy blood group antigens. Both G6PD deficiency and the Duffy Fy (a- b-) phenotype occur with high incidence in persons of African origin.
      (3) Hemoglobin S arises from a point mutation in codon 6 of the β-globin gene and results in a substitution of valine for glutamic acid. At the DNA level, the mutation abolishes a recognition site for the restriction endonuclease *Mst*II. This is the basis for prenatal diagnosis, which can be performed on amniotic cells or on chorionic villus samples.
      (4) Hemoglobin S polymerizes at low oxygen tension, forming tactoids that distort the shape of red cells to elongated, sickle shapes; repeated sickling episodes stiffen red cell membranes, making affected cells more subject to hemolysis; rigid, sickled cells are more likely to obstruct the microvasculature.
      (5) All hemoglobin S disorders are characterized by a positive sickle cell preparation (in vitro sickling of red cells on exposure to reducing agents such as sodium metabisulfite). The sickle cell preparation is positive whenever hemoglobin S is present (e.g., sickle cell anemia, sickle cell trait, sickle C disease, sickle cell thalassemia).
   b. **Sickle cell anemia.** The homozygous form of hemoglobin S leads to sickle cell anemia (sickle cell disease), which is characterized by:
      (1) **Severe hemolytic anemia**
      (2) **Chronic leg ulcers**
      (3) Vaso-occlusive **painful crises** (severe pain in the limbs, back, chest, and abdomen), often precipitated by infection or dehydration

(4) **Repeated infarctions in the lungs and spleen**; the spleen is characteristically congested and enlarged in childhood but becomes progressively smaller through repeated infarcts and fibrosis (**autosplenectomy**).

(5) **Aplastic crises** (distinguished from painful crises), characterized by a precipitous fall in hemoglobin concentration, usually provoked by viral infection such as human parvovirus

(6) **Infectious complications** such as *Salmonella* osteomyelitis

c. **Sickle cell trait.** Hemoglobin S in the heterozygous form leads to sickle cell trait, which is generally without clinical consequence.

2. **Hemoglobin C disorders** are primarily observed in persons of African lineage.
   a. When homozygous, they are characterized by mild hemolytic anemia accompanied by prominent splenomegaly, target cells, and, on occasion, intraerythrocytic crystals.
   b. When heterozygous, they result in disease only when coinherited with other abnormal hemoglobins, most often hemoglobin S.
3. **Hemoglobin E disorders** are prevalent in Southeast Asia.
   a. These disorders have increased significantly in incidence in the United States in recent years and are now more common than hemoglobin S disorders in some urban areas.
   b. Clinical and laboratory manifestations are similar to those of hemoglobin C disorders.

H. Thalassemias

- This heterogeneous group of **genetic disorders** is characterized by deficient production of either α-or β-globin chains of hemoglobin. Heme synthesis is unaffected. They are widespread throughout the world, occurring with high frequency in Africa, India, Southeast Asia, and the Mediterranean area.

1. **β-Thalassemias** are the most common forms of thalassemia found in Mediterranean areas and in the United States. They are caused by defects in the promoter sequence, in introns, or in coding regions of the β-globin gene.
   a. **β-Thalassemia major** is also known as **Mediterranean anemia** or **Cooley anemia.** It results from compound heterozygosity or homozygosity for thalassemic variants of the β-globin gene, and it is characterized clinically by:
      (1) **Marked anemia** resulting from:
         (a) Modest decrease in hemoglobin synthesis
         (b) Marked shortening of red cell life span due to aggregation of insoluble excess α-chains
         (c) Ineffective erythropoiesis
         (d) Relative folate deficiency
      (2) **Marked splenomegaly**
      (3) **Distortion of skull, facial bones, and long bones** because of erythroid marrow expansion
      (4) **Thalassemic red cell morphology** (marked microcytosis, hypochromia, target cells, extensive changes in size and shape)
      (5) **Increased hemoglobin F** ($\alpha_2\gamma_2$) throughout life
      (6) **Generalized hemosiderosis** due to chronic hemolysis, ineffective erythropoiesis, and repeated transfusions
   b. **β-Thalassemia minor** results from heterozygous inheritance of thalassemic variants of the β-globin gene.
      (1) Clinical manifestations include minimal hypochromic microcytic anemia and an **increase in hemoglobin A_2** ($\alpha_2\delta_2$), a normally occurring minor hemoglobin fraction.
      (2) This finding is useful in distinguishing β-thalassemia minor from iron deficiency anemia and the anemia of chronic disease.
   c. **Sickle cell thalassemia** results from coinheritance of hemoglobin S gene and a thalassemic variant of the β-globin gene (compound heterozygosity). It is clinically similar to, but often less severe than, sickle cell anemia.
2. **α-Thalassemias** are the most common forms of thalassemia in Southeast Asia. They are caused by deletions of one or more of the four α-globin genes (see Table 11-2).

TABLE 11-2 ***Examples of Anemias Resulting from Increased Red Cell Destruction***

Type	Mechanisms	Diagnostic Features	Comments
Warm antibody autoimmune hemolytic anemia (primary and secondary forms)	IgG autoantibodies combine with red cell surface antigens; Fc combining site of IgG antibody further reacts with Fc receptor of phagocytic cells	Anemia, spherocytosis, and reticulocytosis; unconjugated hyperbilirubinemia and acholuric jaundice; positive direct Coombs test	Often secondary to lymphocytic neoplasms, Hodgkin disease, or autoimmune disease; sometimes associated with α-methyldopa or penicillin therapy
Hemolytic disease of the newborn (erythroblastosis fetalis)	Maternal alloimmunization to fetal red cell antigens, classically of Rh system; can also be caused by alloimmunization to ABO blood group antigens	Rising titer of maternal anti-Rh antibodies during the latter part of pregnancy; cord blood at delivery contains immature red cell precursors; direct Coombs test positive on cord blood; progressive postnatal increase in unconjugated bilirubin	Prevented by administration of anti-Rh antibody (anti-D IgG) to mother at time of delivery of first and subsequent children, removing Rh-positive red cells from maternal circulation; treated by exchange transfusion to remove unconjugated bilirubin from the serum of a newborn infant to prevent kernicterus
Hereditary spherocytosis	Red cell membrane skeletal protein abnormality	Autosomal dominant inheritance; anemia, spherocytosis, and reticulocytosis; increased mean corpuscular hemoglobin concentration; unconjugated hyperbilirubinemia and acholuric jaundice; splenomegaly; increased erythrocyte osmotic fragility to hypotonic saline	Quantitative deficiency of spectrin due to diverse mechanisms
Glucose-6-phosphate dehydrogenase (G6PD) deficiency	Failure of erythrocyte hexose monophosphate shunt under oxidative stress	Self-limited hemolytic anemia; reduced activity of erythrocyte G6PD	X-linked inheritance
Sickle cell anemia	β-globin hemoglobinopathy (mutation in coding sequence of β-globin gene, GAG [glu] [rightarrow] GTG [val])	Anemia and reticulocytosis; sickle-shaped erythrocytes demonstrable on peripheral blood smear; homozygosity for hemoglobin S demonstrable by electrophoresis	Characterized by severe anemia, recurrent painful and aplastic crises, and nonhealing leg ulcers; recurrent splenic infarcts with progressive fibrosis result in autosplenectomy
β-Thalassemia major (Cooley anemia, Mediterranean anemia)	Diverse mutations in β-globin gene causing decreased synthesis of β-globin chains; aggregation of excess α-chains causes hemolytic anemia and ineffective erythropoiesis.	Severe anemia; thalassemic red cell morphology; increased hemoglobin F	Occurs frequently in Mediterranean populations

(*continued*)

TABLE 11-2 *Continued*

Type	Mechanisms	Diagnostic Features	Comments
α-Thalassemias	Deletion of one or more of the four α-globin genes (α-globin gene is reduplicated in tandem on each chromosome 16)	Differ according to the number of deletions	No clinical abnormalities with one gene deletion; mild-to-moderate thalassemic state with two or three deletions; intrauterine death with four deletions; hemoglobin Barts (γ_4) in fetal life; hemoglobin H (β_4) in adult life

a. In normal persons, there is duplication of the α-globin gene, with a pair of identical α-globin genes on each member of the chromosome 16 pair.

b. Some variants are characterized by increased concentration of hemoglobin Barts (γ_4) or hemoglobin H (β_4).

I. **Hemolytic anemias due to mechanical disruption of circulating erythrocytes**

1. These anemias are associated with **aortic valvular prostheses.** They are also associated with **disseminated intravascular coagulation** and **thrombotic thrombocytopenic purpura.** In these instances, partial occlusion of small vessels is the cause of the mechanical disruption of the erythrocytes. This phenomenon is referred to as **microangiopathic hemolytic anemia.**
2. Characteristics include circulating red cell fragments referred to as **schistocytes** or **helmet cells.**

REVIEW TEST

Directions:** Each of the numbered items or incomplete statements in this section is followed by answers or by completions of the statement. Select the* ***one *lettered answer or completion that is best in each case.*

1. The peripheral blood smear of an anemic 1-year-old child is shown in the illustration. The most likely diagnosis is

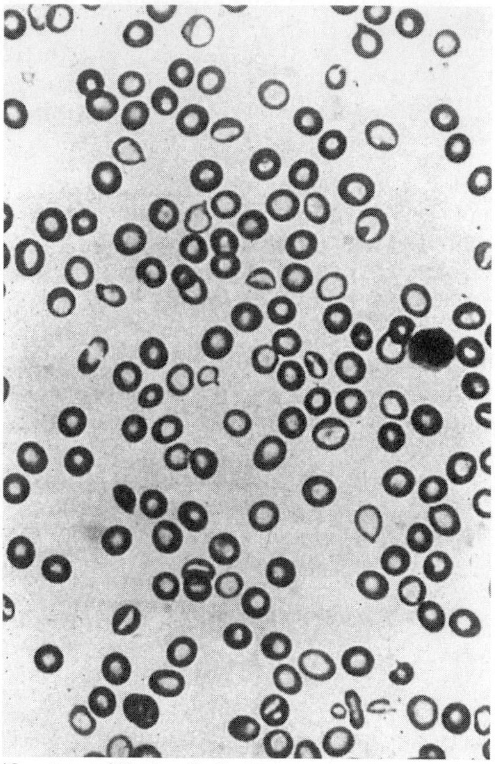

(Courtesy of Dr. Jae O. Ro.)

(A) anemia of chronic disease
(B) aplastic anemia
(C) hereditary spherocytosis
(D) iron deficiency anemia
(E) thalassemia major

2. A patient with severe anemia has a peripheral blood smear with oval macrocytes, hypersegmented neutrophils, and decreased platelets. The most likely cause of the anemia is

(A) a red cell membrane protein defect
(B) an amino acid substitution in the β-globin chain
(C) iron deficiency
(D) marrow hypoplasia
(E) vitamin B_{12} or folate deficiency

3. The patient in question 2 is found to be a severely malnourished alcoholic. The most likely cause of this disorder is

(A) aberrant intestinal bacterial flora
(B) Crohn disease
(C) fish tapeworm infestation
(D) folate deficiency
(E) pernicious anemia

4. A primiparous D-negative (Rh-negative) mother has just delivered a D-positive child. Administration of which of the following substances would be indicated?

(A) Anti-D IgG to child
(B) Anti-D IgG to mother
(C) D-positive red cells to child
(D) D-positive red cells to mother

5. A 62-year-old man presents with pallor, fatigue, and dyspnea on exertion. A complete blood count reveals microcytic hypochromic anemia. The most likely cause of these findings is

(A) dietary deficiency of iron
(B) gastrointestinal bleeding
(C) hemodilution
(D) hemolytic anemia
(E) increased iron requirement

6. A 72-year-old man who has recently had an aortic valve replacement now presents with pallor and fatigue. The red blood cell count is decreased, and schistocytes are reported on examination of a peripheral blood smear. In addition, his indirect (unconjugated) bilirubin is significantly elevated. The cause of the anemia is likely

(A) cold agglutinin disease
(B) dietary deficiency
(C) hereditary spherocytosis
(D) mechanical disruption of red cells
(E) paroxysmal nocturnal hemoglobinuria

7. A 23-year-old African-American man with a history since early childhood of severe anemia requiring many transfusions has nonhealing leg ulcers and recurrent periods of abdominal and chest pain. These signs and symptoms are most likely to be associated with which of the following laboratory abnormalities?

(A) Decreased erythropoietin
(B) Increased erythrocyte osmotic fragility
(C) Schistocytes
(D) Sickle cells on peripheral blood smear
(E) Teardrop-shaped cells

8. The spleen of the patient in question 7 would be expected to be

(A) enlarged
(B) normal sized
(C) shrunken

9. An 18-year-old man is transported to the emergency department within 20 minutes of sustaining a stab wound to the chest. The patient is poorly responsive. Given that he may have lost as much as 1.5 liters of blood at the scene, which of the following is the most likely finding in this patient?

(A) Decreased blood pressure
(B) Decreased hematocrit
(C) Decreased hemoglobin
(D) Decreased red blood cell count
(E) Increased mean corpuscular hemoglobin concentration

10. A 23-year-old man of northern European lineage presents with anemia. His father and paternal aunt had a similar illness that was treated successfully by splenectomy. His peripheral blood smear is similar to that shown in the illustration. Which of the following additional abnormalities is expected?

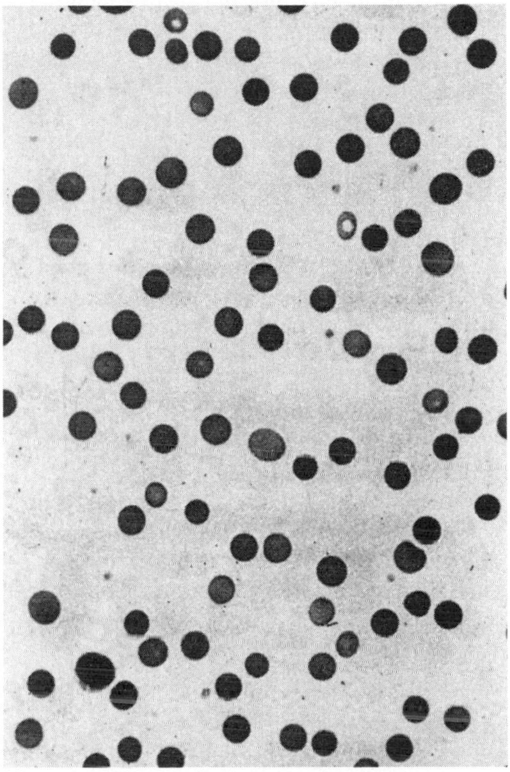

(Courtesy of Dr. Jae O. Ro.)

(A) Bilirubinuria
(B) Decreased mean corpuscular volume
(C) Increased direct (conjugated) serum bilirubin
(D) Polychromatophilic erythrocytes on peripheral blood smear
(E) Positive direct antiglobulin (Coombs) test

11. A 23-year-old woman with epilepsy who is desirous of becoming pregnant is found to be anemic. Examination of a peripheral blood smear reveals oval macrocytes and hypersegmented neutrophils. Neurologic examination is entirely normal. Which of the following is the most likely cause of the anemia?

(A) Alloantibodies directed against fetal red cell antigens
(B) Bone marrow aplasia
(C) Coating of red cells by IgG "warm" autoantibodies
(D) Folate deficiency
(E) Neoplastic replacement of the bone marrow

12. A 56-year-old woman with a history of breast cancer that was treated 5 years ago with lumpectomy and radiation but with no chemotherapy returns with bone pain, fatigue, and weakness. A complete blood count reveals severe anemia as well as decreased white blood cells and platelets. Examination of a peripheral blood smear reveals small numbers of nucleated red cells as well as an occasional "blast" cell and myelocyte. A likely cause of the hematologic abnormalities is

(A) chloramphenicol
(B) *Diphyllobothrium latum* infestation
(C) megaloblastic anemia
(D) myelophthisic anemia
(E) sickle cell anemia

13. A 23-year-old man presented to his primary care physician 2 weeks ago with a nonproductive cough and malaise. He was treated with the antibiotic azithromycin for "walking pneumonia" due to *Mycoplasma pneumoniae*. He now returns with fatigue and pallor. Laboratory studies demonstrate a decreased red blood cell count with polychromatophilia and an increase in indirect (unconjugated) bilirubin. The laboratory findings are most likely due to

(A) acute cold agglutinin disease
(B) aplastic anemia
(C) aplastic crisis
(D) paroxysmal nocturnal hemoglobinuria
(E) warm antibody autoimmune hemolytic anemia

14. Military policy dictates that flight personnel in Iraq receive primaquine chemoprophylaxis for *Plasmodium vivax* malaria on redeploying to a non-malarious area. Several days after beginning such a regimen, a 26-year-old African-American pilot develops anemia, hemoglobinemia, and hemoglobinuria. Special studies will likely reveal an abnormality in which of the following?

(A) Duffy antigen
(B) Glucose-6-phosphate dehydrogenase
(C) Intrinsic factor
(D) *PIG-A*
(E) Spectrin

15. A 28-year-old woman complains of fatigue, dyspnea, and malaise. She also notes that her urine has been reddish-brown, particularly with the first void of the morning. Subsequent studies confirm that she has paroxysmal nocturnal hemoglobinuria. Which of the following best describes the defect leading to this condition?

(A) Anti-intrinsic factor antibodies
(B) Deficiency of the intracellular structural protein spectrin
(C) Impaired synthesis of the cell-surface GPI anchor
(D) Ineffective erythropoiesis
(E) Substitution of a valine for a glutamate residue in the β-globin gene

ANSWERS AND EXPLANATIONS

1-D. The illustration shows hypochromia and microcytosis. Iron deficiency is the most frequent cause of hypochromic microcytic anemia. In infants and preadolescents, iron deficiency is most often nutritional in origin. In young women, the cause is most often related to menstrual blood loss compounded by deficient dietary intake. In men, the usual cause is occult gastrointestinal blood loss.

2-E. Megaloblastic anemia due to deficiency of vitamin B_{12} or folate is characterized by oval macrocytes, hypersegmented neutrophils, and decreased platelets.

3-D. Megaloblastic anemia associated with severe malnutrition is most often due to folate deficiency.

4-B. Administration of anti-D antiserum to a D-negative mother at the time of delivery of a D-positive child prevents maternal alloimmunization by removing fetal red cells from the maternal circulation.

5-B. Iron deficiency anemia is the most common cause of hypochromic microcytic anemia, and gastrointestinal bleeding is the most likely cause of iron deficiency in an adult male. Such a finding warrants a complete workup, including colonoscopy to detect the source of the bleeding. Dietary deficiency of iron and increased iron requirements are common causes of iron deficiency in women of child-bearing age, especially during pregnancy. Hemolytic anemia is usually accompanied by reticulocytosis. The reduced red cell parameters (hemoglobin, red blood cell count, hematocrit) that are observed with hemodilution are not truly representative of anemia, which is formally defined as a reduction in whole body red cell mass.

6-D. Turbulent blood flow over mechanical heart valves can cause shearing of red blood cells, resulting in fragmented cells termed schistocytes. The hemolysis can result in anemia and hyperbilirubinemia. Hereditary spherocytosis causes hemolytic anemia due to an intrinsic defect in the red blood cells. Dietary deficiencies do not cause fragmented red blood cells. Aplastic anemia would result in severe anemia with marked reticulocytopenia.

7-D. Sickle cell anemia is the most common hereditary anemia of persons of African lineage. Leg ulcers and recurring painful crises are characteristic. In sickle cell anemia, in contrast to sickle cell trait, sickle cells are often seen on the peripheral blood smear.

8-C. Repeated episodes of splenic infarction followed by fibrotic healing lead to a fibrotic, shrunken spleen (autosplenectomy) in adult patients with sickle cell anemia. The spleen is enlarged and congested in children with sickle cell anemia.

9-A. Within the first few hours of acute blood loss, findings of hypovolemia predominate, especially with signs of hypovolemic shock such as decreased blood pressure. It is likely that red cell indices (red blood cell counts, hemoglobin, and hematocrit) eventually decrease as a result of hemodilution. Increased mean corpuscular hemoglobin concentration (MCHC) is an unusual finding but is expected in hereditary spherocytosis.

10-D. Spherocytes are present on the peripheral blood smear and, along with the history, strongly suggest a diagnosis of hereditary spherocytosis. Similar cells are also observed in warm antibody autoimmune hemolytic anemia; therefore, these two conditions must be distinguished by means of the direct Coombs test, which is negative in hereditary spherocytosis and positive in warm antibody autoimmune hemolytic anemia. An expected finding would be an increase in indirect (unconjugated) serum bilirubin, not direct (conjugated). The jaundice is acholuric (no bilirubin in the urine, so bilirubinuria would not be expected). The mean corpuscular hemoglobin concentration (MCHC) is often increased. Because hereditary spherocytosis is a normocytic anemia, the mean corpuscular volume is not decreased. Polychromatophilic erythrocytes are an expected finding, as in any hemolytic anemia.

11-D. Phenytoin is a commonly used antiseizure medication that can cause impaired folate absorption, with resultant folate deficiency and megaloblastic anemia. The drug is contraindicated for use during pregnancy, because folate is required during embryogenesis to prevent neural tube defects. Aplastic anemia results in a major failure of erythropoiesis. Myelophthisic anemia occurs in some cancer patients with metastatic disease. Warm antibody hemolytic anemia is manifest by anemia and reticulocytosis, often with spherocytosis. Hemolytic disease of the newborn most commonly occurs with Rh blood group incompatibility between mother and fetus.

12-D. Infiltration of tumor cells from cancers such as those of breast and prostate displaces bone marrow elements, thereby causing myelophthisic anemia. Chloramphenicol causes aplastic anemia in some individuals. *Diphyllobothrium latum* infestation can result in megaloblastic anemia due to vitamin B_{12} deficiency. Sickle cell anemia is more common in black and Mediterranean populations.

13-A. Acute cold agglutinin disease is a form of hemolytic anemia due to autoantibodies to blood group antigens and is sometimes a complication of *Mycoplasma pneumoniae* infection. Aplastic anemia is associated with a variety of toxic exposures, including, among others, the antibiotic chloramphenicol, not azithromycin. Aplastic crises can occur as acute events in the course of hemolytic anemias such as hereditary spherocytosis or sickle cell anemia. Paroxysmal nocturnal hemoglobinuria is an acquired defect that renders red blood cells sensitive to complement-induced lysis. Warm antibody autoimmune hemolytic anemia can be idiopathic or secondary to autoimmune disorders or lymphoid neoplasms.

14-B. Drugs that cause oxidative stress (e.g., primaquine, sulfa-containing drugs) result in intravascular hemolytic anemia in subjects (most often male) with glucose-6-phosphate dehydrogenase (G6PD) deficiency. Current military policy excepts G6PD-deficient persons from the requirement for primaquine chemoprophylaxis or sets up screening criteria for individuals whose G6PD status is unknown. Duffy antigen is a minor red blood cell antigen, the absence of which confers some resistance to malarial infection. Intrinsic factor may be absent in pernicious anemia. *PIG-A* deficiency results in paroxysmal nocturnal hemoglobinuria. Spectrin is deficient in hereditary spherocytosis.

15-C. Paroxysmal nocturnal hemoglobinuria results in an acquired intracorpuscular defect in the ability to synthesize the glycosylphosphatidylinositol (GPI) anchors required for appropriate placement of complement regulatory proteins on the surface of red blood cells. Functional deficiency of such proteins as CD55 and CD59 renders the cells sensitive to complement-mediated lysis. Anti-intrinsic factor antibodies are seen in pernicious anemia. Spectrin is deficient in hereditary spherocytosis. Ineffective erythropoiesis is seen in megaloblastic anemia due to folate or vitamin B_{12} deficiencies. Substitution of valine for glutamic acid in the β-globin gene underlies the defect in sickle cell anemia.

CHAPTER 12

Neoplastic and Proliferative Disorders of the Hematopoietic and Lymphoid Systems

I. Leukemia

A. General concepts

1. Leukemia is a general term for a group of malignancies of either lymphoid or hematopoietic cell origin. The number of circulating leukocytes is often greatly increased.
2. The bone marrow is diffusely infiltrated with leukemic cells, often with encroachment on normal hematopoietic cell development. Consequent failure of normal leukocyte, red cell, and platelet production can result in anemia, infection, or hemorrhage.
3. Infiltration of leukemic cells in the liver, spleen, lymph nodes, and other organs is common.

B. Acute leukemias

1. **General considerations**
   a. A predominance of **blasts** and closely related cells in the bone marrow and peripheral blood is characteristic.
   b. The most common malignancies of the pediatric age group, acute leukemias occur most often in **children**. They exhibit a second incidence peak after 60 years of age.
   c. Cytogenetic abnormalities are frequent. For example, the 9;22 translocation results in a morphologically unique chromosome, the **Philadelphia chromosome (Ph^1).** This abnormality, better known for its association with chronic myelogenous leukemia, is associated with a poorer prognosis when it occurs in acute leukemias.
   d. Without therapeutic intervention, acute leukemia follows a short and precipitous course, marked by anemia, infection, and hemorrhage, and death occurs within 6 to 12 months.
2. **Acute lymphoblastic leukemia (ALL)**
   a. ALL is the most common malignancy of **children.**
   b. A predominance of **lymphoblasts** in the circulating blood and in the bone marrow is characteristic.
   c. ALL is the form of acute leukemia that is most **responsive to therapy.**

d. Further classification into a number of subgroups is based on differences in morphology, cytogenetic changes, antigenic cell-surface markers, or rearrangement of the immunoglobulin heavy-chain or T-cell receptor genes. The form that is most common and most amenable to therapy is characterized by blast cells that are positive for the CD10 marker.

3. **Acute myeloid (myeloblastic) leukemia (AML)**
   a. AML occurs most often in **adults.**
   b. A predominance of **myeloblasts** and early promyelocytes is characteristic.
   c. AML responds to current therapy more poorly than ALL.
   d. Further classification into several subgroups is based on morphology, cytochemical characteristics, surface markers, and genetic alterations.

C. **Chronic leukemias.** These malignancies are characterized by proliferations of lymphoid or hematopoietic cells that are more mature than those of the acute leukemias. The chronic forms have a longer, less devastating clinical course than the acute leukemias but are less responsive to therapeutic intervention.

1. **Chronic lymphocytic leukemia (CLL)**
   a. **General considerations**
      (1) CLL is characterized by proliferation of **neoplastic lymphoid cells** (almost always B cells) with widespread infiltration of the bone marrow, peripheral blood, lymph nodes, spleen, liver, and other organs.
      (2) Leukemic cells of CLL are less capable of differentiating into antibody-producing plasma cells.
      (3) CLL most often occurs in persons older than 60 years of age and more frequently in men.
   b. **Characteristics**
      (1) The leukemic cells closely resemble normal mature peripheral blood lymphocytes and, like these cells, express surface immunoglobulin and pan–B-cell markers such as CD19 and CD20. They are also CD5 positive and CD10 negative.
      (2) The cells are susceptible to mechanical disruption and often appear on the peripheral blood smear as **smudge cells.**
      (3) The peripheral white blood cell count varies from 50,000/μL to 200,000/μL, with a preponderance of leukemic cells.
      (4) Leukemic cells diffusely infiltrate the bone marrow.
   c. **Complications**
      (1) **Warm antibody autoimmune hemolytic anemia**
      (2) **Hypogammaglobulinemia** and increased susceptibility to bacterial infection, often occurring early in the course of this disorder
   d. **Clinical features**
      (1) The clinical course is usually described as indolent, often with few symptoms and minor disability for protracted periods.
      (2) Generalized **lymphadenopathy** and moderate **hepatosplenomegaly** are frequent features.
      (3) Mean survival is 3 to 7 years; treatment relieves symptoms but has little effect on overall survival.
2. **Hairy cell leukemia** is a B-cell disease in which the leukemic cells exhibit characteristic **hair-like filamentous projections.** The cells can be further identified by their **positive staining for tartrate-resistant acid phosphatase (TRAP).**
   a. Hairy cell leukemia most often affects middle-aged men, who present with prominent **splenomegaly** and **pancytopenia.**
   b. The disease has received major attention because of its **dramatic response to several therapeutic agents,** including α-interferon, 2-chlorodeoxyadenosine, and deoxycoformycin.
3. **Chronic myelogenous leukemia (CML)** is a neoplastic clonal proliferation of myeloid stem cells, the precursor cells of erythrocytes, granulocytes, monocytes, and platelets. It is one of the myeloproliferative syndromes.

a. **Molecular changes**
   (1) CML is characterized by a reciprocal chromosomal translocation between chromosomes 9 and 22. The **Philadelphia chromosome** represents a remnant of chromosome 22 with the addition of a small segment of chromosome 9. This cytogenetic change is found in all blood cell lineages (erythroblasts, granulocytes, monocytes, megakaryocytes, B- and T-cell progenitors) but not in the majority of circulating B or T lymphocytes.
   (2) The c-*abl* proto-oncogene on chromosome 9 is transposed to an area on chromosome 22, adjacent to an oncogene referred to as *bcr* (for breakpoint cluster region), forming a new hybrid, or fusion, gene, *bcr-abl.*
   (3) ***Bcr-abl*** codes for a protein (p210) with tyrosine kinase activity, which plays a critical role in the etiopathogenesis of CML.

b. **Characteristics**
   (1) **Marked leukocytosis,** with white blood cell counts varying from 50,000/μL to 200,000/μL
   (2) Leukemic cells in the peripheral blood and bone marrow, mainly **middle-to-late myeloid (granulocytic) precursor cells,** including myelocytes, metamyelocytes, bands, and segmented forms
   (3) Small numbers of blasts and promyelocytes
   (4) The Philadelphia chromosome, found in granulocytic and erythroid precursor cells and in megakaryocytes
   (5) Marked **reduction in leukocyte alkaline phosphatase** activity in the leukemic leukocytes

c. **Clinical features**
   (1) **Prominent splenomegaly** and modestly enlarged liver and lymph nodes
   (2) Peak incidence in middle-age (35–50 years of age)
   (3) Terminates, in most cases, in an accelerated phase leading to so-called blast crisis marked by increased numbers of primitive blast cells and promyelocytes

II. Myeloproliferative Diseases.

This group of clonal proliferations of myeloid stem cells includes chronic myelogenous leukemia, polycythemia vera, chronic idiopathic myelofibrosis (agnogenic myeloid metaplasia), and essential thrombocythemia.

A. Common characteristics
   1. Peak incidence in middle-aged and elderly persons
   2. Proliferation of one or more of the myeloid series (erythroid, granulocytic, and megakaryocytic) cell types
   3. Increase in peripheral blood basophils and nucleated red cells
   4. Increase in serum uric acid
   5. Prominent splenomegaly

B. **Polycythemia vera**
   1. **Clinical characteristics**
      a. **Marked erythrocytosis**
      b. **Moderate increase in circulating granulocytes and platelets**
      c. **Splenomegaly**
      d. Decreased erythropoietin
   2. **Other features**
      a. Sludging of high hematocrit blood often leads to **thrombotic or hemorrhagic phenomena.**
      b. Polycythemia vera often progresses to a late phase in which anemia supervenes. This phase is often marked by bone marrow fibrosis and extramedullary hematopoiesis and an increasing white blood cell count, and it can mimic CML.
      c. Acute leukemia may supervene in approximately 3% of patients, most of whom have received antimitotic drugs or radiation therapy.

3. **Diagnosis**
   a. Polycythemia vera is marked by **decreased erythropoietin,** which distinguishes it from other forms of polycythemia, all of which are associated with increased erythropoietin.
   b. It must be distinguished from **secondary polycythemia,** which is associated with the following:
      (1) **Chronic hypoxia,** associated with pulmonary disease, congenital heart disease, residence at high altitudes, and heavy smoking
      (2) **Inappropriate production of erythropoietin,** associated with androgen therapy, **adult polycystic kidney disease,** and **tumors,** such as renal cell carcinoma, hepatocellular carcinoma, and cerebellar hemangioma
      (3) **Endocrine abnormalities,** prominently including **pheochromocytoma** and adrenal adenoma with **Cushing syndrome**

C. **Chronic idiopathic myelofibrosis (agnogenic myeloid metaplasia, myelofibrosis with myeloid metaplasia)** is characterized by **extensive extramedullary hematopoiesis** involving the liver and spleen and sometimes the lymph nodes. Additional manifestations include proliferation of non-neoplastic fibrous tissue within the bone marrow cavity (**myelofibrosis**). The fibrous tissue replaces normal hematopoietic cells. This late manifestation is often preceded by marrow hypercellularity.

1. **Postulated pathogenetic factors**
   a. Megakaryocytic proliferation may be the primary abnormality; the elaboration of platelet-derived growth factor and of transforming growth factor-β (TGF-β) by platelets and megakaryocytes may be the cause of the fibroblastic proliferation.
   b. Megakaryocytes are spared in the marrow fibrotic process and increase in number, resulting in prominent bone marrow megakaryocytosis and peripheral blood thrombocytosis.
2. **Clinical features**
   a. **Peripheral blood smear**
      (1) **Teardrop-shaped erythrocytes**
      (2) Granulocytic precursor cells and nucleated red cell precursors in variable numbers
   b. **Anemia** and massive **splenomegaly**

D. **Essential thrombocythemia** is characterized by marked **thrombocytosis** in the peripheral blood and **megakaryocytosis** in the bone marrow. Platelet counts in excess of 1,000,000/μL are common (normal value is 150,000–350,000/μL). Additional features include **bleeding and thrombosis.**

III. Non-neoplastic Lymphoid Proliferations

A. **General considerations.** These reactions include acute and chronic nonspecific lymphadenitis occurring in response to a number of infectious agents or immune stimuli.

B. **Infectious mononucleosis**

1. This benign, self-limited disorder is caused by **Epstein-Barr virus** (EBV), which has an affinity for B lymphocytes. It occurs frequently in **young adults.**
2. Circulating **atypical lymphocytes** (reactive CD8+ T lymphocytes) are characteristic.
3. The disorder is marked by a number of serum antibodies, including **anti-EBV antibodies** and **heterophil antibodies** (heterophil agglutinins) directed at sheep erythrocytes; so-called heterophil-negative infectious mononucleosis is most often associated with cytomegalovirus infection.
4. Clinical characteristics are prominent sore throat, fever, generalized lymphadenopathy, and often hepatosplenomegaly. The **spleen is especially susceptible to traumatic rupture.**

IV. Plasma Cell Disorders

A. **General considerations**

1. Plasma cell disorders are neoplastic proliferations of well-differentiated immunoglobulin-producing cells.
2. These disorders include multiple myeloma, Waldenström macroglobulinemia, and benign monoclonal gammopathy, as well as primary amyloidosis and heavy-chain (Franklin) disease.
3. Occurrence is most frequent in persons older than 40–50 years of age.

B. **Multiple myeloma (plasma cell myeloma/plasmacytoma)** is a **malignant plasma cell tumor** usually affecting older persons that typically involves bone and is associated with prominent serum and urinary protein abnormalities.

1. **Bone lesions and protein abnormalities**
   a. The neoplastic cell is an end-stage derivative of B lymphocytes that is clearly identifiable as a plasma cell. The neoplastic cells can easily be identified by bone marrow biopsy or aspiration smears.
   b. The tumor cells produce **lytic lesions in bone,** especially in the skull and axial skeleton.
      (1) The bone lesions appear lucent on radiographic examination, with characteristic sharp borders, and are referred to as **punched-out lesions.** They may be manifest radiographically as diffuse demineralization of bone (**osteopenia**).
      (2) The cause is an osteoclast-activating factor secreted by the neoplastic plasma cells.
      (3) The lesions are often associated with **severe bone pain** and spontaneous fractures.
   c. Multiple myeloma arises from proliferation of a single clone of malignant antibody-producing cells.
      (1) The tumor cells produce massive quantities of identical immunoglobulin molecules demonstrable electrophoretically as a narrow serum band or, after densitometric scanning, as a sharp spike referred to as an **M protein.**
      (2) The M protein in multiple myeloma is most often an IgG or IgA immunoglobulin of either kappa or lambda light chain specificity.
      (3) Synthesis of normal immunoglobulins is often impaired.
      (4) The marked serum immunoglobulin increase is often initially detected by laboratory screening as increased total protein with an increase in serum globulin (**hyperglobulinemia**).
      (5) The urine often contains significant quantities of free immunoglobulin light chains, either kappa or lambda, which are referred to as **Bence Jones protein.**
      (6) As a consequence of hyperglobulinemia, the red cells tend to congregate together in a manner reminiscent of a stack of poker chips (**rouleaux formation**). There is also a marked increase in the erythrocyte sedimentation rate.
2. **Other clinical characteristics of multiple myeloma**
   a. **Anemia** due to neoplastic encroachment on myeloid precursor cells; possible leukopenia and thrombocytopenia
   b. **Increased susceptibility to infection** because of impaired production of normal immunoglobulins
   c. **Hypercalcemia** secondary to bone destruction; in contrast to the increased serum alkaline phosphatase that accompanies most other instances of hypercalcemia, the serum alkaline phosphatase in multiple myeloma is not increased.
   d. **Renal insufficiency with azotemia due to myeloma kidney** (myeloma nephrosis). The renal lesion is characterized by prominent tubular casts of Bence Jones protein, numerous multinucleated macrophage-derived giant cells, and metastatic calcification, and sometimes by interstitial infiltration of malignant plasma cells.
   e. **Amyloidosis** of the primary amyloidosis type

C. **Waldenström macroglobulinemia** is a manifestation of **lymphoplasmacytic lymphoma,** a B-cell neoplasm of lymphoid cells of an intermediate stage between B lymphocytes and plasma cells referred to as **plasmacytoid lymphocytes.** In the case of Waldenström macroglobulinemia, the neoplastic cells produce a monoclonal IgM protein (lymphoplasmacytic lymphomas can also occur without protein production).

1. **Defining characteristics**
   a. **Serum IgM immunoglobulin** of either kappa or lambda specificity occurring as an M protein
   b. **Plasmacytoid lymphocytes** infiltrating the blood, bone marrow, lymph nodes, and spleen
   c. **Bence Jones proteinuria** in about 10% of cases
   d. **Absence of bone lesions**
2. **Clinical features**
   a. Most frequently seen in **men older than 50 years of age**
   b. **Slowly progressive course,** often marked by generalized lymphadenopathy and mild anemia
3. **Complications**
   a. **Hyperviscosity syndrome,** which results from marked increase in serum IgM. Features include **retinal vascular dilation,** sometimes with hemorrhage, confusion, and other central nervous system changes. Sometimes, **emergency plasmapheresis** is required to prevent blindness.
   b. **Abnormal bleeding,** which may be due to vascular and platelet dysfunction secondary to the serum protein abnormality

D. **Benign monoclonal gammopathy (monoclonal gammopathy of undetermined significance, or MGUS)** occurs in 5%–10% of otherwise healthy **older persons.**

1. A monoclonal **M protein** spike of less than 2 g/100 mL, minimal or no Bence Jones proteinuria, less than 5% plasma cells in the bone marrow, and no decrease in concentration of normal immunoglobulins is characteristic.
2. MGUS is most often without clinical consequence.

V. Lymphoid Neoplasms

A. **Hodgkin lymphoma (Hodgkin disease)** is a **malignant** neoplasm with features (e.g., fever, inflammatory cell infiltrates) resembling an inflammatory disorder.

1. **General considerations**
   a. Hodgkin lymphoma characteristically affects **young adults** (predominantly **young men**); an exception is nodular sclerosis, which frequently affects young women.
   b. Associated manifestations often include pruritus, fever, diaphoresis, and leukocytosis reminiscent of an acute infection.
   c. With modern staging and aggressive therapy, a clinical cure is often achieved.
   d. This neoplasm is characterized in all forms by the presence of Reed-Sternberg cells. The diagnosis of Hodgkin lymphoma depends on this histologic finding.
2. **Reed-Sternberg cells** are **binucleated, or multinucleated, giant cells** with eosinophilic inclusion-like nucleoli that may be the actual malignant cells of Hodgkin lymphoma.
   a. Differing numbers are found in varying forms of Hodgkin lymphoma, and the severity of the disease variants is directly proportional to the number of Reed-Sternberg cells found in the lesions.
   b. Conversely, the greater the number of reactive lymphocytes in the Hodgkin lymphoma variant, the better the prognosis.
3. **Classification of Hodgkin lymphoma.** The **World Health Organization (WHO) classification** identifies a number of disease variants (Table 12-1).

a. **Lymphocyte-predominance Hodgkin lymphoma**
   (1) Features include a large numbers of lymphocytes and histiocytes as well as a paucity of Reed-Sternberg cells.
   (2) There is no association with EBV infection.
   (3) Peak incidence occurs in young and middle-aged men.
   (4) The **prognosis is relatively good.**

b. **Lymphocyte-rich Hodgkin lymphoma**
   (1) There is an association with EBV infection in 40% of cases.
   (2) This variant is more common in men than in women.
   (3) The clinical course is moderately aggressive.

c. **Mixed cellularity Hodgkin lymphoma**
   (1) This variant is the one found most often in older persons. It is more common in men than in women.
   (2) Characteristic features include a polymorphic infiltrate of eosinophils, plasma cells, histiocytes, and Reed-Sternberg cells, as well as areas of necrosis and fibrosis.
   (3) There is an association with EBV infection in 70% of cases.
   (4) The clinical course is moderately aggressive.

d. **Lymphocyte depletion Hodgkin lymphoma**
   (1) This variant is the least frequently occurring form of Hodgkin lymphoma.
   (2) Few lymphocytes, numerous Reed-Sternberg cells, and extensive necrosis and fibrosis are apparent.
   (3) There is an association with EBV infection in the great majority of cases; this variant is also more common in persons with human immunodeficiency virus infection.
   (4) This type of Hodgkin lymphoma has the **poorest prognosis** among all the variants.

e. **Nodular sclerosis Hodgkin lymphoma**
   (1) This variant is the most frequently occurring form of Hodgkin lymphoma. Unlike other forms of Hodgkin lymphoma, this variant occurs more frequently in **young women.**
   (2) Nodular division of affected lymph nodes by **fibrous bands** and the presence of **lacunar cells,** Reed-Sternberg cell variants, are characteristic. The neoplasm often arises in the upper mediastinum or lower cervical or supraclavicular nodes.
   (3) There is rarely an association with EBV infection.
   (4) The **prognosis is relatively good.**

4. **Clinical staging: Ann Arbor classification**
   a. This system of classification is based on the degree of dissemination, involvement of extralymphatic sites, and presence or absence of systemic signs such as fever (Table 12-2). It is an essential part of the **diagnostic evaluation** of patients with Hodgkin lymphoma.
   b. Although grading of histopathologic variants roughly correlates with clinical behavior, **prognosis is better predicted by staging** (Ann Arbor classification).

B. **Non-Hodgkin lymphomas.** These **malignant neoplasms** arise from lymphoid cells or other cells native to lymphoid tissue. They originate most frequently within **lymph nodes** or in other lymphoid areas. **Tumor involvement** of the periaortic lymph nodes is frequent.

1. The **WHO classification of lymphoid neoplasms** includes Hodgkin lymphoma and all lymphoid neoplasms, including not only the non-Hodgkin lymphomas but also the lymphoid leukemias and multiple myeloma (see Table 12-1).
2. **Small lymphocytic lymphoma** is a **B-cell lymphoma** that follows an **indolent course** and occurs most often in **older persons.**
   a. Diffuse **effacement of lymph node architecture** by small mature-appearing lymphocytes is characteristic. In addition, **widespread nodal involvement** and involvement of the liver, spleen, and bone marrow frequently occur.
   b. There is a **close relationship to CLL.** In the WHO classification, this disorder is called B-cell chronic lymphocytic leukemia/small lymphocytic lymphoma. The neoplastic cells express surface immunoglobulin and pan–B-cell markers (e.g., CD19 and CD20) and are positive for CD5 but negative for CD10.

TABLE 12-1 ***Proposed World Health Organization (WHO) Classification of Lymphoid Neoplasms (Abbreviated)***

B-Cell Neoplasms
Precursor B-cell neoplasm
Precursor B lymphoblastic leukemia/lymphoma (precursor B-cell acute lymphoblastic leukemia)
Mature (peripheral) B-cell neoplasms
B-cell chronic lymphocytic leukemia/small lymphocytic lymphoma Lymphoplasmacytic lymphoma Hairy cell leukemia Plasma cell myeloma/plasmacytoma Extranodal marginal zone B-cell lymphoma of MALT type Follicular lymphoma Mantle cell lymphoma Diffuse large B-cell lymphoma Burkitt lymphoma/Burkitt cell leukemia
T-cell Neoplasms
Precursor T-cell neoplasm
Precursor T lymphoblastic lymphoma/leukemia (precursor T-cell acute lymphoblastic leukemia)
Mature (peripheral) T-cell neoplasms T-cell granular lymphocytic leukemia Adult T-cell lymphoma/leukemia (HTLV1+) Enteropathy-type T-cell lymphoma Mycosis fungoides (Sézary syndrome)
Hodgkin Lymphoma (Hodgkin Disease)
Classical Hodgkin lymphoma subtypes Lymphocyte-predominance Hodgkin lymphoma Lymphocyte-rich Hodgkin lymphoma Mixed cellularity Hodgkin lymphoma Lymphocyte depletion Hodgkin lymphoma Nodular sclerosis Hodgkin lymphoma

(Modified from Harris NL, Jaffe ES, Diebold J et al: The World Health Organization classification of hematological malignancies report of the Clinical Advisory Committee Meeting, Airlie House, Virginia, November 1997. *Modern Pathology* 13 : 193–207, 2000.)

3. **Follicular lymphoma** is a **B-cell lymphoma,** often following an **indolent course** in **older persons.** It is the **most common form** of non-Hodgkin lymphoma.
   a. Proliferation of **angulated grooved cells** that closely resemble the cells of the lymphoid follicular center, commonly in a follicular (**nodular**) pattern is characteristic. These cells express surface immunoglobulin and B cell markers such as CD19 and CD20, are sometimes positive for CD10, and are CD5 negative.
   b. A **cytogenetic change,** t(14;18) is also characteristic. Expression of ***bcl*-2**, an oncogene also occurs; *bcl*-2 codes for a mitochondrial protein that inhibits apoptosis.
4. **Mantle cell lymphoma** arises from the mantle zone of lymphoid follicles. It is morphologically and immunophenotypically similar to small lymphocytic lymphoma, with slightly different cellular detail.
   a. A translocation, t(11;14), which results in activation of the cyclin D_1 gene (*bcl*-1), is characteristic.

TABLE 12-2 ***Ann Arbor Classification of Hodgkin and Non-Hodgkin Lymphomas***

Stage*	Site of Involvement
I	Involvement of a single lymph node region (I) or involvement of a single extralymphatic organ or site (I_E)
II	Involvement of two or more lymph node regions on the same side of the diaphragm alone (II) or with involvement of limited contiguous extralymphatic organ or tissue (II_E)
III	Involvement of lymph node regions on both sides of the diaphragm (III), which may include the spleen (III_S), limited contiguous extralymphatic organ or site (III_E), or both (III_{ES})
IV	Multiple or disseminated foci of involvement of one or more extralymphatic organs with or without lymphatic involvement

* Stages are further designated on the basis of absence (A) or presence (B) of systemic symptoms. Modified from Carbone PT, et al: Report of the Committee on Hodgkin's Disease Staging. *Cancer Res* 31:1860–1861, 1971.

b. This disorder is most often manifest as a disseminated, aggressive, incurable disease that occurs predominantly in older men.

5. **Extranodal marginal zone B cell lymphoma of MALT type** tends to arise in sites of chronic inflammation or sites of autoimmune disease such as the salivary glands in Sjögren syndrome, the thyroid in Hashimoto thyroiditis, or the stomach in *Helicobacter pylori* gastritis. It is often referred to as a MALToma (MALT = mucosa-associated lymphoid tissue).
6. **Diffuse large B-cell lymphoma** usually presents as a large, often extranodal mass followed by widespread aggressive dissemination. Leukemic involvement is rare. The disease most commonly occurs in **older persons;** however, the age range is wide and many of these lymphomas occur in **children.**
7. **Precursor T lymphoblastic lymphoma/leukemia (precursor T-cell acute lymphoblastic leukemia)** often presents clinically as a **combination of T-ALL and a mediastinal mass.** The disease occurs most often in **children.**
   a. Convoluted-appearing nuclei are characteristic.
   b. The lymphoma most often arises from **thymic lymphocytes.**
   c. The disease rapidly disseminates and **progresses to T-ALL.**
8. **Burkitt lymphoma** is an aggressive **B-cell lymphoma.** The African form frequently involves the maxilla or mandible; the American form usually involves abdominal organs.
   a. There is a close linkage to **EBV infection** (especially in the African variety).
   b. Histologic characteristics include a **"starry-sky"** appearance. As a result of rapid cell turnover, the lesions contain abundant cellular debris that is taken up by non-neoplastic macrophages, resulting in this appearance.
   c. There is a close **relationship to B-ALL** (acute lymphoblastic leukemia of late-stage B-cell origin), which is called Burkitt cell leukemia in the WHO classification.
   d. The lymphoma is associated with a characteristic **cytogenic change,** t(8;14).
      (1) In this translocation, the c-*myc* proto-oncogene located on chromosome 8 is transposed to a site adjacent to the immunoglobulin heavy-chain locus on chromosome 14.
      (2) Increased expression of the c-*myc* gene, presumably caused by the proximity of regulatory sequences of the immunoglobulin heavy chain gene, is characteristic.
9. **Cutaneous T-cell lymphomas**
   a. **Mycosis fungoides**
      (1) Presenting features include an erythematous, eczematoid, or psoriasiform process, progressing to raised plaques and then to a tumor stage.

(2) Histologic characteristics include dermal infiltrates of atypical CD4+ T cells with **cerebriform nuclei.** Small pockets of tumor cells within the epidermis are referred to as **Pautrier microabscesses.**

(3) The disease eventually disseminates to lymph nodes and internal organs.

b. **Sézary syndrome.** This leukemic form of cutaneous T-cell lymphoma is characterized by the combination of skin lesions and circulating neoplastic cells with cerebriform nuclei.

REVIEW TEST

***Directions:** Each of the numbered items or incomplete statements in this section is followed by answers or by completions of the statement. Select the **one** lettered answer or completion that is best in each case.*

1. A 45-year-old woman presents with marked splenomegaly. Her leukocyte count is increased to 300,000/μL. The differential count reveals the presence of small numbers of myeloblasts and promyelocytes, with a predominance of myelocytes, metamyelocytes, bands, and segmented neutrophils. Basophils are also increased in number, as are platelets. The patient is not anemic. Leukocyte alkaline phosphatase is decreased. Which of the following describes a major characteristic of this disorder?

(A) 9;22 translocation
(B) Expansion of mature B lymphocytes within multiple lymph nodes
(C) Hypogammaglobulinemia
(D) Neoplastic cells exhibiting hair-like filamentous projections
(E) Peak incidence at 65 years of age

2. A 3-year-old boy presents with epistaxis and fever. Multiple cutaneous petechiae are evident, and there is generalized enlargement of lymph nodes as well as palpable splenomegaly. The hemoglobin and platelet count are markedly decreased, and the white blood cell count is elevated to 40,000 cells/μL, with a preponderance of lymphoblasts. Which of the following statements best characterizes this disorder?

(A) It is the form of acute leukemia that is most responsive to therapy.
(B) It occurs most often in adults but can occur in children.
(C) Lymphoblastic cells cause damage to normal blood cells, resulting in low cell counts.
(D) The presence of the CD10 marker is indicative of a poorer prognosis.

3. A 60-year-old man is referred because of splenomegaly and generalized lymphadenopathy. The total white blood cell count is markedly elevated, and the differential count reveals a preponderance of mature-appearing lymphocytes. Bone marrow examination reveals a diffuse infiltration with similar-appearing lymphocytes. Which of the following statements best characterizes this disorder?

(A) A progressive increase in the number of myeloblasts and promyelocytes is indicative of acceleration of the disease process.
(B) Bacterial infections are common early in the disease due to hypogammaglobulinemia.
(C) Mean survival is less than 1 year after diagnosis.
(D) Myelofibrosis is a common complication.
(E) The neoplastic lymphoid cells are most often T cells, not B cells.

4. A 70-year-old man presents with severe bone pain and frequent respiratory infections. Serum protein electrophoresis demonstrates an M protein spike in the gamma region. Radiographs of the skull, long bones, and spine demonstrate multiple "punched-out" lesions, and bone marrow aspiration demonstrates large numbers of neoplastic plasma cells. Which of the following statements is true of this disorder?

(A) Although this patient presents at 70 years of age, the average age of presentation is 50 years of age.
(B) Renal insufficiency is a common cause of death.
(C) The M spike is most often an IgM.
(D) The M spike is most often polyclonal in nature.
(E) This disorder is the most common T-cell neoplasm.

5. The peripheral blood smear of an asymptomatic 68-year-old white man exhibiting generalized lymphadenopathy and hepatosplenomegaly is shown in the illustration. Which of the following is the most likely diagnosis?

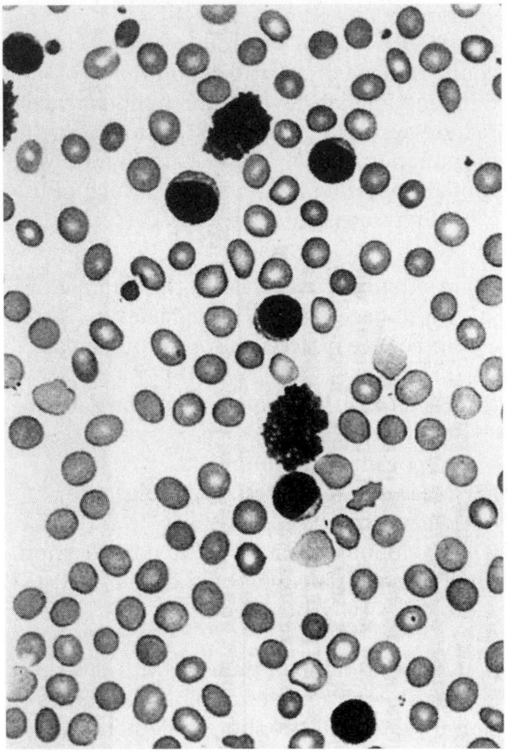

(Courtesy of Dr. Jae O. Ro.)

(A) Acute lymphoblastic leukemia
(B) Acute myeloblastic leukemia
(C) Chronic lymphocytic leukemia
(D) Chronic myelogenous leukemia

6. Radiographic examination of a 65-year-old man with back pain caused by a compression fracture of T12 reveals multiple "punched-out" lytic bone lesions. Which of the following additional abnormalities is likely?

(A) A serum IgG kappa M protein
(B) Hypocalcemia
(C) Increased serum alkaline phosphatase
(D) Marked splenomegaly
(E) Polyclonal urinary light chains

7. Examination of a lymph node from the neck of a 26-year-old man reveals total effacement of architecture in the histologic picture shown below. Which additional studies are needed to confirm the diagnosis?

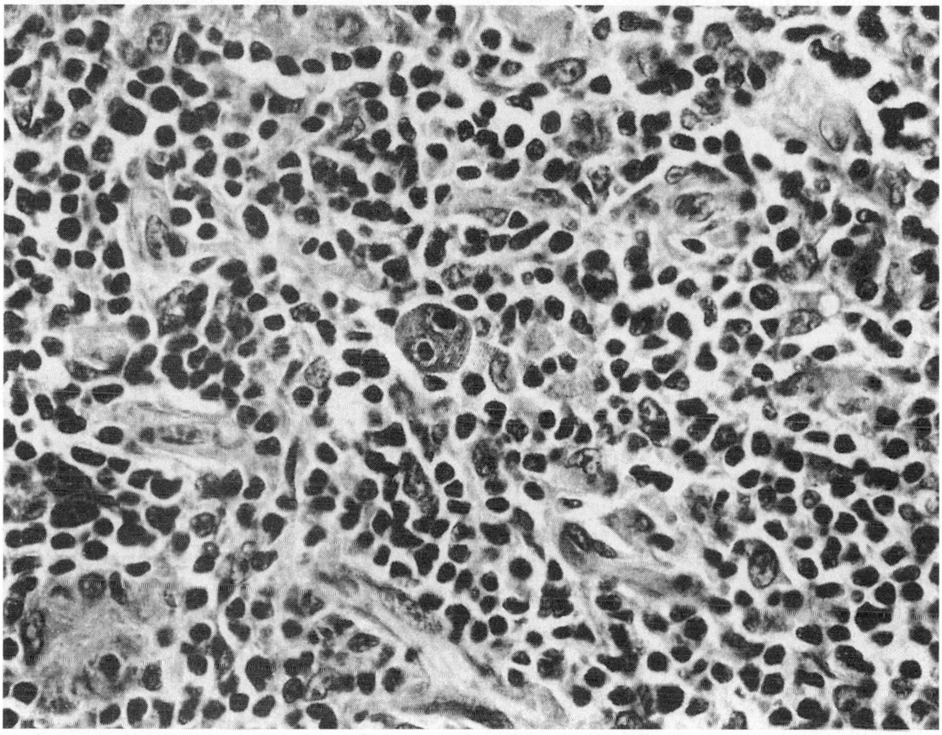

(Reprinted with permission from Golden A, Powell D, Jennings C: Pathology: *Understanding Human Disease*, 2nd ed. Baltimore, Williams & Wilkins, 1985, p 351.)

(A) Angiotensin-converting factor
(B) Gene rearrangement studies
(C) No additional studies
(D) Osteoclastic factor assay
(E) Urine for Bence Jones protein

8. A 55-year-old man presents with abdominal discomfort and fullness. Physical examination is remarkable for a massively enlarged spleen. Attempts at bone marrow aspiration are unsuccessful. A bone marrow core biopsy reveals numerous cells that have a single round nucleus surrounded by a cytoplasm with fine fibrillary projections. A stain for tartrate-resistant acid phosphatase (TRAP) confirms the likely diagnosis. Which of the following statements about this disorder is correct?

(A) The cell surface marker CD3 is almost always demonstrable.
(B) The neoplastic cells stain positive for nonspecific esterase, a marker of monocytic maturation.
(C) The typical patient with this disorder presents with a markedly elevated total leukocyte count.
(D) This is an example of a well-known B-cell disorder.
(E) There is currently no effective therapy for this condition.

9. A 60-year-old man is referred for evaluation of marked erythrocytosis and splenomegaly. Laboratory studies confirm an elevated red blood cell count and additionally demonstrate a moderate increase in circulating granulocytes and platelets. Oxygen saturation studies are normal, and isotopic studies reveal an increase in total red cell mass. Which of the following is characteristic of this disorder?

(A) Frequent association with thrombosis or hemorrhagic phenomena
(B) Increased erythropoietin concentration
(C) Manifestation of Cushing syndrome
(D) Most often secondary to hypoxia
(E) Usual termination in chronic myelogenous leukemia

10. A 23-year-old woman presents with cervical and mediastinal lymphadenopathy. Biopsy of a cervical lymph node reveals a nodular appearance with fibrous bands, effacement of the lymph node architecture, and numerous lacunar cells. Which of the following is characteristic of this disorder?

(A) Benign neoplasm
(B) Frequent association with Epstein-Barr virus infection
(C) Most often a complication of human immunodeficiency virus infection
(D) Peak incidence in early childhood
(E) Relatively favorable clinical course

11. A 60-year-old woman presents with a painless cervical lymph node mass that has been progressively enlarging over the past month. Splenomegaly is noted on abdominal examination. A cervical lymph node biopsy reveals effacement of the architecture by angulated grooved cells in a nodular pattern. Which of the following statements about this disorder is correct?

(A) The findings are those of a benign neoplasm of lymphoid cells.
(B) The findings are those of the least frequently occurring form of non-Hodgkin lymphoma.
(C) The most likely common cytogenetic and molecular change is t(14;18) with increased expression of the oncogene *bcl-2*.
(D) Special stains are required for the diagnosis because the description is that of an anaplastic carcinoma.
(E) This diagnosis cannot be confirmed in the absence of Reed-Sternberg cells.

12. A 10-year-old boy presents with a large abdominal mass. Computed tomography of the abdomen reveals enlarged retroperitoneal and mesenteric lymph nodes. Biopsy of one of the involved lymph nodes shows a "starry-sky" appearance, with prominent debris-containing macrophages. A diagnosis of Burkitt lymphoma is made. Which of the following statements about this disorder is correct?

(A) The American form is most frequently associated with Epstein-Barr virus.
(B) The disorder is considered to be a derivative of Hodgkin lymphoma, lymphocyte depletion subtype.
(C) The most common cytogenetic change is t(8;14), with increased expression of c-*myc*.
(D) The tumor cells are derivatives of T lymphocytes.
(E) The tumor most often has an indolent clinical course.

13. A 50-year-old man presents because of a pruritic rash of several years' duration. The rash is characterized by erythematous, eczematoid patches and raised plaques and is distributed asymmetrically over the chest and abdomen. Biopsy of the plaques reveals atypical CD4+ T cells with cerebriform nuclei. Further marker studies lead to a diagnosis of mycosis fungoides. Which of the following is true of this disease?

(A) The disease eventually disseminates to lymph nodes and internal organs.
(B) The neoplastic cells most commonly display cell markers of CD19 and CD20.
(C) The skin rash most commonly disappears over time.
(D) This disease is caused by a chronic fungal infection in the skin.
(E) This is a benign condition and no further workup is necessary.

ANSWERS AND EXPLANATIONS

1-A. Chronic myelogenous leukemia is almost invariably marked by the finding of the Philadelphia chromosome, a small residual chromosome 22 with the addition of a small segment of chromosome 9, resulting from a 9;22 translocation.

2-A. Acute lymphoblastic leukemia (ALL) is the most common malignancy in children and is the form of acute leukemia that is most responsive to therapy. ALL is characterized by a predominance of lymphoblasts in the circulating blood and in the bone marrow. Other progenitor cells do not mature normally, resulting in neutropenia and thrombocytopenia. CD10-positive ALL is the most frequently occurring form of ALL and is the most amenable to therapy. Thus CD10 is a favorable prognostic marker of this disease.

3-B. The diagnosis is chronic lymphocytic leukemia (CLL). Hypogammaglobulinemia may occur early in the course of the disease, leading to frequent bacterial infections. The mean survival is 3–7 years after diagnosis, although much longer symptom-free survivals are quite common. CLL is characterized by a proliferation of neoplastic mature lymphoid cells, which are almost always B cells.

4-B. The diagnosis is multiple (plasma cell) myeloma, a neoplastic proliferation of malignant plasma cells (mature B cells, not T cells). Death is often caused by renal insufficiency caused by myeloma kidney. The average age of presentation is approximately 70 years of age. IgM myeloma is very uncommon. Both the neoplastic cells and the serum protein spike are monoclonal rather than polyclonal, and the monoclonal spike protein is most frequently an IgG or an IgA.

5-C. The illustration shows predominance of mature-appearing lymphocytes and several cells distorted mechanically in preparation of the blood smear (smudge cells), both characteristic of chronic lymphocytic leukemia (CLL). CLL most often affects older persons, many of whom are asymptomatic for many years. Generalized lymphadenopathy and hepatosplenomegaly are frequent findings.

6-A. Widespread "punched-out" lytic bone lesions in a patient in the older age group are highly suggestive of multiple (plasma cell) myeloma. IgG or IgA M proteins are almost always found in multiple myeloma. Frequent additional laboratory abnormalities include hypercalcemia and urinary excretion of Bence Jones protein (free kappa or lambda monoclonal light chains), red cell rouleaux formation resulting from hyperglobulinemia, and indicators of renal insufficiency.

7-C. The illustration shows mixed cellularity Hodgkin lymphoma. A prominent Reed-Sternberg cell can be seen. The diagnosis is based entirely on the biopsy findings, and there are no confirmatory laboratory tests.

8-D. The diagnosis is hairy cell leukemia, as evidenced by the presentation with splenomegaly, typical cellular morphology, and a positive stain for tartrate-resistant acid phosphatase (TRAP). Hairy cell leukemia is a B-cell disease, and the neoplastic cells are positive for the B cell markers CD19, CD20, and CD22. The most common presentation is in middle-aged men who present with anemia, leukopenia, and thrombocytopenia. The most common physical finding is massive splenomegaly. Hairy cell leukemia is of special interest because of the striking therapeutic efficacy of agents such as α-interferon, 2-chlorodeoxyadenosine, and deoxycoformycin.

9-A. The diagnosis is polycythemia vera (primary polycythemia), one of the myeloproliferative syndromes. The disorder is characterized by prominent erythrocytosis, moderate granulocytosis, and thrombocytosis. Because of hyperviscosity and sludging of blood, there is a frequent association with thrombosis or hemorrhagic phenomena. Marked splenomegaly and decreased erythropoietin are other classic characteristics. Cushing syndrome and hypoxic states are associated with secondary polycythemia, not polycythemia vera. About 3% of patients terminate in acute leukemia, not chronic myelogenous leukemia.

10-E. The diagnosis is Hodgkin lymphoma, nodular sclerosis subtype. This form of Hodgkin lymphoma differs from other forms of Hodgkin lymphoma in being most common in young women, having a relatively favorable clinical course, and having little association with Epstein-Barr virus infection. Lacunar cells are considered a Reed-Sternberg cell variant, and the diagnosis of nodular sclerosis can be based on the finding of fibrous bands and lacunar cells.

11-C. The findings are those of follicular lymphoma, the most frequently occurring form of non-Hodgkin lymphoma. This particular neoplasm is marked by the presence of the 14;18 translocation with increased expression of *bcl*-2, an inhibitor of apoptosis.

12-C. The typical cytogenetic change associated with Burkitt lymphoma is t(8;14) with increased expression of the c-*myc* gene. This disorder is an aggressive B-cell non-Hodgkin lymphoma most commonly affecting children. The African form is characterized by involvement of the maxilla or mandible, whereas the American form usually involves the abdominal organs. Burkitt lymphoma is generally a rapidly growing neoplasm, and the African form has a frequent association with Epstein-Barr virus.

13-A. Mycosis fungoides is a T-cell lymphoma characterized by a rash that may be sited at any cutaneous location. Atypical CD4+ T cells with cerebriform nuclei are found on biopsy. The disorder may remain localized to the skin for many years, but the neoplastic cells eventually disseminate to lymph nodes and other organs. Sézary syndrome, the leukemic form of this cutaneous T-cell lymphoma, is characterized by the combination of skin lesions and circulating neoplastic cells.

CHAPTER 13

Hemorrhagic Disorders

I. Disorders of Primary Hemostasis

A. General considerations

1. Disorders of primary hemostasis are **defects of initial platelet plug formation.**
2. Bleeding from small vessels and capillaries, resulting in mucocutaneous bleeding, is characteristic. **Petechial (pinpoint or punctate) hemorrhages** occur in the skin and mucous membranes, with bleeding and oozing from the nose (epistaxis), gums, and gastrointestinal tract. **Note:** Multiple petechial subcutaneous hemorrhages may sometimes be described as a "rash."
3. Another feature of note is often **prolonged bleeding time**. Other tests, such as the prothrombin time (PT) and activated partial thromboplastin time (APTT or PTT), are characteristically normal.
4. The causes include lesions of the vasculature, thrombocytopenia or platelet dysfunction such as Glanzmann thrombasthenia, or alterations in the plasma proteins required for adhesion of platelets to vascular subendothelium.

B. Lesions of the vasculature.

Usually no laboratory abnormalities are associated with bleeding due to small blood vessel dysfunction, but a **prolonged bleeding time** is sometimes noted. Examples include the following:

1. **Simple purpura** is **easy bruising,** especially of the upper thighs, in otherwise healthy persons.
2. **Senile purpura** is marked by hemorrhagic areas on the back of the hands and forearms of older persons. This condition is presumed to arise from age-dependent atrophy of vascular supportive tissues.
3. **Scurvy** is vitamin C deficiency. Clinical characteristics include:
   - a. Extensive primary hemostatic bleeding with **gingival hemorrhages**
   - b. Bleeding into muscles and subcutaneous tissue
   - c. **Hemorrhagic perifollicular hyperkeratotic papules**, each papule surrounding a **twisted, corkscrew-like hair**
4. **Henoch-Schönlein purpura (allergic purpura)**
   - a. This condition is a form of leukocytoclastic angiitis, hypersensitivity vasculitis resulting from an immune reaction that damages the vascular endothelium.
   - b. Characteristic features include **hemorrhagic urticaria** (palpable purpura) accompanied by **fever, arthralgias, and gastrointestinal and renal involvement.**
5. **Hereditary hemorrhagic telangiectasia (Osler-Weber-Rendu syndrome)** is an autosomal dominant disorder marked by **localized malformations of venules and capillaries** of the skin and mucous membranes, often complicated by **hemorrhage.**

6. **Connective tissue disorders** include **Ehlers-Danlos syndrome,** an inherited disorder caused by abnormalities of collagen or elastin and manifested by vascular bleeding, articular hypermobility, dermal hyperelasticity, and tissue fragility.
7. **Waldenström macroglobulinemia** produces vascular damage from sludging of hyperviscous blood. It can also cause platelet functional abnormalities.
8. **Amyloidosis** can cause **vessel damage.**
9. **Rickettsial and meningococcal diseases** include Rocky Mountain spotted fever and meningococcemia. These disorders involve the vascular endothelium, leading to necrosis and rupture of small blood vessels.

C. **Platelet disorders**

1. **Thrombocytopenia (quantitative platelet dysfunction)**
   a. **General considerations**
      (1) Dominant features include **petechial cutaneous bleeding,** intracranial bleeding, and oozing from mucosal surfaces.
      (2) Characteristics include **decreased platelet count** and **prolonged bleeding time;** bone marrow aspiration reveals decreased megakaryocytes when caused by decreased platelet production and increased megakaryocytes when caused by increased platelet destruction.
      (3) Causes include decreased production, increased destruction, unreplaced loss, or dilution of platelets, brought about by a wide variety of etiologic factors.
   b. **Irradiation, exposure to drugs or chemicals** causes decreased production.
   c. **Acute leukemia** causes decreased production because of replacement of bone marrow by blast cells.
   d. **Myelophthisis** causes decreased production because of bone marrow replacement, usually by tumor cells.
   e. **Aplastic anemia** is often caused by exposure to toxic agents such as benzene. It can also be due to autoimmune destruction by cytotoxic T cells.
   f. **Splenic sequestration** results in loss of circulating platelets.
   g. **Multiple transfusions** result in dilution.
   h. **Disseminated intravascular coagulation (DIC)** results in depletion of platelets.
   i. Thrombocytopenia may be **secondary to other diseases** such as **acquired immunodeficiency syndrome** and **systemic lupus erythematosus**.
   j. **Idiopathic thrombocytopenic purpura (ITP)**
      (1) ITP is also known as immune (or autoimmune) thrombocytopenic purpura.
      (2) In children, ITP is usually an acute, self-limiting reaction to viral infection or immunization. In adults, ITP is a chronic disorder.
      (3) Characteristics include **antiplatelet antibodies** that coat and damage platelets, which are then selectively removed by splenic macrophages. Maternal IgG antibodies in affected mothers can cause fetal thrombocytopenia.
      (4) ITP is diagnosed based on **thrombocytopenia** with normal or **increased megakaryocytes,** no known exposure to thrombocytopenic agents, and lack of palpable splenomegaly.
   k. **Thrombotic thrombocytopenic purpura (TTP)**
      (1) Characteristics include **platelet-derived hyaline microaggregates** in small vessels, **thrombocytopenia,** and **microangiopathic hemolytic anemia**. The microcirculatory lesions produce mechanical damage to red blood cells as they squeeze through the narrowed vessels, resulting in **helmet cells** and **schistocytes.**
      (2) Other features include transient **neurologic abnormalities, renal insufficiency,** and **fever.**
      (3) Causes include deficiency of von Willebrand factor (vWF) metalloprotease (ADAMTS 13). Enzyme deficiency results in accumulation of very-high-molecular-weight multimers of vWF, promoting platelet microaggregate formation.
2. **Platelet functional abnormalities (qualitative platelet dysfunction).** These platelet-mediated bleeding disorders occur in spite of a **normal platelet count.** They result in mucocutaneous bleeding and are often associated with a **prolonged bleeding time.** Causes include:

a. **Defects of platelet adhesion,** as in **von Willebrand disease** or **Bernard-Soulier disease,** an autosomal recessive disorder characterized by unusually large platelets and by lack of a platelet-surface glycoprotein (GPIb-IX-V) needed for platelet adhesion.

b. **Defects of platelet aggregation** can be either acquired or inherited and include the following examples:

(1) Aspirin-induced acetylation and inactivation of cyclooxygenase (both COX-1 and COX-2), which causes **failure of synthesis** of the **platelet aggregant thromboxane A_2**

(2) **Glanzmann thrombasthenia,** inaggregability of platelets due to hereditary deficiency of platelet-surface GPIIb-IIIa, required for formation of fibrinogen bridges between adjacent platelets

II. Disorders of Secondary Hemostasis (Table 13-1)

A. General considerations

1. Disorders of secondary hemostasis are caused by **deficiencies of plasma clotting factors** of the coagulation cascade (see Figure 3-1).

TABLE 13-1 *Laboratory Screening Tests in Selected Hemorrhagic Disorders*

Disorder	Bleeding Time	Platelet Count	PT	APTT	Thrombin Time/ Fibrinogen Assay	Confirmatory Tests or Other Significant Findings
Vascular bleeding	Usually prolonged	Normal	Normal	Normal	Normal	...
Thrombocytopenia	Prolonged	Decreased	Normal	Normal	Normal	Megakaryocytes normal or increased when thrombocytopenia is caused by increased platelet destruction, decreased when due to decreased production
Qualitative platelet defects	Prolonged	Normal	Normal	Normal	Normal	Platelet aggregation and other specialized studies
Classic hemophilia	Normal	Normal	Normal	Prolonged	Normal	Factor VIII assay
Christmas disease	Normal	Normal	Normal	Prolonged	Normal	Factor IX assay
von Willebrand disease	Prolonged	Normal	Normal	Prolonged	Normal	vWF assay
DIC	Prolonged	Decreased	Prolonged	Prolonged	Prolonged	Fibrin and fibrinogen degradation products

APTT = activated partial thromboplastin time; DIC = disseminated intravascular coagulation; PT = prothrombin time; vWF = von Willebrand factor.

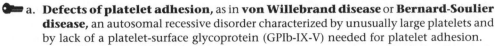

2. Manifestations include **bleeding from larger vessels,** resulting in hemarthroses, large hematomas, large ecchymoses, and extensive bleeding with trauma.
3. Bleeding time or platelet count is not affected (thus distinguishing secondary hemostatic disorders from primary hemostatic disorders).
4. Results may include abnormalities in the **PT,** reflecting deficiencies of fibrinogen or factors II, V, VII, and X; **APTT (or PTT),** reflecting deficiencies of all of the coagulation factors with the exception of factors VII and XIII; and **thrombin time,** reflecting deficiency of fibrinogen. (The whole blood clotting time is an older test that detects the same abnormalities as the APTT.)

B. **Classic hemophilia (hemophilia A, factor VIII deficiency)**
1. This common **X-linked disorder** with worldwide distribution varies in severity, depending on factor VIII activity. Severe cases have less than 1% residual factor VIII activity.
2. Characteristics include bleeding into muscles, subcutaneous tissues, and joints.
3. The disorder is associated with prolongation of the APTT (or PTT) and a normal bleeding time, platelet count, PT, and thrombin time. The prolonged APTT can be corrected in vitro by the addition of normal plasma.

C. **Christmas disease (hemophilia B, factor IX deficiency)**
1. Incidence is approximately one fifth to one tenth that of classic hemophilia.
2. Hemophilia B is **indistinguishable from classic hemophilia** in mode of inheritance and clinical features.

D. **Vitamin K deficiency**
1. In adults, vitamin K deficiency is most often caused by **fat malabsorption** from pancreatic or small-bowel disease.
2. In neonates, vitamin K deficiency causes hemorrhagic disease of the newborn, which is due to **deficient exogenous vitamin K** in breast milk in association with **incomplete intestinal colonization** by vitamin K–synthesizing bacteria.
3. Results include **decreased activity of clotting factors II, VII, IX, and X** and is reflected by **prolongation of the PT and APTT.**

III. Combined Primary and Secondary Hemostatic Defects

A. **von Willebrand disease** is the most common hereditary bleeding disorder.
1. This **autosomal** disorder is marked by **deficiency of vWF,** a large multimeric protein synthesized by endothelial cells and megakaryocytes. **vWF** is a carrier protein for factor VIII (the antihemophilic factor), and the two proteins circulate together as a complex. It also mediates adhesion of platelets to subendothelium at sites of vascular injury, reacting with the subendothelium and the platelet-surface glycoprotein complex GPIb-IX-V.
2. Characteristics include impaired platelet adhesion, prolonged bleeding time, and a functional deficiency of factor VIII.
3. **Dual hemostatic defects**
   a. Deficiency of vWF leads to a **failure of platelet adhesion,** resulting in deficient platelet plug formation manifest clinically by primary hemostatic bleeding and prolonged bleeding time.
   b. A **functional deficiency of factor VIII** occurs as a consequence of the deficit of vWF, its carrier protein. Deficiency is manifest by secondary hemostatic bleeding and prolonged APTT.

B. **Disseminated intravascular coagulation (DIC)**
1. Characteristics include widespread clotting with resultant **consumption of platelets and coagulation factors,** especially factors II, V, and VIII, and **fibrinogen.**
2. Clinical manifestations include **thrombotic phenomena** and **hemorrhage.**

3. Features include microangiopathic hemolytic anemia with fragmented red cells (schistocytes), increased fibrin and fibrinogen degradation (split) products, thrombocytopenia, and prolonged bleeding time, PT, APTT, and thrombin time.
4. Other features are microthrombi in the small vessels of many organs.
5. Causes include **release of tissue thromboplastin** (tissue factor) or **activation of the intrinsic pathway of coagulation,** as well as secondary **activation of the fibrinolytic system.**
6. DIC is seen most commonly in **obstetric complications,** such as toxemia, amniotic fluid emboli, retained dead fetus, or abruptio placentae (premature separation of placenta). It can also result from **cancer,** notably of the lung, pancreas, prostate, or stomach; from tissue damage caused by **infection,** especially gram-negative sepsis; **trauma,** as in chest surgery; or **immunologic mechanisms,** especially immune complex disease or hemolytic transfusion reactions.

C. **Coagulopathy of liver disease**
1. The coagulopathy arises because all coagulation factors except vWF are produced in the liver; therefore, as hepatocellular damage progresses, the **PT, APTT, and thrombin time are prolonged.** In addition, **prolonged bleeding time** due to platelet functional defects or overt thrombocytopenia may occur.
2. In some cases, alleviation may be obtained using **vitamin K derivatives,** which promote carboxylation of glutamyl residues of precursors of factors II, VII, IX, and X.

D. **Dilutional coagulopathy**
1. Causes may include **multiple transfusions** of stored blood deficient in platelets and factors II, V, and VIII.
2. Manifestations often include **persistent bleeding** from surgical wounds.
3. The condition may result in thrombocytopenia or prolonged PT or APTT.

Q REVIEW TEST

***Directions:** Each of the numbered items or incomplete statements in this section is followed by answers or by completions of the statement. Select the one lettered answer or completion that is best in each case.*

1. A 40-year-old woman presents with a "skin rash." Questioning reveals easy bruising on minimal trauma, menorrhagia, and frequent bouts of epistaxis. She has is not taking any medications, and there is no history of toxic exposures. Physical examination reveals multiple petechial hemorrhages most prominently on the dependent portions of the lower extremities. Splenomegaly is not detected. Laboratory studies reveal marked thrombocytopenia, and a bone marrow aspiration reveals increased numbers of megakaryocytes. Which of the following is the most likely mechanism of this disorder?

(A) Antibody-mediated platelet destruction
(B) Disseminated intravascular coagulation, with consumption of platelets and coagulation factors
(C) Intravascular spontaneous lysis of platelets due to increased osmotic fragility
(D) Myeloid stem cell suppression in the bone marrow, with inability to produce platelets
(E) Physical destruction of platelets while negotiating through partially blocked microvasculature

2. A 4-year-old boy presents with recurrent joint pain involving the knees and hips. He had always bruised easily, and recently the parents had seen blood in his urine. A presumptive diagnosis of classic hemophilia (hemophilia A) is made, and coagulation blood tests are performed. Which of the following is the most likely set of findings of coagulation screening tests?

(A) Normal bleeding time, platelet count, and thrombin time; prolonged prothrombin time (PT) and activated partial thromboplastin time (APTT)
(B) Normal bleeding time, platelet count, thrombin time, and APTT; prolonged PT
(C) Normal bleeding time, platelet count, thrombin time, and PT; prolonged APTT
(D) Normal platelet count and thrombin time; prolonged bleeding time, PT, and APTT
(E) Prolonged bleeding time, PT, APTT, and thrombin time; decreased platelet count

3. A 35-year-old woman presents with fever, fatigue, mucocutaneous bleeding, and changing neurologic signs. Laboratory examination reveals thrombocytopenia, anemia and reticulocytosis, as well as increased concentrations of creatinine and urea nitrogen. Examination of a peripheral blood smear reveals many fragmented circulating red cells (helmet cells and schistocytes). The most likely diagnosis is

(A) Bernard-Soulier disease
(B) disseminated intravascular coagulation
(C) idiopathic (immune) thrombocytopenic purpura
(D) thrombotic thrombocytopenic purpura
(E) von Willebrand disease

4. A 25-year-old man has a lifelong hemorrhagic diathesis. The prothrombin time and bleeding time are normal, but the activated partial thromboplastin time is prolonged. The most likely cause of the bleeding disorder is

(A) a platelet functional disorder
(B) factor VII deficiency
(C) factor VIII deficiency
(D) factor IX deficiency
(E) von Willebrand disease

5. A 50-year-old man has been in the medical intensive care unit for septic shock for the past few days. He has now developed rectal bleeding, epistaxis, and gingival bleeding. Disseminated intravascular coagulation is suspected. Which of the following sets of results for a panel of screening tests is most consistent with this diagnosis?

(A) Normal bleeding time, prothrombin time (PT), activated partial thromboplastin time (APTT), thrombin time, and platelet count
(B) Prolonged bleeding time, PT, APTT, and thrombin time; reduced platelet count
(C) Prolonged PT and APTT; normal bleeding time, platelet count, and thrombin time
(D) Prolonged PT and APTT; reduced platelet count; normal bleeding time and thrombin time
(E) Prolonged bleeding time, PT, and APTT; normal platelet count and thrombin time

6. A 14-year-old girl presents with prolonged bleeding from wounds and minor trauma and severe menorrhagia. Family history reveals that her father also has prolonged bleeding from wounds and minor trauma, as does her brother. Which of the following is the most likely mechanism of this patient's disorder?

(A) Absence of platelet glycoprotein IIb-IIIa
(B) Antiplatelet antibodies reacting with platelet surface glycoproteins
(C) Deficiency of factor VIII
(D) Deficiency of factor IX
(E) Deficiency of von Willebrand factor

7. A 60-year-old chronic alcoholic with known alcoholic cirrhosis presents with upper gastrointestinal hemorrhage. Despite prolonged tamponade, bleeding is persistent. A coagulation defect related to the liver disease is suspected. Which of the following abnormalities is most consistent with this possibility?

(A) Deficiency of all clotting factors except for von Willebrand factor
(B) Deficiency of factors II, VII, IX, and X
(C) Deficiency of factors II, V, VII, and X
(D) Deficiency of factors IX, X, XI, and XII
(E) Deficiency of von Willebrand factor

8. A 55-year-old woman with chronic pancreatitis undergoes coagulation screening tests before surgery. The prothrombin time and activated partial thromboplastin time are found to be prolonged. Given the following choices, which of the following is the most likely reason for the abnormal coagulation test results?

(A) Congenital inherited bleeding disorder
(B) Fat malabsorption and vitamin K deficiency
(C) Glutamate deficiency due to impaired digestion of dietary protein
(D) Nutritional vitamin C deficiency
(E) Post-pancreatic carcinoma of the pancreas

9. An 80-year-old woman presents with recent onset of primary hemostatic (mucocutaneous) bleeding. Questioning reveals that she has been maintaining a "tea and toast" diet for the past four months. Her gums are hemorrhagic and spongy in consistency, and gingival bleeding is evident. Perifollicular hyperkeratotic papules, each surrounded by a hemorrhagic halo, are scattered over the lower extremities, and each papule surrounds a twisted, corkscrew-like hair. A nutritional deficiency is suspected. Deficiency of which of the following nutrients is most likely related to the findings in this patient?

(A) Vitamin A
(B) Vitamin B_{12}
(C) Vitamin C
(D) Vitamin K
(E) Protein

10. A 7-year-old boy presents with palpable purpura on the buttocks and legs, fever, abdominal pain and vomiting, arthritis in his knees and ankles, melena, and hematuria. His mother states that he had an upper respiratory illness approximately 1 week ago but has otherwise been well. Blood tests reveal mild renal insufficiency. The most likely cause of the bleeding into the skin observed in this patient is

(A) coagulation factor deficiency
(B) qualitative platelet dysfunction
(C) quantitative platelet dysfunction
(D) vasculitis
(E) vitamin deficiency

11. A 56-year-old physician who has had a recent episode of unstable angina is advised by his cardiologist to take one "baby aspirin" a day because of the antithrombotic effect of aspirin. What is the mechanism by which aspirin acts as an antithrombotic agent?

(A) Acetylation and activation of both cyclooxygenase-1 (COX-1) and cyclooxygenase-2 (COX-2)
(B) Acetylation and inhibition of both COX-1 and COX-2
(C) Selective inhibition of COX-1
(D) Selective inhibition of COX-2

A ANSWERS AND EXPLANATIONS

1-A. Idiopathic (immune) thrombocytopenic purpura is a chronic disease in adults, presumably caused by antibodies that bind to the cell surface of platelets.

2-C. Classic hemophilia (factor VIII deficiency) is an abnormality of the intrinsic pathway of coagulation proximal to the final common pathway, which begins at factor X → Xa activation. This defect leads to a prolonged activated partial thromboplastin time. The other laboratory tests listed remain normal, because the bleeding time is a measure of platelet plug formation, the prothrombin time a measure of the extrinsic pathway of coagulation, and the thrombin time an assay of the conversion of fibrinogen to fibrin. The presumptive diagnosis is confirmed by specific factor VIII assay.

3-D. The classic pentad of thrombotic thrombocytopenic purpura includes fever, microangiopathic hemolytic anemia, thrombocytopenia, renal insufficiency, and neurologic abnormalities. Hyaline microaggregates of platelets in small vessels can be observed on histologic examination. The disorder is caused by deficiency of the enzyme von Willebrand factor (vWF) metalloprotease (also called ADAMTS 13). The enzyme promotes degradation of very-high-molecular-weight multimers of vWF, and the enzyme deficiency results in multimer accumulation in the plasma and consequent platelet microaggregate formation. The enzyme deficiency can be caused by a mutation in the gene that codes for the enzyme, or it can be caused by an antibody inhibiting the enzyme. Treatment is by plasma exchange, and the disorder can be fatal if diagnosis and therapy are delayed.

4-C. The bleeding disorder is most likely factor VIII deficiency. The patient has a disorder of the intrinsic pathway of coagulation (prolonged activated partial thromboplastin time). The abnormality is localized proximal to factor X → Xa activation because the prothrombin time is normal. Significant platelet-related problems such as von Willebrand disease are ruled out by the normal bleeding time. The two most common intrinsic pathway factor deficiencies are factor VIII and factor IX. Of these, factor VIII deficiency occurs 5 to 10 times more frequently than factor IX deficiency and therefore is the most likely cause of the bleeding disorder.

5-B. Disseminated intravascular coagulation (DIC) is characterized by widespread clotting with resultant consumption of platelets, coagulation factors, and fibrinogen, and secondary activation of the fibrinolytic system. Laboratory studies reveal thrombocytopenia; prolonged bleeding time, prothrombin time (PT), activated partial thromboplastin time (APTT), and thrombin time (reflecting decreased fibrinogen); and increased fibrin and fibrinogen split products. In addition, DIC is often marked by microangiopathic hemolytic anemia with circulating fragmented red cells.

6-E. Von Willebrand disease, a disorder transmitted by autosomal modes of inheritance (both dominant and recessive) is the most common hereditary bleeding disorder. There are many variants, all marked by either qualitative or quantitative deficiencies of von Willebrand factor.

7-A. The liver is the site of production of all coagulation factors except von Willebrand factor (vWF), and severe hepatic dysfunction can thus be associated with multiple factor deficiencies, excluding vWF.

8-B. Chronic pancreatitis causes fat malabsorption, because pancreatic lipase is required for fat digestion. Fat malabsorption leads to deficiency of the fat-soluble vitamins A, D, E, and K. Vitamin K is required in the synthesis of clotting factors II, VII, IX, and X as a cofactor for the conversion of glutamyl residues to γ-carboxyglutamates.

9-C. Vitamin C deficiency occurs in infants aged 6–12 months who are fed a diet deficient in citrus fruits or vegetables, or in elderly persons who maintain a "tea and toast" diet. Vitamin C cannot be synthesized by the body, and thus must be supplied by the diet. The body's reserve of vitamin C is approximately 1–3 months with complete dietary absence. Early signs of vitamin C deficiency include those found in this patient.

10-D. The clinical description is that of Henoch-Schönlein purpura, a form of leukocytoclastic angiitis (hypersensitivity vasculitis) resulting from an immune reaction that damages the vascular endothelium.

11-B. Aspirin permanently acetylates the active site of cyclooxygenase (both COX-1 and COX-2), causing enzyme inhibition. This subsequently inhibits synthesis of the prothrombotic agent thromboxane A_2. Thromboxane A_2 causes activation and aggregation of platelets.

CHAPTER 14

Respiratory System

I. Disorders of the Upper Respiratory Tract

A. **Acute rhinitis**

1. **Common cold.** This is the most common of all illnesses and is caused by viruses, especially the **adenoviruses.** It is manifest by coryza ("runny nose"), sneezing, nasal congestion, and mild sore throat.
2. **Allergic rhinitis.** This is mediated by an IgE **type I immune reaction** involving mucosal and submucosal mast cells. It is characterized by increased **eosinophils** in peripheral blood and nasal discharge.
3. **Bacterial infection.** This infection may be superimposed on acute viral or allergic rhinitis by injury to mucosal cilia, which may also occur from other environmental factors.
   a. Most commonly, the cause is streptococci, staphylococci, or *Haemophilus influenzae.*
   b. Fibrous scarring, decreased vascularity, and atrophy of the epithelium and mucous glands may result.

B. **Sinusitis** is **inflammation of the paranasal sinuses** often caused by extension of nasal cavity or dental infection. It results in obstructed drainage outlets from the sinuses, leading to an accumulation of mucoid secretions or exudate.

C. **Laryngitis** is **acute inflammation of the larynx** produced by viruses or bacteria, irritants, or overuse of the voice. It is characterized by inflammation and edema of the vocal cords, with resultant hoarseness.

D. **Acute epiglottitis** is **inflammation of the epiglottis** and may be life-threatening in young children. It is usually caused by *H. influenzae.*

E. **Acute laryngotracheobronchitis (croup)** is acute **inflammation of the larynx, trachea, and epiglottis** that is potentially life-threatening in infants. It is most often caused by **viral infection.** Characteristics include a harsh cough and inspiratory stridor.

II. Tumors of the Upper Respiratory Tract

A. **Malignant tumors of the nose and nasal sinuses**

1. **Nasopharyngeal carcinoma**
   a. This carcinoma is most common in Southeast Asia and East Africa.
   b. The cause is **Epstein-Barr virus.**
2. **Squamous cell carcinoma** is the most frequently occurring malignant nasal tumor.

3. **Adenocarcinoma** accounts for 5% of malignant tumors of the nose and throat.
4. **Plasmacytoma** is a plasma cell neoplasm that, in its extraosseous form, produces tumors in the upper respiratory tract.

B. **Tumors of the larynx**
1. **Singer's nodule.** This small, **benign laryngeal polyp,** usually induced by chronic irritation, such as excessive use of the voice, is associated most commonly with **heavy cigarette smoking.** It is usually localized to the **true vocal cords.**
2. **Laryngeal papilloma**
   a. This **benign neoplasm** is usually located on the true vocal cords.
   b. In adults, the neoplasm usually occurs singly and sometimes undergoes malignant change.
   c. In children, multiple lesions, caused by human papillomavirus, appear. These lesions are benign but often recur after resection.
3. **Squamous cell carcinoma**
   a. This neoplasm is the **most common malignant tumor of the larynx** and is usually seen in men older than 40 years of age; it is often associated with the combination of cigarette smoking and alcoholism.
   b. Initially, it most often presents with persistent hoarseness.
   c. **Glottic carcinoma** arises from the true vocal cords. It is the most common laryngeal carcinoma and has the best prognosis.
   d. **Supraglottic and subglottic carcinomas** are less common and typically have a poorer prognosis.

III. Chronic Obstructive Pulmonary Disease (COPD)

A. **General considerations**
1. COPD is a group of disorders characterized by **airflow obstruction** (Table 14-1).
2. Characteristics include a marked decrease in the 1-second forced expiratory volume (FEV_1) and an increased or normal forced vital capacity (FVC), resulting in a decreased FEV_1:FVC ratio.
3. COPD is often contrasted with restrictive pulmonary disease, a group of disorders characterized by reduced lung capacity due either to chest wall or skeletal abnormalities such as kyphoscoliosis or to interstitial or infiltrative parenchymal disease. In restrictive lung disease, the FEV_1 and FVC are both decreased proportionately, resulting in a normal FEV_1: FVC ratio.

TABLE 14-1 *Pathologic Findings in Chronic Obstructive Pulmonary Disease*

Disorder	Pathologic Findings
Bronchial asthma	Bronchial smooth muscle hypertrophy Hyperplasia of bronchial submucosal glands and goblet cells Airways plugged by viscid mucus containing Curschmann spirals, eosinophils, and Charcot-Leyden crystals
Chronic bronchitis	Hyperplasia of bronchial submucosal glands, leading to increased Reid index, ratio of the thickness of the gland layer to that of the bronchial wall
Pulmonary emphysema	Abnormal dilation of air spaces with destruction of alveolar walls Reduced lung elasticity
Bronchiectasis	Abnormally dilated bronchi filled with mucus and neutrophils Inflammation and necrosis of bronchial walls and alveolar fibrosis

B. **Bronchial asthma**

1. Types include **extrinsic** and **intrinsic asthma.**
   a. **Extrinsic (immune) asthma** is mediated by a **type I hypersensitivity response** involving IgE bound to mast cells. Disease begins in **childhood,** usually in patients with a family history of allergy.
   b. Intrinsic (nonimmune) asthma includes asthma associated with **chronic bronchitis** as well as other asthma variants such as **exercise- or cold-induced asthma.** It usually begins in **adult life** and is not associated with a history of allergy.
2. **Characteristics**
   a. There is marked episodic **dyspnea** and **wheezing expiration** caused by narrowing of the airways. Bronchial asthma is related to increased sensitivity of air passages to stimuli.
   b. Morphologic manifestations include bronchial smooth muscle hypertrophy, hyperplasia of goblet cells, thickening and hyalinization of basement membranes, proliferation of eosinophils, and intrabronchial mucous plugs containing whorl-like accumulations of epithelial cells (Curschmann spirals) and crystalloids of eosinophil-derived proteins (Charcot-Leyden crystals).
3. **Complications** include **superimposed infection, chronic bronchitis,** and **pulmonary emphysema.** Bronchial asthma may lead to **status asthmaticus,** a prolonged bout of bronchial asthma that can last for days and that responds poorly to therapy. Death can result.

C. **Chronic bronchitis**

1. The clinical definition is a productive cough that occurs during at least 3 consecutive months over at least 2 consecutive years.
2. Chronic bronchitis is clearly linked to **cigarette smoking** and is also associated with air pollution, infection, and genetic factors. It may lead to **cor pulmonale.**
3. Typical characteristics include hypersecretion of mucus due to marked **hyperplasia of mucus-secreting submucosal glands.**

D. **Emphysema**

1. **General considerations**
   a. Emphysema is **dilation of air spaces** with destruction of alveolar walls and lack of elastic recoil.
   b. The disease is strongly associated with cigarette smoking.
   c. Clinical characteristics include increased anteroposterior diameter of the chest; increased total vital capacity; and hypoxia, cyanosis, and respiratory acidosis.
2. **Types of emphysema**
   a. **Centrilobular emphysema.** Dilation of the respiratory bronchioles is most often localized to the upper part of the pulmonary lobes.
   b. **Panacinar emphysema**
      (1) Dilation of the entire acinus, including the alveoli, alveolar ducts, respiratory bronchioles, and terminal bronchioles, is most often distributed uniformly throughout the lung.
      (2) It is associated with loss of elasticity and sometimes with genetically determined **deficiency of α_1-antitrypsin** (α_1-protease inhibitor).
   c. **Paraseptal emphysema**
      (1) Dilation involves mainly the distal part of the acinus, including the alveoli and, to a lesser extent, the alveolar ducts. It tends to localize subjacent to the pleura and interlobar septa.
      (2) It is associated occasionally with large subpleural bullae, or blebs.
   d. **Irregular emphysema.** Irregular involvement of the acinus with scarring within the walls of enlarged air spaces is usually a complication of various inflammatory processes.
3. **Complications**
   a. Emphysema is often complicated by, or coexistent with, **chronic bronchitis.**

b. **Interstitial emphysema,** in which air escapes into the interstitial tissues of the chest from a tear in the airways, may occur.

c. Other complications of emphysema may include rupture of a surface bleb with resultant pneumothorax.

4. **Postulated causes.** Emphysema may result from action of proteolytic enzymes such as elastase on the alveolar wall. Elastase can induce destruction of elastin unless neutralized by the antiproteinase-antielastase activities of α_1-antitrypsin.

a. **Cigarette smoking** attracts neutrophils and macrophages, which are sources of elastase. It also inactivates α_1-antitrypsin.

b. **Hereditary α_1-antitrypsin deficiency** accounts for a small subgroup of cases of **panacinar emphysema.** It is caused by variants in the *pi* (proteinase inhibitor) gene, localized to chromosome 14.

(1) The **piZ allele** codes for a structural alteration in the protein that interferes with its hepatic secretion. Hepatic cytoplasmic droplets accumulate, with resultant liver damage.

(2) The **homozygous state (piZZ)** is associated with greatly decreased activity in α_1-antitrypsin, panacinar emphysema, and often hepatic cirrhosis.

E. Bronchiectasis

1. This condition is **permanent abnormal bronchial dilation** caused by chronic infection, with inflammation and necrosis of the bronchial wall.
2. Predisposing factors include **bronchial obstruction,** most often by tumor.
3. Other predisposing factors include **chronic sinusitis** accompanied by postnasal drip. Disease rarely may be a manifestation of **Kartagener syndrome** (**sinusitis, bronchiectasis, and situs inversus**, sometimes with hearing loss and male sterility), caused by a defect in the motility of respiratory, auditory, and sperm cilia that is referred to as **primary ciliary dyskinesia,** an uncommon autosomal recessive syndrome. In this condition, there is a structural defect in dynein arms. Impaired ciliary activity predisposes to infection in the sinuses and bronchi and disturbs embryogenesis, sometimes resulting in situs inversus. **Male infertility** is an important manifestation of ciliary dyskinesia.
4. Bronchiectasis most often involves the lower lobes of both lungs.
5. Characteristics include production of **copious purulent sputum,** hemoptysis, and recurrent pulmonary infection that may lead to **lung abscess.**

IV. Restrictive Pulmonary Disease

A. General considerations

1. Restrictive pulmonary disease is a group of disorders characterized by **reduced expansion of the lung and reduction in total lung capacity.**
2. Examples include abnormalities of the chest wall from **bony abnormalities** or **neuromuscular disease** that restrict lung expansion.
3. Also included are the **interstitial lung diseases,** a heterogeneous group of disorders characterized by interstitial accumulations of cells or noncellular material within the alveolar walls that restrict expansion and often interfere with gaseous exchange. Prominent examples are acute conditions such as the **adult and neonatal respiratory distress syndromes; pneumoconioses** such as coal workers' pneumoconiosis, silicosis, and asbestosis; diseases of unknown etiology such as **sarcoidosis and idiopathic pulmonary fibrosis;** various other conditions such as eosinophilic granuloma, hypersensitivity pneumonitis, and chemical- or drug-associated disorders such as berylliosis or the pulmonary fibrosis associated with bleomycin toxicity; and immune disorders such as **systemic lupus erythematosus, systemic sclerosis (scleroderma)** (see Chapter 5), **Wegener granulomatosis** (see Chapter 9), and **Goodpasture syndrome** (see Chapter 17).

B. **Adult respiratory distress syndrome (ARDS)**

1. ARDS is produced by **diffuse alveolar damage** with resultant increase in alveolar capillary permeability, causing leakage of protein-rich fluid into alveoli.
2. Characteristics include the formation of an **intra-alveolar hyaline membrane** composed of fibrin and cellular debris.
3. The result is severe impairment of respiratory gas exchange with consequent severe hypoxia.
4. Causes include a wide variety of mechanisms and toxic agents, including shock, sepsis, trauma, uremia, aspiration of gastric contents, acute pancreatitis, inhalation of chemical irritants such as chlorine, oxygen toxicity, or overdose with street drugs such as heroin or therapeutic drugs such as bleomycin.
5. ARDS can be a manifestation of the severe acute respiratory syndrome (SARS). The SARS virus is a coronavirus that destroys the type II pneumocytes and causes diffuse alveolar damage.
6. ARDS is initiated by damage to alveolar capillary endothelium and alveolar epithelium and is influenced by the following pathogenetic factors:
   a. Neutrophils release substances toxic to the alveolar wall.
   b. Activation of the coagulation cascade is suggested by the presence of microemboli.
   c. Oxygen toxicity is mediated by the formation of oxygen-derived free radicals.

C. **Neonatal respiratory distress syndrome (hyaline membrane disease)**

1. **General considerations**
   a. Neonatal respiratory distress syndrome is the most common cause of respiratory failure in the newborn and is the most common cause of death in premature infants.
   b. This syndrome is marked by dyspnea, cyanosis, and tachypnea shortly after birth.
   c. This syndrome results from a deficiency of surfactant, most often as a result of immaturity.
2. **Pathogenesis**
   a. **Role of surfactant**
      (1) Surfactant reduces surface tension within the lung, facilitating expansion during inspiration and preventing atelectasis during expiration.
      (2) Surfactant consists primarily of dipalmitoyl lecithin and is secreted by type II pneumocytes.
      (3) **Fetal pulmonary maturity** can be assessed by measuring the ratio of surfactant lecithin to sphingomyelin in the amniotic fluid; the lecithin concentration increases from about the 33rd week of pregnancy, while the sphingomyelin concentration remains stable. A lecithin-sphingomyelin ratio of 2:1 or greater indicates pulmonary maturity.
   b. **Predisposing factors**
      (1) **Prematurity**
      (2) **Maternal diabetes mellitus**
      (3) Birth by **cesarean section**
3. **Pathologic findings**
   a. Lungs are heavier than usual, with areas of atelectasis alternating with occasional dilated alveoli or alveolar ducts.
   b. Small pulmonary vessels are engorged, with leakage of blood products into the alveoli and formation of intra-alveolar **hyaline membranes** consisting of fibrin and cellular debris.
4. **Complications and associated conditions**
   a. **Bronchopulmonary dysplasia,** which appears to be precipitated by treatment with high-concentration oxygen and mechanical ventilation
   b. **Patent ductus arteriosus,** caused by failure of closure of the ductus caused by immaturity and hypoxia
   c. **Intraventricular brain hemorrhage**
   d. **Necrotizing enterocolitis,** a fulminant inflammation of the small and large intestines

D. **Pneumoconioses.** These environmental diseases are caused by **inhalation of inorganic dust particles.** They are exemplified by the following conditions:

1. **Anthracosis** is caused by inhalation of **carbon dust;** it is endemic in urban areas and causes no harm. Characterized by **carbon-carrying macrophages,** it results in irregular black patches visible on gross inspection.
2. **Coal workers' pneumoconiosis** is caused by inhalation of **coal dust,** which contains both carbon and silica.
   a. **Simple coal workers' pneumoconiosis** is marked by **coal macules** around the bronchioles, formed by ingestion of coal dust particles by macrophages. In most cases, it is inconsequential and produces no disability.
   b. **Progressive massive fibrosis** is marked by fibrotic nodules filled with necrotic black fluid. It can result in **bronchiectasis, pulmonary hypertension,** or death from respiratory failure or right-sided heart failure.
3. **Silicosis** is a chronic occupational lung disease caused by **exposure to free silica dust;** it is seen in miners, glass manufacturers, and stone cutters.
   a. This disease is initiated by ingestion of silica dust by alveolar macrophages; damage to macrophages initiates an inflammatory response mediated by lysosomal enzymes and various chemical mediators.
   b. **Silicotic nodules** that enlarge and eventually obstruct the airways and blood vessels are characteristic.
   c. Silicosis is associated with increased susceptibility to tuberculosis; the frequent concurrence is referred to as **silicotuberculosis.**
4. **Asbestosis** is caused by **inhalation of asbestos fibers.**
   a. This disease is initiated by uptake of asbestos fibers by alveolar macrophages. A fibroblastic response occurs, probably from release of fibroblast-stimulating growth factors by macrophages, and leads to **diffuse interstitial fibrosis,** mainly in the lower lobes.
   b. It is characterized by **ferruginous bodies,** yellow-brown, rod-shaped bodies with clubbed ends that stain positively with Prussian blue; these arise from iron and protein coating on fibers. Dense **hyalinized fibrocalcific plaques of the parietal pleura** are also present.
   c. Asbestosis results in marked predisposition to **bronchogenic carcinoma** and to **malignant mesothelioma** of the pleura or peritoneum. Cigarette smoking further increases the risk of bronchogenic carcinoma.

E. **Restrictive lung diseases of unknown etiology**

1. **Sarcoidosis**
   a. Characteristics include **noncaseating granulomas,** often involving multiple **organ systems;** can involve almost any organ system
   b. Occurrence is most frequent in persons of **African lineage.** Sarcoidosis usually becomes clinically apparent during the **teenage or young adult years.**
   c. **Common pathologic changes**
      (1) Interstitial lung disease
      (2) Enlarged hilar lymph nodes
      (3) Anterior uveitis
      (4) Erythema nodosum of the skin
      (5) Polyarthritis
   d. **Immunologic phenomena**
      (1) Reduced sensitivity and often anergy to skin test antigens (characteristically negative result on a tuberculin test)
      (2) Polyclonal hyperglobulinemia
   e. **Clinical abnormalities.** On routine chest radiography, sarcoidosis most often presents with:
      (1) Bilateral hilar lymphadenopathy
      (2) Interstitial lung disease manifest as diffuse reticular densities

TABLE 14-2 *Selected Examples of Interstitial Lung Disease*

Disorder	Description
Hypersensitivity pneumonitis (extrinsic allergic alveolitis)	Interstitial pneumonia caused by inhalation of various antigenic substances; exemplified by inhalation of spores of thermophilic actinomycetes from moldy hay causing "farmer's lung"
Goodpasture syndrome	Hemorrhagic pneumonitis and glomerulonephritis caused by antibodies directed against glomerular basement membranes
Idiopathic pulmonary hemosiderosis	Resembles pulmonary component of Goodpasture syndrome without renal component
Eosinophilic granuloma	Proliferation of histiocytic cells related to Langerhans cells of the skin
Idiopathic pulmonary fibrosis	Immune complex disease with progressive fibrosis of the alveolar wall
Sarcoidosis	Granulomatous disorder of unknown etiology

f. Laboratory findings
   (1) Hypercalcemia and hypercalciuria
   (2) Hypergammaglobulinemia
   (3) Increased activity of serum angiotensin-converting enzyme

g. Definitive diagnosis requires biopsy demonstrating noncaseating granulomas.

2. **Idiopathic pulmonary fibrosis**
   a. This disease is characterized by **chronic inflammation and fibrosis of the alveolar wall.** It begins with alveolitis, progresses to fibrosis, and ends in a distorted fibrotic lung filled with cystic spaces (honeycomb lung).
   b. Death often results within 5 years.

F. **Other interstitial lung diseases** (Table 14-2)
1. **Eosinophilic granuloma**
   a. Morphologic changes involve a localized proliferation of histiocytic cells closely related to the Langerhans cells of the skin. These cells have characteristic cytoplasmic inclusions (**Birbeck granules**) resembling tennis rackets. Other characteristics include prominent monocytes-macrophages, lymphocytes, and eosinophils.
   b. The disease is found in the lung or in bony sites such as the ribs.
   c. Eosinophilic granuloma is often grouped with Hand-Schüller-Christian disease and Letterer-Siwe syndrome as a variant of **histiocytosis X** syndrome.
2. **Hypersensitivity pneumonitis** (see Table 14-2)

V. Pulmonary Vascular Disease

A. **Pulmonary embolism**
1. This is found in more than half of all autopsies.
2. Most often, pulmonary embolism originates from **venous thrombosis** in the lower extremities or pelvis. Rarely, it can be due to nonthrombotic particulate material such as fat, amniotic fluid, clumps of tumor cells or bone marrow, or foreign matter such as bullet fragments.
3. Pulmonary embolism occurs in clinical settings marked by **venous stasis,** including primary venous disease, congestive heart failure, prolonged bed rest or immobilization, and prolonged sitting while traveling. Other predisposing factors include cancer, multiple fractures, and the use of oral contraceptives.

4. These emboli can result in **hemorrhagic, or red, infarcts,** usually in patients with compromised circulation, but embolism can occur without infarction because of the dual blood supply to the lungs.
5. Clinical consequences may vary and range from asymptomatic disease to sudden death.

B. **Pulmonary hypertension**

1. **Primary pulmonary hypertension** is a disorder of **unknown etiology** and poor prognosis that arises in the absence of heart or lung disease.
2. **Secondary pulmonary hypertension** is more common than the primary form.
   a. Most often, the cause is **COPD.** Other causes may be **increased pulmonary blood flow,** as in congenital left-to-right shunt; **increased resistance within the pulmonary circulation,** from embolism or vasoconstriction secondary to hypoxia; or **increased blood viscosity** from polycythemia.
   b. This is a cause of **right ventricular hypertrophy.**

C. **Pulmonary edema** is intra-alveolar accumulation of fluid. It **may be caused by:**

1. **Increased hydrostatic pressure,** as a result of left ventricular failure or mitral stenosis
2. **Increased alveolar capillary permeability,** as in inflammatory alveolar reactions, resulting from inhalation of irritant gases, pneumonia, shock, sepsis, pancreatitis, uremia, or drug overdose
3. **Miscellaneous mechanisms** such as rapid ascent to high altitude

VI. Pulmonary Infection

A. **Pneumonia**

1. **General considerations**
   a. Pneumonia is an inflammatory process of infectious origin affecting the pulmonary parenchyma.
   b. It is characterized by **chills and fever,** productive cough, blood-tinged or **rusty sputum,** pleuritic pain, hypoxia with shortness of breath, and sometimes cyanosis.
   c. If bacterial, it is most characteristically associated with neutrophilic leukocytosis with an increase in band neutrophils ("shift-to-the-left").
2. **Morphologic types of pneumonia.** There are three morphologic and clinical patterns: **lobar pneumonia, bronchopneumonia,** and **interstitial pneumonia** (Table 14-3).
3. **Bacterial pneumonias** (Table 14-4)
   a. **Lobar pneumonia** is most often caused by *Streptococcus pneumoniae* (the pneumococcus). It is characterized by a predominantly **intra-alveolar exudate** and **may involve an entire lobe** of the lung.
   b. **Bronchopneumonia** is caused by a wide variety of organisms. It is characterized by a **patchy distribution** involving **one or more lobes,** with an inflammatory infiltrate extending from the bronchioles into the adjacent alveoli.
4. **Interstitial (primary atypical) pneumonia** is caused by various infectious agents, most commonly ***Mycoplasma pneumoniae*** or **viruses.** It is characterized by **diffuse, patchy inflammation** localized to interstitial areas of alveolar walls.
   a. ***Mycoplasma* pneumonia**
      (1) This is the **most common form of interstitial pneumonia;** it usually occurs in children and young adults, and it **may occur in epidemics.**
      (2) Onset is more insidious compared to bacterial pneumonia and usually follows a mild, self-limited course.
      (3) Characteristics include an inflammatory reaction **confined to the interstitium,** with no exudate in alveolar spaces, and **intra-alveolar hyaline membranes.**
      (4) Diagnosis is by **sputum cultures,** requiring several weeks of incubation, and by complement-fixing antibodies.
      (5) Mycoplasma pneumonia may be associated with **nonspecific cold agglutinins** reactive to red cells. This phenomenon is the basis for a facile laboratory test that can provide early diagnostic information.

TABLE 14-3 ***Morphologic Variants of Pneumonia: Causative Organisms and Characteristics***

Variant	Causative Organism	Characteristics
Lobar pneumonia	Most frequently *Streptococcus pneumoniae* (pneumococcus)	Predominantly intra-alveolar exudate resulting in consolidation May involve the entire lobe If untreated, may morphologically evolve through four stages: congestion, red hepatization, gray hepatization, and resolution
Bronchopneumonia	Many organisms, including *Staphylococcus aureus, Haemophilus influenzae, Klebsiella pneumoniae,* and *Streptococcus pyogenes*	Acute inflammatory infiltrates extending from the bronchioles into the adjacent alveoli Patchy distribution involving one or more lobes
Interstitial pneumonia	Most frequently viruses or *Mycoplasma pneumoniae*	Diffuse, patchy inflammation localized to interstitial areas of the alveolar walls
		Distribution involving one or more lobes

b. **Viral pneumonias** are the most common types of pneumonia in childhood. They are caused most commonly by **influenza viruses,** adenoviruses, rhinovirus, and respiratory syncytial virus; may also arise after childhood exanthems such as rubeola (measles) or varicella (chickenpox); the measles virus produces **giant cell pneumonia,** marked by numerous giant cells and often complicated by tracheobronchitis.

c. **Rickettsial pneumonias: Q fever** is the most common **rickettsial pneumonia;** it is caused by *Coxiella burnetii.* It may infect persons working with infected cattle or sheep, who inhale dust particles containing the organism, or those who drink **unpasteurized milk** from infected animals.

d. **Ornithosis (psittacosis)** is caused by an organism of the genus *Chlamydia,* which is transmitted by inhalation of dried excreta of infected birds.

5. ***Pneumocystis carinii* pneumonia** is the most common **opportunistic infection in patients with acquired immunodeficiency syndrome (AIDS)**; it also occurs in other forms of immunodeficiency.
   a. It is caused by *P. carinii* (recently renamed *Pneumocystis jiroveci*), which is now classified as a fungus.
   b. Diagnosis is by morphologic demonstration of the organism in biopsy or bronchial washing specimens.
6. **Hospital-acquired gram-negative pneumonias**
   a. These pneumonias are often fatal and occur in hospitalized patients, usually those with serious, debilitating diseases.
   b. Causes include many **gram-negative organisms,** including *Klebsiella, Pseudomonas aeruginosa,* and *Escherichia coli.* Endotoxins produced by these organisms play an important role in the infection.

B. **Lung abscess**

1. This is a **localized area of suppuration** within the parenchyma, **usually resulting from bronchial obstruction (often by cancer)** or from **aspiration of gastric contents;** may also be a complication of bacterial pneumonia.

TABLE 14-4 *Important Features of Selected Bacterial Pneumonias*

Organism	Characteristics	Complications
Streptococcus pneumoniae	Most common in elderly or debilitated patients, especially those with cardiopulmonary disease, and malnourished persons	May lead to empyema (pus in the pleural cavity)
Staphylococcus aureus	Often a complication of influenza or viral pneumonias or a result of blood-borne infection in intravenous drug users; seen principally in debilitated hospitalized patients, the elderly, and those with chronic lung disease	Focal inflammatory exudates or abscess formation frequent; may lead to empyema or to other infectious complications, including bacterial endocarditis and brain and kidney abscesses
Streptococcus pyogenes	Often a complication of influenza or measles	Lung abscess
Klebsiella pneumoniae	Most frequent in debilitated hospitalized patients and diabetic or alcoholic patients; high mortality rate in elderly patients	Considerable alveolar wall damage, leading to necrosis, sometimes with abscess formation
Haemophilus influenzae	Usually seen in infants and children but may occur in debilitated adults, most often those with chronic obstructive pulmonary disease	Meningitis and epiglottitis in infants and children
Legionella pneumophila	Infection from inhalation of aerosol from contaminated stored water, most often in air-conditioning systems	

2. Patients predisposed to aspiration by **loss of consciousness** from alcohol or drug overdose, neurologic disorders, or general anesthesia are especially likely to have lung abscesses.
3. Frequent causes include *Staphylococcus, Pseudomonas, Klebsiella,* or *Proteus,* often in combination with anaerobic organisms.
4. Clinical manifestations include fever, foul-smelling purulent sputum, and radiographic evidence of a fluid-filled cavity.

C. **Tuberculosis**
1. **General considerations**
   a. Tuberculosis occurs worldwide, with greatest frequency in disadvantaged groups.
   b. In the pulmonary form, it is spread by inhalation of droplets containing the organism *Mycobacterium tuberculosis* (also referred to as the tubercle bacillus).
   c. In the nonpulmonary form, it is most often caused by the ingestion of infected milk.
2. **Types of tuberculosis**
   a. **Primary tuberculosis is the initial infection, characterized by the primary, or Ghon, complex,** the combination of a peripheral subpleural parenchymal lesion and involved hilar lymph nodes.
      (1) Although granulomatous inflammation is characteristic of both primary and secondary tuberculosis, the Ghon complex is characteristic only of primary tuberculosis. The granuloma of tuberculosis is referred to as a tubercle and is characterized

by central caseous necrosis and often by Langhans giant cells. The calcified lesions are often visible on radiography.

(2) Primary tuberculosis is most often asymptomatic. It usually does not progress to clinically evident disease.

b. **Secondary tuberculosis** usually results from activation of a prior Ghon complex, with spread to a new pulmonary or extrapulmonary site.

(1) Clinical characteristics include progressive disability, fever, **hemoptysis,** pleural effusion (often bloody), and **generalized wasting.**

(2) **Pathologic changes**

(a) **Localized lesions,** usually in the **apical** or posterior segments of the upper lobes. Involvement of **hilar lymph nodes** is also common.

(b) **Tubercle formation.** The lesions frequently coalesce and rupture into the bronchi. The caseous contents may liquefy and be expelled, resulting in **cavitary lesions.** Cavitation is a characteristic of secondary, but not primary, tuberculosis; caseation (a manifestation of partial immunity) is seen in both.

(c) **Scarring and calcification**

(3) **Spread of disease**

(a) Secondary tuberculosis may be complicated by lymphatic and hematogenous spread, resulting in **miliary tuberculosis,** which is seeding of distal organs with innumerable small millet seed-like lesions.

(b) Hematogenous spread may also result in larger lesions, which may involve almost any organ.

(c) Prominent examples of **extrapulmonary tuberculosis** include tuberculous meningitis, Pott disease of the spine, paravertebral abscess, or psoas abscess.

3. **Immune mechanisms in pathogenesis of tuberculosis**

a. The organisms are ingested by macrophages, which process the bacterial antigens for presentation to CD4 T_H1 T cells in the context of class II MHC molecules.

b. The CD4+ T cells proliferate and secrete cytokines, attracting lymphocytes and macrophages.

c. The macrophages ingest and kill some of the tubercle bacilli or are morphologically altered to form epithelioid cells and Langhans multinucleated giant cells.

d. The causes of caseous necrosis remain obscure but most likely include the action of cytokines elaborated by immunologically stimulated cells.

e. Delayed hypersensitivity is marked by a **positive tuberculin skin test result.** The test result is positive in both primary and secondary infection, represents hypersensitivity and relative immunity, and usually remains positive throughout life.

D. ***Mycobacterium avium-intracellulare*** **infection** is an infection with nontuberculous mycobacteria.

1. This infection is seen most often in patients with AIDS and other immunodeficiency diseases.
2. Often, nonpulmonary involvement is a manifestation.

E. **Infections caused by fungi and fungus-like bacteria** (Table 14-5)

1. These infections usually result from inhalation of the organism or from inoculation through the skin.
2. In most instances, they are manifest as inflammatory reactions similar to tuberculosis.

VII. Miscellaneous Disorders of the Lungs

A. **Atelectasis**

1. **Acquired atelectasis** is **alveolar collapse** caused by bronchial obstruction or external compression of lung parenchyma by tumors or by pleural accumulation of fluid.
2. **Atelectasis neonatorum** is failure of alveolar spaces to expand adequately at birth; it occurs in two forms.

TABLE 14-5 *Characteristics of Pulmonary Infections Caused by Fungi and Fungus-like Bacteria*

Disorder	Organism	Characteristics
Actinomycosis	*Actinomyces*, gram-positive anaerobic filamentous bacteria no longer classified as a fungus	Abscess and sinus tract formation Exudate containing characteristic sulfur granules, yellow clumps of the organism
Nocardiosis	*Nocardia*, gram-positive aerobic, filamentous, weakly acid-fast bacteria closely related to *Actinomyces*	Typically opportunistic infection May disseminate to the brain and meninges
Candidiasis	*Candida albicans*	In immunocompromised patients, invasive form produces blood-borne dissemination Pulmonary, renal, and hepatic abscesses and vegetative endocarditis
Cryptococcosis	*Cryptococcus neoformans*	Infection usually begins in the lungs but can also produce cryptococcal meningitis Organism's characteristic encapsulated appearance visualized in India ink preparations
Aspergillosis	*Aspergillus*	Invasive form has predilection for growth into vessels, with consequent widespread hematogenous dissemination
Histoplasmosis	*Histoplasma capsulatum*	Pulmonary manifestations similar to tuberculosis; occurs in primary and secondary forms Results in multiple pulmonary lesions with late calcification Disseminated form, marked by multisystem involvement with infiltrates of macrophages filled with fungal yeast forms
Coccidioidomycosis	*Coccidioides immitis*	Occurs in primary and disseminated forms Fungal spherules containing endospores found within granulomas

a. **Primary atelectasis** is failure of initial aeration of the lungs at birth; the alveoli remain collapsed and respiration is never fully established. It is associated with **prematurity** and **intrauterine fetal anoxia.**

b. **Secondary atelectasis** is collapse of previously aerated bronchi.

B. **Pulmonary alveolar proteinosis** is uncommon and is characterized by accumulation of amorphous, periodic acid–Schiff–positive material in the alveolar air spaces. This material sometimes appears to be surfactant.

VIII. Cancers of the Lung

A. **General considerations.** Most lung tumors are malignant; those that arise from **metastases** from primary tumors elsewhere occur more frequently than those that originate in the lung (Table 14-6).

TABLE 14-6 *Tumors of the Lung*

Type	Location	Characteristics
Bronchogenic carcinoma:		
Squamous cell carcinoma	Central	Appears as a hilar mass and frequently results in cavitation; clearly linked to smoking; incidence greatly increased in smokers; may be marked by inappropriate parathyroid hormone (PTH)-like activity with resultant hypercalcemia
Adenocarcinoma		
Bronchial-derived	Peripheral	Develops on site of prior pulmonary inflammation or injury (scar carcinoma); less clearly linked to smoking
Bronchioloalveolar	Peripheral	Less clearly related to smoking; columnar-to-cuboidal tumor cells line alveolar walls; multiple densities on x-ray, mimicking pneumonia
Small cell (oat cell) carcinoma	Central	Undifferentiated tumor; most aggressive bronchogenic carcinoma; least likely form to be cured by surgery; usually already metastatic at diagnosis; often associated with ectopic production of corticotrophin (ACTH) or antidiuretic hormone (ADH); incidence greatly increased in smokers
Large cell carcinoma	Peripheral	Undifferentiated tumor; may show features of squamous cell or adenocarcinoma on electron microscopy
Other carcinomas of the lung:		
Carcinoid	Major bronchi	Low malignancy, spreading by direct extension into adjacent tissues; may result in carcinoid syndrome
Carcinoma metastatic to the lung	...	Higher incidence than primary lung cancer

B. **Bronchogenic carcinoma**

1. **Etiology and epidemiology**
   a. Bronchogenic carcinoma is the leading cause of death from cancer in both men and women. It is increasing in incidence, especially in women, in parallel with cigarette smoking.
   b. This type of carcinoma is directly proportional in incidence to the number of cigarettes smoked daily and to the number of years of smoking. Various histologic changes, including squamous metaplasia of the respiratory epithelium, often with atypical changes ranging from dysplasia to carcinoma in situ, precede bronchogenic carcinoma in cigarette smokers.
2. **Other etiopathogenic factors**
   a. Air pollution
   b. Radiation; incidence increased in radium and uranium workers
   c. Asbestos; increased incidence with asbestos and greater increase with combination of asbestos and cigarette smoking
   d. Industrial exposure to nickel and chromates
3. **Clinical features**
   a. The 5-year survival rate is less than 10%.
   b. The tumor often spreads by local extension into the pleura, pericardium, or ribs.

c. Clinical manifestations may include cough, hemoptysis, and bronchial obstruction, often with atelectasis and pneumonitis. Other **clinical features** include:

(1) **Superior vena cava syndrome;** compression or invasion of the superior vena cava, resulting in facial swelling and cyanosis along with dilation of the veins of the head, neck, and upper extremities

(2) **Pancoast tumor** (superior sulcus tumor); involvement of the apex of the lung, often with **Horner syndrome** (ptosis, miosis, and anhidrosis); due to involvement of the cervical sympathetic plexus

(3) **Hoarseness** from recurrent laryngeal nerve paralysis

(4) **Pleural effusion,** often bloody; bloody pleural effusion suggests malignancy, tuberculosis, or trauma.

(5) **Paraneoplastic endocrine syndromes,** the most frequent of which is adrenocorticotropic hormone (ACTH) or ACTH-like activity with small cell carcinoma; also of note are the syndrome of inappropriate antidiuretic hormone secretion (SIADH) with small cell carcinoma of the lung and parathyroid-like activity with squamous cell carcinoma.

4. **Classification**

a. Bronchogenic carcinoma is subclassified into squamous cell carcinoma, adenocarcinoma (including bronchioloalveolar carcinoma), small cell carcinoma, and large cell carcinoma; it appears that all share a common endodermal origin despite their morphologic differences.

b. For therapeutic purposes, the bronchogenic carcinomas are often subclassified into small cell carcinoma, which is not considered amenable to surgery, and non-small cell carcinoma, in which surgical intervention may be considered.

REVIEW TEST

***Directions:** Each of the numbered items or incomplete statements in this section is followed by answers or by completions of the statement. Select the **one** lettered answer or completion that is best in each case.*

1. A 3-year-old girl presents to the emergency department with fever, hoarseness, a "seal bark-like" cough, and inspiratory stridor. Her father states that she has had a cold for the past few days, with runny nose, nasal congestion, sore throat, and cough. He is now concerned because her cough has now become loud, harsh, and brassy. Which of the following is the most likely cause of her ailment?

(A) Fungus
(B) Gram-negative bacteria
(C) Gram-positive bacteria
(D) Parasite
(E) Virus

2. A 60-year-old man, a heavy smoker, presents for advice to stop smoking. On physical examination, he is thin and has a ruddy complexion. He has a productive cough and a barrel-shaped chest. He sits leaning forward with his lips pursed to facilitate his breathing. A diagnosis of emphysema is made. Which of the following is the most likely histologic finding in the lungs?

(A) Bronchial smooth muscle hypertrophy with proliferation of eosinophils
(B) Diffuse alveolar damage with leakage of protein-rich fluid into alveolar spaces
(C) Dilation of air spaces with destruction of alveolar walls
(D) Hyperplasia of bronchial mucus-secreting submucosal glands
(E) Permanent bronchial dilation caused by chronic infection, with bronchi filled with mucus and neutrophils

3. A 60-year-old woman with a heavy smoking history presents with chronic productive cough that has been present for 3 consecutive months over the past 2 consecutive years. On physical examination, her skin has a bluish tinge, and she is overweight. The patient is diagnosed with chronic bronchitis. Which of the following is the most likely histologic finding in this patient's lungs?

(A) Bronchial smooth muscle hypertrophy with proliferation of eosinophils
(B) Diffuse alveolar damage with leakage of protein-rich fluid into alveolar spaces
(C) Dilation of air spaces with destruction of alveolar walls
(D) Hyperplasia of bronchial mucus-secreting submucosal glands
(E) Permanent bronchial dilation caused by chronic infection, with bronchi filled with mucus and neutrophils

4. A 65-year-old woman with a significant smoking history presents with cough and shortness of breath. Computed tomography of the chest reveals a central mass near the left mainstem bronchus. Biopsy of the mass is performed. Histologic examination reveals small round blue cells, and a diagnosis of small cell carcinoma is made. Which of the following is a frequent characteristic of this form of lung cancer?

(A) Generally amenable to surgical cure at time of diagnosis
(B) More common in women, and a less clear relation to smoking than other forms of lung cancer
(C) Secretes a parathyroid-like hormone
(D) Secretes either corticotrophin or antidiuretic hormone
(E) Usually in a peripheral rather than in a central location

5. A 23-year-old man presents with radiographic evidence of bilateral hilar lymphadenopathy and interstitial lung disease. A biopsy from the hilar lymph nodes gives findings similar to those shown in the figure. A major characteristic of this disorder is

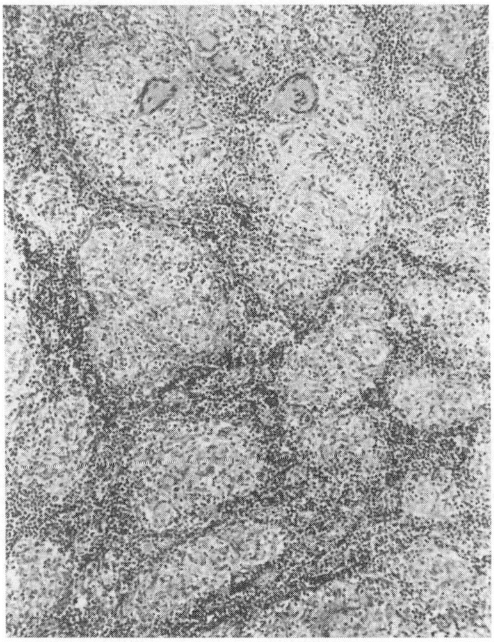

(Reprinted with permission from Golden A, Powell D, and Jennings C: *Pathology: Understanding Human Disease,* 2nd ed. Baltimore, Williams & Wilkins, 1985, p 42.)

(A) a positive test for tuberculin
(B) highest incidence in persons of Asian lineage
(C) hypercalcemia
(D) hypogammaglobulinemia
(E) involvement restricted to the lung

6. An 80-year-old woman, a retirement home resident, has multiple bouts of pneumonia caused by *Streptococcus pneumoniae.* In an attempt to prevent such infections, polyvalent vaccines directed at multiple serotypes of the organism have been administered but have not elicited long-acting immunity. Which of the following is the probable explanation for this phenomenon?

(A) Memory T lymphocytes respond poorly to polysaccharide antigens.
(B) *S. pneumoniae* evades host immune response by forming capsular coatings composed of host proteins and recognized as "self" antigens.
(C) The bacterial capsule binds C3b, facilitating activation of the alternative complement pathway, inducing complement-mediated lysis, and preventing immunization.
(D) The capsular polysaccharides of *S. pneumoniae* have limited hapten potential.
(E) The surface carbohydrate capsule on the surface of the organism acts as an opsonin, facilitating phagocytosis by neutrophils and thus preventing immunization.

7. A 50-year-old man dies of a respiratory illness that had been characterized by dyspnea, cough, and wheezing expiration of many years' duration. Initially episodic, his "attacks" had increased in frequency and at the time of death had become continuous and intractable. At autopsy, which of the following is the most likely histologic finding in the lungs?

(A) Bronchial smooth muscle hypertrophy with proliferation of eosinophils
(B) Diffuse alveolar damage with leakage of protein-rich fluid into alveolar spaces
(C) Dilation of air spaces with destruction of alveolar walls
(D) Hyperplasia of bronchial mucus-secreting submucosal glands
(E) Permanent bronchial dilation caused by chronic infection, with bronchi filled with mucus and neutrophils

8. A 25-year-old man presents with a progressive illness of several days' duration characterized by nonproductive cough, fever, and malaise. A lateral view chest radiograph reveals platelike atelectasis. Elevated titers of cold agglutinins are detected. Which of the following is the most likely type of pneumonia in this patient?

(A) Bacterial pneumonia, most likely caused by *Streptococcus pneumoniae*
(B) Hospital-acquired pneumonia, most likely caused by *Pseudomonas aeruginosa*
(C) Interstitial pneumonia, most likely caused by *Mycoplasma pneumoniae*
(D) *Pneumocystis carinii* pneumonia, most likely related to an immunocompromised state
(E) Viral pneumonia, most likely caused by influenza virus

9. A 60-year-old man presents with fever and chills, productive cough with rusty sputum, pleuritic pain, and shortness of breath for the past several days. A complete blood count reveals neutrophilia and an increase in band neutrophils. A chest radiograph reveals consolidation involving the entire left lower lobe. Which of the following microorganisms is the most likely etiologic agent?

(A) *Haemophilus influenzae*
(B) *Klebsiella pneumoniae*
(C) *Staphylococcus aureus*
(D) *Streptococcus pneumoniae*
(E) *Streptococcus pyogenes*

10. A 46-year-old woman presents with fever, hemoptysis, weight loss, and night sweats. She has never smoked. She recently returned from a month-long trip to Asia. A chest radiograph reveals apical lesions with cavitation in the left lung. A purified protein derivative (PPD) test is placed, and 48 hours later an 18-mm wheal develops. Sputum cultures reveal numerous acid-fast organisms. This patient is put on contact precautions, and a regimen for tuberculosis is started. Which of the following disorders does this patient most likely have?

(A) Acquired immunodeficiency syndrome
(B) Congenital immunodeficiency
(C) Miliary tuberculosis, with seeding of distal organs with innumerable small millet seed-like lesions
(D) Primary tuberculosis, characterized by the Ghon complex
(E) Secondary tuberculosis, resulting from activation of a prior Ghon complex, with spread to a new pulmonary site

11. A 25-year-old African-American woman presents with fatigue, dyspnea, nonproductive cough, and chest pain. She does not smoke. A chest radiograph reveals prominent bilateral hilar lymphadenopathy ("potato nodules") and diffuse reticular densities in the interstitium of the lung. Laboratory studies reveal polyclonal hypergammaglobulinemia, hypercalcemia, and increased serum angiotensin-converting enzyme. Which of the following is the most likely diagnosis?

(A) Acute respiratory distress syndrome
(B) Adenocarcinoma of the lung
(C) Eosinophilic granuloma
(D) Idiopathic pulmonary fibrosis
(E) Sarcoidosis

12. A 60-year-old man presents with dyspnea on exertion and a nonproductive cough. He has never smoked, but he worked as a shipbuilder, with known asbestos exposure approximately 20 years ago. To which of the following conditions is this patient especially predisposed?

(A) Acute respiratory distress syndrome
(B) Goodpasture syndrome
(C) Idiopathic pulmonary fibrosis
(D) Idiopathic pulmonary hemosiderosis
(E) Malignant mesothelioma of the pleura

13. A female infant is born prematurely at 28 weeks' gestation. Shortly after birth, she shows signs of dyspnea, cyanosis, and tachypnea. She is placed on a ventilator for assisted breathing, and a diagnosis of neonatal respiratory distress syndrome (hyaline membrane disease) is made. Which of the following is the cause of this syndrome?

(A) Bronchopulmonary dysplasia
(B) Intraventricular brain hemorrhage
(C) Lack of fetal pulmonary maturity and deficiency of surfactant
(D) Necrotizing enterocolitis
(E) Patent ductus arteriosus

14. A 50-year-old woman has been immobilized in bed for several days after a motor vehicle accident. She had been improving, but this morning she suffered the sudden onset of pleuritic chest pain, hemoptysis, tachypnea, tachycardia, and dyspnea. What is the likely basis of this set of findings?

(A) Arterial thrombus originating in pulmonary blood vessels
(B) Arterial thrombus originating in the lower extremities with migration to pulmonary veins
(C) Deep venous thrombus of the lower extremities with embolization to branches of the pulmonary artery
(D) Mural thrombus originating in the left heart with migration to pulmonary blood vessels
(E) Venous thrombus originating in pulmonary blood vessels

15. The chest radiograph of a 23-year-old medical student reveals a calcified cavitary pulmonary lesion. The tuberculin test is positive, but sputum smears and cultures are negative for *Mycobacterium tuberculosis*. A presumptive diagnosis of secondary tuberculosis is made. If further studies, including a biopsy, were performed, which of the following findings would justify the diagnosis of secondary tuberculosis, as contrasted to primary tuberculosis?

(A) Calcification
(B) Caseating granulomas
(C) Cavitation
(D) Langhans giant cells
(E) Positive tuberculin test result

ANSWERS AND EXPLANATIONS

1-E. This is a classic case of acute laryngotracheobronchitis (croup), an acute inflammation of the larynx, trachea, and epiglottis. The most common cause of croup is a viral (parainfluenza virus type I) infection.

2-C. Emphysema is an example of a chronic obstructive pulmonary disease (COPD). Due to destruction of alveolar walls, a lack of elastic recoil causes air to become trapped in alveoli, and thus airflow obstruction occurs on expiration. In COPD, the forced expiratory volume in one second (FEV_1) is decreased, whereas the forced vital capacity (FVC) is normal or increased. Therefore, patients with COPD have a decreased FEV_1:FVC ratio.

3-D. Chronic bronchitis is an example of a chronic obstructive pulmonary disease. The pathologic hallmark of chronic bronchitis is marked hyperplasia of bronchial submucosal glands and bronchial smooth muscle hypertrophy, which can be quantified by the Reid index, a ratio of glandular layer thickness to bronchial wall thickness.

4-D. Small cell carcinoma of the lung is the most aggressive type of bronchogenic carcinoma. The location of this cancer is usually central. This is an undifferentiated tumor with small round blue cells and is least likely to be cured by surgery because it is usually already metastatic at diagnosis. Associated paraneoplastic syndromes include secretion of adrenocorticotropic hormone and antidiuretic hormone.

5-C. The illustration shows noncaseating granulomas and Langhans giant cells, which, in the clinical setting described, are diagnostic of sarcoidosis. A frequent abnormal laboratory finding is polyclonal hypergammaglobulinemia along with hypercalcemia. Anergy to tuberculin is often demonstrable. The disorder is much more common in persons of African lineage. Patients most often present with lung findings and hilar lymphadenopathy, but any organ system can be involved.

6-A. Antibody responses to the more than 80 differing carbohydrate capsular antigens of the various strains of *Streptococcus pneumoniae* are generally T-cell–independent, and antibody formation is entirely B-cell–mediated. Because of this, memory cells are not formed, and long-lasting immunity is not achieved.

7-A. Bronchial asthma, or hyperreactive airway disease, is a type of chronic obstructive pulmonary disease caused by narrowing of airways. Asthma is manifest morphologically by bronchial smooth muscle hypertrophy, hyperplasia of bronchial submucosal glands and goblet cells, and airways plugged by mucus-containing Curschmann spirals (whorl-like accumulations of epithelial cells), eosinophils, and Charcot-Leyden crystals (crystalloids of eosinophil-derived proteins).

8-C. Interstitial (primary atypical) pneumonia is most commonly caused by *Mycoplasma pneumoniae* or viruses. Interstitial pneumonia is characterized by diffuse, patchy inflammation localized to the interstitial areas of alveolar walls, with no exudate in alveolar spaces, and intra-alveolar hyaline membranes. *M. pneumoniae* infection is associated with the presence of cold agglutinins, which are IgM antibodies that react nonspecifically with all human red blood cells. *Pneumocystis carinii* pneumonia is the most common opportunistic infection in patients with acquired immunodeficiency syndrome or other immunodeficiency disorders. Viral pneumonias are the most common type of pneumonia in childhood, caused most commonly by the influenza virus.

9-D. The most common cause of lobar pneumonia is *Streptococcus pneumoniae*. The organism is also known as the pneumococcus, and the disease entity is often referred to as pneumococcal pneumonia.

10-E. Tuberculosis, at one time a frequent hazard in the United States, is now relatively uncommon except in immunocompromised individuals and persons returning from parts of the world where the disease remains a common problem. Primary tuberculosis is the initial infection by *Mycobacterium tuberculosis*, and is restricted to the primary, or Ghon, complex, a combination of a peripheral subpleural parenchymal lesion and involved hilar lymph nodes. Cavitation and selective localization to the pulmonary apices are characteristics of secondary tuberculosis. Secondary tuberculosis may spread through the lymphatics and blood to other organs, resulting in miliary tuberculosis.

11-E. Sarcoidosis most often presents as a restrictive pulmonary disease that is characterized morphologically by noncaseating granulomas and can involve any organ system. Diagnostic features of note include highest incidence in persons of African lineage, somewhat higher incidence in women, bilateral interstitial pulmonary involvement, prominent hilar lymphadenopathy, polyclonal hypergammaglobulinemia, and hypercalcemia. Increased serum angiotensin-converting enzyme activity is a nonspecific indicator of granulomatous inflammation.

12-E. Asbestosis is caused by inhalation of asbestos fibers, characterized by yellow-brown, rod-shaped ferruginous bodies with clubbed ends that stain positively with Prussian blue. Asbestosis results in a marked predisposition to malignant mesothelioma of the pleura or peritoneum. Exposure to asbestos is also a risk factor for bronchogenic carcinoma as well as for carcinoma of the oropharynx, esophagus, and colon. The risk of bronchogenic carcinoma is greatly increased in cigarette smokers with exposure to asbestos.

13-C. Neonatal respiratory distress syndrome (hyaline membrane disease) is the most common cause of respiratory failure in the newborn and results from a deficiency of surfactant and immature development of the lungs. Surfactant reduces surface tension within the lung, facilitating expansion by inspiration and thus preventing atelectasis during expiration. An indicator of fetal pulmonary maturity is a lecithin:sphingomyelin ratio of approximately 2:1 in the amniotic fluid. Predisposing factors include prematurity, maternal diabetes mellitus, and birth by cesarean section. Known complications of this condition include bronchopulmonary dysplasia, patent ductus arteriosus, intraventricular brain hemorrhage, and necrotizing enterocolitis.

14-C. Pulmonary embolism most often originates from venous thrombosis in the lower extremities or pelvis. An embolus migrates through the venous circulation to the right heart and gets trapped in branches of the pulmonary artery. Pulmonary embolism occurs in clinical settings of venous stasis, such as primary venous disease, congestive heart failure, prolonged bed rest or immobilization, or prolonged sitting while traveling.

15-C. Cavitation occurs only in secondary tuberculosis. Both primary and secondary tuberculosis are characterized by caseating granulomas, often with Langhans giant cells, that heal by scarring and calcification. The skin test result for tuberculin sensitivity is positive in both forms.

CHAPTER 15

Gastrointestinal Tract

I. Diseases of the Mouth and Jaw

A. **Inflammatory disorders**

1. **Herpes labialis** (fever blisters, cold sores) is a common vesicular lesion caused by herpes simplex virus (HSV), most often by HSV type 1 (HSV-1). It tends to recur, with activation by febrile illness, trauma, sunshine, or menstruation.
2. **Aphthous stomatitis** is characterized by painful, recurrent, erosive oral ulcerations.
3. **Oral candidiasis** (thrush, moniliasis) is a local white, membranous lesion caused by *Candida albicans*. It occurs most commonly in debilitated infants and children, immunocompromised patients, and individuals with diabetes.
4. **Acute necrotizing ulcerative gingivitis** (trench mouth, Vincent infection, fusospirochetosis)
   a. This severe gingival inflammation occurs in patients with decreased resistance to infection.
   b. The cause is concurrent infection with symbiotic bacteria, most often *Fusobacterium* species and *Borrelia vincentii*.

B. **Tumors and tumor-like conditions**

1. **Benign tumors of the oral mucosa**
   a. **Papilloma** is the most common benign epithelial tumor of the oral mucosa. It can occur anywhere in the mouth; the most common sites are the tongue, lips, gingivae, or buccal mucosa.
   b. **Fibroma** is most often a non-neoplastic hyperplastic lesion resulting from chronic irritation.
   c. **Hemangioma** occurs most commonly on the tongue, lips, or buccal mucosa.
   d. **Epulis** refers to any benign (usually non-neoplastic) growth of the gingivae. It is most often a reparative growth rather than a true neoplasm.
2. **Leukoplakia** is a clinical term describing irregular white mucosal patches.
   a. These patches result from hyperkeratosis, usually secondary to chronic irritation.
   b. Leukoplakia is usually benign but may represent dysplasia or carcinoma in situ.
3. **Odontogenic tumors**
   a. **Odontoma** is the most common odontogenic tumor. It is a **hamartoma** derived from odontogenic epithelium and odontoblastic tissue.
   b. **Ameloblastoma** (adamantinoma) is an **epithelial tumor arising from precursor cells of the enamel organ.**
      (1) Most frequently, this tumor occurs in the mandible. It usually appears in individuals younger than 35 years of age.
      (2) Although this tumor is benign, it can lead to slow expansion of the jaw because of irregular local extension.

4. **Oral cancer** is most frequently squamous cell carcinoma.
   a. Involvement of the tongue occurs in more than 50% of cases. Carcinoma of the mouth, tongue, and esophagus is often associated with the combined abuse of tobacco and alcohol.
   b. Oral cancer may be associated with irritants such as pipe smoking, chewing tobacco, or betel nuts.

II. Diseases of the Salivary Glands

A. **Sialadenitis.** This **inflammation of the salivary glands** may be caused by infection, immune-mediated mechanisms, or occlusion of the salivary ducts by stones (sialolithiasis).

B. **Acute parotitis.** This condition occurs in mumps but may also be caused by other infectious agents.

C. **Sjögren syndrome.** This condition is most likely of autoimmune origin.
1. Characteristics include **keratoconjunctivitis sicca** (dry eyes), **xerostomia** (dry mouth), and an associated **connective tissue disease,** most often rheumatoid arthritis.
2. Sjögren syndrome is associated with an increased incidence of malignant lymphoma.

D. **Mucocele.** This cyst-like pool of mucus, lined by granulation tissue, develops near a minor salivary gland. It results from mucous leakage caused by rupture of obstructed or traumatized ducts.

E. **Ranula.** This is a **large mucocele, of salivary gland origin,** characteristically localized to the floor of the mouth.

F. **Tumors of the salivary gland** (Table 15-1). The majority of salivary gland tumors occur in the parotid gland.
1. **Pleomorphic adenoma** (mixed tumor) is the most frequently occurring salivary gland tumor. It occurs with greatest frequency in women between 20 and 40 years of age.
   a. This is a **benign** tumor that frequently recurs; it rarely becomes malignant.
   b. It has been called "mixed tumor" because of the presence of myxoid and cartilage-like elements as well as epithelial cells.
   c. Histologically, pleomorphic adenomas vary, but most often they demonstrate irregular masses or anastomosing strands of stellate or fusiform epithelial cells, some forming ducts or tubules, all of which are embedded in a myxoid stroma that may display fibrous, cartilage-like, or hyalinized areas.
   d. The tumor is **most often localized to the parotid gland** (~90%).
   e. Usually, the tumor presents as a firm, nontender swelling.
   f. Often, the tumor is difficult to remove completely because of its proximity to the facial nerve, and it is likely to recur after resection.
2. **Other salivary gland tumors**
   a. **Papillary cystadenoma lymphomatosum** (Warthin tumor)
   b. **Mucoepidermoid tumor**
   c. **Adenoid cystic carcinoma**
   d. **Oncocytoma**

III. Diseases of the Esophagus

A. **Tracheoesophageal fistula.** This congenital disorder is suggested in a newborn by copious salivation associated with choking, coughing, and cyanosis on attempts at food intake. It occurs in three distinct variants:

TABLE 15-1 *Salivary Gland Tumors: Location, Histology, and Characteristics*

Type	Typical Location	Histology	Characteristics
Pleomorphic adenoma (mixed tumor)	Parotid gland; can occur in submandibular or minor salivary glands	Variable mix of epithelial and mesenchyme-like elements	Most common salivary gland tumor; benign; tends to recur after resection; malignant transformation occurs but is rare
Papillary cystadenoma lymphomatosum (Warthin tumor, adenolymphoma)	Parotid gland	Cystic spaces lined by double-layered eosinophilic epithelium, all embedded in lymphoid stroma	Benign
Mucoepidermoid tumor	Parotid gland	Comprised of mucus-producing and epidermoid components and cells intermediate between the two	Behavior varies from benign to highly malignant; tumors with a greater number of epidermoid cells and nonparotid tumors tend to be more aggressive
Adenoid cystic carcinoma	Minor salivary glands	Variable; most characteristic appearance consists of cribriform pattern with masses of small, dark-staining cells arrayed around cystic spaces	Tends to infiltrate perineural spaces and cause pain; slow-growing malignancy with late metastasis
Oncocytoma	Parotid gland	Large, granular-appearing, eosinophilic-staining epithelial cells	Benign; peak occurrence in the elderly

1. In the **most common variant** (90%), the lower portion of the esophagus communicates with the trachea near the tracheal bifurcation. The upper esophagus ends in a blind pouch (esophageal atresia). Maternal polyhydramnios (increased amniotic fluid) is a frequently associated abnormality.
2. The **second most common variant** is characterized by a fistulous connection between the upper esophagus and the trachea; the lower esophageal segment is not connected to the upper esophagus.
3. In a **third variant,** there is a fistulous connection between the trachea and a completely patent esophagus.

B. **Esophageal diverticula** are pouches lined by one or more layers of the esophageal wall.
1. Most commonly, false (**pulsion**) diverticula result from herniation of the mucosa through defects in the muscular layer.
2. Less commonly, true (**traction**) diverticula consist of mucosal, muscular, and serosal layers. Traction diverticula result from periesophageal inflammation and scarring.
3. Esophageal diverticula occur in three characteristic **locations:**
   a. Immediately above the upper esophageal sphincter (**Zenker diverticulum**)
   b. Near the midpoint of the esophagus
   c. Immediately above the lower esophageal sphincter (**epiphrenic diverticulum**)

C. **Achalasia** is persistent contraction of the lower esophageal sphincter and absence of esophageal peristalsis, leading to dilation of the esophagus.

1. The condition is caused by a loss of ganglion cells in the myenteric plexus, which leads to the progressive dilation of the esophagus. One important source (principally in South America) is *Trypanosoma cruzi* infection in Chagas disease. In other cases, ganglion cells are lost for reasons that are not known.
2. Clinical characteristics include difficulty in swallowing.
3. Achalasia can lead to esophageal squamous cell carcinoma in about 5% of subjects.

D. **Esophageal varices.** These **dilated submucosal esophageal veins** that occur secondary to portal hypertension can result in upper gastrointestinal hemorrhage. (The other important causes of upper gastrointestinal hemorrhage are bleeding peptic ulcer and the Mallory-Weiss syndrome, bleeding from esophagogastric laceration as a result of severe retching.)

E. **Inflammatory and related disorders of the esophagus**

1. **Gastroesophageal reflux** is reflux of gastric acid contents into the esophagus.
   a. Characteristics usually include burning pain relieved by antacids. Manifestations often include substernal pain (heartburn).
   b. Most commonly, associated conditions include hiatal hernia and incompetent lower esophageal sphincter. Gastroesophageal reflux is also associated with excessive use of alcohol and tobacco and with increased gastric volume, pregnancy, or scleroderma.
   c. Assuming a recumbent position often precipitates gastroesophageal reflux.
   d. Reflux may cause esophagitis, stricture, ulceration, or columnar metaplasia of esophageal squamous epithelium (Barrett esophagus).
2. **Barrett esophagus** is **columnar metaplasia of esophageal squamous epithelium;** the columnar epithelium is often of the intestinal (specialized) type with prominent goblet cells. This condition is a complication of long-standing gastroesophageal reflux and is a well-known **precursor of esophageal adenocarcinoma.**
3. **Candida esophagitis** (moniliasis)
   a. Associated conditions often include antibiotic use, diabetes mellitus, malignant disease, or immunodeficiency caused by acquired immunodeficiency syndrome or immunosuppressive drugs.
   b. Clinical manifestations are white adherent mucosal patches and painful, difficult swallowing.
4. **Herpetic esophagitis** is caused by HSV-1 infection.
   a. HSV-1 infection tends to occur in immunosuppressed persons.
   b. Characteristics include painful, difficult swallowing.
5. **Less common forms of esophagitis** are caused by cytomegalovirus (CMV) infection, uremia, radiation therapy, or graft-versus-host (GVH) disease.
6. **Esophageal stricture** most often results from prolonged esophageal gastric acid reflux but may also be caused by suicidal or accidental ingestion of corrosive acids or lye. It is marked by progressive dysphagia.

F. **Carcinoma of the esophagus**

1. This aggressive tumor is manifest clinically by **dysphagia,** weight loss, and anorexia. Occasionally, pain or hematemesis occur.
2. In the United States, the incidence of **squamous cell carcinoma** and **adenocarcinoma** is about equal, which differs from the worldwide distribution, in which squamous cell carcinoma is much more frequent. In the United States, the incidence of squamous cell carcinoma is decreasing, and this is thought to be due to a parallel decrease in the use of tobacco and perhaps alcohol. Adenocarcinoma arises most often in aberrant gastric mucosa or submucosal glands or in the metaplastic columnar epithelium of **Barrett esophagus.**
3. **Squamous cell carcinoma arises most frequently in the upper and middle thirds** of the esophagus.
4. **Adenocarcinoma arises most frequently in the lower third** of the esophagus.
5. Pathologic manifestations may include protrusion into the esophageal lumen, with **spread by local extension** into adjacent structures such as the trachea, bronchi, or aorta, or diffuse infiltration into the esophageal wall.

IV. Diseases of the Stomach

A. **Congenital pyloric stenosis**

1. This stenosis is caused by hypertrophy of the circular muscular layer of the pylorus, often leading to a **palpable mass.**
2. The resulting obstruction of the gastric outlet causes episodes of **projectile vomiting** beginning in the first 2 weeks of life. This condition is much more common in boys.
3. The condition is corrected by surgical incision of the hypertrophied muscle.

B. **Gastritis**

1. **Acute (erosive) gastritis**
   a. **Causes**
      (1) Nonsteroidal anti-inflammatory drugs (NSAIDs)
      (2) Cigarette smoking
      (3) Heavy alcohol intake
      (4) Burn injury; **Curling ulcer,** an acute gastric ulcer in association with severe burns
      (5) Brain injury; **Cushing ulcer,** an acute gastric ulcer in association with brain injury
   b. **Characteristics**
      (1) Focal damage to the gastric mucosa, with acute inflammation, necrosis, and hemorrhage
      (2) Manifested as acute gastric ulcers, which are often multiple.
2. **Chronic gastritis** is characterized by chronic mucosal inflammation and atrophy of the mucosal glands.
   a. **Autoimmune gastritis** is associated with the presence of antibodies to parietal cells (and sometimes to intrinsic factor), achlorhydria (lack of gastric acid secretion), pernicious anemia, and autoimmune diseases such as chronic thyroiditis and Addison disease. It is also associated with aging, partial gastrectomy, gastric ulcer, and gastric carcinoma.
   b. ***Helicobacter pylori*–associated gastritis** is the most common form of chronic gastritis.
      (1) There is no association with pernicious anemia, antibodies to parietal cells, or reduced gastric acid secretion.
      (2) Often, increased gastric acid secretion occurs. *H. pylori* is also strongly associated with gastric and duodenal peptic ulcer and is a high suspect in the causality of carcinoma of the stomach and gastric lymphoma of the mucosa-associated lymphoid tissue (MALT) type.
3. **Ménétrier disease** (giant hypertrophic gastritis) is characterized by extreme enlargement of gastric rugae and sometimes by severe loss of plasma proteins from the altered mucosa. Affected patients have an increased risk of stomach cancer.

C. **Peptic ulcer of the stomach**

1. Most often, the stomach ulcer occurs at or near the lesser curvature, in the antral and prepyloric regions.
2. The ulcer is not a precursor lesion of carcinoma of the stomach.
3. Unlike peptic ulcer that occurs elsewhere, peptic ulcer of the stomach is not dependent on increased gastric acid secretion; however, acid and pepsin are believed to play a role, because gastric peptic ulcers rarely occur in association with absolute achlorhydria.
4. Postulated etiopathogenic mechanisms of gastric peptic ulcer production include:
   a. *H. pylori*–mediated processes, in which bacterial ureases and proteases break down glycoproteins in gastric mucus, thus interfering with epithelial protection
   b. Increased permeability of the gastric mucosa to hydrogen ion, resulting in back-diffusion of hydrogen ion with injury to the gastric mucosa
   c. Bile-induced gastritis leading to gastric ulceration

D. **Malignant tumors of the stomach**

1. **Carcinoma of the stomach**

a. **General considerations**
(1) Carcinoma of the stomach is most common after **50 years of age,** with an increased incidence in **men.** It occurs more frequently in persons with **blood group A,** suggesting a genetic predisposition.
(2) Incidence varies greatly from one geographic area to another, with incidence much higher in Japan, Finland, and Iceland.
(3) The incidence is decreasing in incidence in the United States.

b. **Etiologic factors**
(1) ***H. pylori*** is a high suspect.
(2) **Nitrosamines** from dietary amines and nitrites used as food preservatives may play a role. Incidence of the disease is greatly increased in populations who eat large amounts of smoked fish and meat and pickled vegetables.
(3) Increased incidence is also associated with excessive salt intake and a diet low in fresh fruits and vegetables.
(4) Stomach carcinoma is also predisposed by:
(a) Achlorhydria
(b) Chronic gastritis with or without pernicious anemia

c. **Characteristics**
(1) Histologically, stomach carcinoma is almost always **adenocarcinoma.**
(2) Involvement of the distal stomach, along the lesser curvature of the antrum or prepyloric region, is most common; rarely involves the fundus.
(3) Aggressive spread to adjacent organs and the peritoneum and early lymphatic metastasis to regional lymph nodes and the liver occurs.
(4) More distal sites may be involved.
(a) Involvement of a supraclavicular lymph node by metastatic carcinoma of the stomach is referred to as a **Virchow node.**
(b) Bilateral involvement of the ovaries by metastatic carcinoma of the stomach is referred to as **Krukenberg tumors.** The tumor cells often contain abundant mucin, displacing the nucleus to one side and resulting in so-called **signet-ring cells.**

d. **Morphologic variants of stomach carcinoma**
(1) **Intestinal type**
(a) Often, this variant is manifest as polypoid (fungating) carcinoma, which forms a solid mass projecting into the lumen of the stomach. It has a high degree of association with *H. pylori* infection.
(b) The intestinal variant can become ulcerated and must be differentiated from peptic ulcer. Peptic ulcer usually exhibits a smooth base with nonelevated, punched-out margins. In contrast, carcinoma tends to form an ulcer with an irregular necrotic base and firm, raised margins.
(2) **Infiltrating or diffuse carcinoma** (linitis plastica, leather-bottle stomach) is not associated with *H. pylori* infection and is characterized by a thickened, rigid stomach wall, caused by diffuse infiltration of tumor cells with accompanying extensive fibrosis.

2. **Lymphoma** accounts for 4% of malignant gastric tumors. They are of the MALT type, and there is a high association with *H. pylori* infection. The prognosis is better than it is for adenocarcinoma.

V. Diseases of the Small Intestine

A. **Peptic ulcer**
1. Occurrence is most frequent in the first portion of the duodenum, the stomach, or the lower end of the esophagus, all of which are exposed to acid and pepsin.
2. Except for peptic ulcer of the stomach, peptic ulcer is always associated with hypersecretion of gastric acid and pepsin. Ulceration is **closely related to gastric *H. pylori* infection,**

which affects essentially all patients with duodenal ulcer and the majority of patients with gastric ulcer. *H. pylori* increases gastric acid secretion and apparently impairs both gastric and duodenal mucosal defenses.

3. Frequency of occurrence is increased in persons of blood group O, suggesting that genetic factors may play a role.
4. Peptic ulcer is not a precursor of malignancy.
5. Complications often include hemorrhage with melena (black stools containing blood). Other important complications include obstruction and perforation. Peptic ulcer is sometimes associated with:
   a. Intake of **aspirin** or other NSAIDs. The ulcerogenic effect of these drugs may be mediated by inhibition of prostaglandin synthesis.
   b. **Smoking.** The incidence of peptic ulcer is two-fold greater in smokers.
   c. **Zollinger-Ellison syndrome,** increased tendency toward peptic ulcer formation, which is caused by gastric acid hypersecretion due to gastrin-secreting islet cell tumor of the pancreas. Recurrent peptic ulcer or peptic ulcer in aberrant sites such as the jejunum is suggestive of the Zollinger-Ellison syndrome.
   d. **Primary hyperparathyroidism**
   e. **Multiple endocrine neoplasia (MEN) type I** (Wermer syndrome), an autosomal dominant syndrome characterized by pituitary, thyroid, parathyroid, adrenal cortical, and pancreatic islet cell adenomas or hyperplasias associated with hypergastrinemia and peptic ulcer

B. **Crohn disease** (Table 15-2)

1. **General considerations**
   a. This **chronic inflammatory condition** of unknown etiology may affect any part of the gastrointestinal tract but most commonly involves the distal ileocecum, **small intestine,** or **colon.**
   b. Crohn disease tends to affect young people in the second and third decades of life, although no age group is exempt. It occurs most frequently in people of Jewish descent.
   c. The disease can lead to carcinoma involving the small intestine or colon. However, neoplastic transformation is much less frequent in Crohn disease than in ulcerative colitis.
2. **Morphology**
   a. Chronic inflammation involving **all layers** of the intestinal wall (transmural involvement)
   b. **Thickening** of involved segments, with narrowing of lumen

TABLE 15-2 *Comparison of Crohn Disease and Ulcerative Colitis*

Crohn Disease	Ulcerative Colitis
May involve any portion of the gastrointestinal tract, usually the ileocecal region, small intestine, or colon	Affects only colon
Chronic inflammatory reaction extends through the entire thickness of the intestinal wall	Inflammation and ulceration limited to mucosa and submucosa
Lymphocytic infiltrate; noncaseating granulomas; fibrosis; thickening of intestinal wall with narrowing of lumen; fistulous tracts between loops of intestine or between the intestine and other sites; mucosal cobblestone appearance; skip lesions	Crypt abscesses, pseudopolyps
Incidence of secondary malignancy much lower than in ulcerative colitis	Greatly increased incidence of colon cancer in long-standing cases

c. Linear **ulceration** of the mucosa
d. Submucosal edema with elevation of the surviving mucosa, producing a **cobblestone appearance**
e. **Skip lesions** (segments of normal intestine between affected regions)
f. Discrete noncaseating **granulomas** in some cases
g. Submucosal fibrosis

3. **Clinical manifestations**
   a. Abdominal pain and diarrhea
   b. Malabsorption
   c. Fever
   d. Intestinal obstruction resulting from fibrous **stricture**
   e. **Fistulas** between loops of intestine and between the intestine, bladder, vagina, and skin

C. **Meckel diverticulum** is the most common congenital anomaly of the small intestine.
1. Meckel diverticulum is a remnant of the embryonic vitelline duct and is located in the distal small bowel. It may contain ectopic gastric, duodenal, colonic, or pancreatic tissue.
2. The condition is usually asymptomatic but complications, including peptic ulceration in ectopic gastric mucosa with bleeding or perforation, may occur. Occasional associations include:
   a. **Intussusception** (invagination of a proximal segment of bowel into a more distal segment), causing bowel obstruction. Intussusception occurs more often without preexisting bowel pathology and is seen most often in infants and young children.
   b. **Volvulus** (twisting of a portion of the gastrointestinal tract about itself), often causing bowel obstruction

D. **Malabsorption syndromes** (Table 15-3)
1. **Celiac disease** is caused by **sensitivity to gluten** in cereal products.
   a. Clinical manifestations include weight loss, weakness, and diarrhea with pale, bulky, frothy, foul-smelling stools. It is also characterized by **growth retardation** and general **failure to thrive.**
   b. Disease most often becomes **symptomatic in infancy** when cereals are first added to the diet.
   c. Diagnosis involves documentation of malabsorption, small intestinal biopsy demonstrating **blunting of small intestinal villi**, and clinical improvement and restoration of normal intestinal morphology on a **gluten-free diet**.
   d. Incidence increases in association with human leukocyte antigens (HLAs) HLA-B8 and HLA-DW3. This finding and the presence of antibodies directed against gliadin (a glycoprotein component of gluten) and transglutaminase suggest that both **genetic** and **immune-mediated mechanisms** may be involved. These antibody tests may also be used for screening prior to definitive diagnosis by biopsy.
   e. Approximately 10%–15% of cases lead to small intestinal malignancy, most often **enteropathy-type T-cell lymphoma.**
2. **Other malabsorption syndromes** include tropical sprue, Whipple disease, disaccharidase deficiency, abetalipoproteinemia, and intestinal lymphangiectasia. Malabsorption can also be caused by pancreatic insufficiency.

E. **Tumors of the small intestine**
1. **General considerations**
   a. Tumors of the small intestine make up a small percentage of gastrointestinal neoplasms.
   b. The most common malignant tumors are **adenocarcinoma,** lymphoma, and carcinoid.
2. **Carcinoid** occurs most frequently in the **appendix;** it is localized to the small intestine in about 30% of cases.
   a. Although characteristically slow growing, the tumor is of low-grade malignancy; in contrast to other carcinoids, appendiceal carcinoid almost never metastasizes.

TABLE 15-3 *Malabsorption Syndromes*

Disorder	Morphologic Features	Comments
Celiac disease	Flat mucosal surface with marked villous atrophy; increased lymphocytes and plasma cells in lamina propria	Gluten sensitivity
Tropical sprue	Histologic findings vary from no changes to abnormalities similar to those of celiac disease	Tropical disease of probable infectious origin; often responds to antibiotics
Whipple disease	Distinctive PAS-positive macrophages in intestinal mucosa *Tropheryma whippelii* bacilli visualized by electron microscopy	May affect any organ, most commonly small intestine; arthralgias and cardiac and neurologic symptoms are common
Disaccharidase deficiency	No characteristic histologic changes	Deficiency of disaccharidases sited in brush border of mucosal cells of small intestine; lactase deficiency, which leads to milk intolerance, is most frequent
Abetalipoproteinemia	No characteristic features in the intestine; circulating acanthocytes (red cells with spiny projections) suggest the diagnosis	β-lipoprotein deficiency is caused by hereditary deficiency of apoprotein B
Intestinal lymphangiectasia	Generalized dilation of the small intestinal lymphatics	Marked gastrointestinal protein loss with resultant hypoproteinemia and generalized edema

b. Carcinoid, when metastatic to the liver can be manifest as the **carcinoid syndrome**; this syndrome is:
   (1) Caused by the elaboration of vasoactive peptides and amines, especially serotonin
   (2) Manifest clinically by:
      (a) Cutaneous **flushing**
      (b) Watery **diarrhea** and abdominal cramps
      (c) **Bronchospasm**
      (d) **Valvular lesions of the right side of the heart**

3. **Lymphoma** can arise from the abundant lymphoid tissue of the small intestine. It may present with **malabsorption** when there is diffuse involvement.
4. **Adenocarcinoma.** In spite of being rare, it is one of the most common primary malignant tumors of the small intestine.

VI. Diseases of the Colon

A. **Hirschsprung disease** (congenital megacolon) is **dilation of the colon** due to the **absence of ganglion cells** of the submucosal and myenteric neural plexuses; dilation is proximal to the aganglionic segment.

B. **Diverticula** are pulsion (or false) diverticula (pockets of mucosa and submucosa herniated through the muscular layer) that most frequently involve the **sigmoid colon.** They are almost always multiple. Diverticula are most common in older persons.

1. **Diverticulosis** is defined by the presence of multiple diverticula without inflammation.
   a. Occurrence is most common in populations that consume low-fiber diets.
   b. The condition is most often asymptomatic or associated with vague discomfort.
2. **Diverticulitis** refers to inflammation of diverticula.
   a. Older persons are affected.
   b. Complications may include perforation, peritonitis, abscess formation, or bowel stenosis. **Bright red rectal bleeding** is frequent.
   c. Presenting features may include lower abdominal pain and tenderness, fever, leukocytosis, and other **signs of acute inflammation.**

C. **Vascular diseases of the colon**
1. **Ischemic bowel disease**
   a. The cause is **atherosclerotic occlusion** of at least two of the major mesenteric vessels.
   b. Most often affected are the **splenic flexure** and the **rectosigmoid junction,** which lie in the relatively poorly vascularized regions (so-called watershed areas) between areas supplied by the superior mesenteric artery and the inferior mesenteric and internal iliac arteries.
   c. The result is mucosal, mural, or transmural infarction involving the wall of the intestine.
2. **Angiodysplasia** is tortuous dilation of small vessels spanning the intestinal mucosa or submucosa.
   a. Lesions are multiple, most often involving the cecum or ascending colon.
   b. This condition is an extremely **common cause of otherwise unexplained lower bowel bleeding.**
3. **Hemorrhoids** are dilated internal and external venous plexuses in the anal canal. They are predisposed by a low-fiber diet.

D. **Inflammatory disorders of the colon**
1. **Ulcerative colitis**
   a. **General considerations**
      (1) Ulcerative colitis is of unknown etiology.
      (2) It is often grouped along with Crohn disease as **inflammatory bowel disease.** The two disorders are compared in Table 15-2.
      (3) Crohn disease and ulcerative colitis share a similar geographic and racial distribution; some patients have a family history of either ulcerative colitis or Crohn disease.
      (4) Both disorders often demonstrate **extraintestinal manifestations,** which include:
         (a) Polyarthritis
         (b) Uveitis and episcleritis
         (c) Sclerosing cholangitis, a chronic fibrosing inflammatory process of the biliary system leading to chronic cholestasis and sometimes to portal hypertension
         (d) Sacroiliitis
         (e) Skin manifestations, including erythema nodosum and pyoderma gangrenosum
   b. **Characteristics**
      (1) Mucosal inflammation and ulceration **limited to the large intestine;** the rectum is always affected but the entire colon may be involved.
      (2) Inflammatory changes almost entirely **confined to the mucosa and submucosa;** the most characteristic feature is the **crypt abscess,** in which there are infiltrates of neutrophils in the crypts of Lieberkühn.
      (3) **Red, granular appearance** of the mucosa; ulceration may be minimal or quite extensive, with only islands of surviving mucosa remaining.
      (4) **Pseudopolyps,** mucosal remnants of previous severe ulceration
      (5) Chronic **diarrhea** associated with the passage of **blood** and **mucus;** the **most frequent clinical manifestation is bleeding.**

c. **Complications**
   (1) **Toxic megacolon,** a medical emergency in which there is a marked dilation of the colon
   (2) **Perforation** of the colon
   (3) **Carcinoma** of the colon

2. **Pseudomembranous colitis**
   a. This condition is morphologically distinguished by superficial grayish mucosal exudates consisting of necrotic, loosely adherent mucosal debris **(pseudomembrane).**
   b. The cause most often is overgrowth of **exotoxin-producing *Clostridium difficile.*** Fibrinous necrosis of the superficial mucosa is caused by the exotoxin, not by bacterial invasion.
   c. Clinical characteristics include **fever, toxicity, and diarrhea,** most often occurring in patients on **broad-spectrum antibiotic therapy.**

3. **Amebic colitis**
   a. The cause is infection of the colon with *Entamoeba histolytica.*
   b. Flask-shaped ulcers are characteristic.

4. **Cholera**
   a. The cause is infection with *Vibrio cholerae,* a noninvasive toxin-producing bacterium.
   b. Characteristics include toxin-mediated loss of fluid and electrolytes with mucosa of the small bowel and colon remaining normal in appearance.

E. **Tumors**

1. **Benign polyps** (Table 15-4)
   a. **Terminology.** A polyp is a descriptive term for any elevation of the intestinal surface.
      (1) **Pedunculated polyps** are attached by a narrow stem.
      (2) **Sessile polyps** have a broad-based attachment.

TABLE 15-4 *Intestinal Polyps*

Type	Comments
Non-neoplastic polyps	
Hyperplastic polyp	No clinical significance
Inflammatory polyps:	
Lymphoid polyp	Most common site is the rectal mucosa; may be a reaction to local irritation
Inflammatory pseudopolyp	Associated with ulcerative colitis and other inflammatory diseases of the colon; consists of granulation tissue and residual and regenerating mucosa
Hamartomatous polyps:	
Juvenile polyp	Occurs most frequently in children
Peutz-Jeghers polyp	Associated with Peutz-Jeghers syndrome
Neoplastic polyps	
Tubular adenoma	Benign but may undergo malignant change; often multiple; hereditary multiple polyposis syndromes associated with greatly increased risk of malignancy
Tubulovillous adenoma	Morphologically resembles tubular adenoma with additional features similar to those of villous adenoma; greater malignant potential than tubular adenoma
Villous adenoma	Large sessile tumor with velvety surface comprised of finger-like villi; high potential for malignant change

b. **Non-neoplastic polyps**
   (1) **Hyperplastic polyps** can occur anywhere in the colon or small intestine. They have no clinical significance but may be mistaken for an adenomatous polyp.
   (2) **Inflammatory polyps** include **benign lymphoid polyps** and **inflammatory pseudopolyps** consisting of granulation tissue and remnants of mucosa, caused by chronic inflammatory bowel disease.
   (3) **Hamartomatous polyps**
      (a) **Juvenile polyps** occur in the small intestine and colon. They most often occur in children but are also seen in adults.
      (b) **Peutz-Jeghers polyps** occur as part of the Peutz-Jeghers syndrome, which includes hamartomatous polyps of the colon and small intestine and melanotic accumulations in the mouth and on the lips, hands, and genitalia. Peutz-Jeghers polyps have no malignant potential themselves, but the syndrome is associated with increased propensity for adenocarcinoma of the colon (contrary to an older teaching) and malignancy at other sites, such as the stomach, breast, or ovaries.

2. **Adenomatous polyps** are true **neoplasms** rather than benign proliferations of tissue. They are usually **asymptomatic** but can result in rectal bleeding.
   a. **Tubular adenomas**
      (1) These are the **most common** type (75%) of adenomatous polyp.
      (2) These polyps are usually **small** and **pedunculated.**
      (3) They can contain **malignant foci;** the likelihood of malignancy is greater in larger polyps.
   b. **Tubulovillous adenomas**
      (1) These adenomas account for about 15% of adenomatous polyps.
      (2) Tubulovillous adenomas resemble tubular adenomas but have a surface covered by finger-like villi. They are similar histologically to tubular adenomas.
      (3) They are intermediate in malignant potential between tubular adenomas and villous adenomas.
   c. **Villous adenomas**
      (1) These polyps are much less common than tubular adenomas and account for approximately 10% of adenomatous polyps.
      (2) Villous adenomas are usually larger than tubular adenomas, usually sessile and velvety, and are characterized by large numbers of finger-like villi.
      (3) They have the **highest potential for malignancy of all of the adenomatous polyps;** they become malignant in more than 30% of cases.

3. **Multiple polyposis syndromes** are associated with a **greatly increased risk of malignant transformation.**
   a. **Familial polyposis** is an autosomal dominant condition characterized by the presence of numerous adenomatous polyps. **The risk of malignant transformation approaches 100%.**
   b. **Gardner syndrome** is an autosomal dominant condition characterized by the presence of numerous adenomatous polyps along with osteomas and soft tissue tumors.
   c. **Turcot syndrome** is characterized by adenomatous polyps along with tumors of the central nervous system.

4. **Adenocarcinoma of the colon and rectum**
   a. **General considerations**
      (1) Adenocarcinoma of the colon and rectum is one of the most common neoplasms in the Western world. The peak age incidence is in the sixth to seventh decades.
      (2) This form of cancer is associated with increased serum concentration of carcinoembryonic antigen (CEA). Because elevated CEA is not specific for colon cancer, this laboratory determination is most useful for following the course of the disease rather than for making the initial diagnosis.
      (3) The cancer develops through a set of anatomic changes progressing from normal mucosa to adenomatous polyp to carcinoma to metastatic tumor, with a parallel

set of molecular changes in oncogenes and tumor suppressor genes that have been presented as a **model of tumor progression** (see Chapter 6).

b. **Predisposing factors**
   (1) **Adenomatous polyps**
   (2) **Inherited multiple polyposis syndromes**
   (3) **Long-standing ulcerative colitis**
   (4) **Genetic factors;** up to a four-fold increase in incidence is noted among relatives of patients with colon cancer.
   (5) A **low-fiber diet that is high in animal fat;** the disease is less common in much of the Third World, where populations consume a high-fiber diet that is low in animal fat.

c. **Characteristics**
   (1) **Adenocarcinoma** varies in gross presentation according to the region of the colon involved.
   (2) **Carcinoma of the rectosigmoid colon** tends to present in an annular manner, producing early obstruction.
   (3) **Carcinoma of the right colon** usually does not obstruct early and often presents (sometimes quite late) with iron deficiency anemia secondary to chronic blood loss.

VII. Diseases of the Appendix

A. **Acute appendicitis**
   1. Occurrence is most frequent in the second and third decades of life.
   2. The disease is thought to be caused by obstruction of the appendiceal lumen, most often by a fecalith, resulting in bacterial proliferation and invasion of the mucosa.
   3. Gross changes include a congested appendix with a swollen distal half covered by purulent exudate; the lumen also contains a purulent exudate and often a fecalith.
   4. Histologic characteristics include an acute inflammatory infiltrate extending from the mucosa through the full thickness of the appendiceal wall.
   5. Presenting features include anorexia, nausea, and **abdominal pain,** most commonly localized to the **right lower quadrant,** and systemic signs of acute inflammation such as fever.
   6. If untreated by **surgical resection,** appendicitis most often leads to perforation or abscess, or both.

B. **Tumors of the appendix.** The most common appendiceal neoplasm is **carcinoid,** which is usually detected as an incidental finding.

REVIEW TEST

Directions: *Each of the numbered items or incomplete statements in this section is followed by answers or by completions of the statement. Select the* ***one*** *lettered answer or completion that is best in each case.*

1. A 45-year-old woman with long-standing rheumatoid arthritis complains of dry eyes and dry mouth. Bilateral enlargement of the parotids is noted on physical examination. The syndrome described here is best described as

(A) autoimmune
(B) infectious
(C) metabolic
(D) metastatic
(E) primary neoplastic

2. A 40-year-old woman presents with a painless mass anterior to her left ear. The mass had been slowly enlarging over the past year. The mass is firm and nontender. Computed tomography and magnetic resonance imaging reveal a well-circumscribed, homogeneous mass within the left parotid gland. Biopsy reveals anastomosing strands of stellate and fusiform epithelial cells embedded in a myxoid stroma. Which of the following is a characteristic of the lesion?

(A) It is also called papillary cystadenoma lymphomatosum.
(B) It is most often localized to the submandibular gland.
(C) It is the most common malignant salivary gland tumor.
(D) Recurrence often takes place after surgical resection.
(E) Surgical resection should not be performed, because this condition is usually already metastatic on diagnosis.

3. A 45-year-old man complains of "heartburn" and burning epigastric pain, relieved by antacids and triggered by eating spicy or acidic foods or by assuming a recumbent position. The patient smokes two packs of cigarettes a day and consumes several alcoholic drinks each evening. Which of the following is the usual cause of this patient's condition?

(A) Columnar intestinal metaplasia of esophageal squamous epithelium
(B) Excessive acid production in the stomach
(C) Excessive nonsteroidal anti-inflammatory drug use
(D) *Helicobacter pylori* infection
(E) Hiatal hernia and incompetent lower esophageal sphincter

4. A 60-year-old man presents with hematemesis, melena, guaiac-positive stools, and signs of circulatory collapse. He has a 20-year history of burning midepigastric pain and tenderness relieved by food, milk, or antacids. Also, he has been taking high doses of nonsteroidal anti-inflammatory drugs to relieve the pain of long-standing arthritis. Esophagogastroduodenoscopy reveals a peptic ulcer in the upper duodenum. Which of the following is an important association of duodenal peptic ulcer disease?

(A) Barrett esophagus and columnar intestinal metaplasia of esophageal squamous epithelium
(B) Evolution into carcinoma as a likely sequela
(C) *Helicobacter pylori* infection
(D) Hiatal hernia and incompetent lower esophageal sphincter
(E) Pernicious anemia and achlorhydria

5. A 60-year-old Caucasian man with a 5-year history of gastroesophageal reflux disease (GERD) presents with persistent pyrosis (heartburn) and acid regurgitation. He has had similar symptoms for the past 5 years. Because this patient has a long history of GERD, an esophagogastroduodenoscopy is performed to screen for Barrett esophagus, a well-known complication of long-standing GERD. Results reveal that Barrett esophagus is indeed present. Which of the following is true of Barrett esophagus?

(A) A biopsy will show a histologic finding of columnar-to-squamous metaplasia.
(B) It is a known precursor of adenocarcinoma of the esophagus.
(C) It is a known precursor of carcinoma of the stomach.
(D) It is a known precursor of squamous cell carcinoma of the esophagus.
(E) The most common location is the proximal (upper) third of the esophagus.

6. A 65-year-old man presents with dysphagia, weight loss, and anorexia. Physical examination is normal. Esophagogastroduodenoscopy with biopsy of an esophageal lesion is performed, revealing squamous cell carcinoma. Which of the following is true regarding this cancer?

(A) Cigarette smoking and chronic alcohol use are associated risk factors.
(B) Gastroesophageal reflux disease and Barrett esophagus are associated risk factors.
(C) Histologic findings include disordered, back-to-back submucosal glands.
(D) It most frequently arises in the lower third of the esophagus.
(E) This cancer is characterized by an indolent course, and long survival is common.

7. A 10-day-old infant presents with projectile vomiting. His mother states that the infant will actively drink his milk, but he forcefully vomits after each feeding. The infant shows signs of failure to thrive, with weight loss, dehydration, and lethargy. Physical examination reveals a firm, nontender, mobile, "olive-shaped" epigastric mass. Which of the following is the most likely diagnosis?

(A) *Candida* esophagitis
(B) Congenital pyloric stenosis
(C) Esophageal cancer
(D) Gastroesophageal reflux disease
(E) Tracheoesophageal fistula

8. A 25-year-old man presents with low-grade fever, weight loss, fatigue, crampy abdominal pain, episodic diarrhea, and postprandial bloating. Right lower quadrant tenderness is elicited on palpation of the abdomen. A capsule endoscopy reveals thickening of the terminal ileum, edema, marked luminal narrowing, and a cobblestone appearance of the mucosa. Which of the following is a characteristic of this condition?

(A) Additional typical findings include crypt abscesses and pseudopolyps
(B) Inflammation and ulceration limited to mucosa and submucosa with sparing of deeper layers
(C) It can affect any portion of the gastrointestinal tract, but proximal jejunum is most common site of involvement
(D) It can cause fistula formation between loops of affected bowel
(E) It is a benign, self-limited disorder with no complicating sequelae

9. A 70-year-old man presents with fatigue, weight loss, abdominal pain, and overt blood in the stools. A complete blood count reveals anemia with hemoglobin of 10.0 g/dL. A colonoscopy and colon biopsy reveal adenocarcinoma. Which of the following is the most likely predisposing lesion that led to this condition?

(A) Familial adenomatous polyposis syndrome
(B) Hyperplastic polyp
(C) Long-standing ulcerative colitis
(D) Peutz-Jeghers polyp
(E) Tubular adenoma

10. For the past week, a 65-year-old woman has been treated for a severe infection with broad-spectrum antibiotics, and she had recovered well. However, over the past day she has developed foul-smelling, voluminous, greenish, watery diarrhea, as well as abdominal pain and fever. She is diagnosed with pseudomembranous colitis. Which of the following is the mechanism associated with this condition?

(A) Aggregation of bacterial colonies on the lumen, forming pseudomembranes
(B) Bacterial release of exotoxin, inducing necrosis of the mucosa
(C) Physical invasion of bacteria into the superficial mucosa, leading to pseudomembrane formation
(D) Selective killing of *Clostridium difficile* bacteria by antibiotics
(E) Spread of the previous infection to the colon

11. A 20-year-old man presents with severe right lower quadrant abdominal pain, nausea, and anorexia. He states that the abdominal pain started around his umbilicus and has now migrated to the right lower quadrant of his abdomen. Physical examination reveals exquisite tenderness at McBurney point (the point one third of the distance along the line from the right anterior superior iliac spine to the umbilicus). This patient is diagnosed with acute appendicitis. Which of the following is the treatment for this condition?

(A) Antibiotics only, because the appendix is crucial for survival
(B) Surgical resection of the appendix, because appendicitis can lead to appendiceal cancer
(C) Surgical resection of the appendix, because appendicitis can lead to perforation or abscess
(D) "Watch-and-wait" approach over days to see if inflammation subsides

12. A 69-year-old man was seen for vague abdominal distress. The gastric lesion shown in the figure was resected following initial endoscopic discovery. Which of the following statements about this condition is correct?

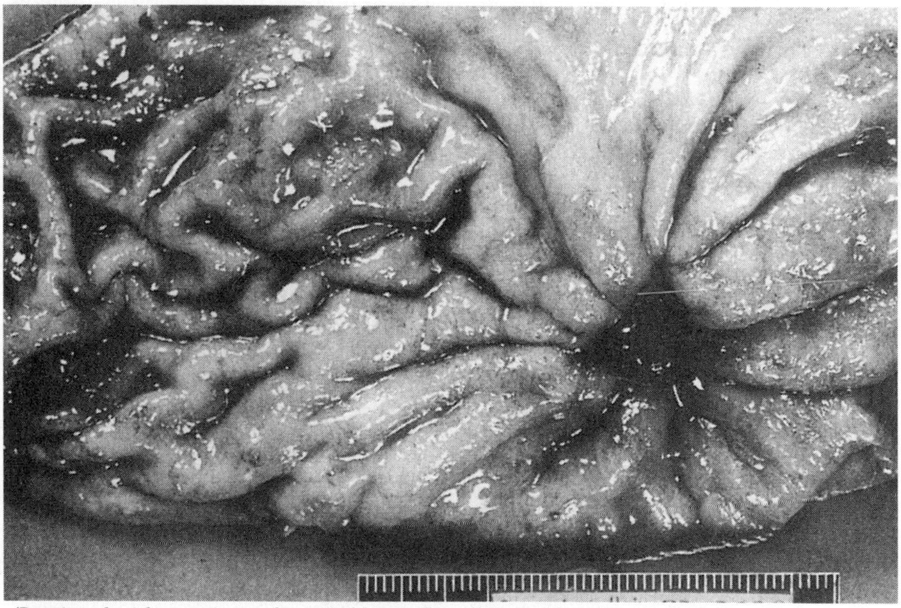

(Reprinted with permission from Golden A, Powell D, and Jennings C: *Pathology: Understanding Human Disease,* 2nd ed. Baltimore, Williams & Wilkins, 1985, p 319.)

(A) It has been decreasing in frequency over the past several decades.
(B) It is more frequent in Japan than in the United States.
(C) It is related to the use of nitrites as food preservatives.
(D) It may result in Krukenberg tumors.
(E) It will most likely heal with conservative management.

13. An elderly woman with chronic constipation dies of a stroke and comes to autopsy. The figure illustrates a portion of her colon. The lesions shown in the figure

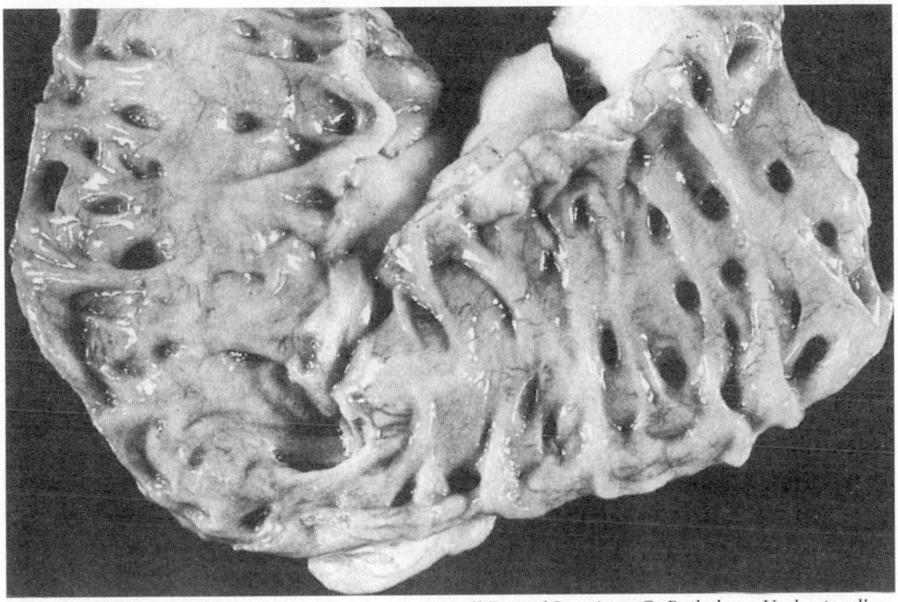

(Reprinted with permission from Golden A, Powell D, and Jennings C: *Pathology: Understanding Human Disease,* 2nd ed. Baltimore, Williams & Wilkins, 1985, p 333.)

(A) Can be complicated by inflammation, perforation, and peritonitis
(B) Is most likely related to a high-fiber diet
(C) Most frequently occurs high in the right side of the colon
(D) Occurs most often in teenagers

14. In a routine colonoscopy, a 76-year-old man is found to have a lesion similar to that shown in the illustration. The lesion shown is a classic example of which of the following?

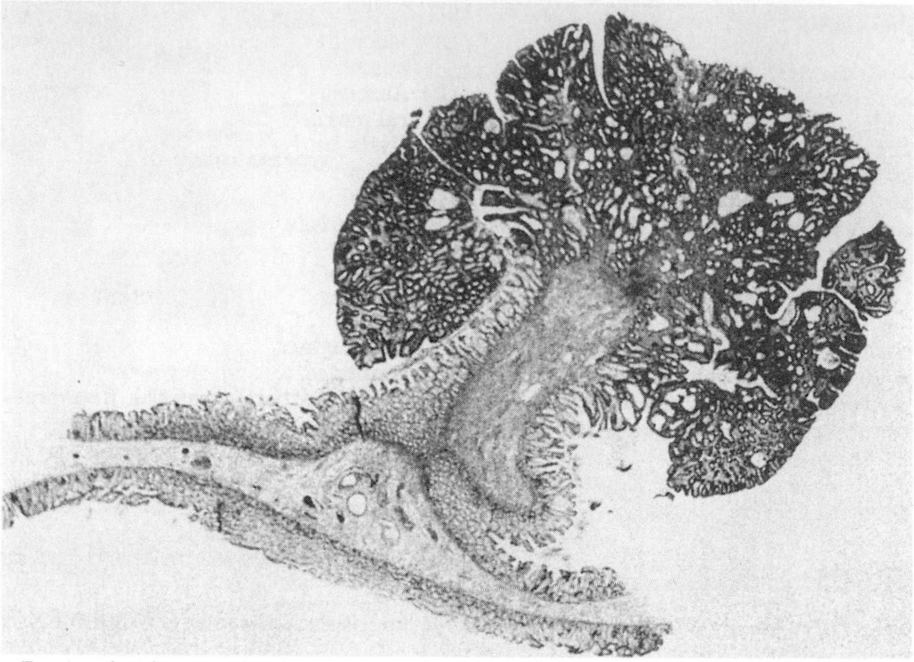

(Reprinted with permission from Golden A, Powell D, and Jennings C: *Pathology: Understanding Human Disease,* 2nd ed. Baltimore, Williams & Wilkins, 1985, p 341.)

(A) Hamartoma
(B) Invasive adenocarcinoma
(C) Peutz-Jeghers polyp
(D) Tubular adenoma
(E) Villous adenoma

ANSWERS AND EXPLANATIONS

1-A. Sjögren syndrome is an autoimmune disorder characterized by keratoconjunctivitis sicca and xerostomia, due to lymphocytic infiltration and parenchymal destruction of the parotid and lacrimal glands in association with a connective tissue disorder such as rheumatoid arthritis. Malignant lymphoma is a frequent complication.

2-D. Approximately 80% to 90% of salivary gland tumors originate in the parotid gland, and of these, approximately 70% are pleomorphic adenomas. The term "mixed tumor" properly applies to this benign tumor, which often demonstrates myxoid and cartilage-like elements in addition to stellate or fusiform epithelial cells. Complete surgical resection is difficult because of the tumor's proximity to the facial nerve, and thus recurrence is frequent.

3-E. This is a classic case of gastroesophageal reflux disease (GERD), which is caused by reflux of gastric acid contents into the lower esophagus. GERD manifests as burning epigastric pain on eating spicy foods or on lying recumbent. The pain is usually relieved by antacids. GERD is most commonly associated with hiatal hernia and an incompetent lower esophageal sphincter, as well as with excessive use of alcohol or tobacco, increased gastric volume, pregnancy, and scleroderma. Barrett esophagus, or columnar intestinal metaplasia of the epithelium of the distal esophagus, is a complication of long-standing GERD.

4-C. Of course, the immediate problem in this patient is life-threatening upper gastrointestinal hemorrhage, an important complication of peptic ulcer disease. Peptic ulcer disease occurs most frequently in the first portion of the duodenum, the lesser curvature of the stomach, or the distal esophagus. Duodenal peptic ulcers are associated with hypersecretion of gastric acid and pepsin and are closely related to gastric *Helicobacter pylori* infection. Apparently, *H. pylori* increases gastric acid secretion and impairs mucosal defenses. Other predisposing factors include aspirin or nonsteroidal anti-inflammatory drug intake, smoking, Zollinger-Ellison syndrome, primary hyperparathyroidism, and multiple endocrine neoplasia type I.

5-B. Barrett esophagus is columnar metaplasia of the esophageal squamous epithelium (squamous-to-columnar). The columnar epithelium is often of the intestinal type with goblet cells. Barrett esophagus is a complication of long-standing gastroesophageal reflux disease and is a precursor of esophageal adenocarcinoma. The most common location is in the distal (lower) third of the esophagus.

6-A. Squamous cell carcinoma of the esophagus is an aggressive cancer with rapid progression and short survival in all stages of disease. It is most common in subjects with a long-term cigarette smoking and alcohol use history. The tumor arises most commonly in the upper and middle thirds of the esophagus.

7-B. Congenital pyloric stenosis is caused by hypertrophy of the circular muscular layer of the pylorus, resulting in a palpable mass in the epigastrium. Hypertrophy of the pyloric musculature leads to obstruction and the characteristic projectile vomiting. This condition most commonly occurs in male infants within the first several days to weeks of life.

8-D. Crohn disease and ulcerative colitis are the two classic inflammatory bowel diseases. Crohn disease is a chronic inflammatory condition that can affect any part of the gastrointestinal tract from mouth to anus, but most commonly involves the distal ileocecum, small intestine, or colon. Morphologically, Crohn disease manifests as transmural inflammation (involving all layers of the intestinal wall), thickening of involved intestine, linear ulceration, a cobblestone appearance, skip lesions (normal intestine between affected regions), and granulomas. Strictures and fistulae may develop, leading to intestinal obstruction. Crohn disease may lead to carcinoma of the small intestine or colon, but much less commonly than ulcerative colitis.

9-E. Adenocarcinoma of the colon most commonly develops through a progression of mutations in oncogenes and tumor suppressor genes in a multistep process. Normal mucosa evolves into a tubular adenoma with malignant potential, which then further evolves into carcinoma (the adenoma-carcinoma sequence). Carcinoma of the rectosigmoid (left-sided) tends to present as early obstruction, with change in bowel habits and decreased caliber of stool, whereas carcinoma of the right colon (right-sided) tends to present late, with iron deficiency anemia due to chronic blood loss from the lesion.

10-B. Pseudomembranous colitis is caused by overgrowth of *Clostridium difficile.* This organism produces exotoxin that induces necrosis of the superficial mucosa, leading to pseudomembrane formation. The bacteria itself does not invade the mucosa. This condition most often occurs in patients with a history of broad-spectrum antibiotic use, because elimination of normal intestinal flora promotes overgrowth of *C. difficile.*

11-C. The inflamed appendix in acute appendicitis should be surgically removed because of possible devastating complications of perforation or abscess.

12-E. The illustration shows a chronic gastric peptic ulcer with characteristic radiating folds of the gastric mucosa starting at the ulcer margins. The lesion has a smooth base and nonelevated, punched-out margins, in contrast to gastric carcinoma, which often has an irregular necrotic base and firm, raised margins. Despite these characteristic findings, the distinction between gastric peptic ulcer and ulcerated carcinoma must be established by biopsy. In contrast to carcinoma, peptic ulcer will usually heal with conservative management.

13-A. The illustration demonstrates diverticulosis of the colon. These lesions are most common in older persons and are found most often in the sigmoid. The incidence of disease is increased in populations that consume low-fiber diets. Although most often asymptomatic, diverticula may become the site of acute inflammation (diverticulitis), sometimes with life-threatening complications, such as perforation and peritonitis.

14-D. The illustration shows a tubular adenoma, which is the most common form of adenomatous polyp. These lesions can be single or multiple, or they can occur as components of various multiple polyposis syndromes. Notable among these syndromes are Gardner (associated with osteomas and soft tissue tumors), Turcot (associated with central nervous system tumors), and familial polyposis. All of the foregoing are associated with an increased incidence of colon malignancy. In contrast, the Peutz-Jeghers polyp is a non-neoplastic hamartomatous lesion. Even though the polyp itself does not transform into colon cancer, the Peutz-Jeghers syndrome is associated with an increased incidence of colon cancer and malignancies elsewhere.

CHAPTER

16

Liver, Gallbladder, and Exocrine Pancreas

I. Diseases of the Liver

A. **Jaundice** (Table 16-1) refers to **yellow discoloration** of skin, sclerae, and tissues caused by hyperbilirubinemia. It is most often associated with hepatocellular disease, biliary obstruction, or hemolytic anemia.

1. **Physiologic jaundice of the newborn** is commonly noted during the **first week of life** but is not usually clinically important. It is characterized chemically by **unconjugated hyperbilirubinemia.**
   a. This form of jaundice results from both increased bilirubin production and a relative deficiency of glucuronyl transferase in the immature liver; these phenomena are exaggerated in premature infants.
   b. Physiologic jaundice of the newborn must be distinguished from neonatal cholestasis, which is due to a wide variety of causes, including extrahepatic biliary atresia, α_1-antitrypsin deficiency, cytomegalovirus infection, and many other conditions.
2. **Congenital hyperbilirubinemias**
   a. **Gilbert syndrome** is extremely **common,** occurring in almost 5% of the population. This familial disorder is characterized by a modest **elevation of serum unconjugated bilirubin;** the liver is otherwise unimpaired, and there are no clinical consequences. The cause is a combination of decreased bilirubin uptake by liver cells and reduced activity of glucuronyl transferase.
   b. **Crigler-Najjar syndrome** is a severe familial disorder characterized by unconjugated hyperbilirubinemia caused by a deficiency of glucuronyl transferase.
      (1) One form leads to early death from kernicterus; damage to the basal ganglia and other parts of the central nervous system are caused by unconjugated bilirubin.
      (2) A less severe form responds to phenobarbital therapy, which decreases the serum concentration of unconjugated bilirubin.
   c. **Dubin-Johnson syndrome** is an autosomal recessive form of conjugated hyperbilirubinemia characterized by defective bilirubin transport. It is characterized by a striking brown-to-black **discoloration of the liver** caused by the deposition of granules of **very dark pigment,** the chemical nature of which is unclear.
   d. **Rotor syndrome** is similar to Dubin-Johnson syndrome, but abnormal pigment is not present.

B. **Acute viral hepatitis** (Table 16-2)

1. **General considerations**
   a. Acute viral hepatitis is characterized by jaundice and extremely high elevations of serum aspartate and alanine aminotransferases.

TABLE 16-1 *Differential Diagnosis of Jaundice*

Type of Jaundice	Hyperbilirubinemia	Urine Bilirubin	Urine Urobilinogen	Other Findings
Hepatocellular	Conjugated and unconjugated	Increased	Normal to decreased	Intrahepatic cholestasis may result in retention of conjugated bilirubin; hepatocellular damage may result in impaired conjugation of bilirubin; enzyme activities of ALT and AST increased; increased alkaline phosphatase indicates intrahepatic obstruction
Obstructive	Conjugated	Increased	Decreased	Alkaline phosphatase and cholesterol increased; ALT and AST variable; with complete obstruction, stools pale and clay-colored and urine urobilinogen undetectable
Hemolytic	Unconjugated	Absent (acholuria)	Increased	Degree of urine urobilinogen increase directly related to increased hemoglobin catabolism

ALT = alanine aminotransferase; AST = aspartate aminotransferase.

TABLE 16-2 *Viral Hepatitis: Causative Agents, Transmission, and Clinical Features*

Virus	Predominant Modes of Transmission	Clinical Features
Hepatitis A virus	Fecal-oral	No carrier state; does not lead to chronic liver disease
Hepatitis B virus (HBV)	Sexual and parenteral	Frequently leads to carrier state or chronic liver disease
Hepatitis C virus	Parenteral	Most frequent cause of transfusion-mediated hepatitis; frequently progresses to chronic liver disease
Delta agent (hepatitis D virus)	Sexual and parenteral	Requires concurrent infection with HBV for replication
Hepatitis E virus	Fecal-oral	Occurs in epidemic form in Third World countries; does not lead to chronic liver disease
Hepatitis G virus	Parenteral	Frequent in blood donors; role as cause of acute or chronic hepatitis is not established

b. The disease may be caused by a variety of viral agents, including Epstein-Barr virus or cytomegalovirus, but usually results from hepatic infection by any of the following viruses, all of which are RNA viruses, with the exception of hepatitis B virus, which is a DNA virus.

2. **Hepatitis A virus (HAV)**
   a. Spread occurs by **fecal-oral transmission; parenteral infection does not occur.**
   b. The incubation period is 15–45 days.
   c. HAV **does not cause a chronic carrier state** or lead to chronic hepatitis; complete recovery almost always occurs. There is no relation to hepatocellular carcinoma.
3. **Hepatitis B virus (HBV)**
   a. HBV consists of a central core containing the viral DNA genome, DNA polymerase, hepatitis B core antigen (HBcAg), and hepatitis B e antigen (HBeAg), and an outer lipoprotein coat containing the hepatitis B surface antigen (HBsAg). The complete virion is known as the Dane particle.
   b. **Transmission is via parenteral, sexual, and vertical (mother to neonate) routes.** There is an increased incidence of HBV infection in male homosexuals.
   c. The incubation period averages 60–90 days.
   d. HBV has a major association with hepatocellular carcinoma.
   e. Infection is associated with a "ground-glass" appearance of hepatocytes.
   f. Disease **can result in a carrier state or in chronic liver disease.** The sequence in which the various antigens or antibodies to these antigens appear in the serum is of clinical significance.
      (1) **HBsAg** appears in serum some weeks before the onset of clinical findings, then decreases and generally persists for a total of 3–4 months. Persistence as detectable serum antigen for more than 6 months denotes the carrier state. HBsAg elicits an antibody response (anti-HBsAg); antibody appears a few weeks after the disappearance of the antigen and indicates recovery as well as immunity to future infection.
      (2) **HBeAg** appears shortly after HBsAg and disappears before HBsAg. It is closely correlated with viral infectivity.
      (3) **Anti-HBcAg** appears about 4 weeks after the appearance of HBsAg, is present during the acute illness, and can remain elevated for several years. It is a marker (along with anti-HBeAg) of hepatitis infection during the "window period" between the disappearance of HBsAg and the appearance of anti-HBsAg.
      (4) **HBV DNA** can also be detected in serum and is an index of infectivity.
4. **Hepatitis C virus (HCV)** is a common cause of what was formerly called non-A, non-B hepatitis.
   a. **Transmission is parenteral.** HCV is a frequent cause of **transfusion-mediated hepatitis** and often leads to a carrier state and chronic hepatitis.
   b. HCV is frequently associated with hepatocellular carcinoma.
5. **Hepatitis D virus (HDV, delta agent)** is a very small, spherical virus consisting of a single RNA strand and the associated delta protein antigen (HDAg), surrounded by a proteinaceous coat of HBsAg. HDV is **replicatively defective,** requiring **simultaneous infection with HBV** for viral replication. It usually causes illness more severe than HBV infection alone.
   a. Transmission is via **sexual or parenteral routes.**
   b. Incidence is especially high in intravenous drug users.
6. **Hepatitis E virus (HEV)** causes an **enterically transmitted** form of viral hepatitis similar to HAV infection that occurs in water-borne epidemic form in underdeveloped countries. HEV has an as yet unknown association with chronic hepatitis or hepatocellular carcinoma, but it has a high incidence of mortality (about 20%) when occuring in pregnancy.
7. **Hepatitis G virus (HGV)** affects 1%–2% of healthy blood donors, but its pathologic significance is questionable. HGV does not lead to chronic hepatitis and has no known relationship to hepatocellular carcinoma.

C. **Chronic hepatitis**

1. Chronic hepatitis is defined by the persistence of abnormalities for more than 6 months. It may result from any of the viral hepatitides except HAV or HEV infection and also from liver damage induced by nonviral agents.
2. **Autoimmune hepatitis** is morphologically indistinguishable from other forms of chronic hepatitis. It is secondary to various immunologic abnormalities. It is clinically marked by hypergammaglobulinemia and anti–smooth muscle antibodies.

D. **Other inflammatory liver disorders**

1. **Neonatal hepatitis** is of unknown etiology.
   a. The presence of multinucleated giant cells is characteristic. There may be bile pigment and hemosiderin within parenchymal cells.
   b. It may cause jaundice during the first few weeks of life.
2. **Other viral infections** may involve the liver along with other organ systems.
   a. **Epstein-Barr virus (EBV)** causes **infectious mononucleosis,** which often has a hepatitic component.
   b. **Cytomegalovirus (CMV)** may involve the liver in infants and immunocompromised persons. Infected liver cells demonstrate characteristic nuclear inclusions surrounded by a halo (owl's eye appearance).
   c. **Herpes simplex virus type 1 (HSV-1)** may involve the liver in infants and immunocompromised persons.
   d. **Yellow fever** characteristically demonstrates a severe hepatitic component marked by midzonal hepatic necrosis. The dying hepatocytes often condense into eosinophilic contracted forms referred to as **Councilman bodies.** Similar inclusions are observed in all of the viral hepatitides and are manifestations of apoptosis.
3. **Leptospirosis,** also known as Weil disease or icterohemorrhagic fever, is caused by *Leptospira* species. This severe infection is characterized by jaundice, renal failure, and hemorrhagic phenomena.
4. ***Echinococcus granulosus*** infestation is caused by ingestion of tapeworm eggs from the excreta of dogs and sheep. It results in **hydatid disease** of the liver, in which large parasitic cysts invade the liver.
5. **Schistosomiasis** is caused by infestation with *Schistosoma mansoni* or *S. japonicum.* The adult worms lodge in the portal vein and its branches. The eggs are highly antigenic and stimulate granuloma formation, with resultant tissue destruction, scarring, and portal hypertension.

E. **Microvesicular fatty liver.** This group of serious disorders is associated with the presence of small fat vacuoles in parenchymal liver cells, which differ from the large fat-containing vacuoles characteristic of fatty change.

1. **Reye syndrome**
   a. This acute disorder of **young children** is characterized by encephalopathy, coma, and microvesicular fatty liver.
   b. Reye syndrome is associated with **aspirin administration** to children with **acute viral infections.**
2. **Fatty liver of pregnancy** is acute hepatic failure during the third trimester of pregnancy associated with microvesicular fatty liver. This condition has a high mortality rate.
3. **Tetracycline toxicity** results in an unpredictable hypersensitivity-like reaction with microvesicular fatty change.

F. **Alcoholic liver disease** is the constellation of hepatic changes associated with excessive alcohol consumption; it varies from fatty change to alcoholic hepatitis and cirrhosis. The most common form of liver disease in the United States, it may be asymptomatic or may be associated with mild-to-severe hepatic inflammation, cirrhosis, or encephalopathy.

1. **Fatty change (steatosis)** is the most frequent morphologic abnormality caused by alcohol and is reversible.

2. **Alcoholic hepatitis**
   a. Characteristics include **fatty change, focal liver cell necrosis, infiltrates of neutrophils,** and the presence of intracytoplasmic eosinophilic hyaline inclusions (**Mallory bodies,** alcoholic hyalin) derived from cytokeratin intermediate filaments; these inclusions are characteristic, but not entirely specific for alcoholic hepatitis.
   b. Alcoholic hepatitis is often associated with irreversible fibrosis that characteristically surrounds central veins and has been referred to as **perivenular fibrosis,** sclerosing hyaline necrosis, or central hyaline sclerosis. This fibrosis can lead to central vein obstruction and fibrosis surrounding individual liver cells and can result in cirrhosis.
3. **Alcoholic cirrhosis**

G. **Cirrhosis** (Table 16-3)
1. **General considerations**
   a. Cirrhosis is a descriptive term for chronic liver disease characterized by generalized disorganization of hepatic architecture with scarring and nodule formation. Liver cell damage, regenerative activity, and generalized fibrosis resulting in a nodular pattern are also characteristic.
   b. Classification can be morphologic, on the basis of nodule size (micronodular, macronodular, and mixed macromicronodular forms).
   c. In all forms, there is an **increased incidence of hepatocellular carcinoma.**
   d. There are numerous etiologic agents, including:
      (1) **Prolonged alcohol intake,** drugs, and chemical agents
      (2) Viral hepatitis, biliary obstruction, and hemochromatosis
      (3) Wilson disease and other inborn errors of metabolism
      (4) Heart failure with long-standing chronic passive congestion of the liver

TABLE 16-3 *Cirrhosis: Types and Features*

Type	Features
Alcoholic (Laennec, nutritional)	Most frequently occurring form of cirrhosis; associated with alcoholism; micronodular pattern evolving in late stages to typical hobnail liver with large, irregular nodules
Postnecrotic (macronodular, posthepatitic)	Large, irregular nodules containing intact hepatic lobules; diverse etiologies; often end result of viral hepatitis, especially hepatitis B
Biliary	
Primary	Probable autoimmune origin; antimitochondrial antibodies; obstructive jaundice
Secondary	End result of long-standing extrahepatic biliary obstruction
Hemochromatosis	
Hereditary (primary)	Familial defect in control of iron absorption; massive accumulation of hemosiderin in hepatic and pancreatic parenchymal cells, myocardium, and other sites; classic triad of cirrhosis, diabetes mellitus, and increased skin pigmentation; cirrhosis micronodular type
Secondary	Caused by chronic iron overload of diverse etiology
Wilson disease	Accumulation of copper in liver, kidney, brain, and cornea; cirrhosis can be micronodular or macronodular; decreased serum ceruloplasmin
Inborn errors of metabolism	Cirrhosis associated with galactosemia, glycogen storage diseases, or α_1-antitrypsin deficiency

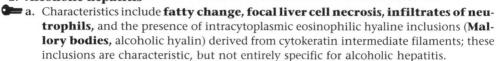

2. **Alcoholic (Laennec, nutritional) cirrhosis** is the prototype for all forms of cirrhosis.
   a. **Clinical manifestations**
      (1) **Findings associated with hepatocellular damage and liver failure** include:
         (a) **Jaundice,** most often mixed conjugated and unconjugated
         (b) **Hypoalbuminemia,** caused by decreased albumin synthesis in damaged hepatocytes
         (c) **Coagulation factor deficiencies,** caused by decreased synthesis; all coagulation factors, with the exception of von Willebrand factor, are synthesized in the liver.
         (d) **Hyperestrinism,** manifest as palmar erythema (liver palms); spider nevi (capillary telangiectases) of the face, upper arms, and chest; loss of body and pubic hair; testicular atrophy; and gynecomastia
      (2) **Consequences of intrahepatic scarring with increased portal venous pressure** include:
         (a) **Esophageal varices,** often leading to upper gastrointestinal hemorrhage
         (b) **Rectal hemorrhoids**
         (c) **Periumbilical venous collaterals** (caput medusae)
         (d) **Splenomegaly**
      (3) **Changes due to both liver cell damage and portal hypertension** include:
         (a) **Peripheral edema, ascites, or hydrothorax,** caused by
            (i) **Increased portal venous pressure,** which leads to increased production of hepatic lymph
            (ii) **Decreased plasma oncotic pressure** secondary to hypoalbuminemia
            (iii) **Retention of sodium and water** as a result of decreased hepatic degradation of aldosterone, activation of the renin-angiotensin system, or both
         (b) **Encephalopathy** (portal-systemic encephalopathy) facilitated by shunting from the portal to the systemic circulation, with direct delivery of neurotoxic substances such as ammonia and other enteric degradation products directly into the systemic circulation. Neurologic manifestations varying from slight confusion to deep coma along with asterixis (flapping tremor of hands) are characteristic features.
   b. **Morphologic abnormalities**
      (1) The liver may be enlarged or small and shrunken.
      (2) The pattern is most often micronodular.
      (3) Hepatic architecture is obscured by fibrous bands surrounding nodules of distorted liver cell plates.
      (4) The fibrous bands contain proliferating bile ducts and inflammatory cells, most often lymphocytes and plasma cells.
      (5) In late stages, the nodules tend to become larger and irregular; this pattern results in a scarred, shrunken liver termed the hobnail liver.
3. **Postnecrotic (macronodular, posthepatitic) cirrhosis**
   a. Morphologic characteristics include broad fibrous bands dividing the liver into **large, irregular nodules,** often containing intact hepatic lobules.
   b. This form of cirrhosis **is often a sequela of chronic active hepatitis; HBV and HCV are the most common viral causes.** In addition, this disease may be caused by noninfectious hepatotoxic agents. Sometimes, it can result from the progression of micronodular alcoholic cirrhosis. Often, the etiology is uncertain (cryptogenic cirrhosis).
   c. Postnecrotic cirrhosis leads to hepatocellular carcinoma more often than other forms of cirrhosis.
4. **Biliary cirrhosis** occurs as a primary, probably autoimmune, disorder and much more frequently as a secondary form due to biliary obstruction.

a. **Primary biliary cirrhosis**
   (1) This form of cirrhosis is most likely of **autoimmune origin.** There is an increased incidence of other autoimmune disorders in affected patients, and **antimitochondrial antibodies** are characteristic.
   (2) Disease is **most common in middle-aged women.**
   (3) Characteristics include **severe obstructive jaundice, itching, and hypercholesterolemia;** hypercholesterolemia leads to cutaneous xanthoma formation.
   (4) Primary biliary cirrhosis is marked by increased parenchymal copper concentration, a finding of unknown significance.

b. **Secondary biliary cirrhosis**
   (1) The cause is **extrahepatic biliary obstruction,** which leads to dilation and increased pressure within intrahepatic bile ducts and cholangioles, further resulting in ductal injury, ductal and periductal inflammation, and resolution by fibrous tissue formation.
   (2) Complications often include ascending cholangitis and bacterial inflammation of the intrahepatic bile ducts.
   (3) Secondary biliary cirrhosis is marked histologically by evidence of bile stasis and by bile lakes, accumulations of bile within hepatic parenchyma.

5. **Primary sclerosing cholangitis** is rare except in association with inflammatory bowel disease, especially ulcerative colitis.
   a. Characteristics include inflammation, fibrosis, and stenosis of intrahepatic and extrahepatic bile ducts. It eventually develops into biliary cirrhosis.
   b. There is an associated increased incidence of cholangiocarcinoma.

6. **Hemochromatosis**
   a. **Hereditary hemochromatosis** is a **familial defect of iron absorption** by the intestinal mucosa.
      (1) This disease has been considered one of the most common autosomal recessive disorders, but this idea has recently been modified. Although the gene defect is common, the penetrance and development of clinical disease is low.
      (2) Hereditary hemochromatosis can be detected and treated successfully before organ damage occurs by screening for increased transferrin iron saturation or, in selected cases, for mutations in the *Hfe* gene on chromosome 6.
      (3) In its fully developed state, characteristics include:
         (a) The **triad of cirrhosis, diabetes mellitus, and increased skin pigmentation,** giving rise to the older term **bronze diabetes**
         (b) Skin pigmentation caused by hemosiderin and melanin deposition
         (c) **Pigment cirrhosis** (micronodular cirrhosis with enormous accumulation of parenchymal hemosiderin demonstrable by Prussian blue staining)
         (d) Marked **increase in serum iron** and modest **reduction in total iron-binding capacity** (TIBC, transferrin). This combination results in **increased transferrin iron saturation.**
         (e) Increased serum ferritin
   b. **Secondary hemochromatosis** is most often associated with a combination of ineffective erythropoiesis and multiple transfusions, such as occurs in thalassemia major. It may also be secondary to various other causes of iron overload.

7. **Wilson disease (hepatolenticular degeneration)** is an **autosomal recessive** disorder of copper metabolism.
   a. A **decreased serum ceruloplasmin** (copper-binding protein) is characteristic. This is probably not a primary defect but it is secondary to increased copper.
   b. Manifestations include **liver disease** that varies from chronic hepatitis to cirrhosis, either micronodular or macronodular in type.
   c. Wilson disease is also marked by the **Kayser-Fleischer ring** circumscribing the periphery of the cornea, representing deposition of copper-containing pigment in Descemet membrane.
   d. In addition, there may be aminoaciduria and glycosuria due to renal tubular damage.
   e. Wilson disease results in an abnormal major **accumulation of copper** in parenchymal cells of the liver and kidney and in the brain and cornea.

f. The disease also results in extrapyramidal motor signs caused by **involvement of the basal ganglia,** especially the putamen of the lenticular nucleus.

8. **Cirrhosis due to inborn errors of metabolism** results from several disorders, including:
   a. α_1-antitrypsin deficiency
   b. Galactose-1-phosphate uridyl transferase deficiency (galactosemia)
   c. Glycogen storage diseases

H. **Vascular disorders of the liver**

1. **Portal hypertension** is characterized by the development of venous collaterals with varices in the submucosal veins of the esophagus, the hemorrhoidal plexus, and other sites. This condition is often classified by the site of portal venous obstruction:
   a. **Prehepatic:** caused by portal and splenic vein obstruction, most often by thrombosis
   b. **Intrahepatic:** caused by intrahepatic vascular obstruction, most often by cirrhosis or metastatic tumor, and more rarely by exotic entities such as schistosomiasis
   c. **Posthepatic:** caused by venous congestion in the distal hepatic venous circulation, most often as a result of constrictive pericarditis, tricuspid insufficiency, congestive heart failure, or hepatic vein occlusion (Budd-Chiari syndrome)
2. **Infarction** is unusual, because the liver has a double blood supply (mesenteric and hepatic).
3. **Budd-Chiari syndrome**
   a. The cause is thrombotic occlusion of the major hepatic veins, resulting in abdominal pain, jaundice, hepatomegaly, ascites, and eventual liver failure.
   b. Budd-Chiari syndrome is most often associated with polycythemia vera, hepatocellular carcinoma, and other abdominal neoplasms; may also occur as a complication of pregnancy.
4. **Congestive heart failure**
   a. In long-standing chronic right-sided heart failure, the cut surface of the liver can assume an appearance referred to as the nutmeg liver, with dark red congested centrilobular areas alternating with pale portal areas.
   b. Eventually, centrilobular fibrosis occurs, resulting in cardiac cirrhosis (cardiac sclerosis). Similar changes may follow long-standing constrictive pericarditis or tricuspid insufficiency.

I. **Hepatic tumors**

1. **Benign tumors**
   a. **Hemangioma** is the most common benign tumor of the liver.
   b. **Adenoma**
      (1) The incidence is apparently related to use of oral contraceptives.
      (2) When the adenoma is subcapsular in location, it may rupture, resulting in severe intraperitoneal hemorrhage.
2. **Malignant tumors**
   a. **Metastatic tumors** account for the majority of hepatic malignancies.
   b. **Hepatocellular carcinoma** is the most common primary malignancy of the liver.
      (1) This hepatic malignancy almost always develops in association with preexisting cirrhosis of any kind, especially when associated with HBV infection.
      (2) Hepatocellular carcinoma has been associated with aflatoxin B_1 contamination of nuts and grains; aflatoxin B_1 is thought to cause specific point mutations in the *p53* gene.
      (3) Frequently, the cancer is marked by increased serum concentration of α-fetoprotein.
      (4) There is a propensity for invasion of vascular channels with hematogenous dissemination.
   c. **Cholangiocarcinoma (bile duct carcinoma)** is less common than hepatocellular carcinoma. This form of hepatic cancer occurs most frequently in the Far East, where it is associated with *Clonorchis sinensis* (liver fluke) infestation.

(1) The cancer originates from intrahepatic biliary epithelium.
(2) Like hepatocellular carcinoma, it has a propensity for early invasion of vascular channels.
(3) Unlike hepatocellular carcinoma, cholangiocarcinoma is not associated with HBV infection or cirrhosis.
(4) Sometimes, it occurs as a late complication of thorium dioxide (Thorotrast) administration.

d. **Hemangiosarcoma (angiosarcoma)**
(1) This form of hepatic cancer is a rare malignant vascular tumor.
(2) It is associated with toxic exposure to polyvinyl (vinyl) chloride, thorium dioxide (Thorotrast), and arsenic.

II. Diseases of the Gallbladder

A. **Cholecystitis**
1. **Acute cholecystitis** is acute inflammation of the gallbladder.
a. The inflammation is most often pyogenic.
b. Clinical manifestations include nausea, vomiting, fever, and leukocytosis associated with right upper quadrant and epigastric pain.
2. **Chronic cholecystitis**
a. Thickening of the gallbladder wall occurs a result of extensive fibrosis.
b. Chronic inflammation is **frequently complicated by gallstones.**

B. **Cholelithiasis (gallstones)** has a higher incidence in women and is often associated with obesity and multiple pregnancies.
1. **Stone types**
a. **Cholesterol stones** are often solitary and too large to enter the cystic duct or the common bile duct.
b. **Pigment stones**
(1) Precipitation of excess insoluble unconjugated **bilirubin** results in their formation.
(2) Association often includes **hemolytic anemia** and bacterial infection.
c. **Mixed stones** account for most stones (75%–80%).
(1) Most of these stones are a mixture of cholesterol and calcium salts.
(2) Mixed stones can often be visualized radiographically because of their calcium content.
2. **Clinical manifestations**
a. **Cholelithiasis** is often silent and asymptomatic.
b. **Fatty food intolerance** is characteristic.
3. **Complications**
a. **Biliary colic** results from impaction of gallstone in cystic or common bile duct.
b. **Common bile duct obstruction** results in obstructive **jaundice** with conjugated hyperbilirubinemia, hypercholesterolemia, increased alkaline phosphatase, and hyperbilirubinuria.
c. **Ascending cholangitis** can result from secondary bacterial infection facilitated by obstructed bile flow.
d. **Cholecystitis,** acute or chronic. There is a reciprocal association between cholecystitis and cholelithiasis (i.e., each predisposes to the other).
e. **Acute pancreatitis**
f. **Gallstone ileus** (intestinal obstruction caused by passage of a large gallstone through the eroded gallbladder wall into the adjacent small bowel)
g. **Mucocele** (distended, mucus-filled gallbladder secondary to chronic cystic duct obstruction)
h. **Malignancy**

C. **Cholesterolosis (strawberry gallbladder)**
   1. Characteristics include yellow cholesterol-containing flecks in the mucosal surface.
   2. There is no association with inflammatory changes and no special association with cholelithiasis.

D. **Tumors**
   1. **Tumors of the gallbladder**
      a. Benign tumors of the gallbladder are rare.
      b. The most common primary tumor of the gallbladder is adenocarcinoma, which is often associated with gallstones.
   2. **Carcinoma of the extrahepatic biliary ducts and the ampulla of Vater** is less common than carcinoma of the gallbladder.
      a. This carcinoma is almost always adenocarcinoma.
      b. Typical presenting features include a progressive, relentless **obstructive jaundice.** Clinical characteristics include the combination of **jaundice** and a **palpably enlarged gallbladder.** Tumors that obstruct the common bile duct result in an enlarged, distended gallbladder; obstructing stones do not **(Courvoisier law)**.

III. Diseases of the Exocrine Pancreas

A. **Acute pancreatitis**
   1. The cause is activation of pancreatic enzymes, resulting in autodigestion of the organ, with **hemorrhagic fat necrosis** and deposition of **calcium soaps,** and sometimes formation of **pseudocysts** (parenchymal cysts not lined with ductal epithelium).
   2. Predisposing factors include **gallstones** and excessive **alcohol** intake.
   3. Clinical manifestations include **severe abdominal pain** and **prostration** closely mimicking an acute surgical abdomen.
   4. There is an association with **increased serum amylase.**
   5. Characteristics include **hypocalcemia** caused by loss of circulating calcium into precipitated calcium–fatty acid soaps.
   6. Acute pancreatitis can be superimposed on chronic pancreatitis.

B. **Chronic pancreatitis**
   1. Morphologic characteristics include **progressive parenchymal fibrosis. Calcification,** which may be visualized using radiography, is frequent. **Pseudocysts** may be evident.
   2. There is almost always an association with **alcoholism.**
   3. Clinical manifestations are extremely variable and include **abdominal and back pain,** progressive disability, and **steatorrhea,** which is a manifestation of pancreatic insufficiency with lipase deficiency. Fat malabsorption may be accompanied by a deficiency of fat-soluble vitamins and can thus lead to such conditions as night blindness (vitamin A deficiency) and osteomalacia (vitamin D deficiency).

C. **Carcinoma of the pancreas** is a common tumor
   1. Incidence is increasing; the carcinoma is more common in smokers.
   2. The carcinoma is almost always adenocarcinoma.
   3. More often, the carcinoma arises in the head of the pancreas, causing obstructive jaundice (see Table 16-1); somewhat less often it originates in the pancreatic body or tail. Carcinoma involving the pancreatic tail can cause islet destruction and secondary diabetes mellitus.
   4. Clinical manifestations may include **abdominal pain radiating to the back,** weight loss and anorexia, sometimes **migratory thrombophlebitis** (Trousseau sign), and frequently common bile duct obstruction resulting in **obstructive jaundice** (often accompanied by a **distended, palpable gallbladder**).
   5. Cancer is often silent before widespread dissemination occurs. Death usually results within 1 year.

REVIEW TEST

Directions:** Each of the numbered items or incomplete statements in this section is followed by answers or by completions of the statement. Select the* ***one *lettered answer or completion that is best in each case.*

1. A neonate has been persistently jaundiced from birth despite aggressive phototherapy and exchange transfusions. Laboratory studies demonstrate significantly elevated unconjugated bilirubin. Tests from an outside laboratory confirm the total absence of glucuronyl transferase activity. The neonate most likely has which of the following condition?

(A) Crigler-Najjar syndrome
(B) Gilbert syndrome
(C) Hemolytic disease of the newborn
(D) Physiologic jaundice of the newborn
(E) Rotor syndrome

2. An 18-year-old man presents to his family physician for a routine physical prior to moving away for college. Other than feeling slightly "stressed" by his soon-to-be new life situation, he has no complaints. A comprehensive metabolic panel reveals a modestly elevated unconjugated bilirubin but a near-normal aspartate aminotransferase and alanine aminotransferase. It is likely that the patient may have which of the following conditions?

(A) Crigler-Najjar syndrome
(B) Dubin-Johnson syndrome
(C) Gilbert syndrome
(D) Infectious mononucleosis
(E) Rotor syndrome

3. A 26-year-old woman presents to her primary care physician with fever, malaise, and "yellow eyes." She denies alcohol abuse but admits to indulging in a dozen raw oysters at happy hour 3 weeks ago. In addition to scleral icterus, physical examination reveals a mildly enlarged liver with tenderness to palpation. Laboratory studies demonstrate a markedly increased aspartate aminotransferase and alanine aminotransferase and increased IgM and anti-hepatitis A titers. Which of the following is the most likely result of this infection?

(A) Cirrhosis
(B) Complete resolution
(C) Establishment of a chronic carrier state
(D) Fulminant hepatitis
(E) Hepatocellular carcinoma

4. A 32-year-old woman seeking to become pregnant visits her physician for a prepregnancy examination. Routine prenatal laboratory testing demonstrates the following profile: HBsAg (−), anti-HBsAg (+), anti-HBcAg (−), anti-HBeAg (−), and HBV DNA (−). Which of the following likely represents the status of the patient?

(A) Hepatitis B carrier
(B) Immunized against hepatitis B
(C) Infected and within the "window period"
(D) Infected with hepatitis B and highly transmissible
(E) Recently infected with hepatitis B

5. A 55-year-old alcoholic man died after an illness characterized by increasing jaundice, ascites, and generalized wasting. Laboratory testing revealed hyperbilirubinemia, hypoalbuminemia, and mildly elevated liver enzymes. The appearance of the liver at autopsy is shown in the figure. The most likely diagnosis is

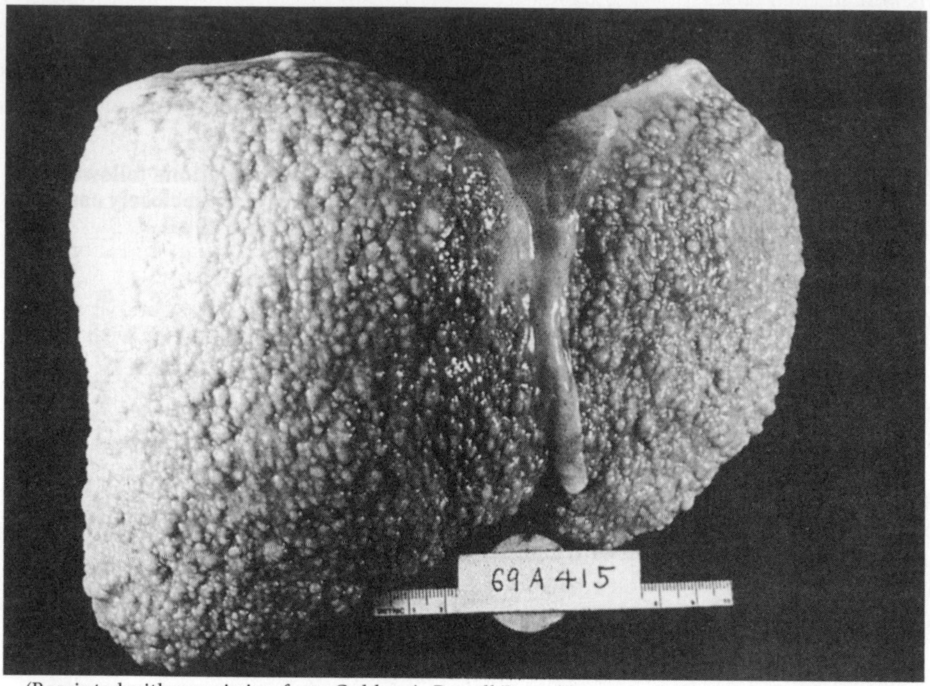

(Reprinted with permission from Golden A, Powell D, and Jennings C: *Pathology: Understanding Human Disease,* 2nd ed. Baltimore, Williams & Wilkins, 1985, p 289.)

(A) α_1-antitrypsin deficiency
(B) cirrhosis
(C) hepatitis A
(D) hepatitis C
(E) multiple metastases

6. While on an international medical rotation, you encounter a pregnant woman in a rural village in India who presents with fever, jaundice, and malaise. The patient unexpectedly expires. This is the second case this month with a similar presentation. Which of the following is the most likely form of hepatitis?

(A) Hepatitis A
(B) Hepatitis B
(C) Hepatitis C
(D) Hepatitis D
(E) Hepatitis E

7. A 56-year-old alcoholic man presents to the emergency department with confusion and lethargy. On physical examination, he is visibly jaundiced with ascites. Laboratory studies reveal increased prothrombin time and prolonged activated partial thromboplastin time as well as significantly increased serum ammonia levels. Given a significantly increased serum ammonia, which of the following physical findings might you expect to see?

(A) Asterixis
(B) Capillary telangiectasias
(C) Caput medusae
(D) Gynecomastia
(E) Palmar erythema

8. A 45-year-old woman presents to her primary care physician with jaundice, pruritus, and periocular and intradigital xanthomas. Her laboratory results indicate a significantly increased alkaline phosphatase as well as a positive test for antimitochondrial antibodies. The most likely cause of her symptoms is

(A) leptospirosis
(B) macronodular cirrhosis
(C) primary biliary cirrhosis
(D) primary sclerosing cholangitis
(E) secondary biliary cirrhosis

9. A 53-year-old man presents to his physician's office for an insurance physical. During the history, you learn that his father had diabetes and died of congestive heart failure. The patient was told it was due to "bronze diabetes." The patient complains only of vague fatigue and arthralgias. You are concerned that the patient may be at risk for hereditary hemochromatosis. Which test would you order to confirm your suspicion?

(A) Antimitochondrial antibodies
(B) α_1-Antitrypsin
(C) Ceruloplasmin
(D) Heterophil antibodies
(E) Transferrin saturation

10. A 13-year-old boy presents to the pediatrician with extrapyramidal signs, including a resting and kinetic tremor. An ophthalmologic examination demonstrates the presence of Kayser-Fleischer rings, and his laboratory studies demonstrate elevated liver enzymes. It is likely that the patient's condition is associated with the accumulation of

(A) copper
(B) Councilman bodies
(C) eosinophilic hyaline inclusions
(D) glycogen
(E) iron

11. A 23-year-old woman is involved in a minor motor vehicle accident, prompting an abdominal computed tomography scan, which was read by the emergency department radiologist as normal with the exception of a questionable mass in the right lobe of the liver. A subsequent fine-needle biopsy confirms the presence of a liver adenoma. Which of the following is associated with the development of this lesion?

(A) Hepatitis B
(B) Hepatitis C
(C) Oral contraceptives
(D) Polycythemia vera
(E) Polyvinyl chloride

12. A 36-year-old man from sub-Saharan Africa presents to the clinic with jaundice and right upper quadrant pain. On examination, the liver is palpably enlarged. Laboratory studies demonstrate an increase in liver enzymes. Computed tomography demonstrates a single large mass in the right lobe of the liver, and serum α-fetoprotein is markedly elevated. Which of the following is likely to have contributed to the patient's condition?

(A) Aflatoxin B_1
(B) *Clonorchis sinensis*
(C) Hepatitis A
(D) Polyvinyl chloride
(E) Tetracycline

13. A 43-year-old multigravida presents with nausea, vomiting, fever, and right upper quadrant pain. On examination, she displays arrested inspiration on palpation of the right upper quadrant (Murphy sign). Her laboratory results reveal neutrophilia with a "left shift." Which of the following is the most likely diagnosis?

(A) Acute cholecystitis
(B) Carcinoma of the ampulla of Vater
(C) Cholangiocarcinoma
(D) Cholesterolosis
(E) Sclerosing cholangitis

14. A 25-year-old obese woman who denies any history of alcohol abuse presents with severe abdominal pain radiating to the back. Laboratory results indicate an increase in serum amylase and lipase, with a marked decrease in calcium. Which of the following likely has caused this condition?

(A) Abetalipoproteinemia
(B) Alcohol
(C) Cholelithiasis
(D) Cystic fibrosis
(E) Mumps

15. A 63-year-old chronic alcoholic presents with weight loss, anorexia, and abdominal pain radiating to the back. Physical examination indicates a palpably enlarged gallbladder, and laboratory studies demonstrate conjugated hyperbilirubinemia. Computed tomography demonstrates a mass in the head of the pancreas. Which of the following is associated with the diagnosis of pancreatic adenocarcinoma?

(A) Asterixis
(B) Gallstone ileus
(C) Murphy sign
(D) Trousseau sign
(E) Whipple triad

A ANSWERS AND EXPLANATIONS

1-A. A total lack of glucuronyl transferase results in Crigler-Najjar syndrome I, which is invariably fatal by 18 months secondary to kernicterus. Gilbert syndrome is typically mild and usually not detected until later in life. Hemolytic disease of the newborn is due to blood group incompatibility between mother and child, and the bilirubinemia is secondary to the inherently decreased glucuronyl transferase with superimposed hemolytic anemia in the child, further overwhelming the conjugation machinery. Neonatal glucuronyl transferase is relatively deficient, although present, in normal infants, contributing to the transient condition termed physiologic jaundice of the newborn. Rotor syndrome is a relatively benign condition resulting in conjugated hyperbilirubinemia.

2-C. Gilbert syndrome is an extremely common cause of clinically insignificant unconjugated hyperbilirubinemia. The hyperbilirubinemia is episodic, with increases related to stress, fatigue, alcohol use, or recurrent infection. Crigler-Najjar syndrome I is often lethal, although Crigler-Najjar syndrome II is compatible with life and often presents with extreme jaundice and neurologic defects secondary to kernicterus. Both Dubin-Johnson syndrome and Rotor syndrome cause conjugated hyperbilirubinemia. Infectious mononucleosis can cause liver damage but would likely be accompanied by malaise and fatigue.

3-B. The patient has a case of hepatitis A (HAV), most likely associated with the consumption of uncooked shellfish. Complete resolution occurs in an overwhelming majority of cases. Although possible, fulminant hepatic failure is unlikely with HAV infection. There is no association of HAV with either cirrhosis or hepatocellular carcinoma, as there is for hepatitis B and C.

4-B. The patient is only positive for antibody to the hepatitis B antigen. This suggests that the patient has been vaccinated for hepatitis B virus (HBV). The vaccine consists of recombinantly produced HBV surface antigen (HBsAg) alone; antibodies to this protein convey immunity. HBsAg would be seen in the serum within the first 3–4 months after initial infection. Antibodies to the core protein (anti-HBcAg) appear during acute illness and between the disappearance of HBsAg and the appearance of anti-HBsAg, the "window period." Anti-HBeAg appears during the window period as well. HBeAg is closely correlated with viral infectivity. HBV viral DNA is also an index of infectivity.

5-B. The figure demonstrates the typical appearance of micronodular cirrhosis, the most common cause of which is alcoholism. Major clinical manifestations include jaundice, ascites, signs of hyperestrinism (palmar erythema, spider telangiectasia, gynecomastia, testicular atrophy), consequences of increased portal venous pressure (esophageal varices, distended abdominal veins [caput medusae], splenomegaly), and consequences of hypoalbuminemia (ascites, peripheral edema).

6-E. Hepatitis E is a common sporadic cause of viral hepatitis in India. It has close to a 20% mortality in pregnant women. Like hepatitis A, it is transmitted enterically. Hepatitis C can be transmitted parenterally, as can hepatitis B and hepatitis D. Hepatitis D requires coinfection with hepatitis B.

7-A. Asterixis is a flapping tremor of the hands associated with hepatic encephalopathy. Failure of the liver to detoxify metabolites absorbed from the gastrointestinal tract leads to accumulation of nitrogenous wastes that are neurotoxic. Caput medusae results from dilation of the periumbilical venous collaterals as a result of portal hypertension and activation of portal-caval anastomoses. Palmar erythema, capillary telangiectasias, and gynecomastia result from the hyperestrinism seen in liver disease with failure of the liver to metabolize estrogen.

8-C. Primary biliary cirrhosis is an autoimmune condition that typically presents in middle-aged women. The itching and hypercholesterolemia are secondary to severe obstructive jaundice. Leptospirosis is a condition caused by a treponemal bacterium that results in jaundice, renal failure, and hemorrhagic phenomena. Macronodular cirrhosis is usually a result of hepatitis B or hepatitis C infection. Primary sclerosing cholangitis is associated with ulcerative colitis and with an increased incidence of cholangiocarcinoma. Secondary biliary cirrhosis is caused by extrahepatic biliary obstruction.

9-E. The recommended screening test for hemochromatosis is serum transferrin saturation, which is increased. Further molecular testing can be performed to look for mutations in the *Hfe* gene on chromosome 6. Early detection and occasional phlebotomy can prevent multiorgan failure attributed to iron accumulation in tissues. Antimitochondrial antibodies are used in the diagnosis of primary biliary cirrhosis. Decreased α_1-antitrypsin levels are associated with liver disease as well as panacinar emphysema. Ceruloplasmin levels are decreased in Wilson disease. Heterophil antibodies occur in infectious mononucleosis due to Epstein-Barr virus.

10-A. Wilson disease is a hereditary condition associated with the accumulation of copper in the liver, brain, and eye. Accumulation of copper in the Descemet membrane of the eye results in the pathognomonic lesion known as the Kayser-Fleischer ring. Accumulation in the liver results in cirrhosis. Accumulation in the brain, specifically in the basal ganglia, results in motor symptoms. Councilman bodies are apoptotic hepatocytes that were first identified in yellow fever. Eosinophilic hyaline inclusions, Mallory bodies, are seen in alcoholic liver disease. Glycogen accumulates in the liver in numerous glycogen storage diseases. Iron accumulates in hemochromatosis.

11-C. Liver adenomas are benign liver tumors commonly associated with oral contraceptive use in young women. They are of concern because they resemble hepatocellular carcinoma. In addition, if they are subcapsular, they can rupture, causing intra-abdominal hemorrhage. Hepatitis B and hepatitis C can lead to hepatocellular carcinoma. Polycythemia vera is associated with thrombosis of the hepatic veins. Polyvinyl chloride predisposes to angiosarcoma of the liver.

12-A. Aflatoxin B_1 is a fungal metabolite found on moldy nuts and grain commonly found in southern Africa. It is a cocarcinogen with hepatitis B, which is nearly endemic to this region of the world. Together they greatly increase the incidence of hepatocellular carcinoma, the most prevalent cancer worldwide. *Clonorchis sinensis* is a parasite associated with the development of cholangiocarcinoma. Hepatitis A has no association with malignancy. Polyvinyl chloride is associated with angiosarcoma of the liver. Tetracyclines can cause microvesicular fatty change in the liver.

13-A. This patient presents with the classic signs of cholecystitis, or inflammation of the gallbladder wall, which is usually due to obstruction of the cystic duct by gallstones. Carcinoma of the ampulla of Vater is closely related to carcinoma of the extrahepatic biliary duct, and presents with jaundice and a palpably enlarged gallbladder, as opposed to stones, which typically do not cause an enlarged gallbladder. Cholangiocarcinoma is a malignancy of the bile ducts. Cholesterolosis, also known as strawberry gallbladder, is noninflammatory in nature. Sclerosing cholangitis is an inflammatory condition of the extrahepatic bile ducts that is often associated with chronic ulcerative colitis.

14-C. The leading cause of pancreatitis, particularly in nonalcoholic patients, is cholelithiasis, or gallstones. Gallstones obstruct the pancreatic ducts, leading to autodigestion of the pancreas by the enzymes it normally secretes into the duodenum (i.e., lipases). These lipids then form soaps (saponify) with calcium, leading to hypocalcemia. Alcohol is another leading cause of pancreatitis. Cystic fibrosis, abetalipoproteinemia, and mumps infection are all less common causes of pancreatitis.

15-D. The Trousseau sign, or migratory thrombophlebitis, is associated with carcinoma of the pancreas. The finding of appearing and disappearing thrombosis can affect up to 10% of patients. Only about 20% of lesions are in the head of the pancreas, where they present relatively early with obstructive jaundice. Asterixis is a flapping tremor associated with hepatic encephalopathy. Gallstone ileus is a complication of cholelithiasis when the gallstone erodes through the gallbladder into the adjacent small bowel. The Murphy sign is associated with acute cholecystitis. The Whipple triad is associated with insulinomas, tumors of the endocrine (rather than exocrine) pancreas.

CHAPTER 17

Kidney and Urinary Tract

I. Congenital Anomalies of the Urinary Tract

A. **Kidney**

1. **Complete or bilateral renal agenesis**
   a. This rare condition is not compatible with life.
   b. Both kidneys are absent.
   c. Resulting conditions include **oligohydramnios,** or decreased amniotic fluid, which occurs because the renal system fails to excrete fluid swallowed by the fetus.
   d. Other resulting conditions include multiple fetal anomalies (e.g., hypoplastic lung, defects in extremities), all caused by oligohydramnios and collectively known as the oligohydramnios, or Potter, sequence. (Hyperhydramnios, or *increased* amniotic fluid, is associated with duodenal atresia or with tracheoesophageal fistula of the type in which the upper esophagus ends in a blind pouch and the lower esophagus communicates with the trachea.)
2. **Unilateral renal agenesis**
   a. One kidney is missing.
   b. This condition is much more common than complete renal agenesis.
3. **Renal ectopia** is the abnormal location of a kidney, frequently in the pelvis (pelvic kidney).
4. **Horseshoe kidney**
   a. This condition refers to two kidneys joined at their lower poles.
   b. It may cause urinary tract obstruction because of impingement on the ureters.

B. **Ureters**. Double ureters may affect the ureters alone or may be part of a duplication of the entire urinary collecting system on one side.

II. Glomerular Diseases (Table 17-1)

A. **Nephrotic syndrome** includes a group of conditions characterized by increased basement membrane permeability, permitting the urinary loss of plasma proteins, particularly low-weight proteins, such as albumin.

1. **Clinical manifestations**
   a. **Massive proteinuria** is generally characterized by excretion of more than 4 grams of protein per day. Unlike disorders with greater disruption of glomerular structure, proteinuria in the nephrotic syndrome is unaccompanied by increased urinary red cells or white cells.
   b. **Hypoalbuminemia** results from proteinuria and is often marked by a serum concentration of less than 3 g/100 mL.

TABLE 17-1 *Glomerular Diseases*

Types	Morphologic Findings
Disorders manifest by nephrotic syndrome	
Minimal change disease (lipoid nephrosis)	No visible basement membrane changes; fused epithelial foot processes; lipid accumulation in renal tubular cells
Focal segmental glomerulosclerosis	No visible basement membrane changes; segmental sclerosis of scattered juxtamedullary glomeruli
Membranous glomerulonephritis	Basement membrane markedly thickened by intramembranous and epimembranous (subepithelial) immune complex deposits; granular immunofluorescence; "spike and dome" appearance
Diabetic nephropathy	Basement membrane markedly thickened; diffuse or nodular mesangial accumulations of basement membrane-like material
Renal amyloidosis	Amyloid protein identified by special stains (e.g., Congo red), birefringence under polarized light, or electron microscopic criss-cross fibrillary pattern
Lupus nephropathy	Immune complex deposition in subendothelial location may manifest as membranous glomerulonephritis
Disorders manifest by nephritic syndrome	
Poststreptococcal glomerulonephritis	Subepithelial electron-dense "humps"; "lumpy-bumpy" immunofluorescence
Rapidly progressive (crescentic) glomerulonephritis	Crescents; antineutrophil cytoplasmic antibody (ANCA)-negative forms with immune complexes or antiglomerular basement membrane antibodies; ANCA-positive (pauci-immune) form with Wegener granulomatosis
Goodpasture syndrome	Linear immunofluorescence caused by antiglomerular basement membrane antibodies
Alport syndrome	Split basement membrane
Other glomerular disorders	
IgA nephropathy (Berger disease)	Mesangial IgA deposits
Membranoproliferative glomerulonephritis	Tram-track appearance; deposits of C3, and dense deposits in one variant

c. **Generalized edema** results from decreased plasma colloid oncotic pressure.
d. **Hyperlipidemia and hypercholesterolemia** are caused by increased hepatic lipoprotein synthesis.

2. **Minimal change disease (lipoid nephrosis)** is seen most often in young children but can also occur in older children and adults. It is the prototype of the nephrotic syndrome.
   a. **Lipid-laden renal cortices** (lipids are intracytoplasmic in tubular cells, particularly in cells of proximal convoluted tubules).
   b. Light microscopy demonstrates normal-appearing glomeruli.
   c. Electron microscopy is normal except for the disappearance or **fusing of epithelial foot processes.**
   d. Most often, this condition responds well to adrenal steroid therapy.
3. **Focal segmental glomerulosclerosis** is clinically similar to minimal change disease but occurs in somewhat older patients. It is characterized by sclerosis within capillary tufts of deep juxtamedullary glomeruli with focal or segmental distribution.

a. **Focal distribution** is involvement of some, but not all, of the glomeruli.
b. **Segmental distribution** is involvement of only a part of the glomerulus.

4. **Membranous glomerulonephritis** is an immune complex disease of unknown etiology.
   a. This disease is a major primary cause of the nephrotic syndrome.
   b. Incidence is highest in teenagers and young adults.
   c. The diagnosis should be suspected when the nephrotic syndrome is accompanied by azotemia (increased concentrations of serum urea nitrogen and creatinine).
   d. Morphologic characteristics include greatly **thickened capillary walls** visible by light microscopy and visible by electron microscopy as a 5- to 10-fold thickening of the basement membrane.
   e. Ultrastructural findings include numerous electron-dense **immune complexes in intramembranous and epimembranous (subepithelial) locations** within and on the basement membrane. This immune complex disease can be mimicked in an animal model resulting from multiple repeated injections of foreign protein.
   f. With special stains, a **"spike and dome" appearance** resulting from the extension of basement membrane between and around the immune deposits is evident; the spikes are basement membrane material, and the domes are immune complex deposits.
   g. Granular deposits of immunoglobulin G (IgG) or C3 are apparent on immunofluorescence. **Granular immunofluorescence** is a general characteristic of immune complex diseases.
   h. Membranous glomerulonephritis is a slowly progressive disorder that shows little response to steroid therapy.
   i. It is seen in 10% of patients with systemic lupus erythematosus (SLE).
   j. Associations sometimes include hepatitis B, syphilis, or malaria infection; drugs, such as gold salts or penicillamine; or malignancy.
   k. The disorder sometimes causes renal vein thrombosis, which was previously thought to be an etiologic factor.
5. **Diabetic nephropathy**
   a. Often, this disease is clinically manifested by the nephrotic syndrome.
   b. Electron microscopy demonstrates a striking increase in thickness of the glomerular basement membrane. Thickening of vascular basement membranes observable by electron microscopy is one of the earliest morphologic changes in diabetes mellitus.
   c. An **increase in mesangial matrix** results in two characteristic morphologic patterns:
      (1) **Diffuse glomerulosclerosis** is marked by a diffusely distributed increase in mesangial matrix.
      (2) **Nodular glomerulosclerosis** is marked by nodular accumulations of mesangial matrix material **(Kimmelstiel-Wilson nodules).**
6. **Renal amyloidosis**
   a. This condition is another cause of the nephrotic syndrome.
   b. Predominantly **subendothelial and mesangial amyloid deposits** are characteristic.
   c. The amyloidosis can be identified by reactivity of amyloid with special stains (e.g., Congo red, crystal violet, thioflavin T) and by birefringence under polarized light. It is also demonstrated by a characteristic criss-cross fibrillary pattern of amyloid by electron microscopy.
   d. Most often, there are associations with chronic inflammatory diseases such as rheumatoid arthritis or plasma cell disorders such as multiple myeloma.
7. **Lupus nephropathy**
   a. This is the renal component of **SLE;** the severity of the renal lesion often determines the overall prognosis in patients with SLE. It is often manifest as the **nephrotic syndrome;** many cases also have major nephritic features.
   b. Lupus nephropathy is classified by the World Health Organization (WHO) into five distinct renal patterns.

(1) **Type I** has no observable renal involvement.

(2) **Type II** is the **mesangial form** of lupus nephropathy.

(a) Focal and segmental glomerular involvement with an increase in the number of mesangial cells and quantitative increase in mesangial matrix is characteristic.

(b) Type II disease results most often in slight proteinuria and minimal hematuria; is usually of little clinical consequence.

(3) **Type III (focal proliferative form)** usually involves less than half of the glomeruli but can cause extensive damage to individual glomeruli.

(4) **Type IV (diffuse proliferative form)** is the prototype of lupus nephropathy and the most severe form of the disease.

(a) Often, there is a combination of the nephrotic and nephritic syndromes.

(b) Almost all of the glomeruli are involved.

(c) Involves includes glomerular changes, such as marked inflammation with small focal thromboses and mesangial proliferation, all resulting in extensive scarring.

(d) Characteristic changes include the **wire-loop abnormality,** a light microscopic finding resulting from immune complex deposition and gross thickening of the glomerular basement membrane, as well as **endothelial cell proliferation,** which is often prominent by electron microscopy. Additional characteristics include marked **subendothelial immune complex deposition;** this is also a major diagnostic feature.

(5) **Type V (membranous form)** is indistinguishable from primary membranous glomerulonephritis.

B. **Nephritic syndrome** is characterized by inflammatory rupture of the glomerular capillaries, with resultant bleeding into the urinary space; proteinuria and edema may be present but usually are mild.

1. **Clinical findings**

a. **Oliguria**

b. **Azotemia**

c. **Hypertension**

d. **Hematuria** results from leakage of red cells directly from glomerular capillaries into the Bowman space. Many of the red cells are aggregated into the shape of the renal tubules and embedded in a proteinaceous matrix forming **red cell casts** that can be observed in the urine; the patient often reports having "**smoky brown urine.**" Red cell casts can degenerate and become pigmented granular casts.

2. **Poststreptococcal glomerulonephritis (acute proliferative glomerulonephritis)** is the prototype of the **nephritic syndrome.** It is an **immune complex disease** with the antigen of streptococcal origin.

a. This disorder most often follows or accompanies infection (tonsillitis, streptococcal impetigo, infected insect bites) with nephritogenic strains of **group A β-hemolytic streptococci.**

b. Complete recovery in almost all children and many adults follows. A very small minority develop rapidly progressive glomerulonephritis.

c. Several laboratory abnormalities are characteristic, including urinary red cells and red cell casts, azotemia, decreased serum C3, and increased titers of antistreptococcal antibodies (antistreptolysin O [ASO], anti-DNAase B, and anticationic proteinase) as evidence of recent streptococcal infection.

d. An **intense inflammatory reaction** involving almost all glomeruli in both kidneys results in:

(1) **Innumerable punctate hemorrhages** on the surface of both kidneys

(2) **Enlarged, hypercellular, swollen, bloodless glomeruli** with proliferation of mesangial and endothelial cells and sometimes neutrophils

(3) Glomerular basement membrane of normal thickness and uniformity despite the extensive inflammatory changes

(4) Characteristic **electron-dense "humps"** on the epithelial side of the basement membrane **(subepithelial localization)**

(5) **"Lumpy-bumpy" immunofluorescence** (extremely coarse granular immunofluorescence for IgG or C3)

3. **Rapidly progressive (crescentic) glomerulonephritis (RPGN)**
   a. By definition, RPGN is the nephritic syndrome that progresses rapidly to renal failure within weeks or months. The disorder is histologically defined by the formation of crescents between the Bowman capsule and the glomerular tuft, which result from deposition of fibrin in the Bowman space and from proliferation of parietal epithelial cells of the Bowman capsule; cells of monocytic origin are often involved.
   b. The etiology is **poststreptococcal** in approximately 50% of cases with immune complex deposition; other immune complex forms of RPGN include, among others, lupus nephropathy and IgA nephropathy.
   c. Antiglomerular basement membrane antibodies (nonstreptococcal) are characteristic in approximately 10% of cases; these cases often present clinically as Goodpasture syndrome.
   d. RPGN can also be of the pauci-immune type, without immune complex deposition or antiglomerular basement membrane antibodies. This third type of RPGN is associated with antineutrophil cytoplasmic antibodies (ANCAs), in contrast with immune complex or antiglomerular basement membrane forms of RPGN, which are ANCA-negative. The ANCA-negative forms of RPGN are designated type I when RPGN is of the antiglomerular basement membrane antibody type and type II when it is of the immune complex type. The ANCA-positive pauci-immune form of RPGN is designated type III.
4. **Goodpasture syndrome (antiglomerular basement membrane disease)**
   a. The cause is antibodies **(antiglomerular basement membrane antibodies)** directed against antigens in glomerular and pulmonary alveolar basement membranes.
   b. Fluorescent antibody studies for IgG demonstrate **linear immunofluorescence**.
   c. Clinical manifestations include:
      (1) **Nephritic syndrome**
      (2) **Pneumonitis with hemoptysis** (hemorrhagic pneumonitis)
      (3) Peak incidence in **men in their mid-20s**
      (4) **RPGN crescentic morphology** with linear immunofluorescence
5. **Focal glomerulonephritis**
   a. This disease is focal and segmental but differs from focal segmental glomerulosclerosis in that the changes are inflammatory and proliferative rather than sclerotic.
   b. Most often this is an immune complex disease, occurring as a manifestation of various disorders, including SLE, subacute bacterial endocarditis, polyarteritis nodosa, Goodpasture syndrome, Wegener granulomatosis, and IgA nephropathy; it can also occur in a primary (idiopathic) form.
6. **Alport syndrome**
   a. This disease is hereditary nephritis associated with nerve deafness and ocular disorders such as lens dislocation and cataracts.
   b. Clinical characteristics include the nephritic syndrome, often progressing to end-stage renal disease by 30 years of age.
   c. The cause is a mutation in the gene for the α_5 chain of type IV collagen.
   d. Irregular glomerular basement membrane thickening with foci of splitting of the lamina densa is seen.

C. **Other glomerular diseases**
   1. **IgA nephropathy (Berger disease)** is an extremely common entity defined by deposition of IgA in the mesangium.
      a. Most frequently, the disease is characterized by benign recurrent hematuria in children, usually following an infection, lasting 1–2 days, and usually of minimal clinical significance.

b. Focal glomerulonephritis may be a presenting feature.
c. IgA nephropathy can be a component of Henoch-Schönlein disease.

2. **Membranoproliferative glomerulonephritis**
   a. Clinical characteristics include slow progression to chronic renal disease.
   b. Histologic characteristics include both basement membrane thickening and cellular proliferation.
   c. Disease is marked by reduplication of glomerular basement membrane into two layers due to expansion of mesangial matrix into the glomerular capillary loops; this results in a characteristic **tram-track appearance** best seen with silver stains.
   d. Disease occurs in two forms:
      (1) **Type I** is an immune complex nephritis associated with an unknown antigen. It has a striking tram-track appearance.
      (2) **Type II (dense deposit disease)** has a tram-track appearance that is not as apparent as that of type I.
         (a) Irregular electron-dense material deposited within the glomerular basement membrane is characteristic. C3 is demonstrable adjacent to but not within the **dense deposits,** and serum C3 is characteristically markedly reduced.
         (b) The possible cause is an IgG autoantibody (C3 nephritic factor) with specificity for the C3 convertase of the alternate complement pathway.

III. Urinary Tract Obstruction

A. This obstruction may occur anywhere in the urinary system.

B. In children, the condition is most often congenital.

C. In adults, the condition is most often acquired, usually occurring as a consequence of renal stones or benign prostatic hyperplasia.

D. Clinical manifestations include:
1. **Renal colic,** which is excruciating pain caused by acute distention of the ureter, usually by the transit of a small stone.
2. **Hydronephrosis,** which is progressive dilation of the renal pelvis and calyces.
3. **Infection,** which is localized proximal to the site of obstruction. It may lead to infection of the renal parenchyma.

IV. Infection of the Urinary Tract and Kidney

A. **General considerations**
1. Incidence of infection of the urinary tract and kidney is greatly increased in women, presumably because of the shorter length of the female urethra; the incidence is increased during pregnancy.
2. This condition can be caused by hematogenous bacterial dissemination to the kidney or by external entry of organisms through the urethra into the bladder; in the latter case infection can spread upward from the bladder into the ureters (vesicoureteral reflux) and through the ureters to the kidney (ascending infection).
3. Most frequently, the infection involves the normal flora of the colon, most often *Escherichia coli.*

B. **Predisposing factors**
1. Obstruction of urinary flow, such as that occurring with urethral obstruction in benign prostatic hyperplasia

2. Surgery on the kidney or urinary tract
3. Catheters inserted through the urethra into the bladder
4. Gynecologic abnormalities

C. **Clinical manifestations**

1. **Urinary frequency:** a compelling necessity to void small amounts of urine at frequent intervals
2. **Dysuria:** painful, burning sensation on urination
3. **Pyuria:** large numbers of neutrophils in the urine
4. **Hematuria:** blood in the urine; urinary red cells are a nonspecific finding in urinary tract infection.
5. **Bacteriuria:** usually defined as more than 10^5 organisms per milliliter of urine; must be distinguished from contamination of urine specimens by external flora

D. **Additional diagnostically significant findings in acute pyelonephritis** (acute infection of the renal parenchyma)

1. **Fever, leukocytosis, flank tenderness, urinary white cells,** and **white cell casts in the urine** (this latter finding is pathognomonic of acute pyelonephritis).
2. Greatly increased frequency in women, especially during pregnancy

E. **Cystitis.** Characteristics include pyuria and often hematuria, but urinary white cell casts are not found.

V. Tubular and Interstitial Disorders of the Kidney

A. **Acute drug-induced interstitial nephritis**

1. Most often the trigger is penicillin derivatives, such as methicillin, and other drugs such as nonsteroidal anti-inflammatory drugs and diuretics.
2. The disease is most likely of immune etiology.
3. **Acute interstitial renal inflammation** is characteristic.
4. The nephritis resolves on cessation of exposure to the inciting drug.

B. **Renal papillary necrosis (necrotizing papillitis)** is ischemic necrosis of the tips of the renal papillae.

1. This form of necrosis is most often associated with **diabetes mellitus,** in which it is related to renal infection and coexisting vascular disease. It is occasionally a catastrophic consequence of **acute pyelonephritis.**
2. Renal papillary necrosis is also associated with long-term persistent abuse of **phenacetin,** most often in association with aspirin and other analgesics. This can lead to **chronic analgesic nephritis,** a chronic inflammatory change characterized by loss and atrophy of tubules and interstitial fibrosis and inflammation. Phenacetin is no longer approved for over the-counter analgesic preparations.

C. **Acute tubular necrosis** is the most common cause of acute renal failure (acute renal shutdown).

1. This condition is reversible. Necrotic renal tubular cells are replaced by new cells in approximately 2 weeks, with complete return of renal function to normal if the patient is maintained on dialysis. Proper medical management results in complete recovery; otherwise the syndrome is potentially fatal.
2. This condition can also lead to cardiac standstill from hyperkalemia, most often during the **initial oliguric phase.** Oliguria from acute tubular necrosis must be distinguished from oliguria due to prerenal causes such as reduced blood volume or dehydration.
3. The acute condition is most frequently precipitated by **renal ischemia,** which is often caused by prolonged hypotension or shock, most often induced by gram-negative sepsis, trauma, or hemorrhage.

4. Another associated condition is crush injury with myoglobinuria. Myoglobinuria also can be observed after intense exercise, but this is not of clinical consequence.
5. Other causes may include direct injury to the proximal renal tubules from mercuric chloride, gentamicin, and several other toxic substances. Ethylene glycol (antifreeze) is extremely toxic when ingested and can result not only in acute tubular necrosis but also in renal oxalosis with massive intratubular oxalate crystal deposition that can be visualized with polarized light.

D. **Disorders of renal tubular function**
1. **Fanconi syndrome**
   a. This manifestation of generalized dysfunction of the proximal renal tubules may be hereditary or acquired.
   b. Impaired reabsorption of glucose, amino acids, phosphate, and bicarbonate is characteristic.
   c. Clinical manifestations include **glycosuria, hyperphosphaturia and hypophosphatemia, aminoaciduria,** and **systemic acidosis.**
2. **Cystinuria**
   a. This impaired tubular reabsorption of cystine is genetically determined.
   b. Clinical manifestations include cystine stones.
3. **Hartnup disease**
   a. This impaired tubular reabsorption of tryptophan is genetically determined.
   b. This condition leads to pellagra-like manifestations.

E. **Chronic pyelonephritis**
1. **Coarse, asymmetric corticomedullary scarring** and deformity of the renal pelvis and calyces occurs; these findings are essential to diagnosis.
2. Characteristics include interstitial inflammatory infiltrate in the early stages and later by **interstitial fibrosis** and **tubular atrophy;** atrophic tubules often contain eosinophilic proteinaceous casts, resulting in an appearance reminiscent of thyroid follicles **(thyroidization of the kidney).**
3. Causes almost always include chronic urinary tract obstruction and repeated bouts of acute inflammation.
4. Consequences include renal hypertension and end-stage renal disease.

VI. Diffuse Cortical Necrosis

A. This disease is acute generalized **ischemic infarction of the cortices** of both kidneys; the medulla is spared. Infarction is patchy in some cases and is compatible with survival.

B. This form of necrosis is most often associated with **obstetric catastrophes** such as abruptio placentae or eclampsia. Diffuse cortical necrosis is also associated with **septic shock** and other causes of vascular collapse.

C. It is thought that the cause is a combination of end-organ vasospasm and disseminated intravascular coagulation.

VII. Nephrocalcinosis

A. This diffuse deposition of calcium in the kidney parenchyma can lead to renal failure.
B. This condition is caused by hypercalcemia such as occurs in hyperparathyroidism or in the milk-alkali syndrome (nephrocalcinosis and renal stones resulting from self-medication for peptic ulcer with milk and absorbable antacids).

C. Nephrocalcinosis can also be caused by hyperphosphatemia. This is usually the cause of the nephrocalcinosis that occurs as a component of renal failure. It is of note that nephrocalcinosis can be both a cause and an effect of renal failure.

VIII. Urolithiasis

- This condition is characterized by calculi (stones) in the urinary tract.
- Incidence is increased in men.

A. **Calcium stones** account for 80%–85% of urinary stones.
1. The stones consist of calcium oxalate or calcium phosphate, or both.
2. They are radiopaque.
3. They are associated with hypercalciuria, which is caused by:
   a. Increased intestinal **absorption of calcium**
   b. Increased primary renal **excretion of calcium**
   c. **Hypercalcemia,** which may be caused by:
      (1) **Hyperparathyroidism** leads to nephrocalcinosis (calcification of the kidney) as well as urolithiasis.
      (2) **Malignancy** leads to hypercalcemia because of osteolytic metastases or ectopic production of parathyroid hormone (often by a squamous cell carcinoma of the lung).
      (3) **Other causes** include sarcoidosis, vitamin D intoxication, and the milk-alkali syndrome.

B. **Ammonium magnesium phosphate stones** are the second most common form of urinary stones.
1. These stones are formed in alkaline urine, which is caused most often by ammonia-producing (urease-positive) organisms, such as *Proteus vulgaris* or *Staphylococcus*
2. They are radiolucent.
3. They can form large **staghorn (struvite) calculi** (casts of renal pelvis and calyces).

C. **Uric acid stones** are associated with hyperuricemia in approximately half of the patients; hyperuricemia can be secondary to gout or to increased cellular turnover, as in the leukemias or myeloproliferative syndromes.

D. **Cystine stones** are almost always associated with cystinuria or genetically determined aminoaciduria.

IX. Cystic Diseases of the Kidney

A. **Adult polycystic kidney disease**
1. This disease manifests clinically between 15 and 30 years of age, even though the genetic defect is present at birth.
2. **Autosomal dominant** inheritance is characteristic. Adult polycystic kidney disease is the most common inherited disorder of the kidney.
3. **Partial replacement of renal parenchyma by cysts** is characteristic. The disease occurs bilaterally; the kidneys are greatly enlarged.
4. This kidney disease is often associated with **berry aneurysm** of the circle of Willis.
5. It is also frequently associated with cystic disease of the liver or other organs.
6. Secondary polycythemia may occur as a result.

7. Clinical manifestations include:
   a. Hypertension
   b. Hematuria
   c. Palpable renal masses
   d. Progression to renal failure

B. **Infantile polycystic kidney disease**
   1. Clinical manifestations include multiple cysts evident at birth. The closed cysts are not in continuity with the collecting system.
   2. Death from this **autosomal recessive** disorder results shortly after birth.

C. **Simple (solitary) renal cyst** is a common lesion that occurs in adults; it is often asymptomatic.

D. **Uremic medullary cystic disease (nephronophthisis)**
   1. This very serious (but uncommon) form of cystic disease affects older children.
   2. It is characterized by cysts in the medulla that may result in renal failure.

E. **Medullary sponge kidney**
   1. Multiple small medullary cysts and impaired tubular function, usually without renal failure, are characteristic; renal stones may form in the dilated ducts.
   2. This disease may be complicated by infection.

F. **Acquired cystic disease**
   1. This disease is associated with long-term dialysis therapy.
   2. Multiple cysts, glomerular and tubular atrophy, and scarring are characteristic.
   3. The incidence of renal cell carcinoma is increased.

X. Renal Failure

A. **General considerations**
   1. Renal failure can be acute or chronic and can result from any of the glomerular or tubulointerstitial lesions discussed in the preceding sections.
   2. **Azotemia of renal origin** is always associated.
   3. In advanced stages, renal failure results in uremia; the term **uremia** denotes the biochemical and clinical syndrome characteristic of symptomatic renal disease.

B. **Major clinical characteristics of uremia**
   1. **Azotemia**
   2. **Acidosis** resulting from the accumulation of sulfates, phosphates, and organic acids
   3. **Hyperkalemia**
   4. **Abnormal control of fluid volume**
      a. An early characteristic is the inability to concentrate urine; a later manifestation is the inability to dilute urine.
      b. Sodium and water retention can result in congestive heart failure.
   5. **Hypocalcemia** caused by failure to synthesize the active form of vitamin D; hypocalcemia can lead to renal osteodystrophy.
   6. **Anemia** caused by decreased secretion of erythropoietin
   7. **Hypertension** caused by hyperproduction of renin

C. **Other clinical characteristics of uremia** include **anorexia,** nausea, and vomiting; **neurologic disorders,** ranging from diminished mental function to convulsions and coma; **bleeding** caused by disordered platelet function; **accumulation in the skin of urochrome** and other urinary pigments; and **fibrinous pericarditis.**

XI. Nonrenal Causes of Azotemia

A. **Prerenal azotemia.** This condition results from **decreased renal blood flow** caused by blood loss, decreased cardiac output, systemic hypovolemia (as in massive burns), or peripheral pooling of blood due to marked vasodilation (as in gram-negative sepsis). It is characterized by increased tubular reabsorption of sodium and water, resulting in oliguria, concentrated urine, and decreased urinary sodium excretion.

1. Measurement of urinary sodium is diagnostically significant in the delineation of the **oliguria of shock.**
   a. Oliguria may be caused by **decreased renal blood flow** with consequent decreased glomerular filtration rate, in which case tubular reabsorption of sodium is maximally increased and urinary sodium is low.
   b. Oliguria may be a manifestation of **acute tubular necrosis,** in which case tubular reabsorption is greatly impaired and urinary sodium is not decreased.
2. The **BUN:creatinine ratio is characteristically greater than 15** due to a combination of both decreased glomerular filtration and increased tubular reabsorption of urea.

B. **Postrenal azotemia** results from **mechanical blockage of urinary flow.**

XII. Tumors of the Kidney, Urinary Tract, and Bladder

A. **Benign tumors of the kidney**

1. **Adenoma**
   a. This tumor is most often small and asymptomatic. It is derived from renal tubules.
   b. It may be a precursor lesion to renal carcinoma.
2. **Angiomyolipoma**
   a. This tumor is a hamartoma consisting of fat, smooth muscle, and blood vessels.
   b. It is often associated with the tuberous sclerosis syndrome.

B. **Malignant tumors of the kidney**

1. **Renal cell carcinoma**
   a. This cancer is the most common renal malignancy.
   b. It is more common in men, occurs most often from 50 to 70 years of age, and has a higher incidence in cigarette smokers.
   c. In some instances, it is associated with gene deletions in chromosome 3; renal cell carcinoma can also be associated with von Hippel-Lindau disease, which is caused by alterations in a gene localized to chromosome 3.
   d. The carcinoma originates in renal tubules. Most often, it arises in one of the renal poles, frequently the upper pole.
   e. Frequently the tumor invades renal veins or the vena cava and can extend up the vena cava. **Early hematogenous dissemination** may occur.
   f. Histologic characteristics include **polygonal clear cells,** sometimes with vestigial tubule formation.
   g. Presenting features may include the **triad of flank pain, palpable mass, and hematuria.** Hematuria is the most frequent presenting abnormality. Renal cell carcinoma may be manifest clinically by any of the following additional findings:
      (1) **Fever**
      (2) **Secondary polycythemia** (results from erythropoietin production)
      (3) **Ectopic production of various hormones or hormone-like substances** (e.g., ACTH, prolactin, gonadotropins, and renin). Paraneoplastic parathyroid-like hormone can cause hypercalcemia.

2. **Wilms tumor (nephroblastoma)**
   a. This cancer is the most common renal malignancy of early childhood.
   b. Incidence peaks in **children 2–4 years of age.**
   c. Wilms tumor originates from primitive metanephric tissue.
   d. Histologic characteristics are varied, with immature stroma, primitive tubules and glomeruli, and mesenchymal elements, such as fibrous connective tissue, cartilage, bone, and, rarely, striated muscle.
   e. Most often, the presenting feature is a **palpable flank mass** (often huge).
   f. Wilms tumor is often associated with deletions of the short arm of chromosome 11. The *WT*-1 and *WT*-2 genes localized to this chromosome are cancer suppressor genes.
   g. The disease can be part of the AGR (or WAGR) complex (**W**ilms tumor, **A**niridia, **G**enitourinary malformations, and mental-motor **R**etardation). This set of anomalies is associated with deletion of the *WT*-1 tumor suppressor gene and other nearby genes.
   h. The disease also can be a part of the Denys-Drash syndrome, which is characterized by abnormalities of the *WT*-1 gene, intersexual disorders, nephropathy, and Wilms tumor.
   i. It can also be associated with hemihypertrophy (gross asymmetry due to unilateral muscular hypertrophy), macroglossia, organomegaly, neonatal hypoglycemia, and various embryonal tumors. This set of anomalies along with Wilms tumor is collectively referred to as the Beckwith-Wiedemann syndrome and is associated with deletion of the *WT*-2 gene. This syndrome is an example of genomic imprinting because the abnormal alleles are always of maternal origin.

C. **Transitional cell carcinoma**
   1. This cancer is the most common tumor of the urinary collecting system and can occur in renal calyces, pelvis, ureter, or bladder. It is often multifocal in origin.
   2. In the renal pelvis, transitional cell carcinoma has been associated with phenacetin abuse.
   3. This carcinoma is likely to recur after removal.
   4. Most often, the presenting feature is **hematuria.**
   5. There is a tendency to spread by local extension to surrounding tissues.
   6. Associatied toxic exposures may sometimes be involved, including the following:
      a. Industrial exposure to benzidine or β-naphthylamine, an aniline dye
      b. Cigarette smoking
      c. Long-term treatment with cyclophosphamide

D. **Squamous cell carcinoma** constitutes a minority of urinary tract malignancies.
   1. This cancer may result from chronic inflammatory processes such as chronic bacterial infection or *Schistosoma haematobium* infection.
   2. It can also be associated with renal calculi.

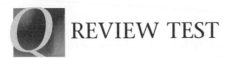

REVIEW TEST

Directions: *Each of the numbered items or incomplete statements in this section is followed by answers or by completions of the statement. Select the one lettered answer or completion that is best in each case.*

1. A 20-year-old woman with the nephrotic syndrome and slowly progressive impairment of renal function marked by azotemia undergoes a renal biopsy. The patient's response to corticosteroid medication has been unimpressive. The appearance of the biopsy is similar to that shown in the figure. The most likely diagnosis is

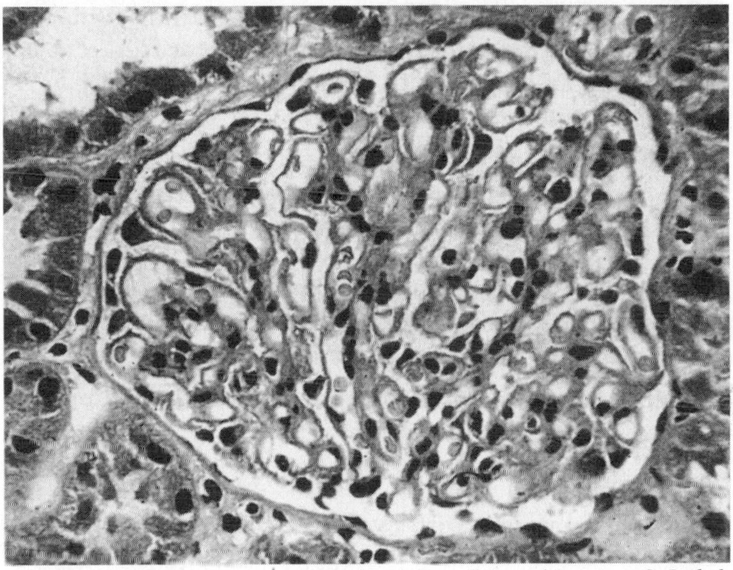

(Reprinted with permission from Golden A, Powell D, and Jennings C: *Pathology: Understanding Human Disease*, 2nd ed. Baltimore, Williams & Wilkins, 1985, p 216.)

(A) focal segmental glomerulosclerosis
(B) membranous glomerulonephritis
(C) minimal change disease
(D) poststreptococcal glomerulonephritis
(E) rapidly progressive glomerulonephritis

2. A 50-year-old man with hypertension and the nephrotic syndrome undergoes a renal biopsy. The appearance of the biopsy is similar to that shown in the figure. Of the following possible additional laboratory findings, which one is most characteristically associated with this lesion?

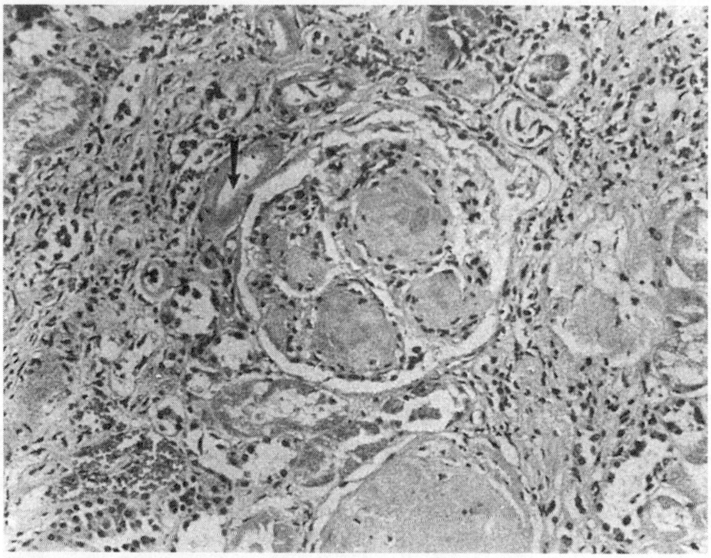

(Courtesy of JB Walter, M.D. Originally published in *Pathology of Human Disease*. Philadelphia, Lea & Febiger, 1989, p 349.)

(A) Decreased creatinine clearance
(B) Fixed specific gravity of urine
(C) Hyperglycemia
(D) Hypocalcemia
(E) Increased blood urea nitrogen

3. A 3-year-old girl presents with generalized edema shortly after recovery from an upper respiratory infection. Laboratory studies reveal marked albuminuria as well as hypoalbuminemia and hyperlipidemia. Prior similar episodes responded to adrenal steroid medication. The most likely diagnosis is

(A) focal segmental glomerulosclerosis
(B) membranous glomerulonephritis
(C) minimal change disease
(D) poststreptococcal glomerulonephritis
(E) rapidly progressive glomerulonephritis

4. A 22-year-old woman presents with fever, malaise, generalized arthralgias, and a skin rash over the nose and malar eminences. Which one of the following possible findings has the greatest relative significance in the overall prognosis for the patient?

(A) Atypical verrucous vegetations of the mitral valve
(B) Glomerular subendothelial immune complex deposition
(C) Immune complexes at the dermal-epidermal junction in skin
(D) Perivascular fibrosis in the spleen
(E) Pleuritis

5. Two weeks after recovery from a severe bout of pharyngitis, an 11-year-old girl is seen because of the acute onset of periorbital edema, hematuria, malaise, nausea, and headache.
Which of the following findings is expected?

(A) Hypotension
(B) Increased antistreptolysin O titer
(C) Marked hypoalbuminemia
(D) Polyuria
(E) Positive urine cultures for β-hemolytic streptococci

6. Expected findings on electron microscopic examination of the glomerulus from the patient in question 5 demonstrate

(A) marked subendothelial immune complex deposition.
(B) marked thickening of the glomerular basement membrane with numerous intramembranous and epimembranous (subepithelial) immune complex deposits.
(C) no changes except for fused epithelial foot processes.
(D) normal-appearing glomerular basement membrane with electron-dense "humps" in subepithelial location.
(E) striking increase in thickness of glomerular basement membrane and diffuse increase in mesangial matrix material.

7. A 28-year-old woman presents with fever, dysuria, urinary frequency, and flank tenderness. The urine contained numerous neutrophils and many white cell casts. Urine protein was moderately increased. A quantitative urine culture revealed more than 10^5 bacteria per milliliter. The most likely causative organism is

(A) *Escherichia coli*
(B) *Haemophilus influenzae*
(C) *Neisseria gonorrhoeae*
(D) *Proteus vulgaris*
(E) *Pseudomonas aeruginosa*

8. A 78-year-old man with long-standing prostatic nodular hyperplasia dies of a stroke. At autopsy, both kidneys demonstrate coarse asymmetric renal corticomedullary scarring, deformity of the renal pelvis and calyces, interstitial fibrosis, and atrophic tubules containing eosinophilic proteinaceous casts. These findings are most suggestive of

(A) Berger disease
(B) chronic analgesic nephritis
(C) chronic pyelonephritis
(D) membranoproliferative glomerulonephritis
(E) renal papillary necrosis

9. A 2-year-old boy with visible abdominal distention is found to have an enormous left-sided flank mass apparently arising from, but dwarfing, the left kidney. The most likely diagnosis is

(A) angiomyolipoma
(B) polycystic kidney
(C) renal cell carcinoma
(D) transitional cell carcinoma
(E) Wilms tumor

10. A syndrome that includes the lesion found in the patient in question 9 has which of the following additional characteristics?

(A) Berry aneurysm of the circle of Willis
(B) Hemihypertrophy
(C) Increased serum uric acid
(D) Marked amplification of genes on the short arm of chromosome 11
(E) Spontaneous regression

11. A 55-year-old man presents with painless hematuria. On cystoscopy, a papillary mass is found in the bladder. Which of the following is a characteristic of this lesion?

(A) Hematuria as a late manifestation
(B) Marked tendency to recur after resection
(C) Much more likely to be benign than malignant
(D) Occurrence only in the bladder and no where else in the urinary tract
(E) Usual presence of distant metastases at the time of diagnosis

12. A glomerular immunofluorescent pattern for IgG similar to that shown in the figure would be expected in which of the following patients?

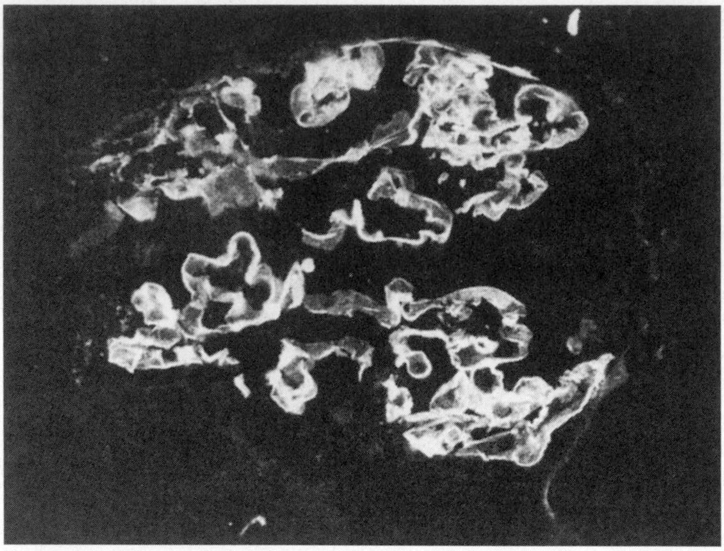

(Reprinted with permission from Walter JB: *An Introduction to the Principles of Disease,* 3rd ed. Philadelphia, WB Saunders, 1992, p 490 [courtesy of Susan Ritchie, M.D., Department of Pathology, The General Division of the Toronto Hospital]).

(A) A 3-year-old girl with recurrent bouts of the nephrotic syndrome
(B) A 9-year-old boy with "smoky" urine 2 weeks after recovery from a streptococcal infection
(C) An 18-year-old woman with the nephrotic syndrome and progressive chronic renal disease
(D) A 25-year-old man with hemoptysis and hematuria
(E) A 26-year-old woman with a "butterfly" rash

13. Enormously enlarged kidneys similar to the one shown in the figure are found at autopsy in a 65-year-old woman. Which of the following is a well-known association or characteristic of this disease process?

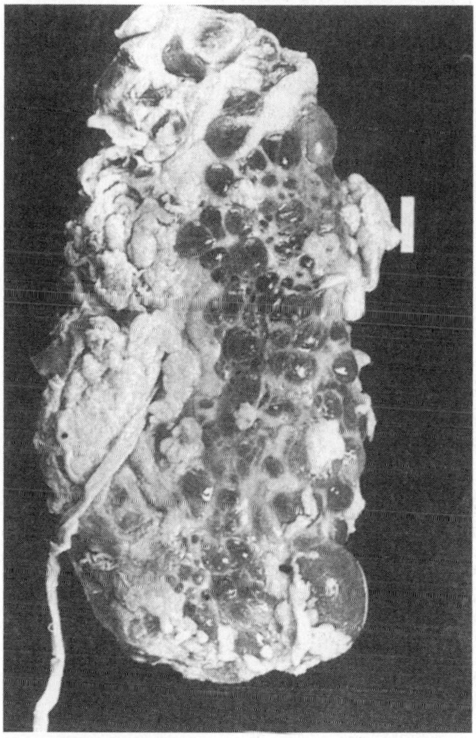

(Courtesy of JB Walter, MD. Originally published in *Pathology of Human Disease*. Philadelphia, Lea & Febiger, 1989, p 700.)

(A) Berry aneurysm of the circle of Willis
(B) Nephrotic syndrome
(C) Polycystic ovaries
(D) Polycythemia vera
(E) X-linked inheritance

14. A 60-year-old woman dies of a tumor that had invaded the renal vein and entered the inferior vena cava. At autopsy, the kidney has the appearance shown in the figure. Which of the following is a characteristic or association of this neoplasm?

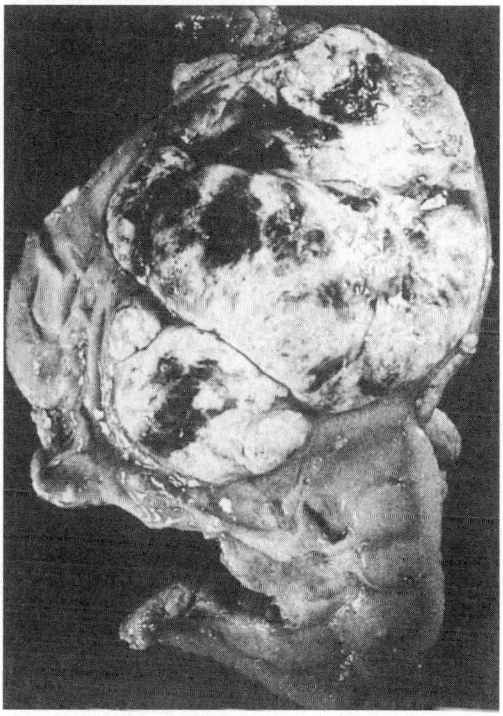

(Reprinted with permission from Golden A, Powell D, and Jennings C: *Pathology: Understanding Human Disease*, 2nd ed. Baltimore, Williams & Wilkins, 1985, p 225.)

(A) Adrenal origin
(B) Hematuria
(C) Hypocalcemia
(D) Tumor cells in the urine
(E) Typical symmetrical bilateral involvement

15. A 4-year-old boy presents with severe proteinuria, hypoalbuminemia, generalized edema, and hyperlipidemia. The patient improves on an empiric trial of corticosteroids, with complete resolution of proteinuria. Which of the following is the most likely diagnosis?

(A) Diabetic nephropathy
(B) Focal segmental glomerulosclerosis
(C) Lupus nephropathy
(D) Membranous glomerulonephritis
(E) Minimal change disease

16. A 25-year-old man presents with generalized edema. Blood tests reveal severe proteinuria, hypoalbuminemia, and hyperlipidemia. The patient does not respond well to a course of corticosteroids. A renal biopsy demonstrates findings indicative of focal segmental glomerulosclerosis. Which of the following best describes the histologic findings in this disorder?

(A) Crescentic formation in glomeruli on light microscopy
(B) Intramembranous and epimembranous immune complex deposits in the glomerular basement membrane on electron microscopy
(C) Nodular accumulations of mesangial matrix material on light microscopy
(D) Sclerosis within capillary tufts that involves only some glomeruli and only parts of affected glomeruli on light microscopy
(E) Wire-loop abnormalities from immune complex deposits and thickening of the glomerular basement membrane on light microscopy

17. A 50-year-old woman with a 20-year history of type 2 diabetes mellitus presents with proteinuria, hypoalbuminemia, edema, and hyperlipidemia. She has not monitored her serum glucose levels over the past several years. Diabetic nephropathy is diagnosed. What is the classic morphologic finding in diabetic nephropathy?

(A) Crescentic formation in glomeruli on light microscopy
(B) Intramembranous and epimembranous immune complex deposits in the glomerular basement membrane on electron microscopy
(C) Nodular accumulations of mesangial matrix on light microscopy
(D) Sclerosis within capillary tufts that involves only some glomeruli and only parts of affected glomeruli on light microscopy
(E) Wire-loop abnormalities from immune complex deposits and thickening of the glomerular basement membrane on light microscopy

18. A 5-year-old boy presents with "tea-colored urine," oliguria, and periorbital edema. He had a sore throat 2 weeks ago that had resolved before his parents sought medical treatment. The patient is found to be hypertensive. Urea nitrogen and creatinine are elevated. Antistreptolysin O titer and anti-DNAase B titer are also elevated. Urine tests are positive for blood and red cell casts. Which of the following is the most likely mechanism for this patient's condition?

(A) Acute bacterial infection of the kidneys
(B) Amyloid deposits
(C) ANCA-positive vasculitis
(D) Antibody against glomerular basement membrane antigens
(E) Immune complex deposits

19. A 5-year-old boy diagnosed with poststreptococcal glomerulonephritis was admitted to the hospital several weeks ago. Over the last several weeks, his clinical state has not improved. Severe oliguria has developed, his serum creatinine has continued to rise, and his glomerular filtration rate has decreased by 50% since his admission to the hospital. Which of the following is the most likely diagnosis?

(A) Alport syndrome
(B) Membranoproliferative glomerulonephritis
(C) Membranous glomerulonephritis
(D) Rapidly progressive glomerulonephritis
(E) Renal papillary necrosis

20. A 25-year-old man presents with hematuria, periorbital edema, hypertension, and hemoptysis. He has also experienced nausea, vomiting, fever, and chills. Serologic testing is positive for antiglomerular basement membrane antibodies. Which of the following is the classic histologic finding in this renal disease?

(A) Linear immunofluorescence
(B) "Lumpy-bumpy" immunofluorescence
(C) "Spike and dome" appearance of the glomerular basement membrane
(D) Subendothelial immune complex deposition
(E) Tram-track appearance of the glomerular basement membrane on electron microscopy

21. A 5-year-old boy presents with hematuria. His mother states that he has had a sore throat for the past 2 days and that he has had hematuria a few times in the past, also concomitantly with a sore throat. She states that his urine usually returns to a normal clear yellow color after a few days. Which of the following is the most likely diagnosis?

(A) Alport syndrome
(B) Goodpasture syndrome
(C) IgA nephropathy
(D) Membranoproliferative glomerulonephritis
(E) Poststreptococcal glomerulonephritis

22. An 18-year-old woman presents with suprapubic pain, urinary frequency, dysuria, and hematuria for the past hour. Urine tests show the presence of pyuria but no white cell casts. Physical examination is remarkable only for suprapubic tenderness on palpation. Which of the following is the most likely diagnosis?

(A) Acute pyelonephritis
(B) Chronic pyelonephritis
(C) Cystitis
(D) Fanconi syndrome
(E) Nephrocalcinosis

23. A 30-year-old man presents with hypertension, hematuria, palpable renal masses, and flank pain. He states that a kidney disease runs in his family, and his mother and maternal grandfather have it. Laboratory abnormalities confirm renal failure. Which of the following is associated with the disorder described here?

(A) Autosomal recessive inheritance
(B) Berry aneurysm of the circle of Willis
(C) Clinical manifestation most commonly at birth
(D) Multiple small medullary cysts in both kidneys
(E) Presence of uric acid stones

24. A 45-year-old man comes to the emergency department in obvious severe pain. He states that he has severe pain in his right flank that extends down to his right groin. The pain is sharp and severe, and it started several minutes earlier. An abdominal radiograph demonstrates the presence of right ureteral urolithiasis. Which of the following is the most likely composition of this patient's stone?

(A) Ammonium magnesium phosphate
(B) Calcium
(C) Cystine
(D) Uric acid

ANSWERS AND EXPLANATIONS

1-B. The diffuse thickening of the walls of the capillary loops seen in the illustration is characteristic of membranous glomerulonephritis, the most frequent cause of the nephrotic syndrome in young adults. Expected associated findings in this immune complex disease include granular immunofluorescence and a characteristic "spike and dome" appearance that is best visualized with special stains. Intramembranous and epimembranous (subepithelial) electron-dense immune complex deposits are seen by electron microscopy.

2-C. The illustration shows nodular glomerulosclerosis (Kimmelstiel-Wilson nodules), the most characteristic glomerular finding in diabetes mellitus. The nodules are accumulations of mesangial matrix-like material.

3-C. The combination of generalized edema, massive proteinuria, hypoalbuminemia, and hyperlipidemia constitutes the nephrotic syndrome, the prototype of which is minimal change disease (lipoid nephrosis). This disorder characteristically occurs in young children and demonstrates intracytoplasmic lipid in the proximal convoluted tubules, a paucity of glomerular abnormalities by light microscopy, and "fusing" (absence) of the epithelial foot processes by electron microscopy.

4-B. The overall prognosis in systemic lupus erythematosus is most closely related to the glomerular lesions in affected patients. These renal lesions are highly variable. In the diffuse proliferative form, almost all of the glomeruli are involved in a marked inflammatory reaction to widespread subendothelial and mesangial immune complex deposition.

5-B. The combination of hematuria (with red cell casts), oliguria, azotemia, and hypertension constitutes the nephritic syndrome, the prototype of which is poststreptococcal glomerulonephritis. An indicator of the prior streptococcal infection is an increased titer of antistreptolysin O. Fluid retention is usually minimal, often limited to periorbital edema, and is the result of reduced renal excretion of salt and water, not hypoalbuminemia. Hypertension, not hypotension, is expected. This disorder is an immune complex disorder, and infection of the kidney does not occur.

6-D. Characteristic electron-dense "humps" on the epithelial side of the basement membrane (subepithelial location) are an extremely important diagnostic feature of poststreptococcal glomerulonephritis. The basement membrane is not thickened in this acute, usually self-limited disorder.

7-A. Organisms involved in urinary tract infections are most often normal flora of the colon, and the most frequent of these is *Escherichia coli.*

8-C. The combination of coarse asymmetric corticomedullary scarring, deformity of the renal pelvis and calyces, and tubular atrophy is characteristic of chronic pyelonephritis. When the atrophic tubules contain eosinophilic proteinaceous casts, the resultant similarity in appearance to thyroid follicles is referred to as "thyroidization." Although an infectious etiology is assumed, the infectious agent is often not demonstrable.

9-E. Wilms tumor is the most common renal neoplasm of children. The tumors are often huge and frequently cause abdominal distention. Renal cell carcinoma and adult polycystic kidney can also present as a large flank mass, but not in a child.

10-B. Associations of Wilms tumor notably include gene deletions localized to the short arm of chromosome 11 (11p13). In some instances, a "two-hit" mechanism of cancer suppressor gene inactivation, similar to that postulated for retinoblastoma, appears to be operative. Other associations of Wilms tumor include congenital aniridia, genitourinary malformations, and mental–motor retardation (the AGR or WAGR complex). Another unusual association is "hemihypertrophy" (gross asymmetry of the body) as part of the Beckwith-Wiedemann syndrome; yet another is the Denys-Drash syndrome, which is characterized by intersexual disorders, nephropathy, and Wilms tumor.

11-B. The majority of urinary tract tumors are transitional cell carcinomas. Following resection, there is a marked tendency to recur. Even benign-appearing transitional cell "papillomas" are usually malignant. These tumors tend to spread contiguously rather than to distal locations. An early sign is hematuria.

12-D. The illustration demonstrates linear immunofluorescence, which is characteristic of disease caused by antiglomerular basement membrane antibodies. In Goodpasture syndrome, antibodies directed against antigens in the basement membranes of the glomeruli as well as the pulmonary alveoli result in both hemorrhagic pneumonitis with hemoptysis and glomerular disease with hematuria.

13-A. Berry aneurysm of the circle of Willis sometimes leading to subarachnoid hemorrhage is a well-known association of adult polycystic kidney disease. Inheritance is by an autosomal dominant mode of inheritance. Secondary polycythemia, not polycythemia vera, is a complication and is caused by increased secretion of erythropoietin.

14-B. The illustration demonstrates a renal cell carcinoma, which most often arises in one of the renal poles, frequently the upper pole. Hematuria is the most frequent presenting sign. The tumor cells have a clear cell appearance, which led to an earlier erroneous concept that this tumor was of adrenal origin and to the older name "hypernephroma." The tumor is often quite large and may result in a palpable mass. Malignant cells are only rarely detected in the urine in renal cell carcinoma.

15-E. Minimal change disease (lipoid nephrosis) is the prototype of the nephrotic syndrome in children, who usually respond well to steroid therapy. Minimal change disease is characterized grossly by lipid-laden renal cortices. Light microscopy reveals normal glomeruli, but electron microscopy demonstrates the fusion of epithelial foot processes.

16-D. Focal segmental glomerulosclerosis has clinical manifestations similar to minimal change disease, but it tends to occur in older patients and does not respond well to steroid treatment. Glomerular hyaline sclerosis occurs in a focal (some, but not all, glomeruli) and segmental (only part of an affected glomerulus) distribution.

17-C. Diabetic nephropathy manifests clinically as the nephrotic syndrome; however, this syndrome is compounded by renal failure and hypertension. Ultrastructural changes include a marked increase in the thickness of the glomerular basement membrane and mesangial accumulation of glycosylated basement membrane-like material. Light microscopy findings include diffuse glomerulosclerosis (a diffuse increase in mesangial matrix) and nodular glomerulosclerosis (nodular accumulations of mesangial matrix).

18-E. The clinical description is that of poststreptococcal glomerulonephritis, the prototype of the nephritic syndrome. An antecedent infection, usually of the pharynx or skin, with a group A β-hemolytic streptococcus occurs approximately 1–2 weeks before the onset of the renal manifestations. Poststreptococcal glomerulonephritis is an immune complex disease, with antigen-antibody-complement complexes localizing to the outside (subepithelial side) of the glomerular basement membrane. An intense inflammatory response is elicited, including chemotactic attraction of neutrophils, release of lysosomal enzymes, partial destruction of basement membrane, and bleeding into the Bowman space.

19-D. The clinical description is that of rapidly progressive glomerulonephritis (RPGN), which is defined as the nephritic syndrome that progresses rapidly to fulminant renal failure within weeks or months. RPGN is classified into three categories: antiglomerular basement membrane (anti-GBM) antibody disease, immune complex deposit disease, and pauci-immune disease (ANCA-positive). Characteristic histologic findings in RPGN include crescents between the Bowman capsule and the glomerular tuft. In approximately 50% of cases of RPGN, the disease is of poststreptococcal etiology. It should be noted, however, that the most common outcome of poststreptococcal glomerulonephritis is complete recovery, and only a small minority of patients progress to RPGN.

20-A. The clinical description is that of Goodpasture syndrome (antiglomerular basement membrane disease), caused by antibodies directed against antigens in the glomerular and pulmonary alveolar basement membranes. Because antigens are an intrinsic component of the basement membrane, labeled antibodies "paint" the surface of the basement membrane, resulting in the characteristic linear immunofluorescent pattern characteristic of this disorder. "Lumpy-bumpy" immunofluorescence is very coarse, granular immunofluorescence found in poststreptococcal immune complex deposit disease. The tram-track appearance is seen in membranoproliferative glomerulonephritis. The "spike and dome" appearance is seen in membranous glomerulonephritis. Subendothelial immune complex deposition is seen in lupus nephropathy.

21-C. IgA nephropathy is the most common glomerular disease and is defined by mesangial deposition of IgA. In its most typical form, the clinical manifestations are limited to a few days of hematuria following an infection. However, there are many etiologic factors, and the condition can vary from one of little import to a severe form of renal disease.

22-C. The clinical description is that of cystitis, which is characterized by pyuria and hematuria but with no white cell casts in the urine. Patients with acute pyelonephritis present with fever, leukocytosis, flank tenderness, urinary white cells, and white cell casts in the urine. Chronic pyelonephritis is almost always the result of chronic urinary tract obstruction and repeated bouts of acute inflammation in the kidneys.

23-B. Adult polycystic kidney disease is the most common inherited disorder of the kidney and is characterized by autosomal dominant inheritance. The disease is characterized by partial replacement of the renal parenchyma with cysts. An important association of adult polycystic kidney disease is berry aneurysm of the circle of Willis.

24-B. Urolithiasis (calculi or stones in the urinary tract) is a very common problem, especially in men. Calcium stones (composed of calcium oxalate or calcium phosphate, or both) account for 80%–85% of urinary stones. Such stones are associated with hypercalciuria, which in turn is caused by increased intestinal absorption of calcium, increased primary renal excretion of calcium, or hypercalcemia. Ammonium magnesium phosphate stones are associated with ammonia-producing (urease-positive) bacteria such as *Proteus vulgaris* or *Staphylococcus*. Uric acid stones are associated with hyperuricemia in 50% of patients and can occur secondary to gout or increased cell turnover (leukemias or myeloproliferative syndromes). Cystine stones are almost always associated with cystinuria, a genetically determined aminoaciduria.

CHAPTER 18

Male Reproductive System

I. Diseases of the Penis

A. Congenital anomalies

1. **Hypospadias** is an anomaly in which the urethral meatus opens on the ventral surface of the penis.
2. **Epispadias** is an anomaly in which the urethral meatus opens on the dorsal surface of the penis. It is less common than hypospadias.

B. Other abnormalities

1. **Phimosis** is an abnormally tight foreskin that is difficult or impossible to retract over the glans penis. This condition may be congenital or result from inflammation or from trauma.
2. **Peyronie disease** is subcutaneous fibrosis of the dorsum of the penis. It occurs in the older age group and is of unknown etiology.
3. **Priapism** is an intractable, often painful erection. This condition is sometimes associated with venous thrombosis of the corpora cavernosa.

C. Inflammatory disorders include a number of sexually transmitted infectious processes.

1. **Balanitis** is inflammation of the glans penis.
   a. This condition is often associated with poor hygiene.
   b. It is rare in circumcised individuals.
2. **Syphilis (lues)**
   a. The infection is caused by spirochetes of *Treponema pallidum,* which are demonstrable by darkfield examination.
   b. Syphilis manifests during the primary stage as **chancre,** an elevated, painless, superficially ulcerated, firm papule. This lesion is most commonly located on the glans penis or prepuce and ordinarily heals within 2–6 weeks. Without treatment, it is followed by secondary and tertiary lues.
3. **Gonorrhea**
   a. The cause is *Neisseria gonorrhoeae,* which appears as an intracellular gram-negative diplococci.
   b. Most often, gonorrhea is manifest by acute purulent urethritis.
   c. Disease can extend to the prostate and seminal vesicles and can also involve the epididymis, but only rarely does it affect the testis.
4. **Chlamydial infection**
   a. This sexually transmitted disease is a common cause of nongonococcal urethritis. It can also cause epididymitis.
   b. Chlamydial infection should be suspected when bacteria are not demonstrated in a purulent urethral discharge.

D. **Neoplasms**

1. **Carcinoma in situ**

a. Bowen disease usually presents as a single erythematous plaque, most often on the shaft of the penis or on the scrotum.

(1) This disease predominantly affects uncircumcised men. The peak incidence is after the fifth decade.

(2) It evolves into invasive carcinoma in fewer than 10% of cases. Additionally, it has been thought to be associated with an increased risk of visceral malignancy; however, this association has recently been disputed.

b. Erythroplasia of Queyrat usually presents as a single erythematous plaque, most often involving the glans penis or prepuce.

(1) This disease occurs predominantly in uncircumcised men. Median incidence is in the fifth decade.

(2) In approximately 10% of cases, the disease progresses to invasive squamous cell carcinoma.

(3) The disease may be a variant of Bowen disease. It is not associated with visceral malignancies.

c. **Bowenoid papulosis**

(1) Histologically, this disease resembles Bowen disease and erythroplasia of Queyrat but is considered to be a distinct entity.

(2) This disease differs from Bowen disease and erythroplasia of Queyrat in terms of clinical presentation, appearing as multiple verrucoid (wart-like) lesions often resembling condyloma acuminatum and containing human papillomavirus (HPV) type 16 viral sequences.

(3) The disease affects a younger age group than Bowen disease and erythroplasia of Queyrat.

(4) The disease is not known to progress to invasive carcinoma but is generally considered to be premalignant.

2. **Carcinoma**

a. Penile cancer is most frequently squamous cell carcinoma.

b. Disease is rare in circumcised men.

c. Incidence is greatly increased in the Far East, Africa, and Central America.

d. Predisposing factors include poor personal hygiene and venereal disease.

e. Disease is often associated with HPV infection types 16, 18, 31, and 33.

II. Diseases of the Testes

A. **Cryptorchidism** is developmental failure of a testis to descend into the scrotum.

1. This condition is associated, even after surgical correction, with a greatly increased incidence of germ cell tumors, especially seminoma and embryonal carcinoma.

2. It is associated with testicular atrophy and sterility.

B. **Torsion of the spermatic cord** compromises blood supply and may result in testicular gangrene.

C. **Hydrocele** is serous fluid filling and distending the tunica vaginalis.

1. This condition is most often idiopathic. Sometimes, it is congenital in origin due to persistence of continuity of the tunica vaginalis with the peritoneal cavity. It can be secondary to infection or to lymphatic blockage by tumor.

2. Usually, hydroceles can be distinguished clinically from solid testicular tumors by physical examination and transillumination.

D. **Hematocele** is an accumulation of blood distending the tunica vaginalis. It is most often caused by trauma, although it is occasionally due to a tumor.

E. **Varicocele** is a varicose dilation of multiple veins of the spermatic cord.

F. **Spermatocele** is a sperm-containing cyst. It is most often intratesticular.

G. **Testicular atrophy**
1. Etiology is often unknown.
2. This condition may be caused by or associated with:
   a. Orchitis, especially mumps orchitis
   b. Trauma
   c. Hormonal excess or deficiency due to:
      (1) Disorders of the hypothalamus or pituitary
      (2) Hormonal therapy, especially with estrogens
      (3) Cirrhosis of the liver
   d. Cryptorchidism
   e. Klinefelter syndrome
   f. Chronic debilitating disease
   g. Old age

H. **Inflammation**
1. **Orchitis**
   a. When bacterial, orchitis is often associated with epididymitis. Orchitis may be caused by syphilis.
   b. When viral, orchitis is most often due to mumps virus.
   c. When bilateral, orchitis may result in sterility due to atrophy of the seminiferous tubules. Serum testosterone is decreased, whereas pituitary follicle-stimulating hormone and luteinizing hormone are increased.
2. **Epididymitis**
   a. This condition is more common than orchitis.
   b. Causes most often include:
      (1) *Neisseria gonorrhoeae*
      (2) *Chlamydia trachomatis*
      (3) *Escherichia coli*
      (4) *Mycobacterium tuberculosis*

I. **Testicular tumors** (Table 18-1) are most often malignant; more than 90% are of germ cell origin.
1. **Seminoma** is a **malignant** germ cell tumor.
   a. This tumor is analogous to dysgerminoma, a tumor of the ovary.
   b. It is the most frequently occurring germ cell tumor, accounting for 40%.
   c. Peak incidence is in the **mid-30s age group.**
   d. Presenting features include painless enlargement of the testis.
   e. Sometimes this tumor is associated with increased serum human chorionic gonadotropin (hCG), the same tumor marker associated with choriocarcinoma and other germ cell tumors.
   f. Seminomas are very **radiosensitive** and can often be cured, even when there are metastasis to abdominal lymph nodes.
2. **Embryonal carcinoma** is a malignant germ cell tumor.
   a. This tumor is analogous to a similar tumor occurring in the ovary.
   b. It is the second most common germ cell tumor, accounting for 20%–30%.
   c. Presenting conditions often include pain or metastasis.
   d. The serum hCG is often increased.
   e. The prognosis is much worse than for seminoma.
3. **Endodermal sinus (yolk sac) tumor** is a malignant germ cell tumor.
   a. This tumor is analogous to endodermal sinus tumor of the ovary.
   b. It has a peak incidence in **infancy and early childhood** and is the most common testicular tumor in this age group.
   c. This tumor causes an **increase in serum α-fetoprotein**, the same tumor marker that is associated with hepatocellular carcinoma.

TABLE 18-1 *World Health Organization Classification of Testicular Tumors*

Types	Comments
Germ cell tumors	
Tumors of one histologic type:	More than 90% of testicular tumors are of germ cell origin
Seminoma	Most frequently occurring germ cell tumor; peak incidence at 35 years of age
Spermatocytic seminoma	Older age group; more favorable prognosis
Embryonal carcinoma	Second most frequently occurring germ cell tumor; often presents with pain or metastasis; somewhat younger age incidence than seminoma
Yolk sac tumor (embryonal carcinoma, infantile type; endodermal sinus tumor)	Peak incidence infancy and early childhood
Polyembryoma	
Choriocarcinoma	
Teratoma	
Mature	Almost always malignant
Immature	
With malignant transformation	Malignant change of one of the tissues within a teratoma (e.g., development of squamous cell carcinoma within epidermoid component)
Tumors of more than one histologic type:	Combinations include mixes of seminoma, embryonal carcinoma, teratoma, and choriocarcinoma
Embryonal carcinoma and teratoma (teratocarcinoma)	
Choriocarcinoma and any other type (specify)	
Other combinations (specify)	
Stromal sex-cord tumors	
Well-differentiated forms:	
Leydig cell tumor	Usually benign; often causes precocious puberty
Sertoli cell tumor	Usually benign; usually no endocrine manifestations
Granulosa cell tumor	
Mixed forms (specify)	
Incompletely differentiated forms	

4. **Teratoma**
   a. This germ cell tumor is derived from two or more embryonic layers.
   b. It is most frequently malignant.
   c. It contains multiple tissue types, such as cartilage islands, ciliated epithelium, liver cells, neuroglia, embryonic gut, or striated muscle.
   d. It can be classified as one of three subtypes:
      (1) **Mature teratoma.** This teratoma is almost always malignant, whereas the corresponding ovarian tumor (dermoid cyst) is almost always benign.
      (2) **Immature teratoma**

(3) **Teratoma with malignant transformation.** This teratoma contains malignant tissue such as squamous cell carcinoma.

5. **Choriocarcinoma** is a malignant germ cell tumor that can occur as an element of other germ cell tumors.
   a. This tumor is analogous to choriocarcinoma of the ovary.
   b. Incidence peaks in the second to third decades.
   c. Histologic characteristics include cells that resemble syncytiotrophoblasts and cytotrophoblasts.
   d. This tumor causes an increase in serum hCG.
6. **Mixed germ cell tumors** consist of varying **combinations of germ cell tumor types.**
   a. Tumors are of **variable prognosis determined by the least mature element.**
   b. Tumors can be **teratocarcinoma,** that is, a combination of teratoma and embryonal carcinoma, which is associated with poor prognosis; can also occur in other combinations, including:
      (1) **Teratoma, embryonal carcinoma, and seminoma**
      (2) **Embryonal carcinoma and seminoma**
7. **Leydig cell (interstitial) tumor** is a non–germ cell tumor derived from testicular stroma.
   a. This tumor is similar to the Sertoli-Leydig cell tumor of the ovary.
   b. It is most often benign.
   c. It is often characterized by intracytoplasmic Reinke crystals. The tumor is characteristically known as androgen-producing but sometimes produces both androgens and estrogens and sometimes corticosteroids.
   d. The tumor is most often associated with precocious puberty in children and with gynecomastia in adults.
8. **Sertoli cell tumor (androblastoma)** is a non–germ cell tumor derived from the sex cord-stroma.
   a. This tumor is also similar to the Sertoli-Leydig cell tumor of the ovary.
   b. It is usually benign.
   c. It is characterized by a paucity of endocrine manifestations.

III. Diseases of the Prostate

A. **Anatomy of the prostate.** This chestnut-sized and -shaped structure surrounds the urethra at the base of the bladder. It is comprised of four groupings of glands, referred to as the periurethral, transitional, central, and peripheral zones.

1. The **periurethral, transitional, and central zones** collectively are equivalent to the older designation of anterior, middle, and lateral lobes and are often the site of benign prostatic hyperplasia (BPH).
2. The **peripheral zone** of glands draining into ducts entering the urethral sinus close to the verumontanum is equivalent to the older designation of posterior lobe; it is the characteristic site for carcinoma.

B. **BPH (benign nodular hyperplasia).** BPH is the most frequent cause of urinary tract obstruction.

1. BPH is extremely common (almost universal) in older men.
2. Although BPH has no relation to prostate cancer, the two conditions can coexist.
3. BPH is directly related to the action of dihydrotestosterone (DHT), a testosterone metabolite. DHT is synthesized from testosterone by the action of 5α-reductase, type 2, and inhibition of this enzyme is one approach to the treatment of BPH.
4. BPH may also be caused by an age-related increase in estrogens (estrogens promote expression of receptors for DHT).
5. Hyperplasia of both glandular and fibromuscular stromal elements is characteristic.

6. BPH is characterized grossly by a rubbery, nodular enlargement of the gland, primarily affecting the inner groupings of glands, especially the **periurethral and transitional zones.**
7. The urethra is compressed side to side, resulting in a vertical slit.
8. Most characteristically, BPH results in **urinary obstruction,** which is manifest by:
   a. Frequency, dysuria, hesitancy (difficulty in starting urination), and urinary tract infection
   b. Incomplete bladder emptying
   c. Distention and muscular hypertrophy of the bladder; in cases of long duration, bands of enlarged bladder muscle form characteristic trabeculae.
   d. Hydroureter and hydronephrosis

C. **Adenocarcinoma** is extremely common.

1. Prostate cancer occurs in the older age group.
2. The course may be indolent or aggressive; this can be predicted by the very useful **Gleason system of grading,** based on differentiation. The tumor is often well differentiated.
3. The tumor arises most often from the peripheral group of glands.
4. Diagnosis is most often by rectal examination.
5. Prostate cancer is associated at an early stage with an **increase in serum prostate-specific antigen (PSA).** Elevations of PSA reflect a complexed form (bound to α_1-antichymotrypsin), which becomes elevated with prostatic cancer, and a free form, which increases with BPH. Thus, an **increased total PSA** with a **decreased fraction of free PSA** suggests malignancy, whereas an increased total PSA with a proportionate increase in the fraction of free PSA suggests BPH.
6. Prostate cancer is characterized by increased serum prostatic acid phosphatase when the tumor penetrates the capsule into adjacent tissues. Although prostatic acid phosphatase is no longer used for detection of early disease because of lack of sensitivity, this enzyme, along with PSA, is useful in the follow-up of disseminated disease.
7. The adenocarcinoma may frequently progress to bony osteoblastic metastasis, which, unfortunately, may be the presenting sign. In this instance, an **increase in serum alkaline phosphatase is often an indicator of osteoblastic lesions and virtually ensures that the osteoblastic tumors originated in the prostate.**
8. When disseminated, the cancer may respond to endocrine therapy because tumor growth is partially related to the activity of androgens.

REVIEW TEST

Directions: *Each of the numbered items or incomplete statements in this section is followed by answers or by completions of the statement. Select the* ***one*** *lettered answer or completion that is best in each case.*

1. A 23-year-old African-American man who is known to have sickle cell anemia presents to the emergency department with a painful erection. The patient explains that the erection had started 3 hours ago. This condition is referred to as

(A) balanitis
(B) hypospadias
(C) Peyronie disease
(D) phimosis
(E) priapism

2. 3-year-old businessman visits his primary care physician complaining of a purulent penile discharge. He had unprotected sex with a woman he met at a conference 1 week ago. Gram stain of the discharge fails to reveal any organisms. Which of the following is the most likely cause of the discharge?

(A) Bowen disease
(B) *Chlamydia trachomatis*
(C) Herpes simplex virus
(D) *Neisseria gonorrhoeae*
(E) *Treponema pallidum*

3. A 5-year-old boy is brought to the pediatrician for a physical examination prior to beginning elementary school. On examination, the boy has only one palpable testis in the scrotum. Further examination reveals a palpable mass in the left inguinal region. This condition is referred to as

(A) cryptorchidism
(B) hydrocele
(C) orchitis
(D) torsion of the spermatic cord
(E) varicocele

4. A 36-year-old man presents to his primary care physician complaining of painless enlargement of the testis. Further laboratory studies reveal an increase in serum human chorionic gonadotropin. Of the following, which of the following is the most likely diagnosis?

(A) Dysgerminoma
(B) Embryonal carcinoma
(C) Seminoma
(D) Teratoma
(E) Yolk sac tumor

5. A 3-year-old boy is brought to the pediatrician because his mother noticed an abnormal mass in his scrotum while changing his diapers. Further workup demonstrates elevated levels of serum α-fetoprotein. Which of the following is the most likely diagnosis?

(A) Choriocarcinoma
(B) Endodermal sinus (yolk sac) tumor
(C) Hepatocellular carcinoma
(D) Leydig cell (interstitial) tumor
(E) Teratoma

6. A 66-year-old man visits his family physician with complaints of urinary frequency, hesitancy, and dysuria. Digital rectal examination reveals an enlarged prostate, and the consistency is rubbery and nodular. Serum prostate-specific antigen is modestly increased. Which of the following is most closely related to the pathogenesis of the likely disorder described here?

(A) Dihydrotestosterone
(B) Estrogen
(C) α-Fetoprotein
(D) Human chorionic gonadotropin
(E) Testosterone

7. A 58-year-old African-American man presents to the emergency department with severe back pain. His history is negative for trauma and he has no other complaints. He denies urinary frequency, hesitancy, or dysuria. A digital rectal examination confirms the presence of a firm, hard, asymmetrical, and stony prostate. Imaging of the spine suggests osteoblastic involvement of the spine at lumbar vertebrae L3–L4. In addition to an increase in PSA, which serum marker might also be elevated?

(A) Alkaline phosphatase
(B) Androgens
(C) Carcinoembryonic antigen-125
(D) α-Fetoprotein
(E) Human chorionic gonadotropin

ANSWERS AND EXPLANATIONS

1-E. Priapism is an intractable, often painful erection associated with conditions such as sickle cell anemia, hypercoagulable states, spinal injuries, and some drugs. Balanitis is associated with poor hygiene and results from inflammation of the glans penis. Hypospadias is an anatomical anomaly wherein the urethral meatus opens on the ventral side of the penis. Peyronie disease results from subcutaneous fibrosis of the dorsum of the penis. Phimosis is an abnormally tight foreskin that is difficult or impossible to retract over the glans penis.

2-B. *Chlamydia trachomatis* is one of the leading causes of urethritis and should be suspected whenever a gonorrhea-like discharge fails to show gram-negative diplococci within neutrophilic phagocytes. It is a sexually transmitted disease that can also cause epididymitis. Bowen disease presents as a single erythematous plaque on the penis or scrotum and may evolve into invasive carcinoma. Herpes simplex virus can cause a vesicular rash on the penis. *Treponema pallidum* causes syphilis, which may present with a painless chancre on the penis.

3-A. Cryptorchidism (undescended testis) predisposes to testicular atrophy and sterility. It is associated with an increased incidence of germ cell tumors of the testis, even if the testis is surgically moved from its ectopic location back to the scrotum. A hydrocele is a serous fluid collection in the scrotum. Orchitis (inflammation of the testis) can result from bacterial or viral infection. A varicocele results from dilation of the veins of the spermatic cord, and the term "bag of worms" aptly describes the abnormality.

4-C. Seminoma is the most common germ cell tumor of the testis. Serum human chorionic gonadotropin levels, elaborated by syncytiotrophoblasts, are elevated in about 15% of cases, but these elevations are not as high as those seen in choriocarcinoma. The tumor is highly radiosensitive and often curable, even when metastatic. Dysgerminoma is analogous to a tumor that occurs in the ovary. Embryonal carcinoma often presents with pain and is the second most common tumor of the testis. Yolk sac tumor is the most common tumor of the testis during infancy and early childhood and is usually accompanied by an increase in serum α-fetoprotein.

5-B. Endodermal sinus (yolk sac) tumor is the most common malignant germ cell tumor of the testis in infancy and early childhood. It is characterized by an increase in serum α-fetoprotein as well as histologically stainable α_1-antitrypsin. Choriocarcinoma is less common in this age group and often results in an increase in human chorionic gonadotropin. Although hepatocellular carcinomas also elaborate α-fetoprotein, this is very unlikely in this patient's clinical setting. Leydig cell tumors are derived from testicular stroma and produce androgens and estrogens, often presenting with precocious puberty. Teratomas contain multiple germ layers and numerous tissues, including hair, teeth, and sebaceous tissue. Unlike the teratomas encountered in women, most teratomas in men are malignant.

6-A. Dihydrotestosterone (DHT) is a major growth factor for prostatic tissue. It is derived from the conversion from testosterone by the action of the enzyme 5α-reductase, type 2. Pharmaceutical inhibition of this enzyme is useful in the medical management of benign prostatic hyperplasia. Estrogens also play an indirect role by stimulating the production of DHT receptors. Human chorionic gonadotropin and α-fetoprotein are serum tumor markers for testicular cancers and bear no relevance to benign prostatic hyperplasia.

7-A. Serum alkaline phosphatase is an indicator of osteoblastic lesions in this advanced and unfortunate patient presentation. Both prostate-specific antigen and serum prostatic acid phosphatase are increased in prostatic cancer. Although prostatic cancers are usually quite androgen-responsive, androgens are not monitored for diagnosis or treatment of prostate cancer. Carcinoembryonic antigen-125 is a tumor marker for ovarian cancer. Serum α-fetoprotein and serum human chorionic gonadotropin are elevated in various germ cell neoplasms of the testis.

CHAPTER 19

Female Reproductive System and Breast

I. Vulva and Vagina

A. Miscellaneous disorders

1. **Bartholin cyst** results from **an obstruction of Bartholin ducts.** The **cyst** can become secondarily infected, most often by *Neisseria gonorrhoeae* or, less often, by *Staphylococcus.*
2. **Vulvar dystrophies** are a group of disorders of **epithelial growth** that often present with leukoplakia, a white, patch-like lesion.
   a. **Histologic forms**
      (1) **Lichen sclerosus** and **hyperplastic dystrophy,** which have no malignant potential
      (2) **Atypical hyperplastic dystrophy,** a premalignant lesion
   b. **Clinical characteristics. Pruritus** and **leukoplakia.** Leukoplakia can be a manifestation of several diverse processes and **should be evaluated by biopsy.**

B. Infectious disorders

1. **Candidiasis (moniliasis)** is the **most common** form of vaginitis.
   a. The cause is *Candida albicans,* a normal component of the vaginal flora.
   b. Associated conditions include diabetes mellitus, pregnancy, broad-spectrum antibiotic therapy, oral contraceptive use, and immunosuppression.
   c. Candidiasis is characterized by white, patch-like mucosal lesions, a thick white discharge, and vulvovaginal pruritus.
2. **Trichomoniasis** is the second most common type of vaginitis.
   a. The cause is *Trichomonas vaginalis.*
   b. Trichomoniasis is most often transmitted by sexual contact.
3. **Bacterial vaginosis (*Gardnerella* vaginitis)** is the most common cause of vaginal discharge. Characteristically, it is a thin, homogeneous vaginal discharge with a malodorous, fishy amine odor, especially on addition of 10% potassium hydroxide.
   a. The cause is a loss of the normal vaginal lactobacilli, a consequent overgrowth of anaerobes (e.g., *Prevotella bivia, Mobiluncus* spp., *Peptostreptococcus* spp.), and a resultant superficial polymicrobial vaginal infection.
   b. This type of vaginitis accounts for many cases formerly classified as nonspecific vaginitis. It is usually transmitted by sexual contact.
   c. Bacterial vaginosis is associated with increased numbers of the facultative anaerobe *Gardnerella vaginalis.*

d. The appearance of "clue cells" (vaginal epithelial cells that have a stippled appearance due to adherent coccobacilli) in Papanicolaou (Pap) smear preparations is characteristic.

4. **Toxic shock syndrome**
   a. This condition was initially associated with the use of highly absorbent tampons. It is caused by exotoxin produced by *Staphylococcus aureus,* which grows in the tampon.
   b. Characteristic features include fever, vomiting, and diarrhea, sometimes followed by renal failure and shock. A generalized rash is followed by desquamation.
5. **Gonorrhea**
   a. The cause is *N. gonorrhoeae.* Gonorrhea is a frequent cause of pelvic inflammatory disease. Other frequent etiologic agents of pelvic inflammatory disease are *Chlamydia trachomatis* and enteric bacteria.
   b. Transmission is by sexual contact.
   c. The disorder can be asymptomatic but infectious. Disease can ascend to infect the endocervix, uterine canal, and fallopian tubes. It is characterized by purulent acute inflammation, initially of the urethra, paraurethral and Bartholin glands, and Skene ducts.
   d. Gonorrhea can result in extragenital infections, including:
      (1) **Pharyngitis** associated with orogenital sexual contact
      (2) **Proctitis** associated with anal intercourse
      (3) **Purulent arthritis,** which is most often monoarticular, involving a large joint, such as the knee, as a consequence of blood-borne infection
      (4) **Ophthalmia neonatorum,** a neonatal conjunctival infection acquired at delivery
6. **Chlamydial infections**
   a. **Chlamydial cervicitis** is the **most common sexually transmitted disease.**
      (1) The cause is certain serotypes of *C. trachomatis.* Chlamydial cervicitis is a frequent cause of pelvic inflammatory disease.
      (2) The disease is most often asymptomatic.
   b. **Lymphogranuloma venereum**
      (1) This disease occurs primarily in the tropics.
      (2) The cause is *C. trachomatis* L1, L2, or L3 serotypes.
      (3) Lymphogranuloma venereum is manifest initially as a small papule or ulcer, followed by superficial ulcers and enlargement of regional lymph nodes, which become matted together. It can lead to rectal stricture as a result of inflammatory reaction and scarring.
7. **Herpes simplex virus (HSV) infections**
   a. HSV type 2 infection accounts for the majority of genital herpes cases and is spread by sexual contact.
   b. HSV infection produces small vesicles and shallow ulcers that can involve the cervix, vagina, clitoris, vulva, urethra, and perianal skin. Multinucleated giant cells with viral inclusions are found in cytologic smears from lesions.
8. **Syphilis**
   a. The cause is *Treponema pallidum.*
   b. Transmission is by sexual contact.
   c. The initial stage manifests as a firm, painless ulcer known as a chancre, which is usually not apparent clinically.
   d. The disease is sometimes manifest during secondary syphilis as condyloma lata, which are gray, flattened, wart-like lesions. **Note:** Condyloma lata should not be confused with condyloma acuminatum (see later).
   e. Syphilis is a hazard during pregnancy because spirochetes can cross the placenta and result in fetal malformation.
9. **Chancroid**
   a. The cause is *Haemophilus ducreyi.*
   b. Transmission is by sexual contact.
   c. This disease is most common in tropical areas; it is rare in the United States.

d. Chancroid is characterized by a soft and painful ulcerated lesion in contrast to the chancre of syphilis, which is firm and painless.

10. **Granuloma inguinale**
   a. The cause is *Calymmatobacterium (Donovania) granulomatis,* a gram-negative rod.
   b. Transmission is probably sexual.
   c. **Donovan bodies,** which are multiple organisms filling large histiocytes, are characteristic and are an important diagnostic histopathologic feature.
   d. An infection appears initially as a papule, which becomes superficially ulcerated. It progresses by adjacent lesions coalescing to form large genital or inguinal ulcerations, sometimes with lymphatic obstruction or genital distortion.

C. **Neoplasms of the vulva** (Table 19-1)
1. **Papillary hidradenoma** is the most common benign tumor of the vulva.
   a. This tumor originates from apocrine sweat glands.
   b. It presents as a labial nodule that may ulcerate and bleed.
   c. Cure is by simple excision.
2. **Condyloma acuminatum**
   a. This benign squamous cell papilloma is caused by **human papillomavirus (HPV),** most frequently HPV types 6 and 11.
   b. Transmission is by sexual contact.
   c. Clinical manifestations include multiple wart-like lesions, **venereal warts,** in the vulvovaginal and perianal regions and sometimes on the cervix.
   d. Histologic characteristics include **koilocytes,** or expanded epithelial cells with perinuclear clearing.
3. **Squamous cell carcinoma** is the most common malignant tumor of the vulva.
   a. This carcinoma has its peak occurrence in older women. It is often preceded by premalignant changes graded as vulvar intraepithelial neoplasia (VIN) 1 through 3. In addition, it may be preceded by vulvar dystrophy.
   b. Squamous cell carcinoma is often associated with HPV infection type 16, 18, 31, or 33. These same HPV strains are associated with squamous cell carcinoma of the vagina and cervix. Other HPV strains are associated with papillomatous lesions elsewhere.
4. **Paget disease of the vulva** is similar to Paget disease of the breast. It is sometimes associated with underlying adenocarcinoma of the apocrine sweat glands.
5. **Malignant melanoma** accounts for approximately 10% of malignant tumors of the vulva.

D. **Neoplasms of the vagina (see Table 19-1)**
1. **Squamous cell carcinoma** is most often due to extension of squamous cell carcinoma of the cervix. The vagina is infrequently the primary site.
2. **Clear cell adenocarcinoma** is a rare malignant tumor.
   a. Incidence is greatly increased in daughters of women who received **diethylstilbestrol (DES)** therapy during pregnancy. Clear cell adenocarcinoma of the cervix and vaginal adenosis may also occur in these patients.
   b. Vaginal adenosis, a benign condition characterized by mucosal columnar epithelial-lined crypts in areas normally lined by stratified squamous epithelium, is thought to be a precursor of clear cell adenocarcinoma.
3. **Sarcoma botryoides** is a rare variant of rhabdomyosarcoma.
   a. This neoplasm occurs in children younger than 5 years of age.
   b. Presenting features include multiple polypoid masses resembling a "bunch of grapes" projecting into the vagina, often protruding from the vulva.

II. Uterine Cervix

A. **Non-neoplastic disorders**
1. **Erosion** is characterized by columnar epithelium replacing squamous epithelium, grossly resulting in an erythematous area. Sometimes it is a manifestation of chronic cervicitis.

TABLE 19-1 *Comparison of Tumors of the Female Reproductive System*

Type	Behavior	Location	Comments
Condyloma acuminatum (venereal wart)	Benign	Vulvovaginal, perianal, sometimes cervical	Most often multiple; etiologic agent HPV (types 6 and 11)
Squamous cell carcinoma	Malignant	Vulva	May be preceded by atypical hyperplastic dystrophy
Clear cell adenocarcinoma	Malignant	Vagina	Peak incidence in teenagers and young women exposed in utero to DES
Squamous cell carcinoma	Malignant	Vagina	Uncommon location for primary squamous cell carcinoma; more often due to extension of squamous cell carcinoma of the cervix
Squamous cell carcinoma	Malignant	Uterine cervix	Squamocolumnar junction most frequent site of origin; often preceded by dysplasia; HPV (types 16, 18, 31, and 33) is suspected to be the etiologic agent
Leiomyoma	Benign	Uterine corpus	Most frequently occurring neoplasm of women; most often multiple; increases in size during pregnancy; regresses with menopause
Endometrial carcinoma	Malignant	Uterine corpus	Peak incidence in older age group; predisposed by estrogen stimulation; incidence increasing
Cystadenoma, serous or mucinous	Benign	Ovary	
Cystadenocarcinoma, serous or mucinous	Malignant	Ovary	Rupture of mucinous form can lead to pseudomyxoma peritonei
Mature teratoma (dermoid cyst)	Benign	Ovary	Most frequent ovarian tumor
Choriocarcinoma	Malignant	Ovary or gestational tissue	Increased hCG in serum and urine
Fibroma	Benign	Ovary	Can be associated with Meigs syndrome (ovarian fibroma, ascites, and hydrothorax)
Granulosa cell tumor	Benign	Ovary	Estrogen-secreting
Krukenberg tumors	Malignant	Ovaries	Metastatic replacement of ovaries with signet-ring cells from primary malignant tumor elsewhere (often from the stomach)

HPV = human papillomavirus; DES = diethylstilbestrol; hCG = human chorionic gonadotropin.

2. **Cervicitis** most often involves the endocervix.
   a. Causes include staphylococci, enterococci, *G. vaginalis, T. vaginalis, C. albicans,* and *C. trachomatis.*
   b. The condition is often asymptomatic. It may be manifest by cervical discharge.
3. **Cervical polyps** are inflammatory proliferations of cervical mucosa; they are not true neoplasms.

B. **Dysplasia and carcinoma in situ**
   1. The squamocolumnar junction is most frequently involved.
   2. There is a major association with **HPV infection** types 16, 18, 31, or 33.
   3. Disordered epithelial growth manifest by loss of polarity and nuclear hyperchromasia, beginning at the basal layer and extending outward, is characteristic.
   4. Dysplasia can progress through mild, moderate, and severe forms to carcinoma in situ and is classified as **cervical intraepithelial neoplasia (CIN),** with subtypes of CIN 1, CIN 2, or CIN 3, depending on the extent of epithelial involvement. CIN 3 (carcinoma in situ) is characterized by atypical changes extending through the entire thickness of the epithelium.

C. **Invasive carcinoma**
   1. **General considerations**
      a. The occurrence peaks in **middle-aged** women.
      b. The cancer is most often **squamous cell carcinoma;** adenocarcinoma accounts for approximately 5% of cases.
      c. Most frequently, the carcinoma arises from preexisting CIN at the squamocolumnar junction. It evolves through a series of increasing epithelial abnormalities proceeding from dysplasia to carcinoma in situ and then to invasive carcinoma.
      d. Since the introduction of the Papanicolaou (**Pap**) cytologic screening test, squamous cell carcinoma has exhibited a striking decrease in mortality.
   2. **Epidemiologic factors** (probable spread by sexual contact)
      a. **Early sexual activity** and **multiple sexual partners** are associated with increased incidence.
      b. Incidence is high in **prostitutes,** rare in celibates, and rare in some Jewish populations. The traditional belief that circumcision of male sexual partners exerts a protective effect has not been confirmed.
      c. Incidence is increased in the economically deprived.
      d. Cigarette smoking is also associated with increased incidence, but the relationship remains unclear.
   3. **Role of HPV**
      a. Dysplastic cells frequently demonstrate **koilocytosis** (as in HPV-induced condyloma acuminatum).
      b. HPV sequences are often integrated into genomes of dysplastic or malignant cervical epithelial cells; HPV types 16, 18, 31, and 33 are most common, as in most malignant genital squamous cell tumors, and are associated with more than 90% of cases. HPV viral proteins E6 and E7 bind and inactivate the gene products of *p53* and *Rb,* respectively.

III. Uterine Corpus

A. **Endometritis**
   1. **Acute endometritis**
      a. The cause is most often *S. aureus* or *Streptococcus* species.
      b. This condition is most often related to intrauterine trauma from instrumentation, intrauterine contraceptive devices, or complications of pregnancy, such as postpartum retention of placental fragments.

2. **Chronic specific (granulomatous) endometritis** is most often tuberculous in etiology.

B. **Endometriosis**

1. The presence and proliferation of ectopic endometrial tissue is characteristic.
2. Causes may include retrograde dissemination of endometrial fragments through fallopian tubes during menstruation, with implantation on the ovary or other peritoneal structures, or blood-borne or lymphatic-borne dissemination of endometrial fragments.
3. The condition is characteristically responsive to hormonal variations of the menstrual cycle.
4. Menstrual-type bleeding occurs into the ectopic endometrium, resulting in blood-filled, or so-called "chocolate," cysts.
5. Endometriosis occurs most often in the pelvic area; the ovary is the most common site, followed by the uterine ligaments, rectovaginal septum, pelvic peritoneum, and other sites.
6. Clinical manifestations include severe **menstrual-related pain.**
7. Endometriosis is non-neoplastic and has no relation to endometrial cancer. It often results in infertility.

C. **Adenomyosis** is characterized by islands of endometrium within myometrium.

D. **Endometrial hyperplasia** is an abnormal proliferation of endometrial glands.

1. The cause is usually **excess estrogen stimulation,** which in turn may be caused by anovulatory cycles, polycystic ovary disease, estrogen-secreting ovarian tumors such as granulosa cell tumor, and estrogen replacement therapy.
2. This condition is most often manifest clinically by **postmenopausal bleeding.**
3. It is sometimes a precursor lesion of endometrial carcinoma; **the risk of carcinoma varies with the degree of cellular atypia.** Simple (cystic or mild) hyperplasias have a low malignant potential, while higher grade (atypical or adenomatous with atypia) hyperplasias have a greater malignant potential.

E. **Endometrial polyp**

1. This **benign** lesion usually occurs in **women older than 40 years of age.**
2. It may result in uterine bleeding.

F. **Leiomyoma (fibroid)**

1. This is the **most common uterine tumor** and the most common of all tumors in women; the incidence is increased in women of African lineage.
2. The tumor is a **benign** neoplasm; putative malignant transformation is rare.
3. Leiomyomas occur in multiple separate foci in most cases.
4. The tumors are **estrogen-sensitive.** They often **increase in size during pregnancy,** and they almost always **decrease in size following menopause.**
5. The tumors may lie within the myometrium (intramural) or in subendometrial (submucous) or subperitoneal (subserous) locations. Leiomyomas, especially if subendometrial, are often manifest clinically by **menorrhagia** (increased menstrual bleeding).

G. **Leiomyosarcoma**

1. This malignant tumor occurs infrequently.
2. It arises de novo and is almost never caused by malignant transformation of a leiomyoma.

H. **Endometrial carcinoma**

1. Endometrial carcinoma is the **most common gynecologic malignancy.** In contrast to carcinoma of the cervix, the incidence of this tumor is increasing. It is increased in incidence in association with nulliparity.
2. Peak occurrence is in **older women,** who are affected more by endometrial carcinoma than by carcinoma of the cervix.

3. Clinical manifestations most often include **postmenopausal bleeding.** This often leads to early diagnosis.
4. The cancer is often preceded by endometrial hyperplasia, especially higher grade dysplasias.
5. Predisposing factors include **prolonged estrogen stimulation,** as occurs with exogenous estrogen therapy or estrogen-producing tumors, as well as obesity, diabetes mellitus, and hypertension; the common factor may be **obesity** because estrone can be synthesized in peripheral adipose tissues.

IV. Fallopian Tubes

A. **Salpingitis**

1. This disorder is most often associated with **inflammation of the ovaries and other adjacent tissue** (pelvic inflammatory disease). It can be caused by trauma such as surgical manipulation.
2. Causes are most often *N. gonorrhoeae,* various anaerobic bacteria, *C. trachomatis,* streptococci, and other pyogenic organisms.
3. Salpingitis can result in **pyosalpinx,** a tube filled with pus, or **hydrosalpinx,** a tube filled with watery fluid; it may also result in a **tubo-ovarian abscess.**

B. **Hematosalpinx** is bleeding into the fallopian tube. It is most often caused by **ectopic pregnancy.**

C. **Fallopian tube tumors**

1. **Adenomatoid tumor** is the most frequent benign tumor of the fallopian tubes.
2. **Adenocarcinoma** most often results from direct extension or metastasis from tumors originating elsewhere.

V. Ovaries

A. **Ovarian cysts**

1. **Follicular cyst**
   a. This cyst is due to distention of the unruptured graafian follicle.
   b. It is sometimes associated with hyperestrinism and endometrial hyperplasia.
2. **Corpus luteum cyst**
   a. This cyst results from hemorrhage into a persistent mature corpus luteum.
   b. It is symptomatically associated with menstrual irregularity, occasionally with intraperitoneal hemorrhage.
3. **Theca-lutein cyst**
   a. This cyst results from **gonadotropin stimulation;** it can be associated with choriocarcinoma and hydatidiform mole.
   b. It is often multiple and bilateral and lined by luteinized theca cells.
4. **Chocolate cyst**
   a. This cyst is a blood-containing cyst resulting from ovarian endometriosis with hemorrhage.
   b. The ovary is the most frequent site of endometriosis.
5. **Polycystic ovary (Stein-Leventhal) syndrome**
   a. This syndrome characteristically occurs in young women.
   b. It is an important cause of infertility.
   c. Clinical characteristics include **amenorrhea, infertility, obesity, and hirsutism.**
   d. Causes may include **excess luteinizing hormone (LH) and androgens.**

e. Polycystic ovary syndrome may be associated with insulin resistance with an increased risk of diabetes mellitus. Hyperinsulinemia may lead to increased ovarian androgen production, which may in turn lead to increased LH.

f. Morphologic characteristics include the following:
   (1) **Markedly thickened ovarian capsule**
   (2) **Multiple small follicular cysts** containing a granulosa cell layer and a luteinized theca interna
   (3) **Cortical stromal fibrosis** with islands of focal luteinization

B. **Ovarian tumors** are categorized according to the World Health Organization **(WHO)** classification, which is based on the **site of origin** of the tumor. The tumors are divided as follows:

1. **Tumors of surface epithelial origin** make up almost three fourths of ovarian tumors. They occur in women older than 20 years of age.
   a. **Serous tumors**
      (1) **Serous cystadenoma.** This benign cystic tumor is lined with cells similar to fallopian tube epithelium. It accounts for approximately 20% of all ovarian tumors and is frequently bilateral.
      (2) **Serous cystadenocarcinoma.** This malignant tumor accounts for approximately **50% of ovarian carcinomas** and is frequently bilateral.
   b. **Mucinous tumors**
      (1) **Mucinous cystadenoma.** This benign tumor is characterized by multilocular cysts lined by mucus-secreting columnar epithelium and filled with mucinous material.
      (2) **Mucinous cystadenocarcinoma**
         (a) This malignant tumor, through rupture or metastasis, can result in **pseudomyxoma peritonei** with multiple peritoneal tumor implants, all producing large quantities of intraperitoneal mucinous material.
         (b) Although mucinous cystadenocarcinoma of the ovary is the most common cause, pseudomyxoma peritonei can also result from mucinous cystadenoma, carcinomatous mucocele of the appendix, and other mucinous tumors.
   c. **Endometrioid tumors** histologically resemble the endometrium. They are usually malignant.
   d. **Clear cell tumors** are **rare** tumors that are almost always malignant.
   e. **Brenner tumors** are rare, benign tumors. They are characterized by small islands of epithelial cells resembling bladder transitional epithelium interspersed within a fibrous stroma.

2. **Tumors of germ cell origin** make up one fourth of ovarian tumors. They account for most ovarian tumors occurring in women younger than 20 years of age.
   a. **Dysgerminoma**
      (1) This tumor is malignant.
      (2) This tumor is analogous to testicular seminoma.
   b. **Endodermal sinus (yolk sac) tumor**
      (1) This tumor resembles extraembryonic yolk sac structures. It produces **α-fetoprotein.**
      (2) This tumor is analogous to endodermal sinus tumor of the testis.
   c. **Teratomas**
      (1) These tumors characteristically demonstrate tissue elements derived from **two or three embryonic layers.**
      (2) Teratomas are observed in three distinct forms:
         (a) **Immature teratoma.** This aggressive malignant tumor includes immature cellular elements.
         (b) **Mature teratoma (dermoid cyst).** This accounts for approximately 20% of ovarian tumors and 90% of germ cell tumors.

(i) The dermoid cyst is the most frequent benign ovarian tumor.

(ii) The cyst is lined by skin, including hair follicles and other skin appendages; other elements often include bone; tooth; cartilage; and gastrointestinal, neurologic, respiratory, and thyroid gland tissues. Radiographically visible focal calcifications may lead to diagnosis.

(iii) The cyst may arise by reduplication of meiotic maternal chromosomes, giving rise to 46,XX cells of maternal origin.

(c) **Monodermal teratoma.** This cyst contains only a single tissue element; for example, the most common is **struma ovarii,** which consists entirely of thyroid tissue and can be hyperfunctional, resulting in hyperthyroidism.

d. **Ovarian choriocarcinoma.** This aggressive malignant tumor secretes **human chorionic gonadotropin (hCG).**

3. **Tumors of ovarian sex cord-stromal origin** account for a small percentage of ovarian neoplasms. Women of all ages are affected.

a. **Thecoma-fibroma group of tumors**

(1) **Fibroma**

(a) This solid tumor consists of bundles of spindle-shaped fibroblasts.

(b) It may be associated with **Meigs syndrome,** a triad of ovarian fibroma, ascites, and hydrothorax.

(2) **Thecoma**

(a) This tumor demonstrates round lipid-containing cells in addition to fibroblasts.

(b) It is occasionally estrogen-secreting.

b. **Granulosa cell tumor**

(1) This **estrogen-secreting** tumor causes precocious puberty.

(2) In adults, it is associated with **endometrial hyperplasia** or **endometrial carcinoma.**

(3) The tumor consists of small cuboidal, deeply staining granulosa cells arranged in anastomotic cords.

(4) **Call-Exner bodies,** small follicles filled with eosinophilic secretion, are an important diagnostic feature.

c. **Sertoli-Leydig cell tumor (androblastoma, arrhenoblastoma).** This **androgen-secreting tumor** is associated with virilism (masculinization).

4. **Tumors metastatic to the ovary** account for approximately 5% of all ovarian tumors.

a. These tumors are frequently of gastrointestinal tract, breast, or endometrial origin.

b. They are called **Krukenberg tumors** when ovaries are replaced bilaterally by mucin-secreting **signet-ring cells;** the site of origin is often the stomach.

VI. Disorders of Pregnancy

A. **Abnormalities of placental attachment**

1. **Abruptio placentae (placental abruption)** is premature separation of the placenta.

a. This is an important cause of antepartum bleeding and fetal death.

b. It is often associated with **disseminated intravascular coagulation (DIC).**

2. **Placenta accreta** is attachment of the placenta directly to the myometrium; the decidual layer is defective.

a. This is predisposed by endometrial inflammation and old scars from prior cesarean sections or other surgery.

b. It is manifest clinically by impaired placental separation after delivery, sometimes with massive hemorrhage.

3. **Placenta previa** is an attachment of the placenta to the lower uterine segment, partially or completely covering the cervical os.

a. This may coexist with placenta accreta.

b. It is often manifest by bleeding.

B. **Ectopic pregnancy**

1. The location is most often in the fallopian tubes. Ectopic pregnancy can also occur in the ovary, abdominal cavity, or cervix.
2. It is most frequently predisposed by chronic salpingitis, often gonorrheal. Other predisposing factors are endometriosis and postoperative adhesions.
3. There is frequently no obvious cause.
4. Ectopic pregnancy is the most common cause of **hematosalpinx.** Tubal rupture may result.

C. **Toxemia of pregnancy.** This disorder is characterized by severe hypertension that most often occurs de novo during pregnancy or complicates preexisting hypertensive disease. Toxemia characteristically occurs during the third trimester, most often in the first pregnancy, and affects the kidneys, liver, and central nervous system. Toxemia of pregnancy occurs in two forms:

1. **Preeclampsia,** a milder form of toxemia characterized by hypertension, albuminuria, and edema. In a variant of preeclampsia, the **HELLP syndrome**, there may be **H**emolysis, **E**levated **L**iver enzymes, and **L**ow **P**latelets.
2. **Eclampsia,** a severe form of toxemia characterized, in addition, by convulsions and DIC; reverses rapidly on termination of pregnancy, but can be fatal.

D. **Other peripartal complications of pregnancy**

1. **Amniotic fluid embolism**
   a. The cause is a tear in the placental membranes and rupture of maternal veins.
   b. This condition is characterized by sudden peripartal respiratory difficulty, progressing to shock and often to death.
   c. Amniotic fluid embolism can cause DIC. It is marked by masses of debris and epithelial squamous cells in the maternal pulmonary microcirculation.
   d. This should not be confused with the amniotic fluid aspiration syndrome, which is a disease of the neonate, not of the mother. This inability to expel amniotic fluid at birth, frequently associated with prematurity, is characterized by squamous epithelial cells of amniotic origin in fetal terminal air spaces and larger bronchi.
2. **Postpartum anterior pituitary necrosis (Sheehan syndrome)**
   a. This condition is a consequence of severe hypotension, most often from blood loss.
   b. It is manifest by the insidious onset, over weeks and months following delivery, of anterior pituitary hypofunction.
3. **Chorioamnionitis**
   a. This condition often follows premature rupture of membranes.
   b. It is usually caused by ascending infection from the vagina or cervix.

E. **Gestational trophoblastic disease** includes disorders characterized by degenerative or neoplastic changes of trophoblastic tissue.

1. **Hydatidiform mole**
   a. The disorder is manifest by enlarged, edematous placental villi in a loose stroma, grossly resembling a bunch of grapes.
   b. It is marked by a diagnostically significant increase in **hCG.** In addition to trophoblastic disease, elevated serum hCG occurs in normal or ectopic pregnancy, gestational choriocarcinoma, and germ cell tumors.
   c. It characteristically occurs in early months of pregnancy and eventuates to **choriocarcinoma** in 2%–3% of cases.
   d. Clinical characteristics include vaginal bleeding and rapid increase in uterine size. A hydatidiform mole can be mistaken for a normal pregnancy, but the uterus is often too large for the supposed state of gestation.
   e. It occurs in two variants:
      (1) **Complete hydatidiform mole:** no embryo is present; 46,XX karyotype, of exclusively **paternal derivation (androgenesis)**

(2) **Partial hydatidiform mole:** embryo is present; triploidy and rarely tetraploidy occur, thought to be due to fertilization of the ovum by two or more spermatozoa. The usual result is 69 chromosomes derived from two paternal and one maternal haploid set.

2. **Gestational choriocarcinoma** is an aggressive malignant neoplasm that occurs more frequently than ovarian choriocarcinoma.
   a. An increased serum concentration of **hCG** is an important diagnostic sign.
   b. Characteristics include **early hematogenous spread** to the lungs.
   c. The tumor is **responsive to chemotherapy.**
   d. Its incidence is greatly increased in Asia and Africa.
   e. It is preceded by:
      (1) **Hydatidiform mole** in 50% of cases
      (2) **Abortion of ectopic pregnancy** in 20% of cases
      (3) **Normal-term pregnancy** in 20%–30% of cases

VII. Breast

A. **Fibrocystic disease** is the most common disorder of the breast.
   1. This disorder is the most common cause of a palpable breast mass in patients between 25 and 50 years of age. It is uncommon before adolescence or after menopause.
   2. Clinical characteristics include lumpy breasts with midcycle tenderness. Fibrocystic disease is usually bilateral.
   3. Disease is postulated to result from increased activity of, or sensitivity to, estrogen or to decreased progesterone activity.
   4. Nonproliferative forms (stromal fibrosis and cyst formation) are not associated with an increased risk of breast cancer. Epithelial hyperplasia (with atypia) or sclerosing adenosis carries a slightly increased risk, and the **risk of cancer is clear when hyperplastic epithelium demonstrates atypia.**
   5. **Morphologic characteristics include:**
      a. **Fibrosis** of varying extent
      b. **Cysts** are grossly visible or may be evident only on histologic examination; they may be filled with fluid, which may appear blue when seen through the cyst wall **(blue dome cyst).**
      c. **Epithelial changes**
         (1) The lining of the epithelium may be flattened, may show **apocrine metaplasia,** or may be hyperplastic.
         (2) Hyperplastic epithelium may show varying degrees of cellular atypia: **adenosis** is the proliferation of small ducts and myoepithelial cells; when combined with fibrosis, it is called **sclerosing adenosis.**

B. **Tumors of the breast**
   1. **Fibroadenoma**
      a. This is the **most common breast tumor in women younger than 25 years of age.**
      b. This tumor is entirely **benign** and is not a precursor of breast cancer.
      c. The lesion is firm, rubbery, painless, and well-circumscribed.
      d. The fibroadenoma is morphologically well-demarcated from adjacent breast tissue; delicate fibrous stroma encloses the epithelial component consisting of gland-like or duct-like spaces lined by cuboidal or columnar cells. The stromal cells are neoplastic, and the ductal epithelial cells are thought to be reactive.
      e. The tumors may be classified into two types:
         (1) **Intracanalicular fibroadenoma:** stroma compresses and distorts glands into slitlike spaces.
         (2) **Pericanalicular fibroadenoma:** glands retain round shape.

2. **Phyllodes tumor**
   a. This tumor is a large, bulky mass of variable malignancy with ulceration of overlying skin.
   b. Cystic spaces containing leaf-like projections from the cyst walls and myxoid contents are characteristic.
3. **Adenoma of the nipple**
   a. This tumor presents with serous or bloody discharge and a palpable mass.
   b. It can be mistaken for malignancy.
4. **Intraductal papilloma**
   a. This is a benign tumor of the major lactiferous ducts that must be distinguished from carcinoma.
   b. It is clinically manifest by serous or bloody discharge.
5. **Carcinoma of the breast** (Table 19-2)
   a. This disease is the second most common malignancy of women (carcinoma of the lung is most common).
   b. It is the most common cause of a breast mass in postmenopausal patients.
   c. Breast cancer occurs most frequently in the **upper outer quadrant** of the breast.

TABLE 19-2 *Abbreviated List of Histologic Types of Carcinoma of the Breast*

Types	Characteristics
Intraductal carcinoma in situ (comedocarcinoma)	Tumor cells fill ducts; tumor cell necrosis results in a cheese-like consistency
Invasive ductal carcinoma (scirrhous carcinoma)	Most common type; characterized by tumor cells arranged in cords, islands, and glands embedded in a dense fibrous stroma; abundant fibrous tissue results in firm consistency
Paget disease of the breast	Eczematoid lesion of the nipple or areola; neoplastic Paget cells, characteristic large cells surrounded by a clear halo-like area, invade the epidermis; underlying ductal carcinoma almost always present
Lobular carcinoma in situ	Clusters of neoplastic cells fill intralobular ductules and acini; may lead to invasive carcinoma (often many years later) in the same or in the contralateral breast; often bilateral at the time of the initial diagnosis
Invasive lobular carcinoma	Often multicentric or bilateral; tends to have cells arranged in a linear fashion ("Indian-file" appearance); better prognosis than that for invasive ductal carcinoma
Medullary carcinoma	Cellular with scant stroma; soft, fleshy consistency; characteristic lymphocytic infiltrate; prognosis better than that for invasive ductal carcinoma
Mucinous (colloid) carcinoma	Pools of extracellular mucus surrounding clusters of tumor cells; gelatinous consistency; prognosis better than that for invasive ductal carcinoma
Inflammatory carcinomas	Lymphatic involvement of skin by underlying carcinoma, causing red, swollen, hot skin resembling an inflammatory process; poor prognosis

d. Sites of metastasis include axillary lymph nodes, lung, liver, and bone.

e. There are several histologic types (see Table 19-2); invasive ductal carcinoma occurs most frequently.

f. Breast cancer demonstrates **estrogen and progesterone receptors** in some tumors but not in others; presence is correlated with a better prognosis and is thought to be a predictor of the efficacy of antiestrogen therapy. Other prognostic indicators are type and size of tumor, extent of lymph node involvement, and DNA ploidy. Hyperexpression of c-*erb*B2 (*HER-2/neu*) is associated with a poorer prognosis.

g. Current regimens of oral contraceptive therapy are not predisposing factors. Conflicting data from some studies indicate a slightly increased risk with high-dose postmenopausal estrogen therapy.

h. **Predisposing factors**

(1) **Age:** incidence increases with increasing age.

(2) **Positive family history:** incidence is greatly increased in **first-degree female relatives** of patients with carcinoma of the breast. Inherited mutations in the *p53, BRCA*-1, or *BRCA*-2 tumor suppressor genes are associated with increased risk. *BRCA*-1 mutations are also associated with ovarian malignancies.

(3) **History of breast cancer in one breast:** associated with increased incidence in the opposite breast

(4) **Early menarche and late menopause:** may be due to increased duration of reproductive life and associated hormonal activity

(5) **Obesity:** possibly due to production of estrogens by adipose tissue

(6) **Nulliparity**

(7) **First pregnancy after 30 years of age**

(8) **Diet high in animal fat:** incidence is five times higher in the United States than in Japan.

(9) **Proliferative fibrocystic disease with atypical epithelial hyperplasia**

REVIEW TEST

Directions: *Each of the numbered items or incomplete statements in this section is followed by answers or by completions of the statement. Select the* ***one*** *lettered answer or completion that is best in each case.*

1. A 24-year-old woman is seen because of high fever, prostration, vomiting, and diarrhea. Her pulse is rapid and thready, and her blood pressure is 60/40 mm Hg. A diffuse generalized macular rash is noted. Culture of which of the following specimens most likely leads to the correct diagnosis?

(A) Sputum
(B) Urine
(C) Stool
(D) Cervical secretions
(E) Cerebrospinal fluid

2. A 56-year-old diabetic woman has recently been treated with a 2-week course of antibiotics for a skin infection. She returns to the clinic for follow-up with a new complaint of a "cottage cheese-like" vaginal discharge with significant vaginal itching. The most likely cause of these symptoms is

(A) *Calymmatobacterium granulomatis*
(B) *Candida albicans*
(C) chancroid
(D) herpes simplex
(E) *Neisseria meningitidis*

3. A 26-year-old woman presents for routine gynecologic examination and Papanicolaou (Pap) smear. A thin, homogenous vaginal discharge is noted, and a sample is taken. When potassium hydroxide is added to a wet mount of the sample, a fishy odor is noted. In addition, the Pap smear reveals the presence of "clue cells." Which of the following organisms is likely to be present in increased numbers?

(A) *Staphylococcus aureus*
(B) *Neisseria gonorrhoeae*
(C) *Candida albicans*
(D) *Trichomonas vaginalis*
(E) *Gardnerella vaginalis*

4. A 35-year-old prostitute is seen in a community health care clinic. About 4 months earlier, she had a painless labial sore and swelling of a right inguinal lymph node, both of which had subsided uneventfully over a period of several weeks. About 3 weeks later she developed fever and a generalized maculopapular skin rash that involved the palms of the hands and the soles of the feet. She has developed a flattened, wart-like labial lesion that is most likely a

(A) chancre
(B) chancroid
(C) condyloma acuminatum
(D) condyloma lata
(E) papillary hidradenoma

5. A 25-year-old woman has cauliflower-shaped perineal lesions that are diagnosed as condyloma acuminatum. The etiologic agent is

(A) herpes simplex virus
(B) *Treponema pallidum*
(C) *Haemophilus ducreyi*
(D) human papillomavirus
(E) *Candida albicans*

6. On routine examination, it is discovered that a 35-year-old woman had been exposed in utero to diethylstilbestrol administered to her mother, who had had a history of recurrent spontaneous abortion. This history suggests that the patient might be at increased risk of

(A) adenomyosis
(B) clear cell adenocarcinoma
(C) lichen sclerosus
(D) sarcoma botryoides
(E) squamous cell carcinoma

7. A 32-year-old woman has been attempting to become pregnant for the past 2 years without success. She also has had extremely painful menstrual cramping of many years' duration. An exploratory laparoscopy demonstrated multiple "power-burn lesions" covering the surface of her ovaries and uterine ligaments. These findings are most likely indicative of which of the following conditions?

(A) Adenomyosis
(B) Endometrial hyperplasia
(C) Endometriosis
(D) Endometritis
(E) Leiomyoma

8. An 18-year-old woman presents for follow-up of an abnormal Papanicolaou smear that revealed an abnormality suggestive of human papillomavirus infection. Which of the following was the likely cytopathologic finding?

(A) Donovan bodies
(B) Koilocytes
(C) Clear cells
(D) Paget cells
(E) Fibroids

9. The cervical lesion shown is similar to that obtained in a cone cervical biopsy from a 28-year-old sexually active woman who had had a "positive" Papanicolaou smear. The type of cervical change seen here is often characterized by

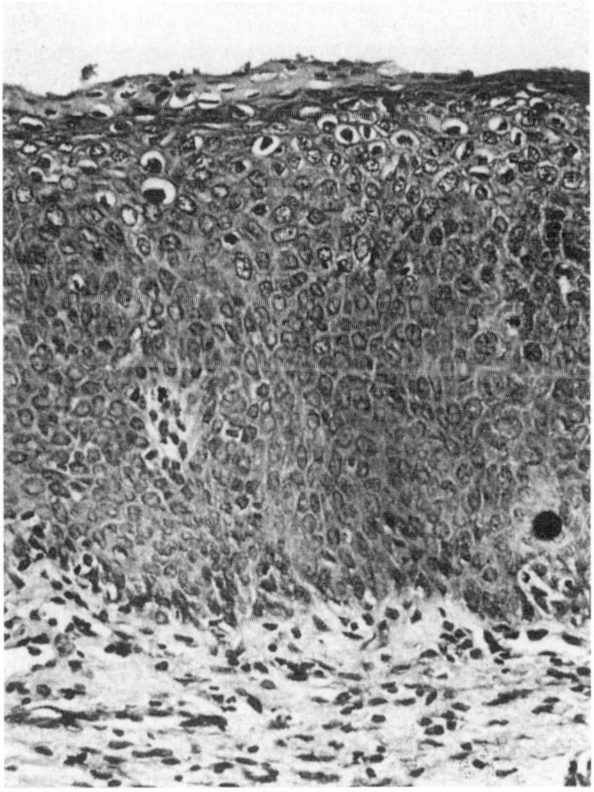

(Reprinted with permission from Golden A, Powell D, and Jennings C: *Pathology: Understanding Human Disease,* 2nd ed. Baltimore, Williams & Wilkins, 1985, p 447.)

(A) local invasion
(B) penetration of the basement membrane
(C) lymphatic spread
(D) genomic integration of human papillomavirus sequences
(E) hematogenous dissemination

10. A 68-year-old postmenopausal woman presents for evaluation of the recent onset of vaginal bleeding, and a diagnosis of endometrial carcinoma is made on endometrial biopsy. Which of the following is a risk factor for this condition?

(A) Endometriosis
(B) Multiparity
(C) Salpingitis
(D) Early sexual activity with multiple partners
(E) Obesity

11. A 28-year-old woman is evaluated for infertility and amenorrhea. She is obese and has significant facial hair in a male distribution. Laboratory studies reveal an increase in serum luteinizing hormone as well as in total serum testosterone and in the testosterone metabolite dehydroepiandrosterone sulfate. A pelvic ultrasound examination would probably reveal which of the following findings?

(A) A mass resembling a bunch of grapes projecting into the vagina
(B) Blood-filled cysts in the ovary
(C) Fluid accumulation in the fallopian tubes
(D) Islands of endometrium within the myometrium
(E) Multiple small follicular cysts on the ovary

12. A 26-year-old woman experiences the sudden onset of left-sided lower abdominal pain with radiation to the back, pelvis, and thigh. Following a negative test for pregnancy, abdominal radiography shows an enlarged left ovary with multiple calcifications. Laparoscopy reveals adnexal torsion and an ovarian tumor. Ovariectomy is performed. The tumor is most likely a

(A) granulosa cell tumor
(B) Brenner tumor
(C) serous cystadenoma
(D) struma ovarii
(E) dermoid cyst

13. A 5-year-old girl begins developing secondary sexual characteristics, including pubic hair growth and breast development. Her concerned parents bring her to the pediatrician for evaluation. An abdominal ultrasound examination reveals an ovarian mass. The mass is resected, and pathologic examination reveals it to be a granulosa cell tumor. Which of the following histologic findings is a characteristic of this type of ovarian tumor?

(A) Signet-ring cells
(B) Call-Exner bodies
(C) Schiller-Duval bodies
(D) Hyperfunctioning thyroid tissue
(E) Transitional cell epithelium

14. Soon after an uncomplicated delivery at 38 weeks' gestation, a mother develops respiratory difficulties and uncontrolled vaginal bleeding progressing to shock, multiorgan failure, and death. At autopsy, masses of debris and epithelial squamous cells are apparent in the pulmonary microcirculation. Which of the following was the likely cause of death?

(A) Sheehan syndrome
(B) Chorioamnionitis
(C) Abruptio placentae
(D) Amniotic fluid aspiration syndrome
(E) Amniotic fluid embolism

15. A 23-year-old woman consults an obstetrician because of the onset of vaginal bleeding in what she considers to be the fifth month of pregnancy. However, examination reveals the uterus to be enlarged to the size of a 7-month pregnancy. Intravaginal ultrasound fails to detect a fetal heartbeat and instead shows a "snowstorm pattern." Human chorionic gonadotropin is markedly elevated. These findings are strongly suggestive of

(A) preeclampsia
(B) eclampsia
(C) placenta accreta
(D) ectopic pregnancy
(E) hydatidiform mole

16. A 65-year-old woman is found to have a 1-cm mass in the upper outer quadrant of the left breast. The most likely cause is

(A) fibrocystic disease
(B) acute mastitis
(C) fibroadenoma
(D) carcinoma
(E) Paget disease of the breast

17. A 50-year-old woman has a lumpectomy following mammographic discovery of a carcinoma of the breast. Which of the following is a well-known characteristic or association of breast cancer?

(A) Low-fat diet
(B) Positive family history
(C) Excessive thinness
(D) Late menarche
(E) Multiparity

18. A 20-year-old woman presents with a solitary discrete, freely movable, firm, rubbery, nontender, well-circumscribed breast lesion. On resection biopsy, the lesion appears similar to that shown in the figure. The most likely diagnosis is

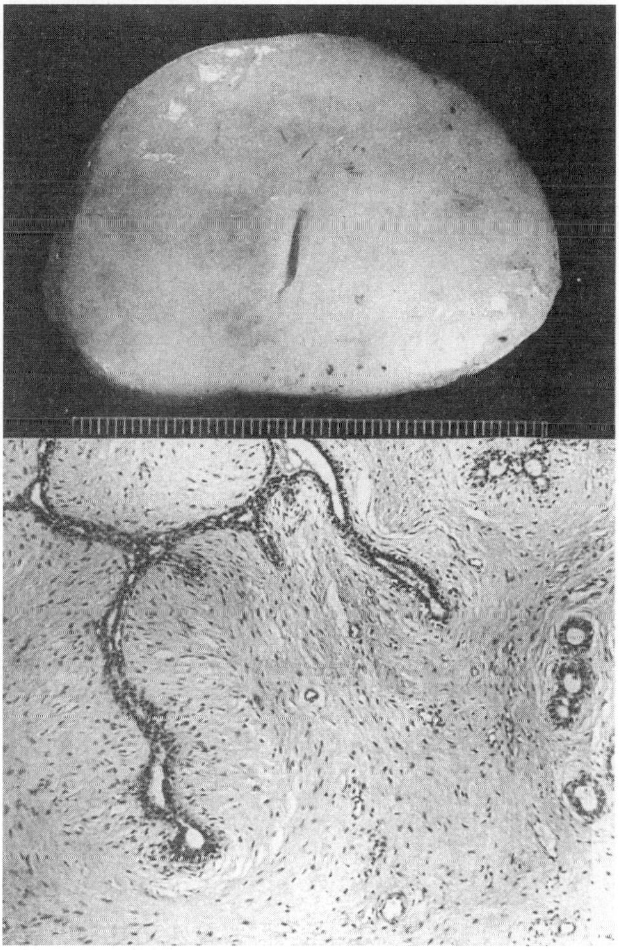

(Reprinted with permission from Golden A, Powell D, and Jennings C: *Pathology: Understanding Human Disease*, 2nd ed. Baltimore, Williams & Wilkins, 1985, p 413.)

(A) fibrocystic disease
(B) fibroadenoma
(C) medullary carcinoma
(D) colloid carcinoma.
(E) intraductal carcinoma

19. A 57-year-old woman who has not seen a physician in more than 20 years now presents with left breast pain. On examination, the left breast is markedly erythematous, swollen, and warm to touch. There is also significant dimpling of the breast (peau d'orange). In addition, the left nipple is completely retracted. Which of the following is the likely diagnosis?

(A) Mastitis
(B) Invasive ductal carcinoma
(C) Medullary carcinoma
(D) Inflammatory carcinoma
(E) Mucinous carcinoma

20. A 27-year-old woman requests a mammogram because both her mother and sister died of metastatic breast cancer before 40 years of age. Which of the following would add to this patient's risk factors for breast cancer?

(A) Multiparity
(B) High-fiber diet
(C) Oral contraceptive use
(D) *BRCA*-1 mutation
(E) Bilateral fibroadenomas

ANSWERS AND EXPLANATIONS

1-D. The association of a severe febrile illness with signs of gastrointestinal dysfunction and a diffuse macular rash is strongly suggestive of toxic shock syndrome. This diagnosis is especially likely if clinical abnormalities are associated with concomitant menstruation and the use of highly absorbent tampons. The clinical abnormalities are due to staphylococcal infection of the tampon, demonstrable in vaginal secretions, and the elaboration of staphylococcal exotoxins. The differential diagnosis includes streptococcal infection, usually pharyngeal, with a scarlatiniform eruption; meningococcemia; endotoxemia associated with various gram-negative organisms; rickettsial infections, and so forth. Except for streptococcal infection, all of these conditions are less likely than toxic shock syndrome.

2-B. *Candida albicans* is a major cause of vulvovaginitis. Many women are carriers of the yeast, and it therefore constitutes normal vaginal flora, although there are many conditions that alter the vaginal microenvironment, including pregnancy, oral contraceptives, and systemic antibiotics, making overgrowth possible. *Calymmatobacterium granulomatis* causes granuloma inguinale. Chancroid results in painful genital ulcers and is caused by the organism *Haemophilus ducreyi*. Herpes simplex virus type 2 can cause genital vesicular lesions. *Neisseria meningitidis* can cause meningitis.

3-E. Bacterial vaginosis is the most common cause of vaginal discharge. Characteristically, the discharge is thin and homogeneous. Addition of 10% potassium hydroxide elicits a fishy amine odor. Usually, increased numbers of *Gardnerella vaginalis* organisms are present and large numbers of "clue cells" are apparent on the Papanicolaou smear. The condition is caused by loss of the normal vaginal lactobacilli, with consequent overgrowth of anaerobes and other bacteria, including *G. vaginalis*. *Neisseria gonorrhoeae* is a common cause of pelvic inflammatory disease. *Candida* causes vulvovaginitis. *Trichomonas vaginalis* is yet another cause of vaginosis, but a wet mount displays flagellated motile organisms.

4-D. The patient presents with a lesion of secondary syphilis known as condyloma lata. The original lesion, the painless ulcer or chancre, is characteristic of primary syphilis. Chancroid is a similar lesion to the primary lesion in syphilis, but instead is painful. Condyloma acuminatum is a similarly named lesion often referred to as a venereal wart and is due to human papillomavirus. Papillary hidradenoma is a common benign tumor of the vulva, presenting as a nodule that may ulcerate and bleed.

5-D. Condyloma acuminatum is a nonmalignant neoplastic-like papillomatous condition that affects epithelium of the perineal, vulval, perianal, and vaginal regions. It is caused by human papillomavirus (HPV, most often HPV 6 and 11). Genital herpes is usually caused by herpes simplex virus type 2. *Treponema pallidum* is a spirochete and the etiologic agent of syphilis. *Haemophilus ducreyi* causes chancroid, a painful, erosive, chancre-like lesion. *Candida* is not a sexually transmitted organism and is often considered normal vaginal flora, although it is an important cause of vulvovaginitis.

6-B. In 1971, it became widely known that there was a danger of development of clear cell adenocarcinoma of the vagina and cervix in young women with a history of in utero exposure to diethylstilbestrol (DES) while their mothers were pregnant. DES has not been administered to pregnant women in this country for more than 30 years.

7-C. Endometriosis, ectopic non-neoplastic endometrial tissue, is an important cause of infertility. The ectopic tissue replicates the cyclic endometrial changes during the menstrual cycle, including sloughing and bleeding. Such ectopic hemorrhage can result in pain, scarring, tubal obstruction, and infertility. Favored sites of endometriosis include pelvic ligaments, ovaries, and rectum. Adenomyosis is a term denoting the presence of endometrial tissue within the myometrium. Endometrial hyperplasia can be a precursor to endometrial carcinoma and manifests with postmenopausal bleeding. Endometritis results from infection of the endometrium. Leiomyomas are benign tumors of the uterus that can also result in painful menses and can contribute to infertility.

8-B. Koilocytes are indicative of human papillomavirus–infected epithelial cells. Viral infection causes intracytoplasmic vacuolation that is apparent in cytopathologic and histopathologic preparations. Donovan bodies represent macrophages stuffed with numerous *Calymmatobacterium (Donovania) granulomatis* organisms. Clear cells are characteristic of clear cell adenocarcinoma of the vagina. Paget cells are characteristic large cells surrounded by a clear, halo-like area that occur in Paget disease of the vulva and Paget disease of the breast. Fibroids are the most common benign tumors of the female reproductive tract.

9-D. The illustration demonstrates dysplasia of the uterine cervix, which is characterized by disordered epithelial growth manifest by loss of polarity and nuclear hyperchromasia beginning at the basal layer and extending outward. In this illustration, the dysplastic changes involve about two thirds of the epithelial thickness and would thus be classified as cervical intraepithelial neoplasia grade 2 to 3. Although mild forms can be reversible, the principal significance of cervical dysplasia is its precursor role in the genesis of invasive cervical carcinoma. Invasion and metastases are not associated with dysplasia but only with fully developed invasive carcinoma. Genomic integration of human papillomavirus DNA sequences, most often types 16, 18, 31, or 33, is associated with cervical dysplasia as well as with frank malignant change.

10-E. Endometrial cancer is the most common gynecologic malignancy, and a major predisposing factor is prolonged and unopposed exposure to estrogen. In the case of obesity, adipose tissue converts androgens into estrogens, fueling the proliferation of endometrial tissue. Similarly, diabetes, nulliparity (not multiparity), and hypertension are also predisposing factors. Early sexual activity with multiple partners is associated with cervical cancer. Salpingitis can predispose to ectopic pregnancy. Endometriosis is a benign condition and has no relation to endometrial cancer.

11-E. The findings are those of the polycystic ovary (Stein-Leventhal) syndrome, an important cause of infertility in young women that is characterized by amenorrhea, infertility, obesity, and hirsutism. Increased levels of luteinizing hormone (LH) and of androgens are often found, and it has been thought that LH may stimulate follicular theca-lutein cells, with consequent hyperproduction of androgens. Alternatively, there has been recent attention to the link of this disorder to the metabolic syndrome and insulin resistance. Hyperinsulinemia may lead to increased ovarian androgen production, which then may lead to increased LH. The syndrome is characterized by multiple small follicular cysts, a markedly thickened ovarian capsule, and cortical stromal fibrosis. A mass resembling a bunch of grapes projecting into the vagina is characteristic of sarcoma botryoides. Blood-filled cysts on the ovary are termed "chocolate cysts" and are associated with endometriosis, another cause of infertility. Fluid accumulation in the fallopian tubes is termed hydrosalpinx. Islands of endometrium in the myometrium are seen in adenomyosis.

12-E. The radiographic calcifications are highly suggestive of a mature teratoma (dermoid cyst). This tumor is composed of all three germ layers and often contains skin, (including adnexal structures such as sebaceous glands and hair follicles), bone, teeth, cartilage, and gastrointestinal, neurologic, respiratory, and thyroid tissues. As the tumor enlarges, it is at risk of torsion. Granulosa cell tumor presents with signs and symptoms of excess estrogen production. Brenner tumor is rare and histologically resembles transitional epithelium of the bladder. Serous cystadenoma is commonly bilateral. Struma ovarii is a monodermal teratoma composed of functional ectopic thyroid tissue.

13-B. A young patient presenting with precocious puberty and an ovarian mass is likely to have a granulosa cell tumor. Call-Exner bodies, small follicles filled with eosinophilic secretion, are an important diagnostic feature. Signet-ring cells are seen in Krukenberg tumors (bilateral metastatic involvement of the ovaries by a signet-ring carcinoma arising in the stomach). Schiller-Duval bodies are seen in dysgerminoma, an ovarian tumor analogous to the male seminoma. Hyperfunctional thyroid tissue is found in struma ovarii, and the Brenner tumor resembles transitional cell epithelium.

14-E. The diagnosis is amniotic fluid embolism, which is characterized by sudden peripartal respiratory difficulty, progressing to shock and often to death. Sheehan syndrome is associated with obstetric blood loss, with resultant pituitary ischemia leading to postpartal hypopituitarism. Chorioamnionitis is infection of the placenta, which can have devastating consequences for both the mother and the child. Abruptio placentae is premature separation of the placenta and can lead to antepartal bleeding and fetal death. Amniotic fluid aspiration can occur in the child and can result in difficulties for the infant, particularly if meconium is aspirated. Amniotic fluid embolism and abruptio placentae are well-known causes of disseminated intravascular coagulation, as are retained dead fetus and toxemia.

15-E. Hydatidiform mole should be suspected when the uterus is enlarged beyond the expected size for the time of the pregnancy. Human chorionic gonadotropin is markedly elevated in this gestational trophoblastic disease. Preeclampsia and eclampsia are forms of toxemia of pregnancy marked by severe hypertension, albuminuria, and edema, with the addition of convulsions and disseminated intravascular coagulation in the latter. Placenta accreta occurs when the placenta adheres directly to the myometrium, leading to severe bleeding at the time of delivery. Ectopic pregnancy is usually discovered early in a suspected pregnancy when ultrasound examination reveals the uterus to be empty.

16-D. The location of the mass in the upper outer quadrant and the patient's age of 65 years suggest that the breast lesion is a carcinoma. A breast mass in a postmenopausal patient is most often a carcinoma.

17-B. A history of breast cancer in first-degree female relatives and a diet high in animal fats are important associations of breast cancer. Associations related to excess estrogen stimulation include high-fat diet, obesity, early menarche, and nulliparity. Additional associations are delayed first pregnancy and exogenous estrogen therapy.

18-B. Fibroadenoma is a benign tumor most often presenting as a single discrete, freely movable lesion, often demonstrating a pattern of compressed glands and young fibrous stroma similar to that shown in the illustration. Fibroadenoma is the most frequent cause of a palpable mass in the breast in women younger than 25 years of age.

19-D. The presentation is that of inflammatory carcinoma of the breast, which typically has an extremely poor prognosis. In this variant, cancer cells have invaded the skin and suspensory ligaments of the breast, causing dimpling and distortion of the normal breast architecture.

20-D. Concern over familial breast cancer is well warranted in this patient, with two first-degree relatives dying of breast cancer at an early age. Both *BRCA*-1 and *BRCA*-2 mutations are major risk factors for the development of breast cancer. Typically, breasts in a younger woman are too dense to be viewed well on normal screening mammograms, although in this case the mammogram and genetic studies are warranted to determine if she too carries the deleterious mutations. There is evidence that a first pregnancy after 30 years of age, early menarche, and late menopause are also contributing factors. A high-fat diet, not a high-fiber diet, is another apparent risk factor. There is no evidence to support that either oral contraceptive use or fibroadenoma is a risk factor for breast cancer.

CHAPTER 20

Endocrine System

I. Pituitary

A. **Anterior pituitary (adenohypophysis)** (Table 20-1)

1. **Anterior pituitary hyperfunction**

a. **Prolactinoma with hyperprolactinemia**

(1) This is the **most common pituitary tumor** (30% of pituitary tumors).

(2) Staining is usually **chromophobic.**

(3) In women, prolactinoma results in **amenorrhea** and **galactorrhea** (inappropriate milk secretion).

(4) It can be caused by hypothalamic lesions or by medications (methyldopa, reserpine) that interfere with dopamine (prolactin-inhibitory factor) secretion. It can also be associated with estrogen therapy.

b. Somatotropic adenoma with hypersecretion of growth hormone

(1) This is the second most common pituitary tumor.

(2) Staining is usually acidophilic (**acidophilic adenoma** is an older name for this tumor).

(3) It causes secondary hyperproduction of somatomedins by the liver. End-organ effects are caused by both growth hormone and somatomedins, especially insulinlike growth factor-I (IGF-I, somatomedin C).

(4) **Gigantism** results if adenoma develops before epiphyseal closure.

(5) **Acromegaly** results if adenoma develops after epiphyseal closure; acromegaly is characterized by overgrowth of the jaws, face, hands and feet, and generalized enlargement of viscera, along with hyperglycemia, osteoporosis, and hypertension.

(6) Other results include local compression effects due to expansion of the tumor within the sella turcica.

c. **Corticotropic adenoma and hypersecretion of adrenocorticotropic hormone (ACTH)** results in increased production of adrenal cortical hormones **(hypercorticism).** This condition is called Cushing syndrome or Cushing disease (these terms are used in variable contexts by different authors).

(1) **Cushing disease**

(a) This condition classically refers to hypercorticism due to a corticotropic adenoma of the pituitary (most often a **basophilic adenoma**).

(b) It also refers to hypercorticism associated with very small, sometimes multiple pituitary adenomas **(basophilic microadenomas).**

(2) **Cushing syndrome**

(a) This condition refers to hypercorticism regardless of cause. It is most often of pituitary and less often of adrenal origin; some authors use the terms adrenal Cushing syndrome and pituitary Cushing syndrome for clarity.

TABLE 20-1 *Pituitary Hyperfunction*

Hormone	Lesion	Classic Staining of Tumor Cells	Manifestations
Prolactin	Prolactinoma	Chromophobic	Amenorrhea and galactorrhea in women; impotence and sometimes galactorrhea in men
Somatotropin (growth hormone)	Somatotropic adenoma	Acidophilic	Gigantism or acromegaly
Corticotropin (ACTH)	Corticotropic adenoma or multiple corticotropic microadenomas	Basophilic	Pituitary Cushing syndrome
Antidiuretic hormone (ADH)	Nonpituitary lesions with ectopic hormone production (small cell carcinoma of the lung)		Water retention with dilutional hyponatremia

(b) The cause may be ectopic ACTH production by various tumors (especially small cell carcinoma of the lung).

2. **Anterior pituitary hypofunction**
   a. **Pituitary cachexia (Simmonds disease)** is **generalized panhypopituitarism.**
      (1) Characteristics include marked wasting.
      (2) Pituitary cachexia can result from any process that destroys the pituitary. It is most frequently caused by:
         (a) **Pituitary tumors**
         (b) **Postpartum pituitary necrosis (Sheehan syndrome)**
            (i) It is caused by ischemic necrosis of the pituitary gland and is characteristically associated with hemorrhage and shock during childbirth.
            (ii) Clinical manifestations are due at first to loss of gonadotropins, then to subsequent loss of thyroid-stimulating hormone (TSH) and ACTH.
   b. **Selective deficiency of one or more pituitary hormones**
      (1) **Deficiency of growth hormone**
         (a) In children, this results in growth retardation (pituitary dwarfism).
         (b) In adults, this may result in increased insulin sensitivity with hypoglycemia, decreased muscle strength, and anemia.
      (2) **Deficiency of gonadotropins**
         (a) In preadolescent children, this results in retarded sexual maturation.
         (b) In adults, this results in loss of libido, impotence, loss of muscular mass, and decreased facial hair in men, and in amenorrhea and vaginal atrophy in women.
      (3) **Deficiency of TSH** results in secondary hypothyroidism.
      (4) **Deficiency of ACTH** results in secondary adrenal failure. It does not result in hyperpigmentation of the skin, probably because of the lack of both ACTH and β-melanocyte-stimulating hormone; this is in contrast to primary adrenal failure (Addison disease), in which ACTH is increased and hyperpigmentation is the rule.

B. **Posterior pituitary (neurohypophysis)**
   1. **Hormones** are synthesized in the hypothalamus and transported via axons to the posterior pituitary.
      a. **Oxytocin** induces uterine contraction during labor and ejection of milk from mammary alveoli.

b. **Antidiuretic hormone (ADH, vasopressin)** promotes water retention through action on the renal collecting ducts.

2. **Syndrome of inappropriate ADH (SIADH) secretion**
   a. SIADH is most commonly caused by ectopic production of ADH by various tumors, especially **small cell carcinoma of the lung.**
   b. SIADH results in retention of water with consequent dilutional hyponatremia, reduced serum osmolality, and inability to dilute the urine.
3. **Deficiency of ADH**
   a. This results in **diabetes insipidus;** is characterized by polyuria, with consequent dehydration and insatiable thirst.
   b. Causes may include tumors, trauma, inflammatory processes, lipid storage disorders, and other conditions characterized by damage to the neurohypophysis or hypothalamus.

C. **Nonfunctioning pituitary tumors**
1. **Nonsecreting pituitary adenomas** are most often chromophobic.
   a. Dysfunction results because of local pressure phenomena.
   b. These tumors are clinically variable; manifestations include hypopituitarism, headache, visual disturbances (**bilateral hemianopsia** [loss of peripheral visual fields due to pressure on optic chiasm]), and palsies caused by cranial nerve damage.
2. **Craniopharyngioma (adamantinoma)**
   a. This benign childhood tumor is derived from remnants of the Rathke pouch. It is not a true pituitary tumor.
   b. It is similar to ameloblastoma of the jaw.
   c. Characteristics include nests and cords of squamous or columnar cells in a loose stroma, closely resembling the appearance of the embryonic tooth bud enamel organ.
   d. This tumor is often cystic; the lining epithelium of flat or columnar cells often expands into papillary projections.
   e. Radiographic detection is often possible because of tumor calcification.

D. **Other causes of pituitary hypofunction**
1. The **empty sella syndrome** is caused by conditions that destroy all or part of the pituitary.
2. The **Nelson syndrome** involves the development of large pituitary adenomas following bilateral adrenalectomy. This is thought to be due to loss of feedback inhibition on growth of preexisting pituitary microadenomas.

II. Thyroid Gland

A. **Thyroid hormones** include **thyroxine (T_4)** and **triiodothyronine (T_3).**
1. Their synthesis depends on sufficient quantities of iodine from dietary sources.
2. The rate of extraction of iodine from the bloodstream and the rate at which T_4 and T_3 are synthesized and released from storage (as thyroglobulin) and secreted into the bloodstream are regulated by pituitary TSH.
3. Feedback mechanisms regulate pituitary production of TSH.
4. Serum T_3 and T_4 are bound to thyroid-binding globulin (TBG).

B. **Congenital anomalies**
1. **Thyroglossal duct cyst** is the most common thyroid anomaly.
   a. This structure is a remnant of the thyroglossal duct.
   b. It does not lead to alterations in thyroid function.
2. **Ectopic thyroid tissue** may be found anywhere along the course of the thyroglossal duct.

C. **Goiter** is a general term for enlargement of the thyroid.

1. **Causes**
   a. **Physiologic enlargement** is not uncommon in puberty and pregnancy.
   b. **Iodine deficiency** occurs in geographic areas in which the diet is deficient in iodine.
   c. **Hashimoto thyroiditis**
   d. **Goitrogens** are foods or drugs that suppress synthesis of thyroid hormones.
   e. **Dyshormonogenesis,** or partial or complete failure of thyroid hormone synthesis, can be caused by various enzyme deficiencies.
2. **Terminology**
   a. **Simple goiter (nontoxic goiter)** is goiter without thyroid hormone dysfunction.
   b. **Toxic goiter** is goiter associated with hyperthyroidism; if the patient is euthyroid or hypothyroid, the term **nontoxic goiter** is appropriate.
   c. **Endemic goiter** is goiter occurring with high frequency in iodine-deficient geographic areas; the term **sporadic goiter** is used for goiter caused by similar mechanisms in non–iodine-deficient areas.
   d. **Nodular goiter** is irregular enlargement of the thyroid, resulting in nodule formation.
      (1) **Nodular colloid goiter** refers to the late stage of simple goiter in which goiter is most often nodular; nodules may be single or multiple (multinodular goiter).
      (2) Most nodules are hypoplastic and do not take up radioactive iodine ("cold" nodules).
      (3) Occasionally nodules are hyperplastic and actively produce thyroid hormone and take up radioactive iodine ("hot" nodules).

D. **Hypothyroidism**
1. **Laboratory abnormalities**
   a. **Decreased serum free T_4, increased serum TSH**
   b. Increased serum cholesterol
   c. Classic thyroid tests now passing into disuse
      (1) **T_3 resin uptake** (also known as thyroid hormone-binding ratio (THBR)
         (a) This is colloquially referred to as "T_3," even though it is not a measure of triiodothyronine.
         (b) This is decreased in hypothyroidism.
         (c) This is inversely proportional to the number of unbound thyroid hormone binding sites on TBG; it is measured by competitive uptake of radioactive T_3 by resin, which competes for unbound sites on TBG.
      (2) **Total T_4** is decreased in hypothyroidism.
2. **Clinical syndromes.** Hypothyroidism is manifest as myxedema in adults or as cretinism in children.
   a. **Myxedema** is more common in women than in men.
      (1) **Causes**
         (a) Therapy for hyperthyroidism with surgery, irradiation, or drugs, which is a common cause of myxedema in the United States
         (b) **Hashimoto thyroiditis**
         (c) Unknown cause. **Primary idiopathic myxedema** is a poorly defined form of myxedema, which may be of autoimmune origin (TSH receptor-blocking antibodies have been identified).
         (d) **Iodine deficiency,** which is the most important cause in non–iodine-deficient geographic regions
      (2) **Clinical characteristics**
         (a) Insidious onset
         (b) Cold intolerance
         (c) Tendency to gain weight because of a low metabolic rate
         (d) Lowered pitch of voice
         (e) Mental and physical slowness
         (f) Menorrhagia
         (g) Constipation
         (h) Abnormal physical findings:

(i) Puffiness of face, eyelids, and hands
(ii) Dry skin
(iii) Hair loss; coarse and brittle hair; scant axillary and pubic hair; thinning of the lateral aspect of the eyebrows
(iv) Increase in relaxation phase of deep tendon reflexes

b. **Cretinism**
(1) **Causes**
(a) Iodine deficiency
(b) Deficiency of enzymes necessary for the synthesis of thyroid hormones
(c) Maldevelopment of the thyroid gland
(d) Failure of the fetal thyroid to descend from its origin at the base of the tongue
(e) Transplacental transfer of antithyroid antibodies from a mother with autoimmune thyroid disease

(2) **Characteristics**
(a) Severe mental retardation
(b) Impairment of physical growth with retarded bone development and dwarfism
(c) Large tongue
(d) Protuberant abdomen

E. Hyperthyroidism (thyrotoxicosis)

1. **Clinical features**
a. Restlessness, irritability, fatigability
b. Tremor
c. Heat intolerance; sweating; warm, moist skin (especially of palms)
d. Tachycardia, often with arrhythmia and palpitation, sometimes with high-output cardiac failure
e. Muscle wasting and weight loss despite increased appetite
f. Fine hair
g. Diarrhea
h. Menstrual abnormalities, commonly amenorrhea or oligomenorrhea
i. **Greatly increased free T_4** and (in Graves disease, see the following) **greatly reduced TSH.** In addition, the less commonly used total T_4 and T_3 resin uptake are both increased.

2. **Graves disease**
a. **General considerations**
(1) Graves disease is hyperthyroidism caused by diffuse toxic goiter.
(2) It occurs more frequently in women than in men.
(3) The incidence is increased in HLA-DR3- and HLA-B8-positive individuals.
(4) Striking exophthalmos (protrusion of the eyes), possibly due to autoimmune mechanisms and independent of thyroid hyperfunction, is characteristic. Manifestations include the signs and symptoms of hyperthyroidism.

b. **Mechanism**
(1) **Thyroid-stimulating immunoglobulin (TSI),** an IgG antibody, reacts with thyroid follicle TSH receptors and stimulates thyroid hormone production.
(2) A similar reaction with **thyroid growth immunoglobulin (TGI)** stimulates glandular hyperplasia and enlargement.
(3) In addition to TSI and TGI, antimicrosomal and other autoantibodies are characteristic.

3. **Other causes of hyperthyroidism**
a. **Plummer disease** is a combination of hyperthyroidism, nodular goiter, and absence of exophthalmos. The "hot" nodules can be adenomas or non-neoplastic areas of nodular hyperplasia.
b. **Pituitary hyperfunction** can cause excess production of TSH and secondary hyperthyroidism.
c. **Struma ovarii** is an ovarian teratoma made up of thyroid tissue; can be hyperfunctional.
d. **Exogenous administration of thyroid hormone**

F. **Thyroiditis**

1. **Hashimoto thyroiditis**
   a. This **autoimmune disorder** occurs more often in women than in men.
   b. It is a common cause of hypothyroidism; may occasionally have an early transient hyperthyroid phase.
   c. Clinical characteristics include a **slow, often inapparent course** and a modestly enlarged and nontender thyroid; the patient is most often euthyroid at first, but transient hyperthyroidism may occur; hypothyroidism develops late when the gland is shrunken and scarred.
   d. Histologic characteristics include **massive infiltrates of lymphocytes with germinal center formation;** thyroid follicles are atrophic and Hürthle cells (epithelial cells with eosinophilic granular cytoplasm) are prominent.
   e. Hashimoto thyroiditis is associated with various **autoantibodies,** most prominently antithyroglobulin, antithyroid peroxidase, anti-TSH receptor, and anti-iodine receptor antibodies.
   f. It may also be associated with an increased incidence of other autoimmune disorders such as pernicious anemia, diabetes mellitus, and Sjögren syndrome; incidence is increased in HLA-DR5- and HLA-B5-positive individuals.
2. **Subacute (de Quervain, granulomatous) thyroiditis**
   a. The disease is more common in women than in men.
   b. Focal destruction of thyroid tissue and granulomatous inflammation is characteristic.
   c. Causes may include a variety of viral infections such as mumps or coxsackievirus.
   d. Subacute thyroiditis follows a self-limited course of several weeks' duration consisting of a flu-like illness along with pain and tenderness of the thyroid, sometimes with transient hyperthyroidism.
3. **Riedel thyroiditis** is characterized by thyroid replacement by fibrous tissue; it is of unknown origin. It can clinically mimic carcinoma.

G. **Benign tumors (adenomas) of the thyroid**

1. These tumors are most often solitary.
2. They present clinically as nodules and can occur in a variety of histologic patterns (e.g., follicular, Hürthle cell).
3. Most often they are nonfunctional, but they can occasionally cause hyperthyroidism.

H. **Malignant tumors of the thyroid**

1. **Papillary carcinoma**
   a. This carcinoma is the **most common thyroid cancer.**
   b. Histologic characteristics include papillary projections into gland-like spaces; tumor cells have characteristic "ground-glass" ("Orphan Annie") nuclei; calcified spheres (psammoma bodies) may be present.
   c. This cancer has a **better prognosis than other forms of thyroid cancer,** even when adjacent lymph nodes are involved.
   d. In some instances, papillary carcinoma can be associated with changes in chromosome 10 (paracentric inversion of chromosome 10 or a reciprocal translocation between chromosomes 10 and 17), which constitutively activate the tyrosine kinase domain of *ret.* These novel fusion genes are referred to as *ret-PTC* (for *ret* and papillary thyroid carcinoma) and are analogous to the *bcr-abl* fusion in chronic myeloid leukemia, which also causes a constitutive activation of a tyrosine kinase domain.
   e. This cancer can be a long-term consequence of prior radiotherapy to the neck.
2. **Follicular carcinoma**
   a. This cancer is characterized histologically by relatively uniform follicles.
   b. It has a poorer prognosis than papillary carcinoma.
3. **Medullary carcinoma**
   a. This cancer originates from C cells of the thyroid.
   b. It produces calcitonin, a calcium-lowering hormone.

c. Histologic characteristics include sheets of tumor cells in an amyloid-containing stroma.
d. Medullary carcinoma can be associated with multiple endocrine neoplasia (MEN) syndrome IIa and IIb (III).
4. **Undifferentiated carcinoma** tends to occur in older patients and has a very poor prognosis.

III. Parathyroid Glands

A. Parathyroid hormone (parathormone, PTH)

1. Secretion is not under pituitary control.
2. The parathyroid glands are responsive to the plasma concentration of ionized calcium; decreased calcium concentration stimulates PTH production.

B. **Hyperparathyroidism** (Table 20-2)

1. **Primary hyperparathyroidism**
   a. Most often, the cause is **parathyroid adenoma;** a few cases are caused by primary **parathyroid hyperplasia;** carcinoma is rarely a cause.
   b. Less often, the cause is **production of PTH-like hormone by nonparathyroid malignant tumors** such as bronchogenic squamous cell carcinoma or renal cell carcinoma.
   c. Primary hyperparathyroidism can occur as part of MEN I and MEN IIa.
   d. **Laboratory findings**
      (1) **Hypercalcemia** and hypercalciuria
      (2) **Decreased serum phosphorus,** decreased tubular reabsorption of phosphorus, and increased urinary phosphorus
      (3) **Increased serum alkaline phosphatase**
      (4) **Increased serum PTH**
   e. **Clinical characteristics**
      (1) **Osteitis fibrosa cystica,** cystic changes in bone due to osteoclastic resorption; it is also known as von Recklinghausen disease of bone; fibrous replacement of resorbed bone may lead to the formation of non-neoplastic tumor-like masses (**"brown tumor"**).

TABLE 20-2 *Hyperparathyroidism*

Causes	Clinical Manifestations	Laboratory Abnormalities
Primary		
Parathyroid adenoma, hyperplasia, or carcinoma; parathyroid hormone-like hormone production by tumors elsewhere; MEN I and MEN IIa	Osteitis fibrosa cystica; metastatic calcification in many tissues; nephrocalcinosis and renal calculi	Increased PTH; hypercalcemia and hypercalciuria; hypophosphatemia and decreased tubular reabsorption of phosphorus; increased alkaline phosphatase
Secondary		
Hypocalcemia (usually due to renal disease)	Diffuse osteoclastic bone disease; metastatic calcification	Increased PTH; hypocalcemia (may be slight); hyperphosphatemia; increased alkaline phosphatase

MEN = multiple endocrine neoplasia syndrome; PTH = parathyroid hormone.

(2) Metastatic calcification affecting various tissues, especially the kidneys (**nephrocalcinosis**)
(3) **Renal calculi,** a frequent complication
(4) Peptic duodenal ulcer; hypercalcemia predisposes to peptic ulcer

2. **Secondary hyperparathyroidism**
   a. Compensatory parathyroid hyperplasia occurs in response to decreased concentration of serum ionized calcium.
   b. The **most common cause is hypocalcemia of chronic renal disease.** Vitamin D conversion by the kidney to biologically active 1,25-$(OH)_2D_3$ (1α,25-dihydroxycholecalciferol) is impeded, resulting in decreased intestinal absorption of calcium; also, the increased serum phosphorus of renal disease induces a reciprocal decrease in serum calcium.
   c. Characteristics include decreased serum calcium, increased serum phosphorus, and increased serum alkaline phosphatase; diffuse osteoclastic bone disease; and metastatic calcification. PTH is increased.
3. **Tertiary hyperparathyroidism**
   a. This persistent parathyroid hyperfunction occurs in spite of correction of hypocalcemia and preexisting secondary hyperparathyroidism.
   b. Often, the cause is development of an adenoma in a previously hyperplastic gland.
4. **1α-hydroxylase deficiency (vitamin D–dependent rickets)**
   a. Impaired hydroxylation of 25-hydroxycholecalciferol is characteristic.
   b. Results include decreased absorption of calcium and increased PTH secretion.

C. Hypoparathyroidism

1. The most common cause is accidental surgical excision during thyroidectomy. In rare instances, this disorder is associated with congenital thymic hypoplasia (DiGeorge syndrome).
2. Severe hypocalcemia manifest clinically by increased neuromuscular excitability and tetany is characteristic.

D. Pseudohypoparathyroidism

1. Pseudohypoparathyroidism is similar to hypoparathyroidism, with decreased calcium, increased phosphate, and increased parathyroid hormone.
2. This disorder is characterized by multihormone resistance involving PTH and the pituitary hormones TSH, luteinizing hormone, and follicle-stimulating hormone.
3. Additional characteristics include **end-organ unresponsiveness of the kidney to PTH,** as well as **shortened fourth and fifth metacarpals and metatarsals, short stature, and other skeletal abnormalities.**
   a. These abnormalities are due to mutations in *GNAS*1, a gene encoding certain G proteins that mediate tissue receptiveness to hormones. Both alleles are expressed in multiple tissues. However, in the kidney and pituitary, there is expression only of the maternally inherited chromosome.
   b. This selective imprinting of the mutant gene (paternal imprinting or silencing) results in maternal inheritance of the end-organ unresponsiveness. The skeletal abnormalities result from inheritance of mutant *GNAS*1 from either parent.
4. Similar skeletal abnormalities, without hormone dysfunction, characterize **pseudopseudohypoparathyroidism,** which requires transmission of a mutant paternal *GNAS*1 allele.

IV. Adrenal Glands (Table 20-3)

A. Cushing syndrome (hypercorticism)

1. **Causes.** Cushing syndrome results from increased circulating glucocorticoids, primarily cortisol.

TABLE 20-3 *Adrenal Endocrine Syndromes*

Syndrome	Usual Anatomic Lesions	Comments
Cortex		
Cushing syndrome (hypercorticism)	Bilateral hyperplasia of adrenal zona fasciculata secondary to hyperactivity of pituitary corticotrophs or to ectopic ACTH-like production by a variety of tumors; adrenal cortical adenoma	May be of pituitary, adrenal, or ectopic origin; can also result from administration of exogenous hormone
Hyperaldosteronism (aldosteronism):		
Primary	Adenoma or hyperplasia of zona glomerulosa	Serum renin decreased
Secondary	Bilateral hyperplasia of zona glomerulosa caused by stimulation of renin-angiotensin system	Serum renin increased; frequently secondary to edema, regardless of the cause
Adrenal virilism	Adenoma, carcinoma, or hyperplasia of zona reticularis	May be due to hyperplasia resulting from congenital enzyme deficiencies such as 21-hydroxylase and 11-hydroxylase
Hypocorticism	Idiopathic adrenal atrophy	Probable autoimmune etiology
	Tuberculosis	Most common cause of Addison disease in prior years
	Infection	Waterhouse-Friderichsen syndrome most often associated with meningococcal infection
Medulla		
Pheochromocytoma	Chromaffin cell tumor; benign or malignant	Tumor secretes catecholamines (epinephrine and norepinephrine) and causes secondary hypertension
Neuroblastoma	Malignant "small blue cell" tumor of adrenal medulla	Catecholamine-secreting malignancy of early childhood; hypertension

a. **Exogenous corticosteroid medication** (most common)

b. **Hyperproduction of ACTH** by corticotrophs of the pituitary

c. **Adrenal cortical adenoma or adrenal carcinoma** (less common than adenoma)

d. **Ectopic production of ACTH** by nonpituitary carcinomas, especially small cell carcinoma of the lung. Hypercorticism is autonomous and cannot be suppressed by exogenous adrenal steroids such as those used in the low- and high-dose dexamethasone suppression tests. Also, the autonomous ACTH stimulation eliminates the normal circadian rhythm of cortisol production.

2. **Morphologic changes in adrenal gland**

a. **Bilateral hyperplasia** of the adrenal zona fasciculata occurs when the syndrome results from ACTH stimulation.

b. **Adrenal cortical atrophy** is seen when exogenous glucocorticoid medication is the cause.

c. **Adrenal cortical adenoma or carcinoma**

(1) Adenoma is more common.

(2) Hypercorticism due to adrenal neoplasms cannot be suppressed by exogenous adrenal steroids in the dexamethasone suppression tests. In contrast, hypercorticism of pituitary origin can usually be suppressed.

(3) In addition to dexamethasone suppression, ACTH determinations are useful diagnostic measures in determining the cause of hypercorticism. ACTH is increased in pituitary hypercorticism and in ectopic ACTH production, and it is low when hypercorticism is of adrenal origin.

3. **Clinical characteristics**
   a. Redistribution of body fat with round moon face, dorsal "buffalo hump," often with relatively thin extremities caused by muscle wasting; skin atrophy with easy bruising and purplish striae, especially over the abdomen; and hirsutism
   b. Muscle weakness, osteoporosis, amenorrhea, hypertension, hyperglycemia, and psychiatric dysfunction

B. **Hyperaldosteronism**

1. **Primary aldosteronism (Conn syndrome)**
   a. The cause is primary hyperproduction of adrenal mineralocorticoids.
   b. This condition usually results from an aldosterone-producing adrenocortical adenoma **(aldosteronoma).** It can also result from hyperplasia of the zona glomerulosa. Rarely it may be caused by adrenocortical carcinoma.
   c. Clinical characteristics include hypertension, sodium and water retention, and hypokalemia, often with hypokalemic alkalosis.
   d. **Decreased serum renin** occurs due to negative feedback of increased blood pressure on renin secretion.
2. **Secondary aldosteronism**
   a. This condition is secondary to renal ischemia, renal tumors, and edema (e.g., cirrhosis, nephrotic syndrome, cardiac failure).
   b. The cause is stimulation of the renin-angiotensin system.
   c. **Serum renin is increased,** in contrast to primary aldosteronism. Renin synthesized in the juxtaglomerular apparatus of the kidney promotes the conversion of angiotensinogen to angiotensin I, which is converted catalytically by angiotensin-converting enzyme (mainly in the lung) to angiotensin II. The release of aldosterone is facilitated by angiotensin II.

C. **Adrenal virilism (adrenogenital syndrome)**

1. **Causes**
   a. **Congenital enzyme defects** lead to diminished cortisol production and compensatory increased ACTH, with resultant adrenal hyperplasia with androgenic steroid production.
      (1) **21-hydroxylase deficiency,** which is most common, can, in its most severe "salt-wasting" form, result in salt loss and hypotension.
      (2) **11-hydroxylase deficiency,** a much less common cause, results in salt retention and hypertension.
   b. **Tumors of the adrenal cortex**
2. **Clinical characteristics.** Adrenal virilism produces virilism in females and precocious puberty in males.

D. **Hypocorticism (adrenal hypofunction)**

1. **General considerations**
   a. Hypocorticism can be of primary adrenal cause or secondary to hypothalamic or pituitary dysfunction.
   b. Deficiency of glucocorticoids (primarily cortisol), often with associated mineralocorticoid deficiency, is characteristic.
2. **Addison disease (primary adrenocortical deficiency)**
   a. This disorder is most commonly due to **idiopathic adrenal atrophy** (autoimmune lymphocytic adrenalitis).
   b. It can also be caused by tuberculosis (formerly most common cause), metastatic tumor, and various infections.

c. Characteristics include hypotension; increased pigmentation of skin; decreased serum sodium, chloride, glucose, and bicarbonate; and increased serum potassium.

3. **Waterhouse-Friderichsen syndrome**
   a. This catastrophic adrenal insufficiency and vascular collapse is due to **hemorrhagic necrosis of the adrenal cortex.**
   b. This syndrome is often associated with **disseminated intravascular coagulation.**
   c. This syndrome is characteristically due to **meningococcemia,** most often in association with meningococcal meningitis.

E. **Tumors of the adrenal medulla**

1. **Pheochromocytoma**
   a. This tumor is derived from **chromaffin cells of the adrenal medulla;** if it is derived from extra-adrenal chromaffin cells, it is called paraganglioma.
   b. Most often this tumor is **benign;** ten percent are malignant.
   c. This uncommon but important cause of surgically correctable hypertension results from hyperproduction of catecholamines (epinephrine and norepinephrine) by the tumor; the hypertension is usually paroxysmal (episodic) but may be persistent.
   d. **Increased urinary excretion of catecholamines and their metabolites (metanephrine, normetanephrine, and vanillylmandelic acid)** is characteristic.
   e. This tumor can also cause hyperglycemia.
   f. Pheochromocytoma can be part of MEN IIa or MEN IIb (III). It can also be associated with neurofibromatosis or with von Hippel-Lindau disease.
2. **Neuroblastoma**
   a. This highly **malignant** catecholamine-producing tumor occurs in **early childhood.**
   b. **Urinary catecholamines** and catecholamine metabolites are the same as in pheochromocytoma.
   c. The tumor causes **hypertension.**
   d. It usually originates in the adrenal medulla and often presents as a large **abdominal mass.**
   e. Occasionally it converts into a more differentiated form termed ganglioneuroma.
   f. The tumor is characterized by **amplification** of the N-*myc* oncogene with thousands of gene copies per cell.
      (1) Amplification results in characteristic karyotypic changes (homogeneously staining regions or double minute chromosomes).
      (2) The number of N-*myc* gene copies is related to the aggressiveness of the tumor.
   g. The malignant cells of neuroblastoma sometimes differentiate into benign cells, and this change is reflected by a marked reduction in gene amplification.

V. Endocrine Pancreas

A. **Diabetes mellitus**

1. **Classification and general features**
   a. **Type 1** (insulin-dependent diabetes mellitus [IDDM], juvenile or ketosis-prone diabetes mellitus)
      (1) **Epidemiologic and etiologic factors**
         (a) Type 1 disease often **begins early in life,** usually before 30 years of age.
         (b) Type 1 disease is less common than type 2 disease.
         (c) Disease is due to **failure of insulin synthesis** by beta cells of the pancreatic islets.
         (d) The cause may be a **genetic predisposition** complicated by **autoimmune inflammation** of islets (insulitis) triggered by a viral infection or environmental factors. Type 1 disease demonstrates a positive family history less frequently than does type 2 disease.

(e) The incidence is greatly increased in individuals with a specific point mutation in the HLA-DQ gene. Incidence is markedly increased in HLA-DR3- and HLA-DR4-positive individuals.

(2) **Characteristics**

(a) Unless insulin is replaced, type 1 diabetes results in marked **carbohydrate intolerance with hyperglycemia,** leading to polyuria, polydipsia, weight loss despite increased appetite, **ketoacidosis,** coma, and death.

(b) Ketoacidosis results from increased catabolism of fat, with production of "ketone bodies" (principally β-hydroxybutyric acid and acetoacetic acid along with small quantities of acetone). It is not limited to diabetic acidosis and, in a much milder form, is seen in starvation.

b. **Type 2** (non–insulin-dependent diabetes mellitus [NIDDM], adult-onset, or ketosis-resistant diabetes mellitus)

(1) **Epidemiologic and etiologic factors**

(a) Type 2 disease is much more common than type 1 disease.

(b) Type 2 disease characteristically begins later in life, most often in **middle age.**

(c) A **positive family history** is more frequent than in type 1 diabetes mellitus.

(d) Type 2 disease is due to **increased insulin resistance** mediated by decreased cell membrane insulin receptors or postreceptor dysfunction. It may also be associated with impaired processing of proinsulin to insulin, decreased sensing of glucose by beta cells, or impaired function of intracellular carrier proteins.

(e) Type 2 disease is most often associated with mild to moderate **obesity.**

(2) **Characteristics**

(a) The plasma insulin concentration is normal and often increased.

(b) Mild carbohydrate intolerance can most often be managed by diet and oral antidiabetic agents; insulin therapy is not usually required.

(c) **Ketoacidosis is unusual** but does occur, characteristically precipitated by unusual stress such as infection or surgery.

c. **Maturity-onset diabetes mellitus of the young (MODY)**

(1) This autosomal dominant syndrome is characterized by mild hyperglycemia and hyposecretion of insulin but no loss of beta cells.

(2) It has an earlier onset than type 2 diabetes mellitus.

(3) It is caused by a diverse group of single gene defects.

d. **Secondary diabetes mellitus** occurs as a secondary phenomenon in pancreatic and other endocrine diseases and pregnancy.

(1) **Pancreatic disease**

(a) **Hereditary hemochromatosis** (bronze diabetes). Characteristics include excess iron absorption and parenchymal deposition of hemosiderin, with reactive fibrosis in various organs, especially the pancreas, liver, and heart.

(b) **Pancreatitis.** Acute pancreatitis is characterized by hyperglycemia; chronic pancreatitis may result in islet cell destruction and secondary diabetes mellitus.

(c) **Carcinoma of the pancreas.** Diabetes mellitus may be the presenting sign.

(2) **Other endocrine diseases**

(a) **Cushing syndrome** produces hyperglycemia as a result of increased gluconeogenesis and impaired peripheral utilization of glucose.

(b) **Acromegaly** produces hyperglycemia due to the anti–insulin-like effect of growth hormone.

(c) **Glucagon hypersecretion** promotes glycogenolysis; is characteristically caused by an islet alpha cell tumor (glucagonoma).

(d) **Other endocrine disorders.** Pheochromocytoma and hyperthyroidism are sometimes associated with hyperglycemia.

(3) **Pregnancy**

(a) Pregnancy may be associated with transient diabetes mellitus **(gestational diabetes);** overt nongestational diabetes sometimes develops later.

(b) Diabetes mellitus is characteristically associated with **increased fetal birth weight** and increased fetal mortality, notably from neonatal respiratory distress syndrome **(hyaline membrane disease).**

(c) When a mother has hyperglycemia, her infant may be born with hyperplasia of the pancreatic islets and hypoglycemia.

2. **Anatomic changes in diabetes mellitus**
   a. **Pancreatic islets**
      (1) **Type 1 diabetes.** Islets are small and beta cells are greatly decreased in number or are absent; **insulitis** marked by lymphocytic infiltration is a highly specific early change for this form of diabetes mellitus.
      (2) **Type 2 diabetes**
         (a) Focal islet fibrosis and hyalinization (due to deposits of **amylin**) are characteristic but not specific.
         (b) Amylin (also known as islet amyloid polypeptide, or IAPP) deposition in the pancreatic islets is characteristic of type 2 diabetes mellitus and is thought to interfere either with the conversion of proinsulin to insulin or with the sensing of insulin by beta cells.
   b. **Kidney**
      (1) Increased width of glomerular basement membrane is the earliest and most common renal manifestation.
      (2) Diffuse diabetic glomerulosclerosis, nodular diabetic glomerulosclerosis (Kimmelstiel-Wilson disease), arteriolar lesions, and exudative lesions such as the fibrin cap or capsular drop are renal manifestations of diabetes mellitus.
      (3) The Armanni-Ebstein lesion (tubular deposition of glycogen) is an uncommon result of prolonged untreated hyperglycemia.
      (4) Pyelonephritis is a frequent complication that may be compounded by renal papillary necrosis.
   c. **Cardiovascular system**
      (1) The incidence of **atherosclerosis** is greatly increased; clinically significant atherosclerotic complications occur at a much earlier age than in the nondiabetic population; the incidence in women, both premenopausal and postmenopausal, is greatly increased.
      (2) **Myocardial infarction** and **peripheral vascular insufficiency** (often with gangrene of the lower extremities) are frequent complications.
      (3) **Capillary basement membrane thickening** occurs in multiple organs and is thought to be due to nonenzymatic glycosylation of membrane protein.
   d. **Eye**
      (1) **Cataract formation** is common.
      (2) Proliferative retinopathy (retinal exudates, edema, hemorrhages, and microaneurysms of small vessels) can lead to blindness.
   e. **Nervous system.** Changes include **peripheral neuropathy** and changes in the brain and spinal cord.
   f. **Liver.** Fatty change is seen.
   g. **Skin**
      (1) **Xanthomas** (collections of lipid-laden macrophages in the dermis)
      (2) **Furuncles** and **abscesses** because of increased propensity to **infection;** frequent **fungal** infections, especially with *Candida*

B. **Endocrine tumors (islet cell tumors)**

1. **Insulinoma (beta cell tumor)** is the most common islet cell tumor.
   a. This tumor can be benign or malignant.
   b. It is characterized by greatly increased secretion of insulin. The problem of distinguishing endogenous insulin production from exogenous insulin (therapeutically or surreptitiously administered) is solved by quantitation of C-peptide, a fragment of the proinsulin molecule split off during the synthesis of insulin. Circulating C-peptide is characteristically increased in patients with insulinoma. In contrast, C-peptide is not

increased by exogenous insulin administration because it is removed during the purification of commercial insulin preparations.

c. Clinical characteristics include the **Whipple triad:**
   (1) Episodic hyperinsulinemia and hypoglycemia
   (2) Central nervous system (CNS) dysfunction temporally related to hypoglycemia (confusion, anxiety, stupor, convulsions, coma)
   (3) Dramatic reversal of CNS abnormalities by glucose administration

2. **Gastrinoma**
   (a) This tumor is often malignant and sometimes occurs in extrapancreatic sites.
   (b) It results in gastrin hypersecretion and hypergastrinemia.
   (c) It is associated with the **Zollinger-Ellison syndrome** (marked gastric hypersecretion of hydrochloric acid, recurrent peptic ulcer disease, and hypergastrinemia).
3. **Glucagonoma (alpha cell tumor)** is a rare tumor.
   a. This endocrine tumor results in **secondary diabetes mellitus.**
   b. It causes a characteristic skin lesion called necrolytic migratory erythema.
4. **VIPoma** is a rare tumor.
   a. This endocrine tumor is marked by secretion of vasoactive intestinal peptide (VIP).
   b. It is associated with **W**atery **D**iarrhea, **H**ypokalemia, and **A**chlorhydria (WDHA) syndrome, also known as Verner-Morrison syndrome or pancreatic cholera.

VI. Multiple Endocrine Neoplasia (MEN) Syndromes

- In this group of autosomal dominant syndromes, more than one endocrine organ is hyperfunctional.
- These conditions may be associated with hyperplasias or tumors.

A. MEN I (Wermer syndrome)

1. This syndrome includes hyperplasias or tumors of the **p**ituitary, **p**arathyroid, or **p**ancreatic islets (3 Ps). In addition, it may include hyperplasias or tumors of the thyroid or adrenal cortex.
2. It may manifest its pancreatic component by the Zollinger-Ellison syndrome, hyperinsulinism, or pancreatic cholera.
3. It is linked to mutations in the *MEN I* gene.

B. MEN IIa (Sipple syndrome)

1. This syndrome includes pheochromocytoma, medullary carcinoma of the thyroid, and hyperparathyroidism due to hyperplasia or tumor.
2. It is linked to mutations in the *ret* oncogene.

C. MEN IIb (MEN III)

1. This syndrome includes pheochromocytoma, medullary carcinoma, and multiple mucocutaneous neuromas or ganglioneuromas.
2. In contrast to MEN IIa, it does not induce hyperparathyroidism.
3. It is linked to different mutations in the *ret* oncogene compared with MEN IIa.

REVIEW TEST

Directions: *Each of the numbered items or incomplete statements in this section is followed by answers or by completions of the statement. Select the* ***one*** *lettered answer or completion that is best in each case.*

1. A 35-year-old woman is seen 6 months after giving birth to a normal infant. She suffered severe cervical lacerations during delivery, resulting in hemorrhagic shock. Following blood transfusion and surgical repair, postpartum recovery has so far been uneventful. She now complains of continued amenorrhea and loss of weight and muscle strength. Further investigation might be expected to demonstrate which of the following findings?

(A) Decreased serum cortisol
(B) Hyperestrinism
(C) Hyperglycemia
(D) Increased hair growth in a male distribution pattern
(E) Increased serum free thyroxine

2. A 10-year-old boy presents with headache and bilateral hemianopsia as well as evidence of increased intracranial pressure and diabetes insipidus. Supersellar calcification is apparent on radiographic examination. Resection of the contents of the sella turcica and parasellar area yields a large tumor with histology closely resembling the enamel organ of the embryonic tooth. The most likely outcome of this lesion is

(A) local invasion and intracranial metastasis
(B) hematogenous metastasis to distal sites
(C) lymphatic spread to distal sites
(D) possible local recurrence with continued pressure-related damage to adjacent structures

3. During a yearlong training program, a 23-year-old female Air Force officer falls in class rank from first place to last place. She has also noted a lower pitch to her voice and coarsening of her hair, along with an increased tendency toward weight gain, menorrhagia, and increasing intolerance to cold. Which of the following laboratory abnormalities is expected?

(A) Increased serum free T_4
(B) Increased serum T_3 resin uptake
(C) Increased saturation of thyroid hormone–binding sites on thyroid-binding globulin
(D) Increased serum thyroid-stimulating hormone
(E) Decreased serum cholesterol

4. A 35-year-old woman presents with amenorrhea and weight loss despite increased appetite. The history and physical examination reveal exophthalmos, fine resting tremor, tachycardia, and warm, moist skin. Laboratory tests for thyroid function would be expected to yield a decreased value for which of the following?

(A) Free T_4
(B) Radioactive iodine uptake
(C) T_3 resin uptake
(D) T_3
(E) Thyroid-stimulating hormone

5. A tumor similar to that shown in the illustration is observed in a biopsy specimen from the thyroid of a 50-year-old woman. An adjacent lymph node is also involved. Which of the following descriptions of this tumor is most appropriate?

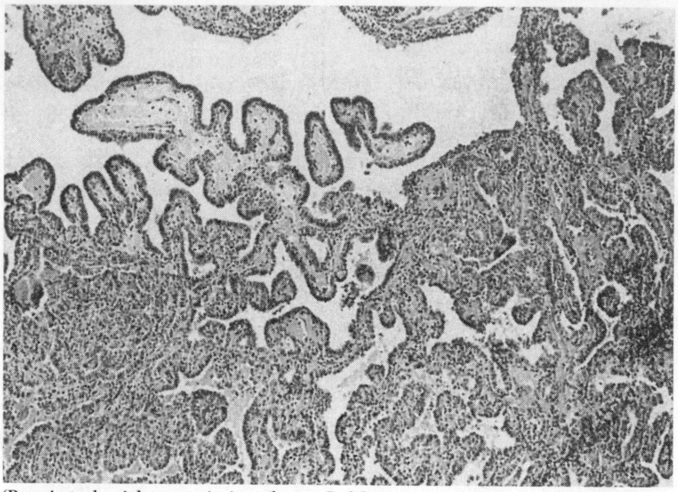

(Reprinted with permission from Golden A, Powell D, and Jennings C: *Pathology: Understanding Human Disease,* 2nd ed. Baltimore, Williams & Wilkins, 1985, p 388.)

(A) Functional tumor resulting in thyrotoxicosis
(B) Slow-growing lesion with relatively good prognosis
(C) Origin from C cells
(D) Calcitonin-producing tumor
(E) Tumor with amyloid-containing stroma

6. After suffering a seizure, a 23-year-old woman is found to have profound hypoglycemia. Determination of which of the following would aid in differentiating exogenous hyperinsulinemia from endogenous hyperinsulinemia?

(A) C-peptide
(B) Gastrin
(C) Glucagon
(D) Proinsulin
(E) Vasoactive intestinal peptide

7. A 34-year-old woman is seen because of unexplained weight gain, selectively over the trunk, upper back, and back of the neck; irregular menstrual periods; and increasing obesity. She is especially concerned about the changing contour of her face, which has become rounder, creating a "moon-faced" appearance. She has also developed purple-colored streaking resembling stretch marks over the abdomen and flanks, as well as increased hair growth in a male distribution pattern. Blood pressure is elevated to 190/100 mm Hg. Blood sugar is elevated. Computed tomography reveals a smooth, homogeneous lesion in the left adrenal gland. Surgery is performed, and the resected adrenal resembled that shown in the figure. The clinical findings and the change in the adrenal gland are most likely related to which of the following?

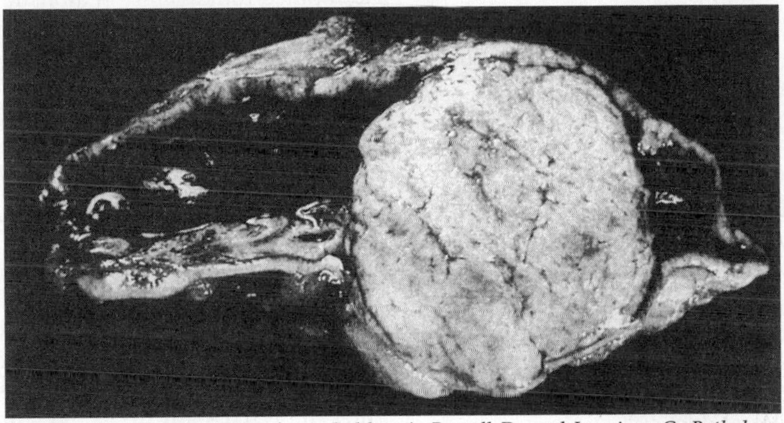

(Reprinted with permission from Golden A, Powell D, and Jennings C: *Pathology: Understanding Human Disease,* 2nd ed. Baltimore, Williams & Wilkins, 1985, p 396.)

(A) Adrenal (glucocorticoid) steroid therapy
(B) Ectopic production of adrenocorticotropin
(C) Hyperproduction of adrenal glucocorticoids
(D) Hyperproduction of hypothalamic corticotropin-releasing factor
(E) Hyperproduction of pituitary corticotropin

8. A 32-year-old woman presents with amenorrhea, galactorrhea, and visual field defects, all of several months duration. Magnetic resonance imaging reveals a hypophyseal mass impinging on the optic chiasm. This is most likely a (an)

(A) prolactinoma
(B) somatotropic adenoma
(C) corticotropic adenoma
(D) craniopharyngioma
(E) acidophilic adenoma

9. A 46-year-old man is referred to an endocrinologist because of the recent onset of diabetes mellitus. However, his overall appearance is striking, and on questioning, he describes marked changes that have been occurring slowly over many years. Comparison with old photographs reveals that he has developed generalized coarseness of his facial features, including frontal bossing, thickening of the nose, prognathism (enlargement and increased prominence of the jaw), and macroglossia (enlargement of the tongue). In addition, he has enlarged extremities, with sausage-like fingers, and he says that he is no longer able to wear his wedding ring and that his shoe size has increased. These findings are characteristic of increased activity of which of the following?

(A) Corticotropin
(B) Dopamine
(C) Insulinlike growth factor-I
(D) Prolactin
(E) Thyroid-stimulating hormone

10. A 36-year-old man is brought to the emergency department by his wife because of lethargy, weakness, and confusion. Serum sodium and serum osmolality are markedly decreased. Urine osmolality is increased. These findings are most likely related to

(A) adenoma of the anterior pituitary
(B) adenoma of the posterior pituitary
(C) bronchogenic carcinoma
(D) diabetes insipidus
(E) Sheehan syndrome

11. A 4-month-old child is brought to the pediatrician for evaluation. The mother received no prenatal care and states that she has "a thyroid condition." The child appears markedly developmentally delayed, with coarse features, macroglossia, and an umbilical hernia. The child likely has which of the following conditions?

(A) Cushing disease
(B) Acromegaly
(C) Diabetes insipidus
(D) Cretinism
(E) Thyroglossal duct cyst

12. A 23-year-old woman presents with tremor, restlessness, heat intolerance, palpitation, and unexplained weight loss. The thyroid is symmetrically enlarged; the pulse is rapid; the skin is moist and warm; and exophthalmos is apparent. This condition is considered to be

(A) autoimmune
(B) congenital
(C) iatrogenic
(D) infectious
(E) nutritional

13. A palpable mass is noted in the right lobe of the thyroid of a 45-year-old man who visits his physician for a periodic checkup. A biopsy is performed and results in a diagnosis of medullary carcinoma of the thyroid. Which of the following histologic features of thyroid disease would most likely be present in this biopsy specimen?

(A) Tumor cells with "Orphan Annie" nuclei
(B) Psammoma bodies
(C) Tumor cells embedded in an amyloid-laden stroma
(D) Infiltrates of lymphocytes with germinal center formation
(E) Replacement of the thyroid with fibrous tissue

14. A 34-year-old man is referred for evaluation of hypertension and persistent hypokalemia in spite of taking oral potassium supplements. Blood pressure is 180/110 mm Hg. Serum sodium is 149 mEq/L (normal 140–148 mEq/L); potassium, 3.3 mEq/L (normal 3.6–5.2 mEq/L); bicarbonate, 29 mEq/L (normal 22–29 mEq/L); chloride, 103 mEq/L (normal 98–107 mEq/L); and urea nitrogen, 23 mg/dL (normal 7–18 mg/dL). Computed tomography demonstrates a 3-cm mass in the right adrenal gland. The most likely diagnosis is

(A) Addison disease
(B) Cushing syndrome
(C) Sipple syndrome
(D) DiGeorge syndrome
(E) Conn syndrome

15. A 14-year-old boy is seen because of increasing weakness, easy fatigability, and weight loss over the past 3 months. In addition, he has recently developed nausea, vomiting, and abdominal pain. His blood pressure is markedly decreased, and he has increased pigmentation of his skin creases. These findings are suggestive of

(A) Cushing syndrome
(B) secondary hyperaldosteronism
(C) osteitis fibrosa cystica
(D) Addison disease
(E) 1α-hydroxylase deficiency

16. A tentatively female newborn has ambiguous genitalia. What appears to be a vagina is associated with a significantly enlarged clitoris resembling a penis. Other findings include hyponatremia, hyperkalemia, and hypotension. Deficiency of which of the following is suggested by these findings?

(A) 11-Hydroxylase
(B) 17-Hydroxylase
(C) 21-Hydroxylase
(D) Amylin
(E) 1α-Hydroxylase

17. An acutely ill 18-year-old female college student is brought to the emergency department by her roommate. The patient is febrile and markedly hypotensive, and her mental status is obtunded. Numerous petechial and purpuric hemorrhages are scattered over the trunk, and aspiration of a lesion reveals neutrophils engulfing gram-negative diplococci. Serum sodium is markedly decreased, and serum potassium is increased. Coagulation testing reveals increased prothrombin time, activated partial thromboplastin time, and fibrin-fibrinogen split products. Which of the following is most likely?

(A) Conn syndrome
(B) Hyperprolactinoma
(C) Neuroblastoma
(D) Waterhouse-Friderichsen syndrome
(E) Sipple syndrome

18. A 26-year-old woman has episodic hypertension with headache, diaphoresis, and palpitation. Which of the following diagnostic procedures would be most useful in evaluating the possibility that a pheochromocytoma might be the cause of these findings?

(A) Serum C-peptide
(B) Serum calcitonin
(C) Serum hemoglobin A1c (glycosylated hemoglobin)
(D) Urinary aldosterone
(E) Urinary vanillylmandelic acid

19. An autopsy is performed on an 8-year-old child with diabetes mellitus of recent onset who has died en route to the hospital following an automobile accident. Which of the following autopsy findings would favor the diagnosis of type 1 diabetes as contrasted to type 2 diabetes?

(A) Amylin deposition in pancreatic islets
(B) Armanni-Ebstein lesion
(C) Insulitis
(D) Kimmelstiel-Wilson nodules
(E) Proliferative retinopathy

20. A 28-year-old man is evaluated for recurrent peptic ulcer disease, apparently refractory to pharmacologic intervention. Serum gastrin is markedly elevated. These findings are most characteristic of which of the following?

(A) Cushing syndrome
(B) Glucagonoma
(C) Whipple triad
(D) Zollinger-Ellison syndrome
(E) Acromegaly

21. A 26-year-old primigravida develops gestational diabetes and remains hyperglycemic during the remainder of her pregnancy. Which of the following abnormalities in the newborn child is likely related to the maternal hyperglycemia?

(A) Ambiguous genitalia
(B) Cretinism
(C) Increased birth weight
(D) Sheehan syndrome
(E) Thyroglossal duct cyst

22. A 15-year-old boy presents to the endocrinologist with multiple mucocutaneous neuromas and a marfanoid habitus (tall with long extremities). His older brother has had a thyroidectomy for medullary carcinoma of the thyroid and later has been diagnosed with bilateral tumors of the adrenal medulla. It is likely that further investigation in both brothers will demonstrate an abnormality in which of the following genes or gene products?

(A) *Bcr-abl*
(B) N-*myc*
(C) *Ret*
(D) Amylin
(E) Insulin-associated polypeptide

A ANSWERS AND EXPLANATIONS

1-A. The history is strongly suggestive of panhypopituitarism due to ischemic necrosis of the pituitary, occurring as a sequela to childbirth complicated by hemorrhagic shock (Sheehan syndrome). This syndrome is clinically dominated by overt evidence of gonadotropin and corticotropin deficiencies along with laboratory evidence of these deficiencies and thyrotropin deficiency. Overt secondary hypothyroidism sometimes occurs.

2-D. The history is that of a craniopharyngioma (adamantinoma), a benign tumor that does not invade or metastasize. However, local effects of this tumor can be quite destructive, and recurrence due to incomplete resection is not uncommon. Local growth and tissue destruction result in both anterior and posterior pituitary dysfunction, and a patient often presents with signs of increased intracranial pressure, sometimes with hydrocephalus and frequently with bilateral hemianopsia (loss of peripheral visual fields) due to impingement on the optic chiasm. Diabetes insipidus is also frequent. Calcification apparent on radiograph is often prominent, facilitating diagnosis.

3-D. The history is strongly suggestive of idiopathic myxedema. Expected laboratory abnormalities include decreased serum free T_4, increased thyroid-stimulating hormone (TSH), and increased cholesterol. Also, because hypothyroidism, with secretion of less thyroid hormone, results in less saturation of binding sites on thyroid-binding globulin (or increased unbound binding sites), the T_3 resin uptake, which is inversely proportional to the number of unbound sites, will be decreased. **Note:** Total T_4 and T_3 resin uptake, although falling into clinical disuse, may still appear in examination questions. The most appropriate test today would be TSH (which is greatly elevated in hypothyroidism) and *free* T_4 (which is greatly reduced in hypothyroidism).

4-E. Graves disease is characteristically associated with decreased thyroid-stimulating hormone (TSH) activity. Thyroid-follicle TSH receptors are stimulated by thyroid-stimulating immunoglobulin, an IgG autoantibody, not by TSH. Laboratory abnormalities in hyperthyroidism include increases in serum T_4, serum T_3, T_3 resin uptake, and radioactive iodine uptake. Total T_4 and T_3 resin uptake are falling into disuse. The best screening tests for Graves disease are free T_4 (elevated in Graves disease) and TSH (greatly decreased in Graves disease).

5-B. The lesion shown is a papillary carcinoma of the thyroid, which is the most common form of thyroid cancer. This tumor most often remains localized to the thyroid and adjacent tissues for many years, even when local lymph nodes are involved. Papillary carcinoma is almost always nonfunctional.

6-A. Distinguishing endogenous insulin production from exogenous insulin (therapeutically or surreptitiously administered) is done by quantitation of C-peptide, a fragment of the proinsulin molecule split off during the synthesis of insulin. Circulating C-peptide is characteristically increased in patients with insulinoma. C-peptide is not increased by exogenous insulin administration because it is removed during the purification of commercial insulin preparations.

7-C. The illustration demonstrates a well-circumscribed adrenal cortical adenoma. Cushing syndrome is a manifestation of hyperproduction of adrenal glucocorticoids, and when of adrenal origin, it is most often caused by adrenal cortical adenoma. Pituitary and hypothalamic causes of Cushing syndrome result in bilateral adrenal cortical hyperplasia. In contrast, Cushing syndrome caused by exogenous steroid medication results in adrenal atrophy.

8-A. The findings described are associated with prolactinoma, the most common hormone-secreting tumor of the pituitary. Hyperprolactinemia results in amenorrhea and galactorrhea. The tumor is generally small. However, about 10% are large enough to impinge on adjacent structures, and bitemporal hemianopsia from pressure on the optic chiasm is common. Somatotropic adenoma (an older name is acidophilic adenoma) secretes growth hormone, causing acromegaly or gigantism, whereas corticotropic adenoma secretes adrenocorticotropic hormone, causing Cushing syndrome of pituitary origin (Cushing disease). Craniopharyngioma is a nonendocrine tumor of Rathke pouch origin that can be locally destructive, indirectly causing panhypopituitarism.

9-C. The findings are those of acromegaly, which is caused by a pituitary somatotropic adenoma. Growth hormone excess causes elevation in concentration of insulinlike growth factor-I (somatomedin C), measurement of which is a reliable indicator of disease activity. The tumor can also produce local effects, the most common of which is bitemporal hemianopsia from pressure on the optic chiasm.

10-C. The description is that of the syndrome of inappropriate antidiuretic hormone secretion, which is excessive release of antidiuretic hormone, most commonly a manifestation of small cell bronchogenic carcinoma. There are numerous other causes, including a variety of tumors, central nervous system disorders, trauma, and infections. The cardinal features are marked decreases in both serum sodium and osmolality, normal urine sodium, and urine osmolality considerably exceeding that of the serum.

11-D. The child exhibits signs of congenital hypothyroidism (cretinism). This disorder can result from many causes, including iodine deficiency, maldevelopment of the fetal thyroid, or transplacental transfer of antithyroid antibodies from a mother with autoimmune thyroid disease (a high possibility in this clinical case). The diagnosis of congenital hypothyroidism is confirmed in infants, as in adults, by decreased serum free T_4 and increased thyroid-stimulating hormone. If maternal antibody transfer is suspected, tests for antithyroid antibody testing can be performed in both the mother and child.

12-A. The patient presents with signs and symptoms of Graves disease, an autoimmune disorder in which patients develop autoantibodies that stimulate thyroid hormone production. As with many other autoimmune disorders, there is an association with certain human leukocyte antigens (HLAs); in the case of Graves disease, it is HLA-DR3 and HLA-B8.

13-C. Medullary carcinoma of the thyroid is a calcitonin-producing tumor of C cells of the thyroid. Calcitonin contributes to amyloid deposition within the tumor. Tumor cells with "Orphan Annie" nuclei and the presence of psammoma bodies are seen in papillary carcinoma of the thyroid. Infiltrates of lymphocytes with germinal center formation are seen in Hashimoto thyroiditis. In Riedel thyroiditis, the thyroid is replaced by fibrous tissue and can clinically mimic carcinoma.

14-E. The combination of hypertension, persistent hypokalemia, and slightly elevated serum sodium is highly suggestive of Conn syndrome (primary aldosteronism, hyperaldosteronism). The diagnosis can be confirmed by demonstration of increased aldosterone, lack of response of aldosterone to sodium loading, and decreased serum renin.

15-D. The clinical findings are suggestive of Addison disease (primary adrenocortical insufficiency). About 70% of cases are now due to autoimmune adrenalitis, but until recently the most frequent cause was tuberculosis. Hyperpigmentation in Addison disease results from compensatory hypothalamic production of proopiomelanocortin, the precursor peptide of both corticotropin and melanocyte-stimulating factor.

16-C. Deficiency of 21-hydroxylase is the cause of the most common of the adrenogenital syndromes. This enzyme deficiency results in decreased cortisol, decreased mineralocorticoids, and an increase in sex hormones, with resultant salt-losing hypotension and virilization (masculinization). Deficiency of 11-hydroxylase causes clinical findings similar to those of 21-hydroxylase deficiency, except for hypertension secondary to increased deoxycorticosterone, which has aldosterone-like activity. Deficiency of 17-hydroxylase results in decreased cortisol, increased mineralocorticoids, and decreased sex hormones. Amylin accumulates in diabetic islets, and 1α-hydroxylase is deficient in vitamin D–dependent rickets (type I).

17-D. The patient presents with signs and symptoms of the Waterhouse-Friderichsen syndrome, a devastating consequence of disseminated meningococcal infection. The disease is characterized by hemorrhagic destruction of the adrenals complicated by disseminated intravascular coagulation.

18-E. Urinary vanillylmandelic acid, a norepinephrine metabolite, is markedly elevated in pheochromocytoma. Serum C-peptide is elevated in insulinoma. Serum calcitonin is sometimes used to screen for medullary carcinoma of the thyroid. Serum hemoglobin A1c is an indicator of long-term blood glucose control in diabetes mellitus. Urine aldosterone is elevated in aldosteronism, both primary and secondary.

19-C. All of the findings listed are characteristic of diabetes mellitus, but only insulitis is specific for type 1 diabetes. Amylin deposition in the pancreatic islets, derived from insulin-associated polypeptide, is found especially in type 2 diabetes mellitus. Armanni-Ebstein lesions (deposition of glycogen in renal tubules) are seen in uncontrolled hyperglycemia, which can occur in either type. Glomerular Kimmelstiel-Wilson nodules are seen in long-standing diabetes, regardless of type. Similarly, proliferative retinopathy is a complication of both forms of diabetes.

20-D. Recurrent intractable peptic ulcer disease is characteristic of the Zollinger-Ellison syndrome with excess gastrin production, most often from a gastrinoma. Cushing syndrome causes an excess of cortisol. Glucagonoma is a rare neuroendocrine tumor of pancreatic alpha cells that can cause hyperglycemia. The Whipple triad (episodic hyperinsulinemia and hypoglycemia causing central nervous system dysfunction reversible by glucose administration) is seen with insulinoma. Acromegaly results from growth hormone excess.

21-C. The most common effect of maternal diabetes mellitus and hyperglycemia on the child is increased birth weight. This also increases the likelihood of obstetric complications, including the need for caesarean section and increased likelihood of brachial plexus injuries. Another complication is hyaline membrane disease. Cretinism results from deficiency of thyroid hormone during fetal development and during postnatal life. Ambiguous genitalia can occur in any of the adrenogenital syndromes. Sheehan syndrome occurs in the mother and has no relationship to diabetes. Thyroglossal duct cysts do not usually result in endocrine complications.

22-C. *Ret* codes for a transmembrane receptor tyrosine kinase that is mutated in the MEN IIa and MEN IIb syndromes as well as in sporadic cases of medullary carcinoma of the thyroid. *Bcr-abl* fusion results from the chromosomal translocation of chronic myelogenous leukemia. N-*myc* is amplified in neuroblastoma. Amylin derived from islet amyloid polypeptide accumulates in the pancreatic islets in type 2 diabetics.

CHAPTER 21

Skin

I. Terminology Relating to Skin Diseases

See Table 21.1 for terms and definitions relating to diseases of the skin.

II. Inflammatory and Vesicular Lesions

A. **Eczematous dermatitis** is a heterogeneous group of pruritic inflammatory disorders.

1. **Etiology**
   a. **Infection**
   b. **Chemicals** (contact dermatitis). Chemicals can directly injure skin or may act as antigens in type IV cell-mediated hypersensitivity reactions, resulting from cooperation of skin macrophages (Langerhans cells) and helper T lymphocytes.
   c. **Atopy (allergy).** Eczematous dermatitis frequently occurs in persons with type I anaphylactic-type hypersensitivities, such as hay fever or bronchial asthma; however, the skin manifestations in these atopic patients are most often caused by type IV rather than type I hypersensitivity.
2. **Morphologic findings** vary depending on the stage of the disorder.
   a. **Acute stage:** spongiosis with vesicle formation
   b. **Chronic stage:** acanthosis, hyperkeratosis, and lichenification; focal lymphocytic dermal infiltrates
   c. **Subacute stage:** intermediate changes between acute and chronic; less spongiosis and vesiculation than in acute; less acanthosis and hyperkeratosis than in chronic eczematous dermatitis

B. **Neurodermatitis (lichen simplex chronicus)**

1. This lesion is clinically indistinguishable from chronic eczematous dermatitis.
2. It produces anatomic changes entirely secondary to scratching. The cause of the pruritus is unknown but may be psychogenic.

C. **Psoriasis**

1. Erythematous papules and plaques with characteristic silvery scaling are typical of this chronic inflammatory process. Lesions are sharply demarcated.
2. Most often, the lesions involve the extensor surfaces of the elbows and knees as well as the scalp and sacral area.
3. Psoriasis is most often nonpruritic. It demonstrates histologic epidermal proliferation with acanthosis and highly characteristic parakeratosis; minute neutrophilic abscesses (Munro abscesses) may be found within the parakeratotic stratum corneum.
4. The condition may be of autoimmune etiology. It can be associated with severe destructive rheumatoid arthritis-like lesions (**psoriatic arthritis**) that most commonly affect the fingers.

TABLE 21-1 *Terms and Definitions Applied Specifically to Skin Disorders*

Term	Definition
Macule	Flat, nonpalpable lesion of a different color than the surrounding skin; less than 1 cm in diameter
Patch	Similar to macule; larger than 1 cm in diameter
Papule	Small, palpable, elevated skin lesion less than 1 cm in diameter
Plaque	Similar to papule; larger than 1 cm in diameter
Vesicle	Small fluid-containing blister
Bulla	Large fluid-containing blister; 0.5 cm or more in diameter
Pustule	Blister containing pus
Crust	Dried exudate from a vesicle, bulla, or pustule
Hyperkeratosis	Increased thickness of the stratum corneum
Parakeratosis	Hyperkeratosis with retention of nuclei of keratinocytes
Acanthosis	Thickening of the epidermis
Spongiosis	Epidermal intercellular edema with widening of intercellular spaces
Acantholysis	Separation of epidermal cells one from the other; cells appear to float within extracellular fluid
Lichenification	Accentuation of skin markings caused by scratching

Terms are arranged in loosely related groups, generally in order of increasing severity.

D. **Varicella (chickenpox)**

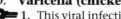

1. This viral infection of childhood is characterized by fever and a generalized vesicular eruption.
2. The varicella-zoster virus may remain latent for years in dorsal root ganglia.
3. Immune individuals may develop herpes zoster (shingles) in adult life. The painful skin eruption of herpes zoster has a characteristic distribution along the dermatomes corresponding to the affected dorsal root ganglia.

E. **Pemphigus vulgaris**

1. This acantholytic disorder occurs most often in persons 30 to 60 years of age.
2. The formation of severe intraepidermal bullae is characteristic. The first lesions often occur in the oral mucosa, and extensive skin involvement follows. Lesions often rupture, leaving large denuded surfaces subject to secondary infection.
3. Prominent intraepidermal acantholysis and sparing of the basal layer occur.
4. This autoimmune disorder is also characterized by IgG autoantibodies directed against the epidermal intercellular cement substance. Antibodies can be demonstrated in serum or by characteristic immunofluorescence encircling the individual epidermal cells.
5. Pemphigus vulgaris can be fatal.

F. **Bullous pemphigoid**

1. This disorder resembles pemphigus vulgaris but is clinically much less severe.
2. Features include subepidermal bullae, with a characteristic inflammatory infiltrate of eosinophils in the surrounding dermis.
3. This is an autoimmune disorder characterized by IgG autoantibodies directed against epidermal basement membrane. Antibodies can be demonstrated in serum or by a characteristic linear band of immunofluorescence along the basement membrane.

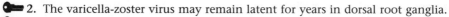

G. **Dermatitis herpetiformis**

1. Incidence is greatest in persons 20 to 40 years of age.
2. This recurrent pruritic blistering disorder usually involves the extensor surfaces of the knees and elbows, scalp, upper back, and sacral area.
3. Dermal microabscesses with neutrophils and eosinophils at the tips of dermal papillae, which become subepidermal blisters, are characteristic. Blisters tend to occur in groups.
4. Deposits of IgA at the tips of dermal papillae occur.
5. Dermatitis herpetiformis is commonly associated with gluten-sensitive enteropathy (celiac disease); both skin lesions and enteropathy improve when patients are placed on gluten-free diets.

H. **Erythema multiforme**

1. As the name suggests, this disorder presents with **multiple types of lesions,** including macules, papules, and vesicles.
2. It is most characteristically associated with a **"target" lesion** resembling an archer's bull's-eye.
3. There is usually **hypersensitivity** to coexistent infectious agents, various drugs, a concomitant connective tissue disorder, or an associated malignancy.

III. Disorders of Pigmentation

A. **Albinism** is a failure of pigment production by otherwise intact melanocytes. It occurs in two variants.

1. **Ocular albinism** is a melanin dysfunction that is limited to the eyes. This condition is an X-linked disorder.
2. **Oculocutaneous albinism** is a melanin synthetic defect that involves the eyes, skin, and hair; it **predisposes to actinic keratosis, basal and squamous cell carcinoma, and malignant melanoma** because of sensitivity of skin to sunlight. Inheritance is most often autosomal recessive. Oculocutaneous albinism is often subclassified as:
   a. **Tyrosinase-negative albinism**, which is failure of conversion of tyrosine to dihydroxyphenylalanine (DOPA), an intermediary in melanin synthesis.
   b. **Tyrosinase-positive albinism.** The mechanisms of deficient melanin synthesis are unknown.

B. **Vitiligo**

1. This acquired loss of melanocytes in discrete areas of skin appears as depigmented white patches.
2. This disorder has no relationship to albinism.
3. Vitiligo may be of autoimmune etiology; it is associated with other autoimmune disorders, such as Graves disease and Addison disease.
4. Antimelanocyte antibodies are sometimes demonstrable. Vitiligo may be caused by destruction of melanocytes by toxic intermediates of melanin production or by neurochemical factors.

C. **Freckle (ephelis)** is produced by an increase of melanin pigment within basal keratinocytes.

D. **Lentigo** is a pigmented macule caused by melanocytic hyperplasia in the epidermis.

E. **Pigmented nevi**

1. **Nevocellular nevus (common mole)**
   a. This lesion is variably classified as a **benign** tumor or hamartoma; nevus cells are derived from melanocytes and ordinarily occur in clusters or nests.
   b. The three most common types are:
      (1) **Junctional nevus:** nevus cells confined to the epidermal–dermal junction

(2) **Compound nevus:** nevus cells both at the epidermal–dermal junction and in the dermis

(3) **Intradermal nevus:** nevus cells confined to clusters within the dermis (these cells are often nonpigmented)

2. **Blue nevus**
   a. This condition is present at birth.
   b. Characteristics include nodular foci of dendritic, highly pigmented melanocytes in the dermis; the blue external appearance results from the dermal location.
3. **Spitz nevus (juvenile melanoma)**
   a. This disorder most often occurs in children.
   b. It is always **benign.** (The term juvenile melanoma is misleading and is falling into disuse.)
   c. It is often characterized by spindle-shaped cells and can be confused with malignant melanoma.
4. **Dysplastic nevus**
   a. This is an atypical, irregularly pigmented lesion with disorderly proliferation of melanocytes, dermal fibrosis, and often subjacent dermal lymphocytic infiltration.
   b. The lesions **may transform into malignant melanoma.**
   c. The disorder is familial in some cases (dysplastic nevus syndrome); these cases exhibit autosomal dominant inheritance and a marked tendency toward conversion to malignant melanoma.
5. **Lentigo maligna (Hutchinson freckle)**
   a. This disorder is a nonfamilial **precursor to lentigo maligna melanoma.**
   b. This irregular macular pigmented lesion on sun-exposed skin is characterized by atypical melanocytes at the epidermal–dermal junction.

IV. Disorders of Viral Origin

A. Molluscum contagiosum

1. This contagious viral disorder occurs most often in children and adolescents.
2. Transmission is by direct contact.
3. This disorder is due to a DNA poxvirus.
4. Umbilicated, dome-shaped papules are characteristic.

B. Verruca vulgaris (common wart)

1. This benign papilloma is caused by certain strains of human papillomavirus (HPV), which are distinct from those associated with gynecologic neoplasms.
2. Vacuolated cells (koilocytes) in the granular cell layer of the epidermis are characteristic.

V. Miscellaneous Skin Disorders

A. Acrochordon (fibroepithelial polyp, skin tag)

1. This extremely common lesion occurs most often on the face near the eyelids, neck, trunk, or axilla.
2. It consists of a central connective tissue core covered by stratified squamous epithelium.

B. Epidermal inclusion cyst

1. This cyst is lined by stratified squamous epithelium and is filled with keratinous material. It has erroneously been called a sebaceous cyst; the sebaceous glands are not involved.
2. It manifests clinically as a dome-shaped nodule that is filled with soft gray-white material.

C. **Dermatofibroma**

1. This benign neoplasm presents as a firm nodule, sometimes with pigmented acanthosis. It is termed fibrous histiocytoma when histiocytes are prominent.
2. Intertwining bundles of collagen and fibroblasts are characteristic.

D. **Dermatofibrosarcoma protuberans.** This slowly growing, well-differentiated malignant neoplasm histologically resembles dermatofibroma. It rarely metastasizes.

E. **Seborrheic keratosis**

1. This extremely common benign neoplasm of older persons is also called senile keratosis.
2. Manifestations include sharply demarcated raised papules or plaques with a typical pasted-on appearance; lesions occur on the head, trunk, and extremities.

F. **Keratoacanthoma**

1. This disorder is generally considered to be a benign neoplasm that closely resembles squamous cell carcinoma.
2. It regresses spontaneously without therapy.

G. **Actinic keratosis**

1. This **premalignant** epidermal lesion is caused by chronic excessive exposure to sunlight.
2. Characteristics include rough, scaling, poorly demarcated plaques on the face, neck, upper trunk, or extremities.

H. **Acanthosis nigricans**

1. This disorder is sometimes a **marker of visceral malignancy** (stomach, lung, breast, uterus).
2. Acanthosis and hyperpigmentation, most often involving flexural areas, are characteristic.

I. **Xanthoma**

1. This disorder is most often associated with hypercholesterolemia.
2. Characteristics include yellowish papules or nodules composed of focal dermal collections of lipid-laden histiocytes.
3. Xanthoma occurs most frequently on the eyelids (xanthelasma); it can also occur as nodules over tendons or joints.

J. **Hemangioma** is sometimes considered to be a hamartoma rather than a neoplasm.

1. **Major forms**
   a. **Capillary hemangioma:** small, blood-filled capillaries lined with a single layer of endothelium. Capillary hemangioma occurs in three variants:
      (1) **Port-wine stain:** purple-red area on the face or neck
      (2) **Strawberry hemangioma:** bright-red raised lesion
      (3) **Cherry hemangioma:** small, dome-shaped red papule
   b. **Cavernous hemangioma:** large, endothelial-lined spaces in the dermis and subdermis
2. **Other manifestations.** Hemangiomas occur rarely as part of:
   a. **Sturge-Weber syndrome**
      (1) This disorder involves port-wine stain of the face, ipsilateral glaucoma, vascular lesions of ocular choroidal tissue, and extensive hemangiomatous involvement of meninges.
      (2) Clinical manifestations include convulsions, mental retardation, and retinal detachment.
   b. **von Hippel-Lindau disease** involves multiple vascular tumors and other tumors and cysts that are widely scattered throughout many organ systems.

K. **Granuloma pyogenicum**
   1. This vascular pedunculated lesion is characterized by numerous capillaries and edematous stroma. It is common in skin or mucous membranes.
   2. It often develops following trauma.

L. **Keloid**
   1. This abnormal proliferation of the connective tissue, with deranged arrangement of collagen fibers, results in large, raised, tumor-like scars.
   2. This condition occurs in genetically susceptible individuals, more frequently in those of African lineage.
   3. It often follows trauma to the skin, such as ear-piercing or surgical wounds.
   4. It tends to recur after resection.

VI. Skin Malignancies

A. **Squamous cell carcinoma** is a common malignant skin tumor.
   1. This disorder is most often locally invasive; fewer than 5% of tumors metastasize. Excision is usually curative.
   2. It is associated most often with excessive exposure to sunlight; it occurs most frequently in sun-exposed areas such as the face and back of the hands; in contrast to basal cell carcinoma, squamous cell carcinoma tends to involve the lower part of the face. It is also associated with chemical carcinogens, such as arsenic, and radiation or radiologic exposure.
   3. It frequently originates in a preexisting actinic keratosis.
   4. Squamous cell carcinoma most often presents as a scaling, indurated, ulcerated nodule. Invasion of dermis by **sheets and islands of neoplastic epidermal cells,** often with **keratin "pearls"** is characteristic.

B. **Basal cell carcinoma** is the most common of all malignant skin tumors.
   1. This disorder tends to involve sun-exposed areas, most frequently the head and neck; in contrast to squamous cell carcinoma, tends to involve the upper part of the face.
   2. It grossly presents as a pearly papule, often with overlying telangiectatic vessels.
   3. It is characterized by clusters of darkly staining basaloid cells with a typical **palisade arrangement of the nuclei** of the cells at the periphery of the tumor cell clusters.
   4. Basal cell carcinoma can be locally aggressive, ulcerate, and bleed; however, it almost never metastasizes. It is almost always cured by surgical resection.

C. **Malignant melanoma**
   1. **General considerations**
      a. The incidence is increasing. Malignant melanoma is most common in fair-skinned persons.
      b. This disorder arises from melanocytes or nevus cells.
      c. It is most often associated with **excessive exposure to sunlight.**
   2. **Growth phases**
      a. **Radial (initial phase)**
         (1) Growth occurs in all directions but is predominantly lateral within the epidermis and papillary zone of the dermis.
         (2) Lymphocytic response is prominent.
         (3) Melanomas in the radial growth phase do not metastasize; clinical cure is frequent.
      b. **Vertical (later phase)**
         (1) Growth extends into the reticular dermis or beyond.
         (2) Prognosis varies with the depth of the lesion.
         (3) Lymphatics or hematogenous metastasis may occur.
   3. **Clinical variants**
      a. Malignant melanomas have a better prognosis when characterized by a long period of radial growth than when associated with an early vertical growth phase.

b. The most important clinical variants include:

(1) **Lentigo maligna melanoma** occurs on sun-exposed skin. The radial growth phase predominates initially; most often develops from preexisting lentigo maligna (Hutchinson freckle).

(2) **Superficial spreading melanoma** is the most common of the variants. The lesion is irregularly bordered with variegated pigmentation; most frequent locations are the trunk and extremities. Radial growth phase predominates.

(3) **Nodular melanoma** begins with the vertical growth phase. It has the **poorest prognosis** of the clinical variants.

(4) **Acral-lentiginous melanoma** most often appears on the hands and feet of dark-skinned persons.

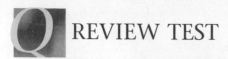

REVIEW TEST

Directions: *Each of the numbered items or incomplete statements in this section is followed by answers or by completions of the statement. Select the* ***one*** *lettered answer or completion that is best in each case.*

1. A 70-year-old retired farm worker is seen for evaluation of a pearly appearing papule on the face just below and lateral to the left eye. The lesion is covered by small telangiectatic vessels. An excisional biopsy is performed, and the microscopic appearance is similar to that seen in the figure. Which of the following is characteristic of this disorder?

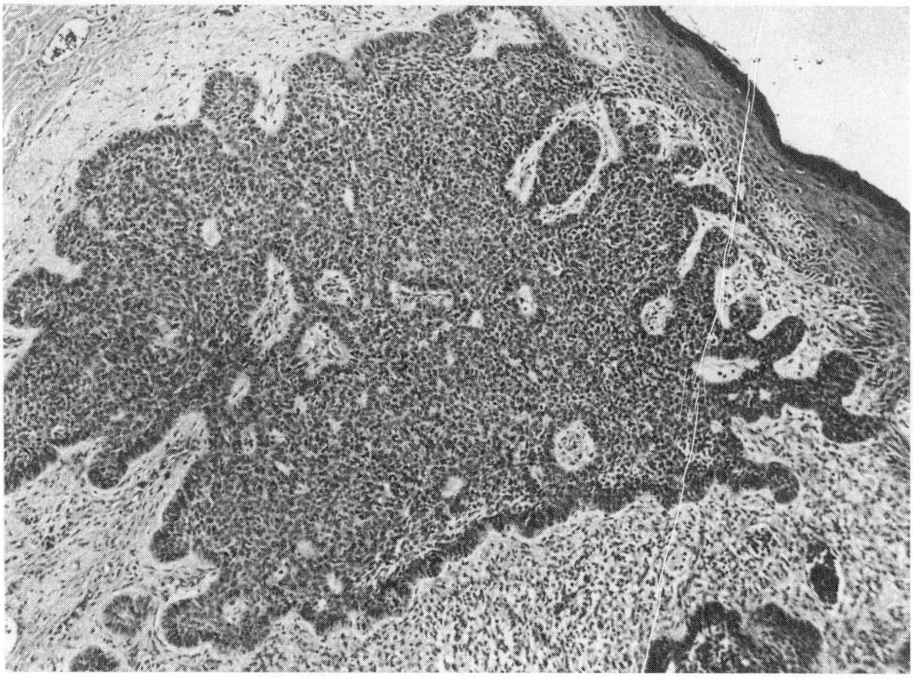

(Reprinted with permission from Golden A, Powell D, and Jennings C: *Pathology: Understanding Human Disease,* 2nd ed. Baltimore, Williams & Wilkins, 1985, p 508.)

(A) Distal metastases common at the time of initial diagnosis
(B) Frequent origin in a preexisting actinic keratosis
(C) Hamartomatous non-neoplastic lesion
(D) Most frequent occurrence on head or neck

2. A scaling, ulcerated lesion develops on the forearm of a 45-year-old fisherman. Excisional biopsy is performed, and the histologic appearance is similar to that shown in the figure. Which of the following is most applicable to this lesion?

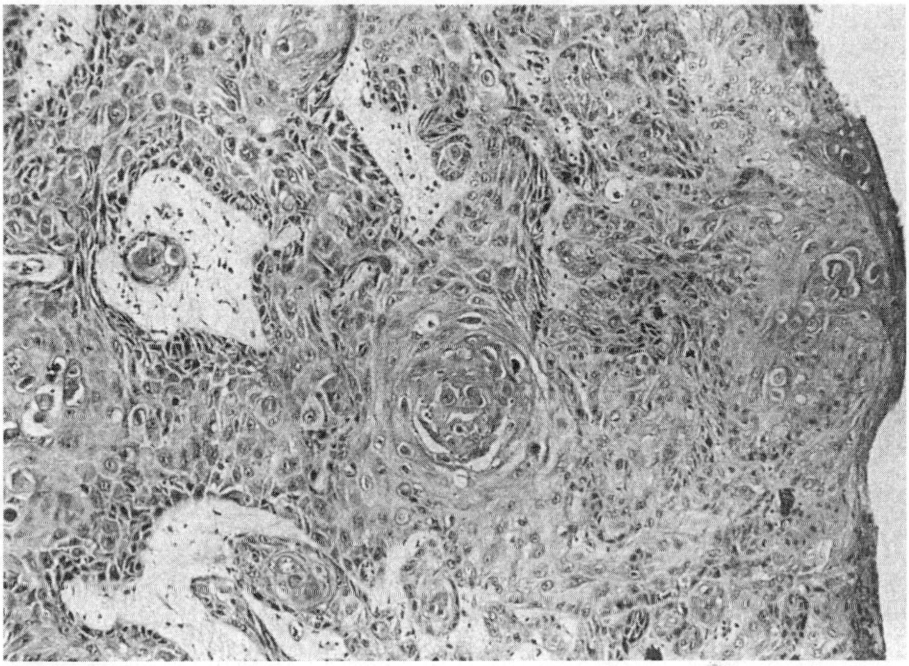

(Reprinted with permission from Golden A, Powell D, and Jennings C: *Pathology: Understanding Human Disease,* 2nd ed. Baltimore, Williams & Wilkins, 1985, p 506.)

(A) Distal metastases almost always occur
(B) Indicative of an underlying visceral malignancy
(C) Predilection for sun-exposed areas
(D) Uncommon skin tumor

3. A 20-year-old woman presents with a skin rash. The rash is localized to the extensor surfaces of her elbows and knees, and is composed of multiple well-demarcated circular to oval-shaped plaques and papules covered by a silvery scale overlying reddened erythematous skin. The silvery scale can be scraped off, revealing inflamed skin underneath. She states that several family members have a similar rash. Which of the following is the most likely diagnosis?

(A) Neurodermatitis (lichen simplex chronicus)
(B) Psoriasis
(C) Pemphigus vulgaris
(D) Bullous pemphigoid
(E) Dermatitis herpetiformis

4. An 8-year-old boy presents with an intensely pruritic vesicular rash and fever. Several playmates have had similar findings. The etiology of this common infectious exanthem is

(A) autoimmune
(B) bacterial
(C) fungal
(D) parasitic
(E) viral

5. A 25-year-old man presents with a skin rash of "target" lesions on the palms of the hands, the soles of the feet, and the arms and legs. The rash is composed of macules, papules, and vesicles. The dermatologist makes a diagnosis of erythema multiforme. Which of the following is the probable etiology of this condition?

(A) Physical scratching of the skin
(B) IgG autoantibodies directed against the epidermal intercellular cement substance
(C) IgA antibody deposits localized to the tips of dermal papillae
(D) Hypersensitivity to multiple concomitant infectious agents or drugs
(E) Chemical exposure

6. An 80-year-old man presents with sharply demarcated, light brown, flat macules varying markedly in size. The lesions have the appearance of being "stuck on" or "pasted on," and they are particularly numerous on the trunk. Microscopically, sheets of small basaloid cells with some melanin production are seen. Keratin production occurs at the surface, and numerous small keratin-filled cysts are apparent. Which of the following is the likely diagnosis?

(A) Seborrheic keratosis
(B) Dermatofibroma
(C) Keratoacanthoma
(D) Actinic keratosis
(E) Acanthosis nigricans

7. A 25-year-old woman presents with concern about a mole on her abdomen. The mole is small, round, symmetric, and dark-colored, and has sharply defined borders. It is diagnosed as a common mole. This lesion is properly termed a

(A) nevocellular nevus
(B) blue nevus
(C) Spitz nevus
(D) dysplastic nevus
(E) lentigo maligna

8. A 20-year-old woman presents with depigmented white patches of skin on the face, neck, and hands. She has a past history of Graves disease. Which of the following is the most likely diagnosis?

(A) Ocular albinism
(B) Oculocutaneous albinism
(C) Vitiligo
(D) Freckle
(E) Verruca vulgaris (common wart)

9. A 70-year-old man presents with a scaling, indurated, ulcerated nodule on the back of his left hand. He states that the nodule has been growing larger over time. The patient has had much direct sun exposure in the past. Which of the following is the most likely histologic finding in this patient's skin lesion?

(A) Invasion of the dermis by sheets and islands of neoplastic epidermal cells, often with "keratin pearls"
(B) Clusters of darkly staining basaloid cells, with a palisading arrangement of the nuclei of the cells at the periphery of the clusters
(C) Malignant melanocytes with numerous mitotic figures
(D) Abnormal proliferation of the connective tissue, with deranged arrangement of collagen fibers

10. A 55-year-old man presents with a large, black-colored, asymmetric skin lesion with ill-defined borders on his back. He reports a family history of malignant melanoma. Which of the following clinical variants of malignant melanoma has the poorest prognosis?

(A) Lentigo maligna melanoma
(B) Superficial spreading melanoma
(C) Nodular melanoma
(D) Acral-lentiginous melanoma

ANSWERS AND EXPLANATIONS

1-D. The basal cell carcinoma shown in the figure has typical palisading of the nuclei of the cells at the periphery of the tumor cell clusters. Unlike squamous cell carcinoma, this tumor does not originate in preexisting actinic keratosis.

2-C. The lesion shown in the figure is a well-differentiated squamous cell carcinoma demonstrating sheets of neoplastic epidermal cells with keratin "pearls," a very common skin tumor. There is a marked predilection for sun-exposed areas, and most lesions occur on the lower part of the face or the back of the hands. Metastasis occurs in fewer than 5% of cases, because most of these lesions are discovered early and are cured by ablative therapy.

3-B. Psoriasis is a chronic inflammatory skin disease characterized by erythematous plaques covered with a silvery scale. Histologic findings include epidermal proliferation with acanthosis, parakeratosis, and Munro abscesses (minute neutrophilic abscesses). Psoriasis is sometimes associated with a rheumatoid arthritis–like condition termed psoriatic arthritis.

4-E. Chickenpox (varicella), caused by the varicella-zoster virus, is a viral infection of childhood characterized by fever and a predominantly vesicular rash. Following overt varicella, the virus can remain latent for years in dorsal root ganglia and reappear several years later as herpes zoster (shingles).

5-D. Erythema multiforme manifests as a variegated group of lesions: macules, papules, and vesicles. The most characteristic of these is the "target" lesion. The disorder is thought due to hypersensitivity, often to coexistent stimuli such as infectious agents or drugs, or to a concomitant connective tissue disorder or an associated malignancy.

6-A. Seborrheic keratosis is an extremely common benign neoplasm occurring in older persons. This neoplasm is manifest by sharply demarcated, raised papules or plaques with a "pasted-on" appearance on the head, trunk, and extremities.

7-A. A nevocellular nevus (common mole) is a benign tumor or hamartoma. Nevus cells are derived from melanocytes and ordinarily occur in clusters or nests. A dysplastic nevus is an atypical, irregularly pigmented lesion with disorderly proliferation of melanocytes, dermal fibrosis, and lymphocytic infiltration. Dysplastic nevi may transform into malignant melanoma. Lentigo maligna is characterized by atypical melanocytes at the epidermal-dermal junction and is a precursor to lentigo maligna melanoma.

8-C. Vitiligo is an acquired loss of melanocytes in discrete areas of skin that appear as depigmented white patches. Vitiligo has no relationship to albinism. It is sometimes associated with autoimmune disorders, such as Graves disease, Addison disease, and antimelanocyte antibodies.

9-A. This is a case of squamous cell carcinoma of the skin. Squamous cell carcinoma is a common skin tumor associated with excessive sun exposure. Clusters of darkly staining basaloid cells with a palisading arrangement of nuclei are characteristic of basal cell carcinoma. Malignant melanocytes are found in malignant melanoma. A keloid is a tumor-like scar resulting from abnormal proliferation of connective tissue with deranged arrangement of collagen fibers.

10-C. Malignant melanoma arises from melanocytes or nevus cells, is most often associated with excessive sun exposure, and is most common in fair-skinned persons. Of the clinical variants of malignant melanoma, nodular melanoma has the worst prognosis. Malignant melanomas have a better prognosis when characterized by a long period of radial (superficial) growth, as opposed to early vertical growth (as in nodular melanoma).

CHAPTER 22

Musculoskeletal System

I. Diseases of Skeletal Muscle

A. **Muscle atrophies**

1. **Denervation atrophy** is associated with muscle denervation.
   a. This type of change involves both type I (red) and type II (white) fibers, which may appear small and angular on cross section. **Target fibers,** which have a central darker area reminiscent of the bull's-eye of a target, may also be seen.
   b. After reinnervation occurs, **fiber-type grouping,** a cluster of type I fibers adjacent to a cluster of type II fibers, may be seen. This contrasts with the mixture of individual type I and type II fibers characteristic of normal muscle.
2. **Disuse atrophy** is associated with prolonged immobilization. It is characterized histologically by **angular atrophy,** primarily of type II fibers.

B. **Muscular dystrophies**

1. **General considerations**
   a. This group of genetically determined, progressive disorders is characterized by degeneration of skeletal muscle and profound wasting and weakness. They are differentiated by age of onset, muscle groups involved, and mode of inheritance.
   b. Increased serum activities of creatine kinase (CK) and other muscle enzymes derived from degenerating muscle fibers are characteristic.
   c. Nonspecific degenerative changes on muscle biopsy are also characteristic. Although nonspecific, the muscle biopsy findings are helpful in distinguishing dystrophies from abnormalities secondary to denervation or from entities characterized by specific morphologic changes
2. **Duchenne muscular dystrophy** is the most common and most severe of the muscular dystrophies.
   a. This type of dystrophy occurs almost entirely in male children.
   b. It begins with weakness in the proximal muscles of the extremities, commencing at about 1 year of age and progressing to immobilization, wasting, muscle contracture, and death in the early teens, most often due to pneumonia caused by weakness of respiratory muscles.
   c. The cause is a deficiency of dystrophin.
   d. The dystrophy exhibits **X-linked inheritance;** as many as one third of cases resulting from de novo mutation. Various deletions or point mutations occur involving segments of the dystrophin gene, which is located on the short arm of the X chromosome. The mutations are variable but are constant within families and lead characteristically to a DNA coding frameshift, with resultant formation of stop codons and total failure of dystrophin synthesis.

e. Histologic characteristics include random variation in muscle fiber size, necrosis of individual muscle fibers, and replacement of necrotic fibers by fibrofatty tissue.
f. Laboratory characteristics include **increased serum CK.**
g. Duchenne muscular dystrophy presents initially in proximal muscles of the extremities.
h. It is characterized later by **compensatory hypertrophy** of distal sites, such as the calf muscles, followed eventually by **pseudohypertrophy** (increased fibrous tissue and adipose tissue).

3. **Becker muscular dystrophy**
   a. Becker muscular dystrophy is clinically similar to, but less severe than, Duchenne muscular dystrophy.
   b. It is also caused by an abnormality in dystrophin; the molecule is truncated and presumably less functional. The dystrophin abnormality is caused by segmental deletions within the gene that do not cause a coding frameshift.
4. **Facioscapulohumeral muscular dystrophy**
   a. This dystrophy demonstrates autosomal dominant inheritance.
   b. It is associated with a slowly progressive, nondisabling course and an almost normal life expectancy.
   c. It sequentially involves the muscles of the face, scapular area, and humerus.
5. **Limb-girdle dystrophy**
   a. This disorder demonstrates autosomal recessive inheritance.
   b. It involves the proximal muscles of the shoulder, pelvic girdle, or both.
6. **Myotonic dystrophy**
   a. This disorder demonstrates an autosomal dominant mode of inheritance.
   b. Characteristics include a weakness associated with **myotonia** (inability to relax muscles once contracted).
   c. Associated features include **cataracts** as well as with **testicular atrophy** and baldness in men.
   d. It is an example of a disorder caused by an increased number of trinucleotide repeats. Normal individuals have less than 30 CTG repeats in the myotonin protein kinase gene, whereas patients with myotonic dystrophy can have from 50 to 1000 repeats. In addition, the number of trinucleotide repeats increases with each generation (anticipation), with a corresponding earlier age of onset and more severe manifestations.

C. **Congenital myopathies with specific histologic changes.** These disorders are often characterized by floppy infant syndrome, marked hypotonia at birth. They can be distinguished from dystrophies by the combination of specific histologic changes, often with normal serum creatine kinase.

1. **Central core disease**
   a. A loss of mitochondria and other organelles in the central portion of type I muscle fibers occurs.
   b. This disease is characterized by muscle weakness and hypotonia, but affected infants eventually become ambulatory.
2. **Nemaline myopathy**
   a. This disease demonstrates tangles of small rod-shaped granules predominantly in type I fibers.
   b. It varies clinically from a mild, nonprogressive disease to severe weakness ending in death from respiratory failure.
3. **Mitochondrial myopathies**
   a. These diseases demonstrate non-Mendelian inheritance.
   b. They are mediated by maternally transmitted mitochondrial DNA abnormalities (most often deletions).
   c. They may be characterized by a ragged red appearance of muscle fibers and by various mitochondrial enzyme or coenzyme defects. For example, the Kearns-Sayre syndrome is characterized by ophthalmoplegia, pigmentary retinopathy, heart block, cerebellar ataxia, and an exclusively **maternal mode of transmission.**

D. **Myasthenia gravis**

1. This autoimmune disorder is caused by **autoantibodies to acetylcholine receptors** of the neuromuscular junction.
2. It is three times more frequent in women than in men.
3. Characteristics include muscle weakness intensified by muscle use, with recovery on rest.
4. Clinical manifestations include effort-associated weakness involving the extraocular and facial muscles, muscles of the extremities, and other muscle groups.
5. Presenting features frequently include ptosis or diplopia, or difficulty in chewing, speaking, or swallowing. This disease can be complicated by respiratory failure.
6. Myasthenia gravis improves dramatically with administration of drugs with anticholinesterase activity, an important diagnostic finding.
7. The disorder is frequently associated with tumors of the thymus or with thymic hyperplasia.

E. **Lambert-Eaton syndrome**

1. This paraneoplastic disorder (most commonly associated with small cell carcinoma of the lung) has clinical manifestations similar to those of myasthenia gravis.
2. The cause is a defect in the release of acetylcholine by nerve cells.
3. It may be due to acquired autoantibodies that react with presynaptic voltage-gated calcium channels.

II. Diseases of Bone

A. **Metabolic bone disease** is usually characterized by osteopenia (diffuse radiolucency of bone) or alterations in serum calcium, phosphorus, and alkaline phosphatase (Table 22-1).

1. **Osteoporosis** is characterized by a **decrease in bone mass.**
   a. The cause may be impaired synthesis or increased resorption of bone matrix protein.
   b. It results in bone structures inadequate for weight bearing; fractures commonly occur, especially compression fractures of the vertebrae that cause spinal deformity (most typically kyphosis) and shortened stature.
   c. Radiographic characteristics include diffuse radiolucency of bone.
   d. Clinical associations include:
      (1) **Postmenopausal state** (estrogen deficiency is a presumptive cause)
      (2) **Physical inactivity**
      (3) **Hypercorticism**
      (4) **Hyperthyroidism**
      (5) **Calcium deficiency**
2. **von Recklinghausen disease of bone (osteitis fibrosa cystica)**
   a. The cause is primary or secondary **hyperparathyroidism.**
   b. Widespread osteolytic lesions are characteristic.
   c. von Recklinghausen disease of bone may manifest as "**brown tumor**" of bone, cystic spaces that are lined by multinucleated osteoclasts and filled with vascular fibrous stroma, often with brown discoloration resulting from hemorrhage.

TABLE 22-1 *Blood Chemistries in Metabolic Bone Disease*

Bone Disease	Calcium	Phosphorus	Alkaline Phosphatase
Osteoporosis	Normal	Normal	Normal or decreased
Von Recklinghausen disease of bone	Increased	Decreased	Increased
Osteomalacia and rickets	Decreased or normal	Variable	Increased or normal
Paget disease of bone	Normal	Normal	Markedly increased

d. Diffuse radiolucency of bone mimicking osteoporosis may sometimes be evident.
e. Laboratory manifestations of hyperparathyroidism, high serum calcium, low serum phosphorus, and high serum alkaline phosphatase occur.

3. **Osteomalacia**
a. The cause is **vitamin D deficiency in adults.**
b. Defective calcification of osteoid matrix is characteristic.
c. Diffuse radiolucency, which can mimic osteoporosis, is characteristic radiographically.
d. When secondary to renal disease, osteomalacia is called **renal osteodystrophy.**

4. **Rickets**
a. This disorder is caused by **vitamin D deficiency in children.**
b. Decreased calcification and excess accumulation of osteoid lead to increased thickness of the epiphyseal growth plates and other skeletal deformities.
c. Clinical manifestations include:
(1) **Craniotabes:** thinning and softening of occipital and parietal bones
(2) **Late closing of fontanelles**
(3) **Rachitic rosary:** thickening of the costochondral junctions that results in a string-of-beads-like appearance
(4) **Harrison groove:** depression along the line of insertion of the diaphragm into the rib cage
(5) **Pigeon breast:** caused by protrusion of the sternum
(6) **Decreased height:** caused by a spinal deformity

5. **Paget disease of bone (osteitis deformans)** is most common in the elderly.
a. This disorder is of unknown etiology; a viral etiology is suggested by ultrastructural intranuclear inclusions in osteoclasts; studies suggest the possible role of a slow virus infection by a paramyxovirus.
b. **Abnormal bone architecture** caused by **increases in both osteoblastic and osteoclastic activity** is characteristic.
c. Paget disease of bone most commonly involves the spine, pelvis, calvarium of the skull, femur, and tibia.
d. Clinical manifestations may include a **marked increase in serum alkaline phosphatase** (a manifestation of osteoblastic activity) and normal serum calcium and phosphorus.
e. This disorder can be **monostotic** (involving only one bone) or **polyostotic** (involving multiple bones).
f. **Morphologic phases**
(1) **Osteolytic phase:** osteoclastic resorption predominates.
(2) **Mixed osteoblastic and osteolytic phase:** new bone formation leads to a characteristic **mosaic pattern.**
(3) **Late phase:** bone density is increased; trabeculae are thick; and mosaic pattern is prominent.
g. **Complications**
(1) **Bone pain resulting from fractures:** although bone is thick, it lacks strength; fractures can lead to deformity.
(2) **High-output cardiac failure** can result from multiple functional arteriovenous shunts within highly vascular early lesions.
(3) **Hearing loss** is caused by narrowing of the auditory foramen or direct involvement of the bones of the middle ear.
(4) **Osteosarcoma** occurs in approximately 1% of cases. **Note:** Except for its occurrence in Paget disease, osteosarcoma most often affects younger people.

B. **Other non-neoplastic diseases of bone**

1. **Scurvy**
a. The cause is **ascorbic acid (vitamin C) deficiency.**
b. Scurvy is characterized by bone lesions leading to **impaired osteoid matrix formation.** This, in turn, is caused by the failure of the proline and lysine hydroxylation required for collagen synthesis.

c. Manifestations include the following bone changes:
   (1) **Subperiosteal hemorrhage** (often painful)
   (2) **Osteoporosis** (especially at the metaphyseal ends of bone)
   (3) **Epiphyseal cartilage not replaced by osteoid**

2. **Achondroplasia** is one of the most common causes of dwarfism.
   a. This autosomal dominant disorder is caused by a mutation in the fibroblast growth factor receptor 3 (*FGFR3*) gene, which is located at 4p16.3.
   b. Short limbs with a normal-sized head and trunk are characteristic. Additional features include narrow epiphyseal plates and bony sealing off of the area between the epiphyseal plate and the metaphysis; the failure of elongation results in short, thick bones.
3. **Fibrous dysplasia**
   a. This disorder is characterized by replacement of portions of bone with fibrous tissue.
   b. It is of unknown etiology.
   c. There are three main types:
      (1) **Monostotic fibrous dysplasia:** solitary lesions that are often asymptomatic but can result in spontaneous fractures with pain, swelling, and deformity.
      (2) **Polyostotic fibrous dysplasia:** multiple sites are involved; it can be associated with severe deformity.
      (3) **McCune-Albright syndrome:** polyostotic fibrous dysplasia, precocious puberty, café-au-lait spots on skin, and short stature, occurring in very young girls. The skin manifestations have irregular borders, sometimes likened to the "coast of Maine." The disorder is usually caused by a postzygotic somatic cell mutation of the *GNAS*1 gene, which codes for a G protein, and is thus genetic but often not hereditary.
4. **Aseptic (avascular) necrosis**
   a. This disorder is most often of unknown etiology. It most often results from infarction caused by interruption of arterial blood supply.
   b. It can be secondary to trauma or to embolism of diverse types, such as thrombosis, decompression syndrome or "the bends," and sickle cell anemia.
   c. In growing children, avascular necrosis may involve a variety of characteristic sites, including the head of the femur **(Legg-Calvé-Perthes disease)**, the tibial tubercle **(Osgood-Schlatter disease)**, or the navicular bone **(Köhler bone disease)**.
5. **Osteogenesis imperfecta**
   a. This disorder is characterized by multiple fractures occurring with minimal trauma **(brittle bone disease)**.
   b. The cause is a group of specific gene mutations, all resulting in defective collagen synthesis, which results in generalized connective tissue abnormalities affecting the teeth, skin, eyes, and bones.
   c. **Blue sclerae** from translucency of thin connective tissue overlying the choroid are often present.
   d. The several clinical types vary greatly in severity. In the most common type, an autosomal dominant variant, blue sclerae and multiple childhood fractures are prominent clinical findings.
6. **Osteopetrosis (marble bone disease, Albers-Schönberg disease)**
   a. This disorder is characterized by greatly increased density of the skeleton.
   b. The cause is failure of osteoclastic activity.
   c. Osteopetrosis is associated with multiple fractures in spite of increased bone density. In addition, it is associated with anemia as a result of decreased marrow space, and with blindness, deafness, and cranial nerve involvement because of narrowing and impingement of neural foramina.
   d. It occurs in two major clinical forms: an autosomal recessive variant that is usually fatal in infancy and a less severe autosomal dominant variant.
7. **Pyogenic osteomyelitis**
   a. **Etiology**
      (1) In **children,** pyogenic osteomyelitis occurs most often as a result of blood-borne spread from an infection located elsewhere. *Staphylococcus aureus* is the most com-

mon organism; group B β-streptococci or *Escherichia coli* are frequent in newborns; *Salmonella* is frequent in association with sickle cell anemia.
(2) In **adults,** the disorder occurs usually as a complication of compound fracture or a sequela of surgery.
(3) In **intravenous drug users,** the disorder is often a result of *Pseudomonas* infection.

b. **Characteristics**
(1) Pyogenic osteomyelitis is an acute pyogenic infection of bone.
(2) It most often initially involves the metaphysis; the distal end of the femur, proximal end of the tibia, and proximal end of the humerus are the most common sites.

c. **Course**
(1) In the acute stage, pyogenic osteomyelitis may resolve with antibiotic therapy.
(2) The disorder may compress vasculature with pyogenic exudate, resulting in ischemic necrosis of bone and marrow; necrotic bone **(sequestrum)** acts as a foreign body and as a locus for persistent infection.
(3) Subperiosteal dissection by pyogenic exudate may further impair blood supply; pus can rupture into surrounding tissues and form sinuses draining through skin.
(4) A sleeve of new bone formation **(involucrum)** may surround the infected necrotic area, which may be localized by a surrounding wall of granulation tissue (Brodie abscess).
(5) The disorder may be complicated by secondary (reactive systemic) amyloidosis.

8. **Tuberculous osteomyelitis**
a. This disorder is secondary to tuberculous infection located elsewhere.
b. It characteristically occurs in:
(1) **Vertebrae (Pott disease);** vertebral collapse can lead to spinal deformity.
(2) **Hip**
(3) **Long bones, especially the femur and tibia**
(4) **Bones of the hands and feet**

9. **Histiocytosis X** can occur in various sites, including bone.
a. This group of disorders is characterized by proliferation of histiocytic cells that closely resemble the Langerhans cells of the epidermis; **Birbeck granules,** tennis racket-shaped cytoplasmic structures, are characteristic markers of these cells; distinctive surface antigens also characterize these Langerhans-like cells.
b. Histiocytosis X includes the following variants:
(1) **Letterer-Siwe disease** (acute disseminated Langerhans cell histiocytosis)
(a) This disease is an aggressive, usually fatal, disorder of infants and small children.
(b) Characteristics include hepatosplenomegaly, lymphadenopathy, pancytopenia, pulmonary involvement, and recurrent infections as a result of widespread histiocytic proliferation.
(2) **Hand-Schüller-Christian disease** (chronic progressive histiocytosis)
(a) This disease has a better prognosis than Letterer-Siwe disease.
(b) It usually presents before 5 years of age.
(c) Characteristics include histiocytic proliferation mixed with inflammatory cells in bone, especially the skull; liver; spleen; and other tissues.
(d) Clinical manifestations include the classic triad of skull lesions, diabetes insipidus, and exophthalmos caused by involvement of the orbit.
(3) **Eosinophilic granuloma**
(a) This disease has the best prognosis within the group; fatalities are rare, and lesions sometimes heal without treatment.
(b) This disease can present as a solitary bone lesion; extraskeletal involvement is most often limited to the lung.
(c) Histiocytic proliferation mixed with inflammatory cells, including ordinary macrophages, lymphocytes, and many eosinophils is characteristic.

C. **Bone tumors**

1. **General considerations**

   a. The most frequently occurring **benign** tumors of bone are **osteochondroma and giant cell tumor.**

   b. The most frequently occurring **malignant** tumors of bone are **osteosarcoma, chondrosarcoma, and Ewing sarcoma;** this excludes **metastatic carcinoma** and **multiple myeloma,** which are **more common than primary bone tumors.**

   c. Table 22-2 presents a comparison of several important bone tumors.

2. **Benign bone tumors**

   a. **Osteochondroma (exostosis)** is the most common benign tumor of bone.

      (1) This bone growth is covered by a cap of cartilage projecting from the surface of a bone.

      (2) It occurs most frequently in men younger than 25 years of age.

      (3) It may be a hamartoma rather than a true neoplasm.

      (4) The tumor most often originates from the metaphysis of long bones, with the lower end of the femur or the upper end of the tibia being favored locations.

      (5) It rarely undergoes transition to chondrosarcoma; malignant transformation is more frequent in multiple familial osteochondromatosis, a rare hereditary variant characterized by multiple lesions.

TABLE 22-2 *Notable Features of Selected Bone Tumors*

Type	Description	Most Frequent Location	Incidence
Benign			
Osteochondroma (exostosis)	Cartilage-capped subperiosteal bony projection from bone surface	Lower end of the femur and upper end of the tibia	Males under age 25
Giant cell tumor	Tumor characterized by multinucleated giant cells and fibrous stroma	Epiphyses of the long bones, especially at the lower end of the femur and the upper end of the tibia	Females ages 20–40
Enchondroma	Intramedullary cartilaginous neoplasm	Bones of the hands and feet	No special age or sex incidence
Osteoma	Tumor of dense mature bone	Skull or facial bones; often protrudes into a paranasal sinus	Males of any age
Osteoid osteoma	Neoplastic proliferation of osteoid and fibrous tissue	Near the end of the diaphysis of the femur or tibia	Males under age 25
Osteoblastoma	...	Within vertebrae	...
Malignant			
Osteosarcoma (osteogenic sarcoma)	Osteoid- and bone-producing neoplasm	Tibia and femur near the knee	Males ages 10–20
Chondrosarcoma	Cartilaginous tumor	Pelvic bones, proximal and distal femur, proximal tibia, ribs, vertebrae	Males ages 30–60
Ewing sarcoma	Undifferentiated "small blue cell" tumor	Long bones, pelvis, scapulae, and ribs	Males under age 15

b. **Giant cell tumor**
(1) This disorder is characterized by oval or spindle-shaped cells intermingled with numerous multinuclear giant cells.
(2) The peak incidence is in persons between 20 and 40 years of age. It is somewhat more common in women than in men.
(3) The tumor occurs most often on the epiphyseal end of long bones; more than 50% occur about the knee.
(4) On radiography, it has a characteristic "soap bubble" appearance.
(5) Although this tumor is benign, it is a locally aggressive tumor and often recurs after local curettage.

3. **Malignant bone tumors**
a. **Osteosarcoma (osteogenic sarcoma)**
(1) This is the **most common primary malignant tumor of bone.**
(2) The peak incidence is in males 10 to 20 years of age.
(3) The tumor occurs most frequently in the **metaphysis of long bones;** the proximal portion of the tibia and most distal portion of the femur (**about the knee**) are preferred sites.
(4) **Clinical characteristics** include:
(a) Pain and swelling and occasionally pathologic fracture
(b) A two- to three-fold increase of serum alkaline phosphatase
(c) Lifting of the periosteum by the expanding tumor, which creates a characteristic radiologic appearance known as the **Codman triangle.** Another radiologic sign is a spiculated **"sunburst" pattern** of growth.
(d) Early hematogenous spread to the lungs, liver, and brain
(5) **Predisposing factors**
(a) Paget disease of bone, fibrous dysplasia, chondroma, osteochondroma
(b) Ionizing radiation
(c) Bone infarcts
(d) Familial retinoblastoma (in these patients, surgical cure of the primary ocular tumor is often followed by the later development of osteosarcoma, presumably due to loss of the *Rb* suppressor gene locus on chromosome 13)

b. **Chondrosarcoma**
(1) This is a **malignant cartilaginous tumor.**
(2) The peak incidence is in men 30 to 60 years of age.
(3) The neoplasm may arise as a primary tumor or from transformation of preexisting cartilaginous tumors, especially multiple familial osteochondromatosis or multiple enchondromatosis.
(4) Characteristic sites of origin include the pelvis, spine, or scapula; the proximal humerus or proximal femur; and femur or tibia near the knee.

c. **Ewing sarcoma**
(1) This extremely anaplastic **"small blue cell" malignant tumor** has a morphologic resemblance to malignant lymphoma.
(2) It occurs most often in long bones, ribs, pelvis, and scapula.
(3) It has a peak incidence in boys younger than 15 years of age.
(4) It follows an extremely malignant course with early metastases.
(5) It responds to chemotherapy.
(6) In early stages, Ewing sarcoma may clinically mimic acute osteomyelitis.
(7) It is characterized by an 11;22 chromosomal translocation identical to that found in peripheral neuroectodermal tumor (a soft tissue neoplasm of neural crest origin) and olfactory neuroblastoma and is most likely closely related to these lesions.

III. Diseases of Joints (Table 22-3)

A. **Arthritides of probable autoimmune origin**
1. **Rheumatoid arthritis**
- This chronic inflammatory disorder primarily affects the synovial joints.

TABLE 22-3 *Distinctive Features of Selected Arthritides and Related Disorders*

Type	Etiology	Incidence	Most Frequent Site	Notable Features
Rheumatoid arthritis	Autoimmune	Women ages 20–50	Joints of the hands, knees, and feet; proximal interphalangeal and metacarpophalangeal joints	Subcutaneous nodules; rheumatoid factor (IgM anti-IgG)
Ankylosing spondylitis	Probably autoimmune; may have genetic component	Young men	Spine and sacroiliac joints	Almost all patients positive for HLA-B27 antigen
Osteoarthritis (degenerative joint disease)	Mechanical injury ("wear-and-tear"); may have a genetic component?	After age 50; somewhat more frequent in women	Weight-bearing joints; distal and proximal interphalangeal joints	Osteophytes; Heberden and Bouchard nodes; joint mice
Gout	Hyperuricemia with deposition of urate crystals in multiple sites	Men older than age 30	Metatarsophalangeal joint of the great toe	Tophi; urate nephropathy and nephrolithiasis
Gonococcal arthritis	Infection with *Neisseria gonorrhoeae*	Variable	Knee, wrist, small joints of the hands	Often monoarticular
Hypertrophic osteoarthropathy	Secondary manifestation of chronic lung disease, cyanotic heart disease, and various nonpulmonary systemic disorders	Variable, depending on the primary disorder	Fingers, radius, and ulna	Clubbing of the fingers; periostitis

- It is most common in women between 20 and 50 years of age.

a. **Pathogenetic factors**
   (1) Rheumatoid arthritis is likely of **autoimmune origin,** with interplay of genetic and environmental factors.
   (2) It is often characterized by the presence of serum **rheumatoid factor,** an immunoglobulin (most often IgM) with anti-IgG Fc specificity, which is highly characteristic of, but not specific for, rheumatoid arthritis.
   (3) It occurs most often in HLA-DR4-positive individuals.

b. **Morphology.** Rheumatoid arthritis manifests most characteristically by **synovitis.** The disease progresses as follows:
   (1) Earliest changes include an **acute inflammatory reaction** with edema and an inflammatory infiltrate, beginning with neutrophils and followed by lymphocytes and plasma cells.
   (2) **Hyperplasia and hypertrophy** of the synovial lining cells eventuate into numerous finger-like villi.
   (3) Granulation tissue (**pannus**) extends over articular cartilage; extension of pannus to subchondral bone results in erosion and cyst formation, leading to deformities of both cartilage and bone.

(4) **Scarring, contracture, and deformity** result from destructive inflammation of ligaments, tendons, and bursae.
(5) Subcutaneous **rheumatoid nodules** develop in approximately one third of patients.

c. **Clinical course**
(1) **Episodic changes**
(a) Fatigue, malaise, anorexia, weight loss, fever, and myalgia
(b) Swelling of the joints and stiffness, especially in the morning or after inactivity
(c) Polyarticular and symmetric joint involvement
(2) **Chronic joint changes**
(a) **Proximal interphalangeal** and **metacarpophalangeal** joints of the hands are frequent sites.
(b) **Ulnar deviation** of fingers results from synovitis of ligaments.
(c) **Minimal radial deviation** of the wrist may occur.
(3) **Extra-articular manifestations**
(a) Pleural and pericardial effusions
(b) Anemia of chronic disease
(c) Vasculitis
(d) Lymphadenopathy
(e) Pulmonary involvement
(f) Neurologic abnormalities
(g) Secondary reactive amyloidosis

d. **Variants of rheumatoid arthritis**
(1) **Sjögren syndrome** with rheumatoid arthritis
(2) **Felty syndrome:** splenomegaly, neutropenia, and rheumatoid arthritis
(3) **Still disease (juvenile rheumatoid arthritis),** often preceded or accompanied by generalized lymphadenopathy and hepatosplenomegaly and an acute onset marked by fever

2. **Seronegative arthritis (spondyloarthropathies)**

a. **Characteristics**
(1) Absence of rheumatoid factor
(2) Extremely high incidence in **HLA-B27**-positive individuals
(3) Peripheral arthritis
(4) Sacroiliitis

b. **Types**
(1) **Ankylosing spondylitis:** HLA-B27 association is most striking with this entity (as many as 90% of patients). This chronic condition affects the spine and sacroiliac joints and can lead to rigidity and fixation of the spine as a result of bone fusion (ankylosis).
(2) **Reiter syndrome:** urethritis, conjunctivitis, and arthritis; is often associated with venereal or intestinal infection.
(3) **Psoriatic arthritis** occurs in approximately 10% of patients with psoriasis.
(4) **Arthritis associated with inflammatory bowel disease:** peripheral arthritis or ankylosing spondylitis complicating ulcerative colitis or Crohn disease.

B. **Osteoarthritis (degenerative joint disease)** is the most common form of arthritis.

1. This chronic noninflammatory joint disease is characterized by degeneration of articular cartilage accompanied by new bone formation subchondrally and at the margins of the affected joint.
2. The incidence is greater in women, most often beginning after 50 years of age.
3. Osteoarthritis is most often related to mechanical trauma to the affected joints ("wear-and-tear" arthritis). **Characteristic morphologic changes** include:

a. Loss of elasticity, pitting, and fraying of cartilage; fragments may separate and float into synovial fluid.
b. **Eburnation:** polished, ivory-like appearance of bone, resulting from erosion of overlying cartilage

c. **Cystic changes** in subchondral bone
d. **New bone formation,** resulting in:
    (1) Increased density of subchondral bone
    (2) **Osteophyte** (bony spur) formation at the perimeter of the articular surface and at points of ligamental attachment to bone
e. **Osteophytes fracturing** and floating into synovial fluid (along with fragments of separated cartilage; these particles are called **joint mice**)
f. **Heberden nodes:** osteophytes at the distal interphalangeal joints of the fingers
g. **Bouchard nodes:** osteophytes at the proximal interphalangeal joints of the fingers

4. **Types**
    a. **Primary osteoarthritis** occurs without known cause. It may result from a complex interplay of genetic predisposition with a variety of mechanical or inflammatory mechanisms.
    b. **Secondary osteoarthritis** occurs in joints damaged by known mechanisms, including mechanical factors, metabolic disorders such as ochronosis, and inflammatory disorders.

C. **Arthritides of metabolic origin**

1. **Gout**
    a. **General considerations**
        (1) **Deposition of urate crystals** in several tissues, especially the joints, results from **hyperuricemia.**
        (2) An intense inflammatory reaction begins with opsonization of crystals by IgG, followed by phagocytosis by neutrophils, and eventuating in the release of proteolytic enzymes and inflammatory mediators from the phagocytic cells.
        (3) The disorder is manifest by an inflammatory response that leads to extremely painful acute arthritis and bursitis.
        (4) The disorder occurs most frequently in the metatarsophalangeal joint of the great toe. Acute gouty arthritis in this characteristic location is known as **podagra.**
        (5) A large meal or alcohol intake, both of which may increase hyperuricemia, often precipitate an exacerbation of the disorder.
        (6) Gout eventually leads to the formation of nodular **tophi,** which are located about joints, in the helix and the antihelix of the ear, in the Achilles tendon, and in other sites. Tophi consist of urate crystals in a protein matrix surrounded by fibrous connective tissue, all demonstrating a foreign body giant cell reaction.
        (7) Gout often leads to **urate nephropathy** characterized by interstitial deposition of urate crystals and obstruction of collecting tubules by urate crystals and by formation of urate and calcium stones.
        (8) The diagnosis is based on the finding of hyperuricemia along with urate crystals and neutrophils in synovial fluid or with biopsy evidence of tophaceous deposits; urate crystals are negatively birefringent under polarized light.
    b. **Primary gout** is the most common form. Characteristics include:
        (1) Hyperuricemia without evident cause. No single enzyme defect has been demonstrated.
        (2) Most common form in middle-aged men
        (3) A marked familial predisposition
    c. **Secondary gout** is much less common. It is characterized by hyperuricemia with evident cause, such as:
        (1) **Leukemia, multiple myeloma, and myeloproliferative syndromes,** with increased cellular turnover
        (2) Decreased urate excretion because of chronic renal disease or intake of various drugs
        (3) **Lesch-Nyhan syndrome:** hyperuricemia with severe neurologic manifestations, including self-mutilation, due to X-linked hypoxanthine-guanine phosphoribosyltransferase (HGPRT) deficiency

2. **Chondrocalcinosis (pseudogout)**
   a. The cause is calcium pyrophosphate dihydrate crystal deposition, which elicits an inflammatory reaction in cartilage.
   b. Pseudogout clinically resembles gout.

D. **Infective arthritis** is characterized by purulent synovial fluid.
   1. **Gonococcal arthritis** is the most common form of bacterial arthritis.
      a. This disorder is most often **monoarticular.**
      b. The arthritis most frequently involves the **knee;** other favored sites are the wrist and small joints of the hand.
   2. **Lyme disease**
      a. The cause is infection with the spirochete *Borrelia burgdorferi,* which is most often transmitted by *Ixodes dammini,* a tick.
      b. A skin lesion, erythema chronicum migrans, a slowly spreading lesion with prominent erythematous margins and central fading ("bull's-eye" lesion), is characteristic.
      c. Most characteristically, the disorder leads to polyarticular arthritis as a late sequela; typically involves the knees and other large joints. It can also lead to myocardial, pericardial, or neurologic changes as late sequelae.
      d. Diagnosis is by demonstration of IgM serum antibodies to *B. burgdorferi.*
      e. Response to early treatment with antibiotics is good.

E. **Miscellaneous joint diseases**
   1. **Hypertrophic osteoarthropathy**
      a. This disorder is associated with systemic disorders such as chronic lung disease, congenital cyanotic heart disease, cirrhosis of the liver, and inflammatory bowel disease.
      b. This chronic condition may manifest as **clubbing of the fingers** (the most obvious abnormality) and, more frequently, as associated **periostitis** at the distal end of the radius and ulna.
      c. Presenting features may also include painful swelling and tenderness of the peripheral joints.
   2. **Ganglion cyst.** This small cystic nodule arising in the tendon sheath or the joint capsule of the wrist is thought to be caused by myxoid degeneration of connective tissue.

IV. Soft Tissue Tumors

A. **General considerations**
   1. Tumors originate in fibrous connective tissue, adipose tissue, skeletal muscle, joint tissue, and the peripheral nervous system.
   2. Tumors most often require diagnostic adjuncts such as special stains, electron microscopy, or immunohistochemistry (studies for S-100, desmin, vimentin, and cytokeratin are most commonly used).

B. **Examples of soft tissue tumors**
   1. **Rhabdomyosarcoma**
      a. This malignant tumor of skeletal muscle is the most common soft tissue sarcoma of children.
      b. It may arise in other soft tissues.
      c. There are several variants, including pleomorphic rhabdomyosarcoma, embryonal rhabdomyosarcoma, and alveolar rhabdomyosarcoma.
   2. **Synovial sarcoma**
      a. This highly malignant soft tissue tumor most often originates in tissue adjacent to a joint rather than in a joint cavity.
      b. It often occurs in the lower extremities.
      c. A biphasic growth pattern in which both epithelial and spindle cells occur is characteristic.

3. **Fibrous histiocytoma** is a benign tumor consisting of a mixture of fibroblasts and histiocytes.
4. **Malignant fibrous histiocytoma** is the most common soft tissue sarcoma of late middle and old age.
5. **Fibrosarcoma** is a malignant tumor of fibroblasts characterized by spindle-shaped cells demonstrating a herringbone pattern.
6. **Lipoma** is a benign tumor of mature adipose tissue. It is the most common soft tissue tumor.
7. **Liposarcoma** is a malignant tumor of adipose tissue.

REVIEW TEST

***Directions:** Each of the numbered items or incomplete statements in this section is followed by answers or by completions of the statement. Select the **one** lettered answer or completion that is best in each case.*

1. A 4-year-old boy develops weakness of proximal lower back and extremity muscles, manifest by lordosis, a waddling gait, and the need to push on his knees in order to stand (Gower sign). Examination reveals proximal muscle weakness and bilateral enlargement of the calves. His younger brother has begun to display similar findings, as has his older half-brother, who has the same mother. Serum creatine kinase is markedly elevated. Which of the following is characteristic of this disorder?

(A) Aberrant protein coded by a very small gene sequence on the Y chromosome
(B) Autosomal dominant mode of inheritance
(C) Mitochondrial inheritance
(D) Regression of findings in late adolescence and adult life
(E) Total absence or marked decrease of an important gene product

2. A 40-year-old woman presents with ptosis, diplopia, and dysarthria that fluctuate in intensity and tend to worsen as the day progresses. Edrophonium (an acetylcholinesterase inhibitor) is administered, and after a minute, there is a striking improvement in muscle strength. Which of the following is characteristic of this disorder?

(A) Tangles of small rod-shaped granules in type I muscle fibers
(B) Autoantibodies to acetylcholine receptors
(C) Multiple CTG trinucleotide repeats
(D) Hypothalamic dopamine-mediated inhibition
(E) Paraneoplastic manifestation of small cell lung cancer

3. An 88-year-old woman with marked kyphosis and loss of height that had been gradually progressive over many years experiences the sudden onset of acute back pain following a sudden change in position. Radiographic examination demonstrates generalized osteopenia and a fracture of a lower thoracic vertebra. Which of the following is an association or characteristic of the patient's generalized bone disorder?

(A) Increased serum calcium and phosphate levels
(B) Postmenopausal state and estrogen deficiency
(C) Physical inactivity
(D) Hypothyroidism
(E) Excessive calcium intake

4. A 3-year-old boy, an inner city resident, has multiple bony abnormalities, including bowlegs and knock-knees, thickening of the skull with frontal bossing, knobby deformities of the costochondral junctions and at the ends of the long bones, distortion of the rib cage with flaring over the diaphragm, and pigeon-breast deformity. A decrease in which of the following is characteristic of this condition?

(A) Bony osteoblastic activity
(B) Calcification of osteoid
(C) Release of parathyroid hormone
(D) Serum alkaline phosphatase activity
(E) Synthesis of osteoid

5. When ordering academic attire for a recent graduation, a 65-year-old university professor is surprised to find that his hat size has increased. Shortly thereafter in a routine checkup, serum alkaline phosphatase activity is found to be markedly elevated. Serum calcium and phosphorus are normal. Examination reveals enlargement of the skull with frontal bossing and enlarged maxilla, and hearing loss is evident. Which of the following abnormalities is associated with the bone disorder suggested by these findings?

(A) "Brown tumor"
(B) Defective calcification of osteoid matrix
(C) Mosaic pattern of bone
(D) Polyostotic fibrous dysplasia with severe deformity
(E) Subperiosteal hemorrhage and osteoporosis

6. A 2-year-old boy presents with his third bone fracture within the past several months. There is no history or evidence of trauma. Several close family members have been similarly affected. The child is small for his age, and the sclerae are tinged a bluish color. Radiographs reveal generalized osteopenia and evidence of multiple fractures, both old and new. Which of the following is the usual mode of inheritance of this disorder?

(A) Autosomal dominant
(B) Autosomal recessive
(C) X-linked dominant
(D) X-linked recessive
(E) Mitochondrial

7. A 17-year-old boy presents with pain and swelling about the left knee for the past month. He thought that this condition resulted from an old football injury and that it would resolve without incident. However, the pain has persisted and is severe enough to cause him to limp. Radiographs of the knee demonstrate a lifting of the periosteum and a spiculated "sunburst" pattern in the distal femur. Which of the following is the most likely diagnosis?

(A) Osteosarcoma
(B) Chondrosarcoma
(C) Ewing sarcoma
(D) Giant cell tumor
(E) Knee sprain

8. A 40-year-old woman presents with symmetric stiffness and swelling of the proximal interphalangeal joints of the hands and of the metacarpophalangeal joints, as well as fatigue, malaise, and myalgia. Symptoms are worse in the morning or after extended inactivity and improve with movement and use throughout the day. Ulnar deviation of the fingers symmetrically on both hands is noted. Which of the following is the most likely etiology of this condition?

(A) Autoimmune disease
(B) Mechanical injury ("wear and tear")
(C) *Neisseria gonorrhoeae* infection
(D) Secondary manifestation of chronic lung disease or cyanotic cardiac disease
(E) Urate crystal deposition

9. A 60-year-old woman presents with deep, achy joint pain in her fingers. She states that the pain gets worse with extensive use of her fingers. Physical examination reveals reduced range of motion and crepitus, with pain noted asymmetrically in the distal interphalangeal (DIP) joints, proximal interphalangeal joints, and metacarpophalangeal joints. Heberden nodes are noted on the DIP joints of one hand. Which of the following is the most likely etiology of this condition?

(A) Autoimmune disease
(B) Mechanical injury ("wear and tear")
(C) *Neisseria gonorrhoeae* infection
(D) Secondary manifestation of chronic lung disease or cyanotic cardiac disease
(E) Urate crystal deposition

10. A 50-year-old man presents with recurrent episodes of acute excruciating pain, swelling, and redness of his right great toe, all following a large meal that was accompanied by copious consumption of alcohol. In the past, others in his family have had similar symptoms. The metatarsophalangeal joint of the right great toe is erythematous, edematous, and tender. Which of the following is the most likely etiology of this condition?

(A) Autoimmune disease
(B) Mechanical injury ("wear and tear")
(C) *Neisseria gonorrhoeae* infection
(D) Secondary manifestation of chronic lung disease or cyanotic cardiac disease
(E) Urate crystal deposition

A ANSWERS AND EXPLANATIONS

1-E. The clinical picture is that of Duchenne muscular dystrophy, the most common and most severe of the muscular dystrophies. This X-linked disorder is characterized by failure of synthesis of dystrophin, most often because of deletion of one or many exons in the *DMD* gene. Patients manifest with proximal muscle weakness, progressing to muscle necrosis. Serum creatine kinase is markedly increased. Compensatory hypertrophy is followed by pseudo-hypertrophy, in which necrotic muscle is replaced by fat and connective tissue. Most patients become wheelchair-bound and die of respiratory or cardiac failure in their late teenage years or in their early twenties.

2-B. Myasthenia gravis is an autoimmune disorder caused by autoantibodies to postsynaptic acetylcholine receptors of the neuromuscular junction. The disease commonly presents as ptosis, diplopia, and difficulty chewing, speaking, or swallowing. Respiratory failure from diaphragmatic weakness can occur. Marked improvement with cholinesterase inhibitors is characteristic. For unexplained reasons, myasthenia gravis is associated with thymic hyperplasia or thymoma.

3-B. Osteoporosis is characterized by a decrease in bone mass due to loss of bone matrix, and it is unassociated with abnormalities in mineral metabolism. This condition is the most common bone disorder in older persons. It occurs most commonly in elderly women and is associated with the postmenopausal state and estrogen deficiency. Characteristics include fractures, kyphosis, and shortened stature. Predisposing factors include physical inactivity, hypercorticism, hyperthyroidism, and calcium deficiency. Serum calcium and phosphate levels are typically normal.

4-B. The child has rickets, which is caused by failure of action of calcitriol (1,25-dihydroxycholecalciferol), the active form of vitamin D. The bony abnormalities in rickets are caused by failure of osteoid matrix to calcify, leading to excess accumulation of osteoid, increased thickness of the epiphyseal growth plates, and other skeletal deformities. Many of the effects of calcitriol deficiency are mediated by increased release of parathyroid hormone (PTH). Parathyroid hormone stimulates bony osteoblastic activity, which is mirrored by an increase in serum alkaline phosphatase.

5-C. A mosaic pattern of bone caused by increases in both osteoblastic and osteoclastic activity is characteristic of Paget disease of bone (osteitis deformans). Serum alkaline phosphatase is markedly increased. Hearing loss is common (from narrowing of the auditory foramen and compression of the VIIIth cranial nerve), and an increase in hat size due to frontal bossing is often noted.

6-A. Osteogenesis imperfecta (or brittle bone disease) is an autosomal dominant disorder characterized by multiple fractures with minimal trauma. It is caused by mutations in either of the genes (*COL1A*1 or *COL1A*2) that code for type I collagen and is manifest by connective tissue abnormalities affecting the bones, teeth, skin, and eyes. The sclerae can appear blue due to translucency of the thin connective tissue overlying the choroid. The disorder occurs in several variants defined by the age of onset and the severity of the fractures. In the less obvious cases, the principal differential diagnostic consideration is child abuse.

7-A. Osteosarcoma is the most common primary malignant tumor of bone. The most common presentation is in adolescents, with pain, swelling, and occasionally pathologic fracture in the proximal tibia or distal femur (about the knee). The characteristic radiologic findings include the Codman triangle (lifting of the periosteum of the bone caused by the expanding tumor) and a spiculated "sunburst" pattern of growth.

8-A. This is a case of rheumatoid arthritis. Rheumatoid arthritis is a chronic inflammatory autoimmune disorder that primarily affects the synovium, especially in the proximal interphalangeal and metacarpophalangeal joints of the hands. Ulnar deviation of the fingers results from synovitis of the ligaments. In the synovium, an acute inflammatory reaction is followed by hyperplasia and hypertrophy of the synovial lining cells, granulation tissue (pannus) development over the articular cartilage, and scarring, contracture, and deformity from chronic inflammation.

9-B. This is a case of osteoarthritis (degenerative joint disease), the most common form of arthritis. Osteoarthritis is a chronic noninflammatory joint disease most often related to mechanical trauma and long-term use of affected joints ("wear-and-tear" arthritis). Osteoarthritis is characterized by eburnation (polished, ivory-like appearance of bone, due to erosion of overlying cartilage), cystic changes in subchondral bone, and new bone formation. Osteophytes (bony spurs) can form at the distal interphalangeal joints (Heberden nodes) or at the proximal interphalangeal joints (Bouchard nodes).

10-E. This is a case of gout. Gout is characterized by deposition of monosodium urate crystals in joints and other tissues as a result of hyperuricemia. Gouty arthritis most commonly affects the metacarpophalangeal joint of the great toe (podagra). Primary gout, the most common type of gout, is characterized by hyperuricemia without evident cause. Secondary gout, much less common, is characterized by hyperuricemia due to evident cause, such as leukemia, multiple myeloma, myeloproliferative syndromes, or Lesch-Nyhan syndrome (hypoxanthine guanine phosphoribosyl transferase deficiency).

CHAPTER 23

Nervous System

I. Congenital Disorders

A. **Neural tube defects**

1. This group of disorders is characterized by failure of closure of the neural tube. The resulting defects can involve the vertebrae or skull with or without involvement of the underlying meninges, spinal cord, or brain.
2. These disorders are characteristically associated with increased concentration of α-fetoprotein in amniotic fluid or maternal serum. They are also linked with maternal folic acid deficiency.
3. Neural tube defects include:
   a. **Spina bifida:** failure of posterior vertebral arches to close
   b. **Spina bifida occulta:** spina bifida with no clinically apparent abnormalities; vertebral arch defect most often limited to one or two vertebrae
   c. **Spina bifida cystica:** spina bifida complicated by herniation of meninges through a defect
   d. **Meningocele:** herniated membranes consisting of meninges only
   e. **Meningomyelocele:** portion of spinal cord included in herniated tissue
   f. **Anencephaly:** marked diminution (sometimes absence) of fetal brain tissue; usually associated with the absence of overlying skull.

B. **TORCH complex** is a group of infections transmitted from the mother to the fetus with similar clinical manifestations.

1. TORCH stands for **TO**xoplasma, **R**ubella, **C**ytomegalovirus, and **H**erpes simplex virus (and others such as congenital syphilis).
2. TORCH involves the heart, skin, eye, and central nervous system (CNS) and causes chorioretinitis. Characteristics include microcephaly and focal cerebral calcification.

C. **Hydrocephalus**

1. This condition denotes increased volume of cerebrospinal fluid (CSF) within the cranial cavity.
2. In infants, it is associated with (sometimes marked) enlargement of the skull.
3. Hydrocephalus is most often caused by obstruction to the CSF circulation by mechanisms such as congenital malformations, inflammation, and tumors. It can also result from overproduction of CSF by choroid plexus papilloma (rare).
4. It can also occur as **hydrocephalus ex vacuo** without obstruction or increased CSF production in disorders characterized by decreased cerebral mass, such as ischemic brain atrophy or advanced Alzheimer disease.
5. Hydrocephalus occurs in these forms:
   a. **Internal hydrocephalus:** the increased volume of CSF is entirely within the ventricles

b. **External hydrocephalus:** the increased volume of CSF is confined to the subarachnoid space
c. **Communicating hydrocephalus:** free flow of CSF between the ventricles and the subarachnoid space
d. **Noncommunicating hydrocephalus:** obstructed flow of CSF from the ventricles to the subarachnoid space

D. Arnold-Chiari malformation

1. This is a downward displacement of the cerebellar tonsils and medulla through the foramen magnum.
2. Arnold-Chiari malformation results in pressure atrophy of displaced brain tissue.
3. In addition, it causes hydrocephalus as a result of obstruction of the CSF outflow tract.
4. Presence of a thoracolumbar meningomyelocele is almost always characteristic.

E. **Agenesis of the corpus callosum** can be asymptomatic and is often found in association with other abnormalities.

F. Fetal alcohol syndrome

1. This is associated with excessive maternal alcohol intake during pregnancy.
2. Characteristics include facial abnormalities and developmental defects such as microcephaly, atrial septal defect, mental and growth retardation, and other anomalies.

G. Tuberous sclerosis syndrome

1. This disorder includes autosomal dominant nodular proliferation of multinucleated atypical astrocytes forming tubers (small white nodules scattered in the cerebral cortex and periventricular areas). It also includes adenoma sebaceum of the skin and angiomyolipoma of the kidney.
2. Seizures and mental retardation beginning in infancy are characteristic.

II. Cerebrovascular Disease (Table 23-1)

- This is the most common group of CNS disorders; it ranks after heart disease and cancer as the third major cause of death in the United States.

A. Infarction

1. This disorder is more frequent than hemorrhage.
2. It is characterized by liquefactive necrosis leading to cyst formation.
3. Causes include arterial occlusion from:
   a. **Thrombosis,** most often caused by atherosclerosis
   b. **Embolism,** from cardiac mural thrombi, vegetations of infected endocarditic valves, clumps of tumor cells, bubbles of air, or droplets of fat. Embolism is much less common than thrombosis.
4. Infarction results in clinical manifestations that depend on the site of vascular obstruction and extent of collateral circulation; the **carotid bifurcation and the middle cerebral artery are the most frequent sites of thrombotic occlusion,** and the **middle cerebral artery is the most frequent site of embolic occlusion.** Arterial obstruction in this site causes contralateral paralysis as well as motor and sensory defects and aphasias.
5. When infarction is caused by an obstruction of small vessels, it can result in small lesions that are recognizable as lacunae (small pits) on healing. Clinical manifestations of **lacunar strokes** are focal and are most often purely sensory or motor. Pure motor lacunar stroke most often results from lesions affecting the internal capsule. Pure sensory lacunar stroke most often results from lesions affecting the thalamus.

TABLE 23-1 *Cerebrovascular Disease*

Type	Principal Predisposing Factors	Common Sites
Infarction		
Thrombosis	Atherosclerosis	Arterial obstruction of the internal and external carotid arteries at origin in the neck, vertebral and basilar arteries, and vessels branching from the circle of Willis, especially the middle cerebral artery
Embolism	Cardiac mural thrombi, valvular vegetations, fat emboli	Middle cerebral artery most frequent site of embolic occlusion
Hemorrhage		
Intracerebral	Hypertension, coagulation disorders, hemorrhage within a tumor	Can result from rupture of Charcot-Bouchard aneurysms, which result from long-standing hypertension
Subarachnoid	Rupture of a congenital berry aneurysm; likelihood of rupture compounded by hypertension	Circle of Willis and bifurcation of the middle cerebral artery

B. **Hemorrhage**

1. **Intracerebral hemorrhage** consists of bleeding into the brain substance.
   a. Most frequently, the cause is hypertension, which is often complicated by minute dilations at small artery bifurcations. These **Charcot-Bouchard aneurysms** may be sites of hemorrhagic rupture.
   b. Most often, it occurs in the basal ganglia/thalamus; other favored sites include the pons, cerebellum, and frontal lobe white matter.
2. **Subarachnoid hemorrhage** consists of bleeding into the subarachnoid space.
   a. This is frequently associated with **berry aneurysm** of the circle of Willis.
   b. Causes include arteriovenous malformations, trauma, or hemorrhagic diatheses.

C. **Transient ischemic attacks (TIAs)**

1. These brief episodes of impaired neurologic function are caused by temporary disturbance of cerebral circulation.
2. TIAs are not associated with permanent damage but are considered precursors to more serious occlusive events.

III. Head Injuries

A. **Causes.** Head injuries result from **penetrating wounds,** which, in addition to brain damage, can predispose to infection. Other causes include **nonpenetrating injuries;** brain injury at the site of impact is referred to as **coup** injury; injury on the opposite side of the brain from the site of impact is **contrecoup** injury; contusions characterize both coup and contrecoup injuries.

B. **Epidural hematoma**

1. This hematoma is an arterial hemorrhage associated with **skull fracture** and most often with laceration of branches of the **middle meningeal artery.**
2. Clinical characteristics include a short period of consciousness (lucid interval) followed by rapidly developing signs of cerebral compression.

3. Epidural hematoma is amenable to emergency surgical intervention because bleeding into the brain substance itself does not occur.

C. **Subdural hematoma**

1. The cause is venous bleeding, most often from **bridging veins** joining the cerebrum to venous sinuses within the dura.
2. Clinical characteristics include **gradual signs of cerebral compression** occurring hours to days or even weeks after head injury; venous hemorrhage typically arrests early, but the volume of the hematoma gradually increases as a result of osmotic imbibement of water, resulting in a slowly enlarging tumor-like mass.

IV. Infections

A. **Portals of entry of infection into the CNS**

— **Note:** No lymphatics enter the CNS.

1. **Hematogenous spread** is most common.
2. **Trauma**
3. **Local spread from paranasal sinuses, dental infections, and so forth.**
4. **Via peripheral nerves**

B. **Pyogenic meningitis**

1. Clinical manifestations include fever, headache, prostration, and nuchal rigidity.
2. Peak incidence is in children (almost 75% of cases), with a second high incidence peak in the elderly.
3. Resulting conditions include reactive fibroblastic arachnoiditis, with scarring, obliteration of the subarachnoid space, and hydrocephalus caused by impedance of the flow of CSF.
4. Pyogenic meningitis can also lead to leptomeningeal venulitis with venous occlusion and hemorrhagic infarcts, as well as brain abscess.
5. Purulent exudate in the subarachnoid space is characteristic. **CSF findings** of diagnostic significance include:
   a. **Numerous neutrophils**
   b. **Decreased glucose** (less than two thirds of the serum glucose concentration)
   c. **Increased protein**
6. **Etiology**
   a. In neonates and infants, pyogenic meningitis is most frequently caused by group B streptococci, *Escherichia coli,* and *Listeria.*
   b. In older infants, children, and young adults, the disease is most frequently caused by *Streptococcus pneumoniae* (pneumococcus) and *Neisseria meningitidis.*
   c. *N. meningitidis* occurrence may be sporadic or epidemic and may be accompanied by meningococcemia secondary to a primary infection in the nasopharynx.
   d. Meningococcemia can also be associated with purpuric skin lesions and is sometimes complicated by the **Waterhouse-Friderichsen syndrome** (hemorrhagic destruction of the adrenal cortex, acute hypocorticism with circulatory collapse, and disseminated intravascular coagulation).
   e. In older adults, the disease is most frequently caused by *S. pneumoniae* and gram-negative rods.

C. **Cerebral abscess** can result from penetrating skull injuries or from spread of infection originating elsewhere; sources of infection include the paranasal sinuses or middle ear (the most common source), bronchopulmonary infections, infective endocarditis, and other sites.

D. **Tuberculosis** occurs as tuberculosis of the brain substance or as tuberculous meningitis. It is secondary to tuberculous infection occurring elsewhere in the body.

E. **Fungal infection**
1. Most often, the cause is *Cryptococcus neoformans, Coccidioides immitis, Aspergillus,* or *Histoplasma.*
2. These infections can involve the brain substance or the meninges.
3. It is often associated with impaired resistance to infection.

F. **Toxoplasmosis**
1. This parasitic infection of the brain is caused by *Toxoplasma gondii.*
2. In neonates, the disease is **transmitted transplacentally** from the infected mother.
3. It is also spread by ingestion of foods contaminated by animal urine or feces; household pets, especially **cats,** are frequent reservoirs.
4. In newborns, the disease results in hydrocephalus, mental retardation, and other **neurologic abnormalities;** characteristic **periventricular calcifications** are demonstrable radiographically; the cerebral cortex, basal ganglia, and retinae as well as the heart, lungs, and liver are sites of involvement.
5. In adults, the disease is most often manifest as lymphadenitis; CNS involvement may occur in immunosuppressed persons.

G. **Viral infection**
1. **Viral infection** can be limited to the meninges or can involve the brain or spinal cord.
   a. **Viral meningitis (lymphocytic or aseptic meningitis)**
      (1) The cause is a variety of viral agents.
      (2) Clinical manifestations include fever, headache, and nuchal rigidity.
      (3) CSF demonstrates an increase in lymphocytes, moderately increased protein, and normal glucose concentration.
   b. **Meningoencephalitis and encephalitis**
      (1) These disorders have the following morphologic changes in the brain substance:
         (a) **Perivascular cuffing** (infiltrate of mononuclear cells within Virchow-Robin spaces)
         (b) **Inclusion bodies** in neurons or glial cells (a frequent but not invariable finding)
         (c) **Glial nodules** as a result of nonspecific proliferation of microglia
      (2) These disorders can present as brain stem disease (e.g., poliomyelitis, which even more characteristically exhibits prominent involvement of the spinal cord).
2. **Examples of viral infection**
   a. **Arbovirus encephalitides**
      (1) **St. Louis encephalitis:** reservoir, horses and birds; mosquito vector; disease varies from an asymptomatic state to severe meningoencephalitis.
      (2) **Eastern equine encephalitis:** associated with a high mortality rate; reservoir, horses and birds.
      (3) **Western equine encephalitis:** less severe than Eastern equine encephalitis.
   b. **Herpes simplex encephalitis**
      (1) This disorder is most common in teenagers and young adults.
      (2) It is an uncommon complication of herpes simplex virus infection but is nonetheless the most common agent of severe viral encephalitis.
   c. **Poliomyelitis** is characterized by degeneration and necrosis of anterior horn cells of the spinal cord.
   d. **Rabies**
      (1) This disorder is spread by the bite of such animals as dogs, raccoons, foxes, squirrels, skunks, and bats; saliva contains the virus.
      (2) Results include severe encephalitis with increased excitability of the CNS; it is characterized by violent muscle contractions and convulsions after minimal stimuli.
      (3) The disorder is aborted by active immunization during the interval between the bite and the projected onset of clinical manifestations; it is usually fatal once clinical signs develop.

(4) Histologic characteristics include neuronal degeneration, perivascular accumulations of mononuclear cells in the brain stem and spinal cord, and characteristic eosinophilic intracytoplasmic inclusions **(Negri bodies)** in the hippocampus and Purkinje cells of the cerebellum.

e. **Cytomegalovirus infection**

(1) This disorder generally affects immunosuppressed persons.

(2) Results include encephalomyelitis as well as in lesions of the kidneys, liver, lungs, and salivary glands.

(3) Giant cells with **eosinophilic inclusions** involving both the nucleus and cytoplasm are characteristic.

(4) In infants, cytomegalovirus may be characterized in severe cases by mental retardation, microcephaly, chorioretinitis, and hepatosplenomegaly; periventricular calcification within the brain is demonstrable.

f. **Human immunodeficiency virus (HIV) infection**

(1) HIV can cause nervous system dysfunction before the onset of immunodeficiency.

(2) This disorder may affect the brain, spinal cord, or peripheral nervous system by direct HIV infection. Cells of monocyte-macrophage origin are vehicles for viral entry into the nervous system and may serve as the viral reservoir.

(3) It may facilitate opportunistic infection or tumor development within the nervous system, both mediated by immunodeficiency.

(4) Most often, HIV infection results in AIDS dementia complex, although other clinical syndromes also occur; difficulty concentrating, memory impairment, slowness of thinking, depression, personality changes, lethargy, and difficulty with balance, coordination, and motor function are all frequently seen; downhill course with progressive dementia is characteristic.

H. **Prion diseases**

1. **General considerations**

a. Prion diseases are thought to be caused by **prions,** infectious protein particles termed prion protein (PrP). Prions are considered infectious and transmissible, devoid of DNA or RNA, and resistant to heating and other methods used for inactivation of common infectious agents.

b. These disorders are anatomically defined by the finding of **spongiform encephalopathy** (spongiosis), which is characterized by clusters of small cysts in CNS gray matter along with a striking absence of inflammatory response.

c. Another defining feature is a **long incubation period** (thus the older classification within the group of "slow virus diseases") and a progressive course.

d. Prion diseases include kuru, Creutzfeldt-Jakob disease, the Gerstmann-Sträussler-Scheinker syndrome, and fatal familial insomnia in humans, and bovine spongiform encephalopathy (mad cow disease), scrapie, and mink-transmissible encephalopathy in animals.

e. Transmission is thought to be by exposure to (most commonly by ingestion of) prion-containing animal (or human) tissue, particularly, but not exclusively, brain. For example, it is thought that prion-containing beef products from animals slaughtered during the presymptomatic phase of mad cow disease may present a danger of a variant form of Creutzfeldt-Jakob disease in humans.

2. **Kuru**

a. In the past, this disease was transmitted by ritual ingestion of human brain by cannibals of New Guinea.

b. Morphologic features include loss of neurons, gliosis, and striking spongiosis in the cerebrum, cerebellum, and spinal cord; cerebellar atrophy is often present.

c. Characteristics include cerebellar degeneration with marked tremor, ataxia, slurred speech, and progressive mental deficiency, followed by death within a few months.

3. **Creutzfeldt-Jakob disease (subacute spongiform encephalopathy)**

a. This disease exhibits morphologic changes similar to those of kuru; spongiosis is prominent.

b. It is believed to be a potential hazard to health workers who work with brain specimens. It has also been putatively transmitted by corneal transplantation.
c. In a variant form, Creutzfeldt-Jakob disease appears to have been transmitted to humans by ingestion of beef products from cattle affected by mad cow disease.
d. Characteristics include ataxia, rapidly progressive dementia, and early death.

I. **Slow virus infections**
1. **Subacute sclerosing panencephalitis**
a. The cause is persistent infection with an **altered measles virus;** patients are infected in infancy but an asymptomatic interval of several years is followed by neurologic manifestations in late childhood or early teenage years.
b. The disease is slowly progressive and is usually fatal.
c. Characteristics include lack of M component of measles virus, a protein required for extracellular spread of virus; this deficiency may explain the slow nature of infection. CSF contains oligoclonal immunoglobulins against viral proteins but lacks "anti-M."
2. **Progressive multifocal leukoencephalopathy**
a. Most often, the cause is the JC polyoma type of **papovavirus,** which preferentially infects oligodendrocytes, thus causing demyelination.
b. Characteristics include rapidly progressive multiple foci of demyelination in the brain, and it is associated with abnormal oligodendrocytes and astrocytes.
c. Progressive multifocal leukoencephalopathy is often associated with **leukemia or lymphoma** or with immunodeficiency.

V. Demyelinating Diseases

- These disorders are characterized by **destruction of myelin with relative preservation of axons.**

A. **Multiple sclerosis**
1. **Epidemiology**
a. Multiple sclerosis is by far the most common of the demyelinating diseases.
b. This disease most often begins between 20 and 30 years of age.
c. This disease is more common in women.
2. **Etiology**
a. The etiology is unknown; immune or viral factors are suspected but unproven causes.
b. Multiple sclerosis is thought to be multifactorial in origin, with both **environmental and genetic factors** playing a role, a view supported by the following:
(1) Frequent occurrence of increased CSF immunoglobulin, often manifest as **multiple oligoclonal bands** on electrophoresis, suggests that viral or immune factors may play a role.
(2) Increased incidence in association with certain HLA haplotypes (A3, B7, DR2, and DW2) suggests that immune factors may play a role.
(3) Highest incidence occurs in persons of northern European ancestry.
(4) Incidence is directly proportional to the geographic distance from the equator; predisposition remains when persons move to a low-incidence geographic site if the move is made after 15 years of age.
3. **Morphologic changes**
a. Changes are **confined to the CNS;** peripheral nerves are not affected.
b. Characteristics include depletion of myelin-producing oligodendrocytes, with multiple focal areas of demyelination (plaques) that are irregularly scattered in the brain and spinal cord; the optic nerve, brain stem, and **paraventricular** areas are favored sites; helper CD4+ and cytotoxic CD8+ T lymphocytes and macrophages infiltrate plaques; reactive gliosis occurs later.

4. **Clinical manifestations**
   a. Multiple sclerosis follows a highly variable clinical course depending on the site of involvement.
   b. Characteristics include **exacerbations** with long asymptomatic **remissions** and often a progressive course, leading to invalidism with mental deterioration.
   c. This disease manifests by early findings: weakness of the lower extremities, visual disturbances and retrobulbar pain, sensory disturbances, and possible loss of bladder control.
   d. The classic Charcot triad (nystagmus, intention tremor, and scanning speech), which is significant for diagnosis, may occur.

B. **Acute disseminated encephalomyelitis**
1. This disease follows viral illnesses such as measles, mumps, rubella, and chickenpox and is often known as **postinfectious encephalitis.**
2. It may be a manifestation of a delayed hypersensitivity reaction.
3. The course varies from a complete recovery to a fatal outcome.
4. Characteristics include widespread demyelination.

C. **Guillain-Barré syndrome**
1. This acute inflammatory demyelinating disease primarily involves **peripheral nerves.**
2. Incidence is highest in young adults.
3. This disease is often preceded by viral infection, immunization, or allergic reactions.
4. Guillain-Barré syndrome is generally considered to be of autoimmune etiology.
5. Clinical manifestations include **ascending muscle weakness and paralysis** beginning in the lower part of the lower extremities and ascending upward; respiratory failure and death can occur but most patients recover.
6. Guillain-Barré syndrome causes **albumino-cytologic dissociation** of CSF, a greatly increased protein concentration with only modest increase in cell count, which is an important diagnostic finding.

VI. Degenerative Diseases (Table 23-2)

A. **Alzheimer disease** is the most important cause of dementia. This disease was formerly viewed as premature senility occurring in middle-aged persons (presenile dementia); the entity now includes dementia at any age if associated with characteristic clinical and pathologic findings.

1. **Clinical findings**
   a. Slow, progressive intellectual deterioration during the course of several years, including:
      (1) Loss of recent memory, the most frequent early sign
      (2) Loss of long-term memory and other intellectual functions, leading to inability to read, count, or speak
   b. Motor problems, contractures, and paralysis, which are sometimes terminal events
2. **Morphologic abnormalities**
   a. **Neurofibrillary tangles:** intracytoplasmic bundles of filaments, derived in part from microtubules and neurofilaments, occur within neurons, especially in the cerebral cortex.
   b. **Neuritic (senile) plaques:** swollen eosinophilic nerve cell processes occurring in spherical focal collections within the cerebral cortex, hippocampus, and amygdala. A central amyloid core with a distinctive peptide structure is characteristic.
   c. **Granulovacuolar degeneration:** intraneuronal cytoplasmic granule-containing vacuoles occurring within the pyramidal cells of the hippocampus
   d. **Amyloid angiopathy:** amyloid deposition in and about vessels
   e. **Hirano bodies:** intracytoplasmic proximal dendritic eosinophilic inclusions consisting of actin
   f. **Generalized cerebral atrophy with moderate neuronal loss** is most prominent in frontal and hippocampal areas; sulci are widened because of narrowing of the gyri.

TABLE 23-2 *Degenerative Brain Disease*

Type	Clinical Presentation	Occurrence	Anatomic Changes
Alzheimer disease	Progressive dementia	Sporadic form presents at age 60 or later; familial form may present as early as age 40	Generalized cerebral atrophy; neurofibrillary tangles, neuritic (senile) plaques, granulovacuolar degeneration, Hirano bodies; decreased number of neurons in the nucleus basalis of Meynert
Pick disease	Progressive dementia	More frequent in women	Cerebral atrophy with gliosis and loss of cortical neurons, especially affecting temporal and frontal lobes; Pick bodies within some neurons, especially in the horn of Ammon
Huntington disease	Chorea and athetoid movements, progressive motor deterioration, wasting	Autosomal dominant disorder with delay of onset of clinical abnormalities until age 30–40	Atrophy, neuronal depletion, and gliosis of the caudate nuclei, putamen, and frontal cortex
Idiopathic Parkinson disease (paralysis agitans)	Parkinsonism	Usually presents after age 50	Neuronal depletion and depigmentation of cells of the substantia nigra and locus ceruleus; Lewy bodies
Amyotrophic lateral sclerosis (ALS)	Rapidly progressive upper and lower motor neuron failure, leading to death, most often from respiratory failure	Middle-aged men	Degeneration of lateral corticospinal tracts and anterior motor neurons of spinal cord

3. **Lack of specificity of morphologic abnormalities**
   a. Similar morphologic changes are associated with aging.
   b. Patients with Down syndrome who survive to 40 years of age and older often exhibit Alzheimer-like findings.
   c. Neurofibrillary tangles are observed in postencephalitic Parkinson disease.
4. **Etiology** is unknown.
   a. **Abnormal amyloid gene expression** is the most favored etiologic concept today.
      (1) Aggregates of **Aβ40 amyloidogenic peptide** constitute the amyloid of neuritic plaques and nearby cerebral vessels.
      (2) The *APP* gene on chromosome 21 codes for amyloid precursor protein, a precursor to the Aβ peptide.
      (3) Several mutations in the APP gene have been linked to familial Alzheimer disease.
      (4) In addition, increased gene copy number has been demonstrated in some patients with the sporadic form of Alzheimer disease.
      (5) Alzheimer-like abnormalities occur in trisomy 21 (Down syndrome).
   b. **Other genetic abnormalities**
      (1) **Inheritance of the ε4 allele of apoprotein E** (chromosome 19). The ε4 allele occurs with greater frequency in patients with Alzheimer disease.

(2) **Mutations in genes coding for presenilins.** Presenilin-1 (chromosome 14) and presenilin-2 (chromosome 1) have been linked to many kindreds with familial early-onset Alzheimer disease.

c. **Choline acetyltransferase deficiency.** The brain content of the enzyme and its product, acetylcholine, is decreased, especially in the cerebral cortex and hippocampus. Acetylcholine plays a role in learning, and drugs that block its action adversely affect short-term memory.

d. **Alterations in the nucleus basalis of Meynert.** There is a marked reduction in the number of neurons within the nucleus; neuritic plaques may represent degenerating neuronal processes from this site.

5. **Other causes of dementia**

a. **Multi-infarction dementia** is the second most frequent cause of dementia after Alzheimer disease; it is caused by cerebral atherosclerosis.

b. **Alcohol encephalopathy (Wernicke disease)**

(1) The cause is the combined effects of alcohol and thiamine deficiency.

(2) Morphologic features include marked atrophy or demyelination affecting the cerebral cortex, pons, cerebellar vermis, **mamillary bodies,** and other paramedian masses of gray matter in the brain stem and diencephalon.

(3) Clinical manifestations may include the Wernicke triad (confusion, ataxia, and ophthalmoplegia).

c. **Binswanger disease** (subcortical leukoencephalopathy) is associated with hypertension. It is characterized by the presence of multiple lacunar infarcts and progressive demyelination limited to the subcortical area, with characteristic sparing of the cortex.

d. **Pick disease**

B. Pick disease

1. This disorder clinically resembles Alzheimer disease.
2. It is more frequent in women.
3. Characteristics include marked cortical atrophy, especially of the temporal and frontal lobes, by swollen neurons, and by Pick bodies, round intracytoplasmic inclusions consisting of neurofilaments.

C. Huntington disease

1. This disease is an **autosomal dominant,** fatal, progressive degeneration and atrophy of the striatum **(caudate nucleus and putamen)** and frontal cortex with neuronal depletion and gliosis.
2. It is characterized by the **delay of clinical abnormalities until 30 to 40 years of age;** course extends 15 to 20 years, beginning with athetoid movements, followed by progressive deterioration leading to hypertonicity, fecal and urine incontinence, anorexia and weight loss, and eventually dementia and death.
3. Cholinergic and GABA-ergic neurons are especially affected.
4. Huntington disease is marked by **increased numbers (more than the normal 11–34) of CAG trinucleotide repeats** within the *HD* (huntingtin) gene on the short arm of chromosome 4. Paternal transmission results in an increased number of CAG repeats and correspondingly earlier onset of disease manifestations in successive generations (anticipation; see Chapter 4).
5. This disease may be related to a failure in the up-regulation of transcription of brain-derived neurotrophic factor (BDNF), a prosurvival factor for the neurons of the striatum. The transcription of BDNF is apparently decreased in the presence of the huntingtin gene with increased numbers of CAG repeats.

D. Idiopathic Parkinson disease (paralysis agitans)

1. This disease appears clinically most often after 50 years of age.
2. Histologic manifestations include **depigmentation of the substantia nigra** and locus ceruleus; damaged cells contain highly characteristic eosinophilic intracytoplasmic inclusions **(Lewy bodies)**.

3. Idiopathic Parkinson disease damages neuronal pathways from the substantia nigra to the corpus striatum, resulting in **dopamine depletion of the corpus striatum;** therapy with L-dopa, a dopamine precursor, is often effective.
4. Idiopathic Parkinson disease is the most common cause of **parkinsonism,** a group of disorders characterized by resting pill-rolling tremor, masked (expressionless) facies, slowness of movements, muscular rigidity, and festinating (shuffling) gait. Other causes of parkinsonism include:
   a. **Von Economo encephalitis,** an infectious disorder that appeared transiently from 1915 to 1918 concurrent with the influenza pandemic, caused **postencephalitic parkinsonism,** most often in older persons affected by that pandemic.
   b. **Trauma,** especially repeated trauma as may occur in boxers
   c. **Drugs and toxins,** especially dopamine antagonists such as MPTP (methyl-phenyl-tetrahydropyridine), a contaminant in illicit street drugs
   d. **Shy-Drager syndrome,** parkinsonism with autonomic dysfunction and orthostatic hypotension

E. **Motor neuron disease**
1. **Amyotrophic lateral sclerosis (ALS, Lou Gehrig disease)**
   a. **Degeneration of upper and lower motor neurons** is characteristic.
   b. Amyotrophic lateral sclerosis is the most common form of motor neuron disease.
   c. Morphologic characteristics include degeneration and atrophy of the lateral corticospinal tracts as well as of the anterior motor neurons of the cord.
   d. Results include denervation atrophy of musculature.
   e. Clinical manifestations include symmetric atrophy and fasciculation (lower motor neuron signs) as well as hyperreflexia, spasticity, and pathologic reflexes (upper motor neuron signs).
   f. Clinical onset occurs in early middle age, with a **rapid course leading to death** (most often from respiratory failure) in 1 to 6 years.
2. **Other forms of motor neuron disease**
   a. **Progressive bulbar palsy:** brain stem and cranial nerve involvement predominate; characteristic findings include difficulty in swallowing and speaking and termination in respiratory failure.
   b. **Werdnig-Hoffmann syndrome (infantile progressive spinal muscular atrophy)** is an autosomal recessive lower motor neuron disease that manifests clinically in infancy.

VII. Ocular Disorders

A. **Conjunctivitis**
1. This disease is most commonly caused by adenovirus infection.
2. It is also frequently caused by bacterial infection.

B. **Retinopathy of prematurity (retrolental fibroplasia)**
1. The disease is due to toxicity of therapeutic oxygen, most often administered because of neonatal respiratory distress syndrome (hyaline membrane disease).
2. It leads to blindness.

C. **Diabetic retinopathy** is a major cause of blindness.
1. **Nonproliferative (background) retinopathy**
   a. Manifestations include microaneurysms, dilation of veins, hemorrhages, soft (cotton-wool) exudates (microinfarcts), and hard exudates (deposits of protein that have leaked from damaged capillaries), all of which can be viewed with the ophthalmoscope.
   b. The retinopathy also includes increased capillary permeability, edema, and diffuse thickening of basement membranes (microangiopathy).

c. The disorder is related to the duration of the disease, occurring in most patients with diabetes mellitus after 10 years.

2. **Proliferative retinopathy**

a. New retinal vessel formation (neovascularization) and fibrosis, both extending into the vitreous, is characteristic.

b. This disorder can lead to hemorrhage and retinal detachment.

D. **Retinitis pigmentosa**

1. This disorder is characterized by hereditary (usually autosomal recessive) night blindness with progressive loss of central vision.
2. It is caused by early loss of rods and later loss of cones.
3. Clinical manifestations include retinal pigmentation, which can be seen with the ophthalmoscope.

E. **Macular degeneration of the aged (senile macular degeneration)**

1. This disorder is a major cause of impaired vision in the elderly.
2. It is characterized by loss of central vision and pigmentary changes or hemorrhage in the macula.
3. It is often bilateral.

F. **Glaucoma**

1. **Open-angle glaucoma**

a. This is the most common form of glaucoma.

b. It is characterized by gradually increasing intraocular pressure, leading to visual impairment and, eventually, blindness.

2. **Angle-closure (congestive) glaucoma**

a. This form of glaucoma is caused by narrow anterior chamber angle.

b. It is manifest by an increase in intraocular pressure on dilation of pupil.

G. **Retinoblastoma** is a malignant retinal tumor of childhood.

1. The tumor is sporadic in approximately 60% of cases; sporadic cases are unilateral and monocentric in origin.
2. It is familial in approximately 40% of cases; familial cases are frequently bilateral and multicentric in origin.
3. It demonstrates homozygous deletion of the *Rb* gene (located on chromosome 13 at band q14).
4. The tumor is the prototype of the "two-hit" hypothesis of Knudson.

a. **First deletion** ("hit") is inherited in germ line cells in familial cases or occurs as a somatic mutation in sporadic cases.

b. **Second deletion** ("hit") results from somatic mutation in both familial and sporadic cases.

c. **Both deletions** are required for tumor development.

VIII. Tumors (Table 23-3)

A. **General considerations**

1. Most tumors are intracranial; tumors of the spinal cord are much less frequent.
2. In adults, the majority of intracranial tumors are supratentorial.
3. In children, the majority of intracranial tumors are infratentorial.
4. CNS tumors are the second most common form of malignancy in children (only leukemia is more frequent).
5. Primary malignant CNS tumors rarely metastasize.
6. Benign intracranial tumors can result in devastating clinical consequences due to compression phenomena.

TABLE 23-3 *Selected Central Nervous System Tumors*

Type	Predominant Incidence	Most Frequent Site	Characteristics
Glioblastoma multiforme	Older persons	Cerebral hemispheres	Highly malignant, rapidly growing tumor; most common primary intracranial neoplasm
Meningioma	More frequent in women	Convexities of cerebral hemispheres, parasagittal region, falx cerebri, sphenoid ridge	Benign tumor external to the brain and usually resectable; second most common primary intracranial neoplasm
Medulloblastoma	Young children	Cerebellum	Highly malignant tumor; common intracranial tumor of children
Neuroblastoma	Children	Cerebral hemispheres	Less common than adrenal and other peripheral neuroblastomas; linked to marked amplification of N-*myc* oncogene
Retinoblastoma	Young children; occurs in familial and sporadic forms	Retina; bilateral and multifocal in familial form, unilateral and unifocal in sporadic form	Most common eye tumor of young children; linked to *Rb* gene deletion or inactivation
Neurilemmoma (schwannoma)	Middle and later life	Eighth cranial nerve (when schwannoma is intracranial)	Acoustic schwannoma, common intracranial tumor, ranking third after glioblastoma multiforme and meningioma; most often benign and usually resectable
Metastatic tumors	Variable	From primary sites in the lung, breast, skin, kidney, gastrointestinal tract, and thyroid	More common than primary central nervous system tumors

7. Metastatic tumors to the brain are found more frequently than primary intracranial neoplasms; in order of frequency, the most common primary intracranial tumors in adults are glioblastoma multiforme, meningioma, and acoustic neuroma. The most common primary intracranial tumors in children are cerebellar astrocytoma and medulloblastoma.

B. **Glioblastoma multiforme**

1. This disorder is the **most common primary intracranial neoplasm.**
2. Peak occurrence in the late middle-age group.
3. This neoplasm is associated with marked anaplasia and pleomorphism; pronounced vascular changes with endothelial hyperplasia occur. Areas of necrosis and hemorrhage are surrounded by a **"pseudopalisade" arrangement** of tumor cells.
4. It originates most often in the cerebral hemisphere.
5. Prognosis is very poor; death occurs in less than 1 year.

C. **Oligodendroglioma**
1. This neoplasm presents as a slow-growing tumor in the middle-age group.
2. Morphologic characteristics include:
    a. Closely packed cells with large round nuclei surrounded by a clear halo of cytoplasm ("fried egg" appearance)
    b. Site of origin in the cerebral hemispheres
    c. Tumor divided into groups of cells by delicate capillary strands
    d. Foci of calcification

D. **Ependymoma**
1. This neoplasm most frequently occurs in the fourth ventricle.
2. Peak incidence is in childhood and adolescence.
3. Histologic characteristics include tubules or rosettes with cells encircling vessels or pointing toward a central lumen; tumor cells characteristically demonstrate blepharoplasts, rod-shaped structures near the nucleus representing basal bodies of cilia.
4. Results may include papillary growths that obstruct flow of CSF and lead to hydrocephalus.

E. **Meningioma**
1. This is the **second most common primary intracranial neoplasm.**
2. This a **benign, slowly growing tumor.**
3. This neoplasm most often occurs after 30 years of age. It occurs more frequently in women than in men.
4. The neoplasm originates in arachnoidal cells of the meninges; the tumor is external to the brain and can often be successfully removed surgically.
5. This neoplasm occurs most frequently in the convexities of the cerebral hemispheres and the parasagittal region; other common locations include the falx cerebri, sphenoid ridge, olfactory area, and suprasellar region.
6. Histologic characteristics include a whorled pattern of concentrically arranged spindle cells and laminated calcified psammoma bodies.

F. **Medulloblastoma**
1. This is one of the most common neoplasms of childhood.
2. It is a highly **malignant tumor of the cerebellum.**
3. Histologic characteristics include sheets of closely packed cells with scant cytoplasm arranged in a rosette or perivascular pseudorosette pattern.

G. **Neuroblastoma**
1. This neoplasm is closely related to neuroblastoma of the adrenal medulla or sympathetic ganglia.
2. This is much less common than peripheral neuroblastoma.
3. Amplification of the N-*myc* oncogene (multiple copies demonstrable either as homogeneously staining regions or as extrachromosomal double minute chromatin bodies) is characteristic; a greater degree of amplification correlates with worse prognosis.

H. **Hemangioblastoma**
1. This neoplasm occurs most frequently in the cerebellum.
2. It may be associated with similar lesions in the retina and other organs as part of von Hippel-Lindau disease.
3. It sometimes produces erythropoietin, leading to secondary polycythemia.

I. **Neurilemmoma (schwannoma)**
1. This benign, slowly growing encapsulated tumor arises from Schwann cells.
2. When intracranial, it is most frequently localized to the eighth cranial nerve (**acoustic neuroma,** acoustic schwannoma); acoustic neuroma is the **third most common primary intracranial neoplasm.**
3. It also originates frequently in posterior nerve roots and peripheral nerves.

4. It is characterized histologically by one of two patterns:
   a. **Antoni A:** interlacing bundles of elongated cells with palisading nuclei
   b. **Antoni B:** looser, less cellular pattern than Antoni A

J. **Neurofibroma**
   1. This neoplasm occurs as solitary or multiple tumors of peripheral nerves derived from Schwann cells.
   2. It may be part of von Recklinghausen neurofibromatosis.

K. **Metastatic tumors**
   1. These tumors are more common than any of the primary intracranial neoplasms.
   2. They originate most frequently from primary sites in lung, breast, skin, kidney, gastrointestinal tract, and thyroid.

REVIEW TEST

***Directions:** Each of the numbered items or incomplete statements in this section is followed by answers or by completions of the statement. Select the **one** lettered answer or completion that is best in each case.*

1. A 75-year-old woman appears well after slipping on wet pavement and striking the right side of her head. When questioned, she says that she does not remember the fall. Subsequently she complains of persistent headache and confusion. Magnetic imaging studies reveal a subdural hematoma over the lateral aspect of the right cerebral hemisphere. Which of the following is a well-known association or characteristic of this disorder?

(A) Bleeding from arteries of the circle of Willis
(B) Rapidly progressive cerebral compression
(C) Characteristically caused by venous hemorrhage
(D) Laceration of branches of middle meningeal artery
(E) Causally associated with hypertension

2. A 2-year-old child presents with fever, headache, prostration, and nuchal rigidity. The cerebrospinal fluid (CSF) is cloudy, and microscopic examination reveals innumerable neutrophils. The CSF protein is increased, and glucose is decreased. The most likely etiologic agent is

(A) *Escherichia coli*
(B) *Haemophilus influenzae*
(C) group B streptococci
(D) *Streptococcus pneumoniae*
(E) *Staphylococcus aureus*

3. A 40-year-old woman who has had progressive localizing signs of central nervous system compression fully recovers following resection of an intracranial neoplasm. These clinical findings are highly suggestive of a specific diagnosis. Assuming that this diagnosis is correct, which of the following is most characteristic?

(A) Extracranial metastases
(B) "Fried egg" appearance of tumor cells
(C) Multiple areas of necrosis and hemorrhage within the tumor
(D) Origin in arachnoidal cells of the meninges
(E) Tumor cells arranged in a rosette pattern

4. The figures shown here are representative of the gross and microscopic appearance of an autopsy specimen from a 55-year-old woman who had a 1-year history of progressive headache and seizures leading to aphasia. The diagnosis is

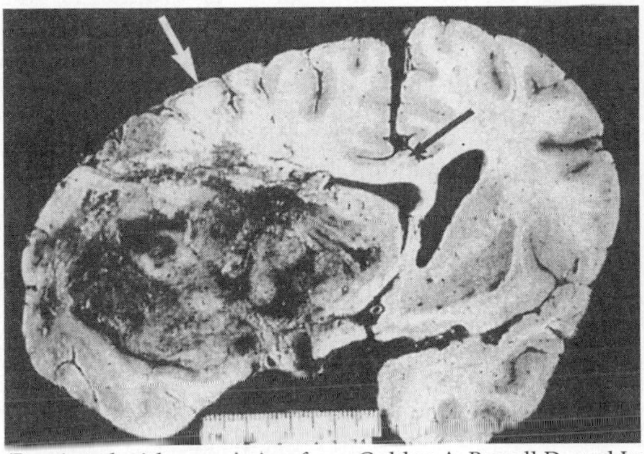

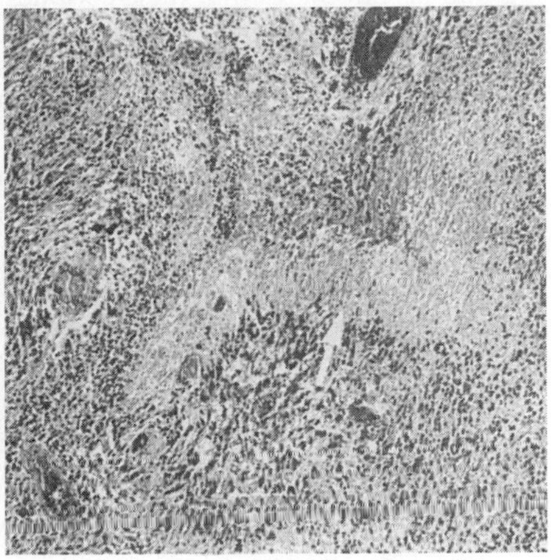

(Reprinted with permission from Golden A, Powell D, and Jennings C: *Pathology: Understanding Human Disease*, 2nd ed. Baltimore, Williams & Wilkins, 1985, p 266, p 267.)

(A) ependymoma
(B) glioblastoma multiforme
(C) medulloblastoma
(D) meningioma
(E) oligodendroglioma

5. A newborn girl is found to have herniation of both the spinal cord and meninges through a defect in the vertebral arch of the spinal column. Her mother had not had prenatal care and had not taken nutritional supplements during pregnancy. Which of the following best describes this defect?

(A) Spina bifida occulta
(B) Meningocele
(C) Meningomyelocele
(D) Anencephaly

6. Following a bar fight, a 22-year-old man is brought unconscious to the emergency department. Several minutes earlier, he had been hit on the head with a heavy iron club and had been briefly unconscious, but had then apparently recovered. One or two minutes later, he had again lost consciousness. Which of the following is the most likely diagnosis?

(A) Epidural hematoma
(B) Subarachnoid hemorrhage
(C) Subdural hematoma
(D) Transient ischemic attack
(E) Stroke

7. A 60-year-old woman with chronic atrial fibrillation is seen in the emergency department because of acute onset of marked weakness of her right arm, drooping of the left side of her face, and verbal aphasia. T_2-weighted magnetic resonance imaging reveals a cerebral infarct. Assuming that the lesion has been caused by embolization from the left atrium, which vessel is the most likely site of embolic arrest?

(A) Right middle cerebral artery
(B) Left middle cerebral artery
(C) Right anterior cerebral artery
(D) Left anterior cerebral artery
(E) Right posterior cerebral artery

8. A 25-year-old woman presents with brief episodes of loss of vision in her left eye, paresthesias (sensory loss), and clumsiness in her hands. She states that these episodes come and go. Magnetic resonance imaging of the head reveals paraventricular plaques of demyelination in the central nervous system white matter. A cerebrospinal fluid (CSF) tap is performed. The patient is diagnosed with multiple sclerosis. Which of the following is the most likely finding in the CSF?

(A) Acellular, with normal glucose and normal protein
(B) Albumino-cytologic dissociation, with markedly increased protein but only modestly increased cell count
(C) Increased immunoglobulin, manifesting as multiple oligoclonal bands on electrophoresis
(D) Increased neutrophils, with decreased glucose and increased protein

9. A 70-year-old man presents with loss of memory for recent events. He has forgotten his grandchildren's names, and he has been unable to manage his personal finances. Also, he has lost his way while driving to familiar locations. Which of the following is the most likely diagnosis?

(A) Alzheimer disease
(B) Amyotrophic lateral sclerosis
(C) Creutzfeldt-Jakob disease
(D) Huntington disease
(E) Parkinson disease

10. A 45-year-old man presents with involuntary facial grimaces and movements of the fingers. His mother had had similar symptoms beginning at about the same age. Her disorder had progressed to dancing movements, writhing of the arms and legs, and eventually coma and death. His maternal grandfather had had a similar disorder but at an age older than the mother. Which of the following is most characteristic of this disease?

(A) Degeneration of upper and lower motor neurons
(B) Dopamine depletion and depigmentation of the substantia nigra
(C) Increased number of trinucleotide repeats in a gene on chromosome 4
(D) Neurofibrillary tangles and amyloid plaques in the cerebral cortex
(E) Pick bodies, characterized by round intracytoplasmic inclusions consisting of neurofilaments

11. Several years ago, a 60-year-old woman had presented with bradykinesia, rigidity, a resting pill-rolling tremor in her right hand, and "mask-like," expressionless facies. She currently presents with gait problems, taking short, shuffling steps and losing her balance easily. Which of the following is the most likely diagnosis?

(A) Alzheimer disease
(B) Amyotrophic lateral sclerosis
(C) Creutzfeldt-Jakob disease
(D) Huntington disease
(E) Parkinson disease

12. A 60-year-old man, a suicide victim, comes to autopsy. Before dying, he had been despondent after being informed that he had an extremely aggressive brain tumor. There had been a recent onset of headache, seizures, and mental status changes, and magnetic resonance imaging (MRI) had demonstrated an infiltrating neoplasm invading the cerebral hemispheres and crossing the midline, with areas of necrosis and abnormal blood vessels. The autopsy confirms the MRI findings and also demonstrates hemorrhage and a pseudopalisade arrangement of tumor cells. The tumor is most likely a (an)

(A) ependymoma
(B) glioblastoma multiforme
(C) meningioma
(D) neurilemmoma (schwannoma)
(E) oligodendroglioma

ANSWERS AND EXPLANATIONS

1-C. Subdural hematoma is characteristically caused by venous bleeding, most often from veins that join the cerebrum to venous sinuses within the dura. The venous hemorrhage typically arrests early, but the volume of the hematoma gradually increases because of osmotic imbibement of water. This results in a slowly enlarging tumor-like mass characterized clinically by gradual signs of cerebral compression occurring hours to days or even weeks after head injury.

2-D. Pyogenic meningitis in older infants and young children is most frequently caused by *Streptococcus pneumoniae* or *Neisseria meningitidis.* In newborns, the most likely agents are group B streptococci, *Escherichia coli,* and *Listeria;* in young adults, the most frequent agent is *N. meningitidis.* In older adults, especially those with impaired resistance to infection, the most common etiologic agents are *S. pneumoniae* and gram-negative rods.

3-D. Meningioma is the second most common primary intracranial neoplasm of adults, second only to glioblastoma multiforme. Because this slowly growing benign tumor arises from the arachnoidal cells of the meninges, it is actually external to the brain and is frequently amenable to surgical resection and complete cure.

4-B. The lesion shown in the illustrations is a glioblastoma multiforme, the most frequently occurring primary neoplasm of the central nervous system. Characteristic features include the intracerebral location, prominent hemorrhage and necrosis, and the pseudopalisading appearance of the pleomorphic tumor cells.

5-C. A meningomyelocele is a neural tube defect in which both the meninges and spinal cord are included in the herniated tissue. A meningocele is a defect in which the herniated membranes consist only of meninges, and spina bifida occulta does not manifest any apparent abnormalities. Anencephaly is the diminution or absence of fetal brain tissue. In neural tube defects, an increase in α-fetoprotein in both the maternal serum and the amniotic fluid is noted.

6-A. An epidural hematoma is an arterial hemorrhage between the dura and the skull, most often resulting from skull fracture and laceration of the middle meningeal artery. Epidural hematomas are characterized clinically by a short period of consciousness (lucid interval) followed by loss of consciousness and signs of cerebral compression. A subdural hematoma is venous hemorrhage underneath the dura, resulting from laceration of the bridging veins. Subdural hematomas are characterized clinically by gradual signs of cerebral compression occurring hours, days, or weeks after injury. Subarachnoid hemorrhage is commonly associated with rupture of a berry aneurysm in the circle of Willis. A transient ischemic attack is a brief episode of impaired neurologic function caused by a brief disturbance in cerebral circulation.

7-B. The middle cerebral arteries are the most common sites of cerebral embolic occlusion in general, and in this instance, the involvement is almost certainly left-sided. Middle cerebral artery lesions are manifest by contralateral upper extremity weakness and ipsilateral facial weakness. Also, in right-handed individuals, the left side of the cerebral cortex is usually dominant, and verbal aphasias are caused by left-sided lesions in the great majority of cases. Anterior cerebral artery occlusions cause contralateral lower extremity weakness and altered mental status. Posterior artery occlusions cause contralateral homonymous hemianopsia (e.g., right-sided posterior artery occlusion causes left visual field loss).

8-C. Multiple sclerosis is the most common demyelinating disease and is characterized by destruction of myelin with relative preservation of axons. The classic cerebrospinal fluid (CSF) electrophoretic finding is that of multiple oligoclonal bands of immunoglobulin. Also, the incidence of multiple sclerosis is increased in association with HLA haplotypes A3, B7, DR2, and DW2, suggesting that immune factors may play a role. The disease is associated with plaques scattered irregularly throughout the central nervous system. Common sites are the optic nerve, brain stem, and paraventricular areas. Although characterized by exacerbations and remissions, the course is progressive, leading to increasing disability. Albumino-cytologic dissociation in the CSF is characteristic of Guillain-Barré syndrome. Increased neutrophils, decreased glucose, and increased protein are characteristics of bacterial meningitis.

9-A. Alzheimer disease is a major cause of dementia and is characterized by relatively slow, progressive memory loss followed in later stages by motor problems, contractures, and paralysis. Morphologic findings in Alzheimer disease include neurofibrillary tangles within neurons in the cerebral cortex, neuritic (senile) amyloid plaques, Hirano bodies, and generalized cerebral atrophy.

10-C. This is a case of Huntington disease, an autosomal dominant, fatal, progressive degeneration and atrophy of the striatum (caudate nucleus and putamen). The disorder is characterized by an increased number of trinucleotide (CAG) repeats in the HD (huntingtin) gene on the short arm of chromosome 4. Degeneration of the upper and lower motor neurons is characteristic of amyotrophic lateral sclerosis. Dopamine depletion and depigmentation of the substantia nigra is characteristic of Parkinson disease. Neurofibrillary tangles and amyloid plaques are found in Alzheimer disease. Pick bodies can be found in Pick disease, which clinically resembles Alzheimer disease.

11-E. Parkinson disease, or parkinsonism, is characterized by a resting pill-rolling tremor, masked facies, slowness of movements, muscular rigidity, and a festinating (shuffling) gait. Parkinsonism can be idiopathic or due to trauma, drugs, toxins (e.g., methyl-phenyl-tetrahydropyridine), or to the Shy-Drager syndrome. In the past, a major cause was von Economo encephalitis.

12-B. Glioblastoma multiforme is the most common primary intracranial neoplasm. This brain tumor has a very poor prognosis, with death occurring in less than 1 year.

CHAPTER 24

Interpretation of Diagnostic Tests: Laboratory Statistics

I. General Considerations

- Laboratory results can be interpreted (often by comparison to reference ranges) as positive or negative.

A. **Positive results.** These can be further divided into true-positive results and false-positive results.

1. A **true-positive (TP) result** is a positive test result for a person with the appropriate disease.
2. A **false-positive (FP) result** is a positive test result for a healthy person.

B. These definitions depend on determination of the presence or absence of the disease by criteria other than the laboratory test (e.g., through biopsy).

C. **Negative results.** Similarly, these can be divided into true-negative results and false-negative results.

1. A **true-negative (TN) result** is a negative test result in a healthy person.
2. A **false-negative (FN) result** is a negative test result in a person with the appropriate disease.

II. Sensitivity and Specificity (Table 24-1)

A. **General considerations**

1. These concepts describe quantitatively the ability of a test to correctly identify populations of persons with and without a particular disease.
2. They are independent of the **prevalence** of the disease, which is the occurrence of a disorder or trait in a given population, often expressed as a ratio, such as 1:10,000.
3. They are also independent of the **incidence** of the disease, which is the occurrence of new cases in a defined interval of time.

B. **Sensitivity**

1. Sensitivity measures the **extent to which a laboratory test is positive in patients** (i.e., correctly identifies persons with the appropriate disease).
2. It is the ratio (expressed as a percentage) of TP results to all results in persons with the disease (TP + FN).

TABLE 24-1 ***Frequently Used Laboratory Computations***

Standard deviation	$\sqrt{\frac{\Sigma(X-\overline{X})^2}{n-1}}$ or $\sqrt{\frac{\Sigma X^2 - \frac{(\Sigma X)^2}{n}}{n-1}}$ where Σ = sum of $X - \overline{X}$ = difference of each observation from the mean n = number of observations
Sensitivity	$\frac{TP}{TP + FN} \times 100$ where TP = true positives FN = false negatives
Specificity	$\frac{TN}{TN + FP} \times 100$ where TN = true negatives FP = false positives
Positive predictive value	$\frac{TP}{TP + FP} \times 100$
Negative predictive value	$\frac{TN}{TN + FN} \times 100$
Coefficient of variation	$\frac{\text{Standard deviation}}{\text{Mean}} \times 100$

FN = false negative; FP = false positive; TN = true negative; TP = true positive.

3. Ideally, sensitivity should be very high when a procedure is used as a screening test, because it is desirable to identify as many persons as possible with the disease. For most analytic procedures (i.e., when abnormal results are higher rather than lower), the point of maximum sensitivity is the lowest test value that detects subjects with the disease.

C. **Specificity**

1. Specificity measures **the extent to which a laboratory test is negative in healthy persons** (i.e., correctly identifies persons who do not have the appropriate disease).
2. It is the ratio of TN results to all results of persons free of the disease (TN + FP).
3. Ideally, specificity should be very high when a procedure is used as a confirmatory test, because it is desirable to exclude as many people as possible who do not have the disease. For most analytic procedures, the point of maximum specificity is the highest test value that correctly identifies all subjects without the disease.

III. Positive and Negative Predictive Values (see Table 24-1)

- These value describe quantitatively the likelihood that a positive or negative result in an individual is correctly predictive of the presence or absence of the disease.
- They are dependent on the prevalence of the disease (in contrast to sensitivity and specificity).

A. **Positive predictive value**

1. This value is a measure of the **likelihood that a person with a positive test result actually has the disease**.
2. It is the ratio of TP results to all positive results (TP + FP).

B. **Negative predictive value**

1. This value is a measure of the **likelihood that a person with a negative test result is actually free of the disease.**
2. This is the ratio of TN results to all negative results (TN + FN).

IV. Variation

A. **Physiologic variation**
1. This type of variation describes variable laboratory results unrelated to disease processes.
2. It is called **diurnal variation** when laboratory results vary systematically according to the time of day.
3. It is called **day-to-day variation** when results vary from day to day.
4. In some instances, it is influenced by variable factors such as diet, exercise, posture, or the effects of smoking, alcohol, medications.

B. **Analytic variation: precision (reproducibility)**
1. This type of variation describes the **variability of repeated laboratory measurements on identical specimens** over a specified time span. The measurements are most often repeated at daily intervals, thus assessing daily variability.
2. It is quantitatively described by the **coefficient of variation** (CV) (see Table 24-1).
   a. The CV is defined as the **ratio of the standard deviation to the mean of the values in the series** and is an inverse measurement of precision. Thus, tests with a low CV are very precise (e.g., hemoglobin, hematocrit) and tests with a high CV are less precise (e.g., most serum enzyme measurements).
   b. It is desirable to attain a high degree of precision if a test is used to monitor progression of a disease or the effects of therapy (e.g., successive measurements of a cancer marker in a patient with a known tumor).
   c. To be analytically useful, the CV ideally should not exceed 25% of the physiologic variation.

REVIEW TEST

***Directions:** Each of the numbered items or incomplete statements in this section is followed by answers or by completions of the statement. Select the* **one** *lettered answer or completion that is best in each case.*

1. A worker in a research laboratory is developing a new diagnostic procedure making use of a newly discovered marker protein for ovarian cancer. The laboratory has at its disposal 1000 preserved serum samples from patients who are known to have had this tumor. The percentage of the samples that test positive with this new procedure is referred to as the

(A) sensitivity
(B) specificity
(C) precision
(D) accuracy
(E) predictive value

2. Conversely, the same laboratory has at its disposal 1000 similarly preserved serum samples from normal subjects who are known not to have had ovarian cancer. The ability of the new procedure to correctly identify these individuals as normal is referred to as

(A) sensitivity
(B) specificity
(C) precision
(D) accuracy
(E) predictive value

Questions 3–7: Questions 3 through 7 refer to the following scenario:
A biotechnology company has just released a new blood screening test for ovarian cancer. The test is positive in 90% of all women with ovarian cancer and negative in 80% of women without ovarian cancer. The prevalence of ovarian cancer in the study population of 1000 women is 30%.

3. What is the sensitivity of this test?

(A) 32.5%
(B) 66%
(C) 80%
(D) 90%
(E) 95%

4. What is the specificity of this test?

(A) 32.5%
(B) 66%
(C) 80%
(D) 90%
(E) 95%

5. What is the positive predictive value of this test?

(A) 32.5%
(B) 66%
(C) 80%
(D) 90%
(E) 95%

6. What is the negative predictive value of this test?

(A) 32.5%
(B) 66%
(C) 80%
(D) 90%
(E) 95%

7. A physician participating in this study finds that one of his patients has a positive test result. What is the likelihood that this patient has ovarian cancer?

(A) 66%
(B) 80%
(C) 90%
(D) 95%

8. A urologist is using prostate-specific antigen (PSA) measurements to monitor the progress of one of his patients, a 73-year-old-man who has high-grade prostatic intraepithelial neoplasia. At a prior office visit, the PSA had been 6 ng/mL (normal less than 4 ng/mL). At the current visit, PSA is 6.2 ng/mL. Which of the following laboratory measurements is most useful to the urologist in assessing the significance of the change in PSA?

(A) Accuracy
(B) Coefficient of variation
(C) Positive predictive value
(D) Sensitivity
(E) Specificity

9. A medical student participating in a summer fellowship program begins to work on an inborn error of metabolism referred to as Z disease. In the course of his investigations, he develops a diagnostic procedure for the disorder. A survey of unaffected normal subjects demonstrates the Z test to always be negative in this group. However, the Z test is found to be positive in 160 of 1000 subjects from a geographically isolated population group in which the prevalence of the disorder (as assessed by clinical features) is known to be 20%. What is the sensitivity of the test?

(A) 65%
(B) 70%
(C) 75%
(D) 80%
(E) 85%

Questions 10–12: Questions 10 through 12 refer to the following scenario:
A newly established physician in a small community is asked to advise a local committee that is designing a set of physical standards for potential volunteer firefighters. He is told that firefighters must test negative for a new blood chemistry test, the S test, which predicts susceptibility to smoke inhalation damage. It is known (for unexplained reasons) that susceptibility to smoke damage is uncommon in brown-eyed persons, more common in green-eyed persons, and very common in blue-eyed persons. The S test is found to have a sensitivity of 99% and a specificity of 99%. The S test is further evaluated in three highly selected population subgroups, each with differing eye colors (and thus with different prevalences of susceptibility to smoke inhalation damage).

10. What is the likelihood that the S test will correctly identify a potential firefighter as one with an unacceptable sensitivity to smoke inhalation damage if the applicant is *brown-eyed* (prevalence of susceptibility in this group is known to be 1 in 1000)?

(A) 1%
(B) 9%
(C) 50%
(D) 92%
(E) 99%

11. What is the likelihood that the S test will correctly identify a potential firefighter as one with an unacceptable sensitivity to smoke inhalation damage if the applicant is *green-eyed* (prevalence of susceptibility is known to be 1 in 100)?

(A) 1%
(B) 9%
(C) 50%
(D) 92%
(E) 99%

12. What is the likelihood that the S test will correctly identify a potential firefighter as one with an unacceptable sensitivity to smoke inhalation damage if the applicant is *blue-eyed* (prevalence of susceptibility is known to be 1 in 10)?

(A) 1%
(B) 9%
(C) 50%
(D) 92%
(E) 99%

13. A screening program is started test potential blood donors for human immunodeficiency virus infection. Two screening tests are under consideration, and you are asked for your opinion on the use of these testing procedures. Test A has a known sensitivity of 99.9% and a specificity of 99.9%. Test B has a sensitivity of only 90%, but has a specificity of 100%. Which of the following should be your advice on the use of these procedures for screening?

(A) For screening purposes, Test A should be used instead of Test B, since it has the higher sensitivity.
(B) For screening purposes, Test B should be used instead of Test A, since it has the higher specificity.

ANSWERS AND EXPLANATIONS

1-A. Sensitivity is defined as the ability of a test to be positive in patients with a specific disease; it is the percentage of known positives who actually test positive. It is calculated by dividing the number of positive results in patients (true positives, or TP) by the total number of patients (true positives plus false negatives, or TP + FN).

2-B. Specificity is defined as the ability of a test to be negative in healthy persons; it is the percentage of known negatives who actually test negative. It is calculated by dividing the number of negative results in healthy persons (true negatives, or TN) by the total number of healthy persons (true negatives plus false positives, or TN + FN).

3-D. Sensitivity is defined as the probability that a test will be positive in individuals who are already known to have disease (ovarian cancer) and is stated to be 90%.

4-C. Specificity is defined as the probability that a test will be negative in individuals who are already known to be healthy (no ovarian cancer) and is stated to be 80%.

5-B. The positive predictive value is the probability that a woman with a positive test actually has the disease in question. In this example, there are 410 women (270 true positives [90% of 300] + 140 false positives [20% of 700]) who had a positive test result. The ratio of true positives (TP) to all positives (TP + FP) is 270/410, or 66%.

6-E. The negative predictive value is the probability that a woman with a negative test does *not* have the disease in question. In this example, there are 590 women (560 true negatives [TN] [80% of 700] + 30 false negatives [FN] [10% of 300]) who had a negative test result. The ratio of TN to all negatives (TN + FN) is 560/590, or 95%.

7-A. This question is actually the same as question 5, just expressed in more familiar terms. The likelihood that this patient actually has ovarian cancer is determined by the predictive value of a positive result, which in this instance is 66%.

8-B. If a test is used to monitor progressive changes in a patient, the test results must be highly reproducible, that is, have a high degree of precision. The coefficient of variation (CV), a measure of precision, describes the variability of repetitive measurements on the same sample. For most laboratory procedures, precision is determined by successive daily measurements on a stored, properly preserved sample. The standard deviation of the repetitive measurements is divided by the mean of the values, yielding the CV. The rule is that the more reproducible the test, the lower the CV.

9-D. Sensitivity, the ability of a test to be positive in patients with a specific disease, is expressed as the ratio of true positives to the total number of patients known to have the disease. In this example, the number of true positive results is the same as the total number of positive results because the test is stated to always be negative in healthy persons; that is, the specificity is 100%, and there are no false positives. Thus, the sensitivity is (160/ [0.2 × 1000]) × 100, or 80%. In perhaps simpler terms, a population of 1000 with a prevalence of 20% has 200 persons with the disease. One hundred sixty test positive. Thus, the sensitivity is 160/200 × 100, or 80%.

10-B. A population arbitrarily set at 100,000 (to avoid the use of decimal fractions) includes 100 potential firefighters with unacceptable smoke damage susceptibility (0.1% of 100,000) and 99,900 individuals resistant to smoke damage (100,000 – 100). Of the 100 applicants, 99 test positive (99% of 100). Of the 99,900 unaffected persons, 999 test positive ([100 – 99]% of 99,900). The total number of positive results is thus 99 (true positives) + 999 (false positives). The predictive value of a positive result is then 99/(99 + 999), or approximately 9%.

11-C. A similar computation yields a predictive value of a positive result of 50%.

12-D. In this very high prevalence subgroup, the predictive value of a positive result is 92%. These three examples illustrate the profound effect of prevalence on the usefulness of a diagnostic test. Although these examples are centered on a fictitious laboratory-based employment standard, the real-life corollary is the usefulness of screening procedures in medical practice. A test procedure is more likely to be useful when directed to patients who have a high likelihood of the disorder, as dictated by good clinical judgment, than when used in an indiscriminate, unselective fashion.

13-A. Tests designed to screen for disease should be highly sensitive in order to capture everyone in the population with the disease. If a test is highly sensitive, then a negative result essentially rules out disease. Test B should be used as a confirmatory test. If a test is highly specific, then a positive result essentially rules in disease.

Comprehensive Examination

1. During a pre-employment evaluation for an executive position, a 35-year-old man is found to have a serum calcium of 12.4 mg/100 mL (normal 9–11), a serum phosphorus (phosphate) of 2.0 mg/100 mL (normal 3.0–4.5), a serum alkaline phosphatase of 150 U/L (normal 20–70), and a serum parathyroid hormone (PTH) of 800 pg/mL (normal 225–650). If untreated, the likely lesion responsible for these findings will result in consequences mediated by which of the following mechanisms?

(A) Liquefactive necrosis
(B) Apoptosis
(C) Metastatic calcification
(D) Oxygen toxicity
(E) Amyloid deposition

2. After a football injury, a 16-year-old boy survives a ruptured spleen, hemorrhagic shock, and profound hypotension. However, a period of severe oliguria follows; so the boy undergoes a kidney biopsy. Which one of the following renal tubular changes found represents irreversible cellular injury?

(A) Fatty change
(B) Formation of cell blebs
(C) Formation of myelin figures
(D) Nuclear pyknosis
(E) Swelling of organelles

3. A 65-year-old woman fell and sustained a pelvic fracture. After a short period of rapidly progressive mental confusion and respiratory insufficiency, the woman died. Numerous conjunctival petechiae were noted. These abnormalities were most likely due to which one of the following conditions?

(A) Epidural hematoma
(B) Aspiration pneumonia
(C) Fat embolization
(D) Acute tubular necrosis
(E) Saddle embolus occluding bifurcation of pulmonary arteries

4. An Rh-positive neonate born to an Rh-negative mother has severe anemia and rapidly progressive jaundice. An older sibling, now also known to be Rh-positive, was delivered by a neighbor at home. The mother is unaware of any prior special testing or therapy related to anemia, jaundice, or "Rh problems." Which of the following mechanisms underlies the clinical scenario described here?

(A) Activation of sensitized CD4+ T cells with release of cytokines
(B) "Graft-versus-neonate" response of immunologically incompetent newborn
(C) Immunoglobulin (Ig)E-mediated degranulation of mast cells and basophils
(D) Immune complex deposition with secondary inflammatory reaction
(E) Interaction of IgG antibodies with intrinsic cell-surface antigens

5. A 17-year-old girl develops an acute syndrome characterized by low-grade fever, lassitude, pharyngitis, generalized lymphadenopathy, and a palpable liver and spleen. A peripheral blood smear reveals the presence of "atypical lymphocytes." A heterophil test for antibodies reacting with sheep erythrocytes is negative. Infection with which one of the following viruses is most likely?

(A) Cytomegalovirus (CMV)
(B) Epstein-Barr virus (EBV)
(C) Measles virus
(D) Papillomavirus
(E) Parvovirus

6. A 70-year-old man is found to have a papillomatous neoplasm of the bladder. Even though the lesion is extremely well-differentiated, the pathologist makes a diagnosis of transitional cell carcinoma grade I (urothelial neoplasm of low malignant potential). The distinction of "malignant" from "benign" in this instance was most likely based on which of the following known general characteristics of this type of lesion?

(A) Appearance of oncofetal antigens
(B) Chromosomal aneuploidy
(C) Loss of contact inhibition in tissue culture
(D) Clinical behavior
(E) Ultrastructural alterations

7. A 24-year-old nonsmoker who does not consume alcohol is found to have both pulmonary emphysema and cirrhosis of the liver. A sister and several close relatives also have had similar findings. This history suggests that this patient's illness may be caused by deficiency of

(A) α_1-antitrypsin.
(B) galactokinase.
(C) glucose-6-phosphatase.
(D) glucocerebrosidase.
(E) phenylalanine hydroxylase.

8. Upper and lower gastrointestinal endoscopic examinations are performed on a 45-year-old man. A lesion is found and the patient is told that the lesion has NO malignant potential. Of the following choices, which is the lesion that was most likely found?

(A) Colorectal villous adenoma
(B) Crohn disease
(C) Duodenal peptic ulcer
(D) Familial multiple polyposis
(E) Ulcerative colitis

9. A 60-year-old man presents with progressive bone deformity and pain, progressive hearing loss, and increasing skull size. Workup revealed generalized increased bone density with cortical thickening, normal serum calcium and phosphorus, and markedly elevated serum alkaline phosphatase. Biopsy revealed a characteristic "mosaic" pattern. Which one of the following tumors is a known complication of the disorder suggested by this scenario?

(A) Ewing sarcoma
(B) Giant cell tumor
(C) Metastatic duct carcinoma of the breast
(D) Multiple enchondromas
(E) Osteosarcoma

10. A 50-year-old woman had a partial colectomy performed for adenocarcinoma of the sigmoid colon, with apparent complete and uneventful recovery. At followup visits, her physician is particularly interested in changes that may occur in which of the following laboratory measures?

(A) Human chorionic gonadotropin (hCG)
(B) α-fetoprotein (AFP)
(C) Vanillylmandelic acid (VMA)
(D) Carcinoembryonic antigen (CEA)
(E) Estriol

11. A 21-year-old basketball player died suddenly during a game. Autopsy revealed hypertrophy of the left ventricular wall, especially of the ventricular septum. Histologically, the myocardial fibers were arranged in a disorganized pattern. Which of the following best characterizes this disorder?

(A) Can be a manifestation of primary amyloidosis
(B) Can be a result of myocarditis
(C) Is often associated with alcohol abuse
(D) Is often associated with coronary artery disease
(E) Often demonstrates autosomal dominant inheritance

12. A 40-year-old woman in the 30th week of gestation presents to the emergency room because she has vaginal bleeding and lower abdominal pain. The uterus is tender to palpation and there are signs of fetal distress. Because of hematuria and rectal bleeding, disseminated intravascular coagulation (DIC) is suspected. Which of the following findings would be most supportive of the diagnosis of DIC?

(A) Increased fibrin degradation products
(B) Decreased activated partial thromboplastin time (APTT)
(C) Decreased prothrombin time (PT)
(D) Normal thrombin time
(E) Thrombocytosis

13. A 10-day old infant has high fever, nuchal rigidity, and photophobia. A lumbar puncture is performed to obtain cerebrospinal fluid (CSF) for analysis. Which of the following is the most likely CSF finding?

(A) Decreased protein, decreased glucose
(B) Decreased protein, increased glucose
(C) Increased protein, decreased glucose
(D) Increased protein, increased glucose
(E) Normal protein, decreased glucose

14. In an experimental model, an autopsy study of a rat exposed to toxic doses of carbon tetrachloride (CCl_4) revealed fatty change and necrosis of hepatocytes. The mechanism of cell injury exemplified here is

(A) activation of apoptosis.
(B) acute phase reaction.
(C) arrest of cell cycle.
(D) free radical injury.
(E) thrombosis and ischemia.

15. A 48-year-old man with early-stage colon cancer undergoes a partial resection of the colon. Molecular analysis reveals that the tumor tissue harbors a mutation in codon 12 of the *ras* oncogene. The mutant gene codes for a ras protein product that has

(A) decreased GTPase activity.
(B) decreased reverse transcriptase activity.
(C) increased protein phosphatase activity.
(D) increased responsiveness to growth factors.
(E) increased tyrosine kinase activity.

16. A 68-year-old woman presents with fever, chills, and cough productive of blood-tinged sputum. Fluid aspirated from the right pleural space would most likely

(A) be clear and straw-colored in appearance.
(B) contain large numbers of neutrophils.
(C) have a glucose content somewhat higher than the serum glucose.
(D) have a protein content of less than 1 g/dL.
(E) have a specific gravity of 1.012.

17. Prior to the birth of a stillborn infant, decreased amniotic fluid (oligohydramnios) for gestational age was demonstrated on ultrasound examination. Which of the following autopsy findings of the stillborn is most consistent with this maternal–fetal abnormality?

(A) Infection with *Toxoplasma gondii* plus microcephaly, hydrocephaly, chorioretinitis, and microphthalmia
(B) Infection with rubella virus along with microcephaly and heart malformations
(C) Infection with CMV plus microcephaly, hepatitis, and intracranial calcifications
(D) Microcephaly, facial anomalies, and a number of CNS anomalies as well as a history of major maternal alcohol abuse
(E) Bilateral renal agenesis and hypoplasia of one lung

18. A 45-year African-American man has marked splenomegaly. This finding is unusual and unexpected in which of the following disorders?

(A) Infectious mononucleosis
(B) Sickle cell anemia
(C) Chronic myelogenous leukemia
(D) Hereditary spherocytosis
(E) Agnogenic myeloid metaplasia (idiopathic myelofibrosis)

19. A 68-year-old man presented with painless hematuria. Cystoscopic examination revealed a papillary tumor. Excisional biopsy was performed, and the diagnosis of transitional cell carcinoma was made. Which of the following is a well-known association of this type of cancer?

(A) Early hematogenous spread
(B) Exposure to aflatoxin
(C) Long-term use of methyldopa, an antihypertensive agent
(D) Industrial exposure to aniline dyes such as β-naphthylamine
(E) *Schistosoma haematobium* infection

20. A 16-year-old girl with short stature, rounded face, and shortening of the fourth and fifth metacarpals and metatarsals has hypocalcemia and hyperphosphatemia. She has multiple calcifications involving the basal ganglia, vasculature, and other sites. PTH varies from normal to increased, and administration of PTH does not result in phosphaturia. These findings are characteristic of which of the following?

(A) Primary hyperparathyroidism
(B) Secondary hyperparathyroidism
(C) Tertiary hyperparathyroidism
(D) Hypoparathyroidism
(E) Pseudohypoparathyroidism

21. A 56-year-old woman presents with bone pain, diffuse demineralization of bone, hypercalcemia, anemia, hypergammaglobulinemia, proteinuria, and normal serum alkaline phosphatase. This set of findings is most suggestive of

(A) Ewing sarcoma.
(B) hyperparathyroidism.
(C) multiple myeloma.
(D) osteomalacia.
(E) Paget disease of bone.

22. A biopsy of a "cold" nodule from the left lobe of the thyroid from an otherwise asymptomatic 30-year-old woman is found to demonstrate a malignant proliferation of C cells and an amyloid stroma that stains positively with a Congo red stain. This tumor is referred to as which of the following types of carcinoma?

(A) Epidermoid
(B) Follicular
(C) Medullary
(D) Papillary
(E) Undifferentiated

23. A 55-year-old woman who died suddenly at home was found at autopsy to have suffered a rupture of the left ventricle. Which one of the following myocardial changes is the most frequent cause of this catastrophic event?

(A) Abscess formation and tissue destruction due to infective endocarditis
(B) Fatty change due to interaction of diphtheria exotoxin and carnitine
(C) Inflammation associated with Aschoff bodies
(D) Inflammation due to coxsackie B infection
(E) Necrosis due to coronary artery obstruction

24. A 4-year-old boy is seen after he suddenly develops a fever, abdominal pain and tenderness, hematuria, and palpable purpuric skin lesions on his buttocks and the extensor surfaces of the arms and legs. The most likely diagnosis is

(A) Henoch–Schönlein purpura.
(B) idiopathic (immune) thrombocytopenic purpura (ITP).
(C) Kawasaki disease.
(D) polyarteritis nodosa.
(E) thrombotic thrombocytopenic purpura (TTP).

25. A 65-year-old man is found to have the combination of increased skin pigmentation, cirrhosis of the liver, and diabetes mellitus. Which pattern of serum iron and total iron-binding capacity (TIBC) is most consistent with the familial illness suggested by these findings?

(A) Serum iron increased, TIBC increased
(B) Serum iron increased, TIBC decreased
(C) Serum iron normal, TIBC increased
(D) Serum iron decreased, TIBC increased
(E) Serum iron decreased, TIBC decreased

26. A 45-year-old woman dies several days after a partial small bowel resection for repair of a volvulus. The surgery had apparently gone well, but shortly afterward she developed intractable fever, hypotension, multiorgan failure, and marked respiratory distress. Just prior to death, chest radiographs showed complete "whiteout" of both lungs. At autopsy, both lungs were found to have collapsed or distended alveoli, many of which were lined with fibrin-rich hyaline membranes. The cause of these pulmonary findings is best characterized as

(A) aspiration.
(B) diffuse alveolar damage.
(C) generalized atelectasis.
(D) lobar consolidation.
(E) pneumothorax.

27. A 6-month-old boy with hypertension is found to have a very large tumor arising in the left adrenal gland. Microscopically, the tumor consists of sheets of "small round blue cells" with minimal cytoplasm. Some of the cells contain pink cytoplasm and nucleoli, suggesting differentiation toward ganglion cells, and neurosecretory granules are visualized by electron microscopy. Urinary VMA is markedly increased. Which of the following is a major characteristic of this neoplasm?

(A) Characteristic gene deletions on chromosome 5
(B) Highly differentiated form of malignant ganglioneuroma
(C) Posterior cranial fossa origin with metastasis to both adrenals
(D) Serotonin production
(E) Spontaneous differentiation in some instances

28. A 34-year-old man, who is positive for human immunodeficiency virus (HIV), and a resident of the Ohio–Mississippi River valleys region, developed a systemic illness characterized by hepatosplenomegaly and generalized lymphadenopathy. Which of the following microscopic descriptions of organisms from a resected lesion is most consistent with a presumptive diagnosis of disseminated histoplasmosis?

(A) Budding yeast forms surrounded by empty haloes
(B) Cup-shaped forms demonstrable by silver stain within a foamy amorphous intra-alveolar exudate
(C) Intracavitary mycelial forms
(D) Minute fungal yeast forms within phagocytes
(E) Thick-walled spherules filled with endospores

29. In a 44-year-old man with hemoptysis and hematuria, a linear pattern of glomerular immunofluorescence for IgG is observed in a renal biopsy. The most likely associated laboratory finding is a positive test for antibodies directed to

(A) streptolysin O.
(B) C3 convertase.
(C) glomerular basement membranes.
(D) hepatitis B virus.
(E) Sm (Smith) nuclear antigen.

30. After being picked up by the police, a runaway adolescent girl became increasingly somnolent, lapsing into a deep coma 72 hours later. Her respirations were rapid and deep, and she appeared to be severely dehydrated. Laboratory studies revealed a marked reduction in serum bicarbonate and a significant anion gap, as well as neutrophilic leukocytosis. The most likely additional laboratory abnormality is

(A) a blood urea nitrogen (BUN):creatinine ratio of less than 1:10.
(B) decreased serum cortisol.
(C) decreased serum thyroxine (T_4).
(D) increased CSF protein with no parallel increase in cell count.
(E) increased serum glucose.

31. A 65-year-old alcoholic is found to have megaloblastic anemia. He has no neurologic abnormalities. Serum and erythrocyte folate are markedly decreased, and serum vitamin B_{12} is normal. Which of the following is an expected characteristic of this form of anemia?

(A) Decreased susceptibility to malaria
(B) Hypochromic erythrocytes
(C) Increased mean corpuscular hemoglobin concentration (MCHC)
(D) Increased mean corpuscular volume (MCV)
(E) Suppressed β-chain synthesis

32. A 56-year-old man collapsed at work and died 20 minutes later in the emergency room while blood was being drawn.The patient's history revealed an episode of prolonged chest discomfort 3 months earlier. Which of the following is least likely?

(A) Death from arrhythmia
(B) Fibrotic scar in the ventricular septum
(C) Loss of myocardial striations and beginning infiltration with neutrophils
(D) Normal values for serum creatine kinase, troponin I, and myoglobin
(E) Severe atherosclerotic narrowing of the anterior descending branch of the left coronary artery with overlying thrombus formation

33. A 25-year-old man is seen because he has a purulent urethral discharge. Microscopic examination reveals the presence of gram-negative diplococci within neutrophilic phagocytes. Which of the following structures is most resistant to infection with the likely organism responsible for this man's findings?

(A) Urethra
(B) Prostate
(C) Seminal vesicles
(D) Epididymis
(E) Testes

34. In the diagnostic workup of a 42-year-old man with chronic malabsorption and diarrhea, bacillary forms within periodic acid Schiff (PAS)-positive macrophages in the lamina propria of the small intestinal mucosa were demonstrated by electron microscopy. This finding is characteristic of

(A) celiac disease.
(B) Crohn disease.
(C) disaccharidase deficiency.
(D) tropical sprue.
(E) Whipple disease.

35. In a laboratory exercise, a 23-year-old female pathology student was found to have a prolonged bleeding time and a prolonged APPT. Her platelet count was normal. These findings are strongly suggestive of

(A) Christmas disease.
(B) classic hemophilia.
(C) congenital afibrinogenemia.
(D) Glanzmann thrombasthenia.
(E) von Willebrand disease.

36. A 67-year-old man, a heavy smoker, is seen because of dyspnea and cough. A chest X-ray reveals abnormal densities, and a computed tomography (CT) scan is suggestive of a neoplasm involving the pleura. A biopsy confirms the diagnosis of mesothelioma. Other than cigarette smoke, this finding suggests exposure which other toxin?

(A) Aflatoxin B_1
(B) Asbestos
(C) Diethylstilbestrol (DES)
(D) Ionizing radiation
(E) β-Naphthylamine

37. Cytologic findings consistent with carcinoma of the endometrium are found during diagnostic evaluation of a 65-year-old woman with uterine bleeding. Which of the following is associated with this condition?

(A) Arsenic exposure
(B) *BRCA* mutations
(C) Endometriosis
(D) Prolonged exposure to estrogens
(E) Sexual promiscuity

38. A 3-year-old boy is brought to the clinic because of fever and "fussiness," and he is diagnosed as having acute otitis media. In this acute inflammatory reaction, which of the following cells would have reached the site of inflammation first?

(A) Basophils
(B) Lymphocytes
(C) Monocytes–macrophages
(D) Neutrophils
(E) Plasma cells

39. A 4-year-old girl with a known chromosomal defect is seen because of fever and a skin rash. The rash consists of numerous small petechial hemorrhages with predominant involvement of the lower extremities. Her platelet count is markedly reduced, and the total white count is markedly increased. A blood smear and bone marrow aspirate reveal large numbers of undifferentiated blast cells, which by flow cytometry are found to be positive for the CD10 antigen. This complication occurs most frequently in association with which one of the following chromosomal disorders?

(A) Cri du chat syndrome
(B) Down syndrome
(C) Fragile X syndrome
(D) Klinefelter syndrome
(E) Turner syndrome

40. A renal biopsy taken from a 23-year-old woman with nephrotic syndrome prominently features glomerular immune complex deposits. Of the following disorders that affect the glomerulus, which is suggested by the findings?

(A) Amyloidosis
(B) Diabetic nephropathy
(C) IgA nephropathy
(D) Minimal change disease (lipoid nephrosis)
(E) Membranous glomerulonephritis

41. A rubbery, well-encapsulated, freely movable mass is found in the breast of a 20-year-old woman. Which of the following is most likely?

(A) Fibroadenoma
(B) Fibrocystic disease
(C) Intraductal papilloma
(D) Paget disease
(E) Phyllodes tumor

42. A 38-year-old woman is found to have episodic headache, palpitation, and diaphoresis, along with severe hypertension. She is also found to have hyperglycemia, but diabetes mellitus has been ruled out. These findings suggest an endocrine tumor secreting which of the following hormones?

(A) Antidiuretic hormone (ADH)
(B) Catecholamines
(C) Insulin
(D) PTH
(E) Prolactin

43. A 32-year-old woman was evaluated for severe watery diarrhea. Diagnostic testing revealed achlorhydria and reduced concentrations of serum potassium. Imaging studies revealed the presence of a pancreatic tumor. Special stains will most likely reveal the pancreatic tumor to be which of the following?

(A) Alpha-cell tumor (glucagonoma)
(B) Beta-cell tumor (insulinoma)
(C) Gastrinoma
(D) Somatostatinoma
(E) VIPoma

44. A 25-year-old woman experiences the sudden onset of fever, chills, right flank pain, and right-sided costovertebral angle tenderness. Her urinary sediment contains numerous gram-negative bacilli. Which of the following additional urinary findings would help establish the likely diagnosis?

(A) Broad waxy casts
(B) Decreased protein
(C) Decreased volume
(D) Red cell casts
(E) White cell casts

45. A 10-day-old boy with projectile vomiting and a palpable midepigastric mass most likely has
(B) infantile polycystic kidney.
(C) intussusception.
(D) tracheoesophageal fistula.
(E) Wilms tumor.

46. A volunteer physician in a village in Rwanda sees a 45-year-old man who has an aortic diastolic murmur and a "water-hammer" pulse. Blood pressure is 200/70. Which of the following associated abnormalities is most likely?

(A) Aneurysm of ascending aorta
(B) Cerebral infarct
(C) Gangrene of small bowel
(D) Mural thrombosis
(E) Myocardial infarct

47. Three days after being admitted to the hospital for treatment of a gunshot wound, a 29-year-old man suffered the onset of acute respiratory distress, and diffuse bilateral infiltrates were seen in both lung fields on chest X-ray. A lung biopsy revealed the presence of intra-alveolar edema along with hyaline membrane formation. These findings are indicative of

(A) bacterial pneumonia.
(B) viral pneumonia.
(C) diffuse alveolar damage.
(D) pulmonary hypertension.
(E) left-sided heart failure.

48. In a pre-employment examination, a 23-year-old woman is found to have laboratory values consistent with mild anemia, and a blood smear is reported as demonstrating hypochromia and microcytosis. Which of the following determinations would be most useful in demonstrating that these findings were manifestatons of β-thalassemia minor, as contrasted to other causes of hypochromia and microcytosis?

(A) Hemoglobin A_{1c}
(B) Hemoglobin A_2
(C) Hemoglobin value on routine complete blood count (CBC)
(D) Histochemical demonstration of α-chain aggregates
(E) Microscopic examination of peripheral blood smear

49. A 50-year-old, HIV-positive man has Hodgkin disease. Lymph nodes on both sides of the diaphragm are involved, as are the liver and bone marrow. Histologic examination of an involved node reveals a diffuse infiltrate with large numbers of Reed-Sternberg cells with many bizarre sarcomatous variants. Tests for Epstein-Barr proteins are positive. From this description, which Hodgkin disease variant is most likely?

(A) Lymphocyte predominance
(B) Mixed cellularity
(C) Lymphocyte depletion
(D) Nodular sclerosis

50. A 20-year-old man is found to have hemolytic anemia with jaundice and splenomegaly. A younger brother is found to be similarly affected, and his mother had had a history of splenectomy. Which of the following abnormalities is an expected finding in this patient?

(A) Increased haptoglobin
(B) Unconjugated hyperbilirubinemia
(C) Increased urine bilirubin
(D) Decreased reticulocytes
(E) Marrow erythroid hypoplasia

51. A 10-year-old girl presents with an orange-red, dome-shaped papule on her right leg. Her parents state that the papule has grown from a tiny dot to over a centimeter in length in just a few months. Following biopsy, the dermatologist reassures the parents, stating that although the papule superficially resembles malignant melanoma, it is actually a benign lesion without malignant potential. Which of the following is the likely diagnosis?

(A) Acanthosis nigricans
(B) Actinic keratosis
(C) Dysplastic nevus
(D) Juvenile melanoma
(E) Xeroderma pigmentosum

52. A 40-year-old woman presents with grayish pigmentation of the skin in a large region covering her entire posterior neck and axillae. The hyperpigmented areas started out as smaller macules but have now progressed to form palpable plaques. At times the hyperpigmented areas are pruritic. Which of the following is an important association of this skin lesion?

(A) Hypercholesterolemia
(B) Marker of visceral malignancy
(C) Tends to recur after resection
(D) Convulsions, mental retardation, and retinal detachment
(E) Viral infection

53. A 35-year-old man with a known history of severe chronic alcohol abuse presents with low-grade fever, jaundice, hepatomegaly, leukocytosis, and markedly abnormal liver function tests. Aspartate aminotransferase (AST) and alanine aminotransferase (ALT) are both elevated. An expected histologic finding in this condition is

(A) effacement of the normal liver architecture by diffuse fibrosis and abnormal regenerating nodules.
(B) Mallory hyaline inclusions, macrovesicular steatosis, and neutrophilic infiltration.
(C) multiple giant cells.
(D) nests or cords of well-differentiated cells separated by dense collagen lamellae.
(E) parenchymal deposition of hemosiderin.

54. A 16-year-old boy is referred to a dermatologist by an emergency room physician. The patient has had an intractable, severe, itching, burning, pruritic rash of the hands and lower extremities that has lasted several hours. Earlier in the day he had hiked through a wooded area filled with brush but was unaware of any direct contact with plants or other possible irritants. A skin biopsy revealed many infiltrating T cells and macrophages, suggesting an immune hypersensitivity reaction. Which type of reaction is most likely?

(A) Type I (immediate or anaphylactic) hypersensitivity
(B) Type II (antibody-mediated or cytotoxic) hypersensitivity
(C) Type III (immune complex) hypersensitivity
(D) Type IV (cell-mediated) hypersensitivity

55. A 19-year-old boy is seen because of bilateral enlargement of the kidneys. His father, paternal uncle, and several other family members have similar abnormalities. Which of the following aneurysms is frequently associated with this disorder?

(A) Berry aneurysm of the circle of Willis
(B) Dissecting aneurysm
(C) Fusiform aneurysm of the abdominal aorta
(D) Saccular aneurysm of the thoracic aorta

56. A 30-year-old African-American woman presents with bilateral hilar lymphadenopathy and reticular densities in both lung fields. Which of the following is a defining characteristic of the disorder suggested by these findings?

(A) Abnormalities restricted to lung and hilar lymph nodes
(B) Hypocalcemia
(C) Impaired synthesis of immunoglobulins
(D) Marked hyperreactivity to tuberculin
(E) Noncaseating granulomas

57. A 25-year-old woman is struck in the left breast in a "steering wheel" injury in what appeared to be a minor auto accident. After several days of pain and tenderness, she noted the persistence of a "lump" at the site of the injury. After excision biopsy, amorphous basophilic material was noted within the mass. The amorphous material is an example of

(A) apocrine metaplasia.
(B) dystrophic calcification.
(C) enzymatic fat necrosis.
(D) granulomatous inflammation.
(E) mammary dysplasia.

58. A 56-year-old man was recently diagnosed with early-stage colon cancer. He has no known family history of colon cancer. Which of the following known risk factors is most likely to have contributed to the development of this form of cancer?

(A) A diet low in fiber and high in fat
(B) Aflatoxin B_1 ingestion
(C) *Helicobacter pylori* infection
(D) Hepatitis B infection
(E) Tobacco and alcohol abuse

59. A 49-year-old man has a recent diagnosis of small cell carcinoma of the lung. Which of the following is an important characteristic of this form of lung cancer?

(A) Ectodermal origin
(B) Frequent peripheral location
(C) Less association with cigarette smoking than other forms of lung cancer
(D) Paraneoplastic hyperparathyroidism
(E) Poorly amenable to surgery

60. A 45-year-old man presents with a form of bacterial infection in which the invading microorganisms are opsonized prior to their engulfment by phagocytic cells. Of the following complement components or groups of components, which is most likely involved?

(A) C3a and C5a
(B) C3b
(C) C4a
(D) C5a alone
(E) C5b-9

61. A 67-year-old man, a two-pack-a-day smoker since age 18, has had a productive cough over the past 20 years. Although continuous through the years, there have been episodic exacerbations of these symptoms, which have worsened during the past 4 or 5 years, lasting 3 or 4 months at a time. Arterial pO_2 is decreased and pCO_2 is increased. Total lung capacity measurements are normal. These findings are most suggestive of which of the following pulmonary disorders?

(A) ARDS
(B) Bronchial asthma
(C) Bronchogenic carcinoma
(D) Chronic bronchitis
(E) Panacinar emphysema

62. A 56-year-old man who had been receiving intravenous antibiotics for severe cellulitis develops fever, toxicity, and severe diarrhea. This scenario suggests which of the following disorders?

(A) Celiac sprue
(B) CMV infection
(C) Pseudomembranous colitis
(D) Ulcerative colitis
(E) Whipple disease

63. A 54-year-old carpenter was brought to the hospital by ambulance after he was involved in a high-speed automobile chase that terminated in a collision into the trunk of a tree. On admission to the hospital, his skin was cold and clammy, his pulse was rapid and thready, and his blood pressure was 60 systolic and 40 diastolic. His blood alcohol was 0.29 g/dL (presumptive level for drunkenness is 0.08). In spite of blood transfusions, he died during an emergency laparotomy that revealed a ruptured spleen and a slightly enlarged liver. Microscopic examination of the liver at autopsy revealed intracytoplasmic clear vacuoles displacing the intact nuclei of the hepatocytes to the periphery of the cells. Special stains will most likely demonstrate that the vacuolar material is

(A) bilirubin.
(B) fat.
(C) glycogen.
(D) hemosiderin.
(E) water.

64. A 5-year-old boy is seen because he has recurrent hemarthroses and a large painful hematoma involving the soft tissues of his right thigh. Given the following choices, which is the most likely cause of the bleeding?

(A) Ascorbic acid deficiency
(B) Christmas disease
(C) Disseminated intravascular coagulation (DIC)
(D) Rocky Mountain spotted fever
(E) Primary thrombocytopenia

65. A 43-year-old woman has a recent diagnosis of Hashimoto thyroiditis. This disease's autoimmune nature is suggested by which of the following features?

(A) Association with human leukocyte antigen (HLA)-DR5 and HLA-B5
(B) Atrophy of thyroid follicles
(C) Palpable thyroid
(D) Presence of Hürthle cells
(E) Signs and symptoms of hypothyroidism

66. An autopsy is performed on a 60-year-old man with a history of sustained ethanol abuse. There had been a history of progressive dementia with marked memory loss manifest by a tendency to fabricate false accounts of recent events. Additionally, confusion, ataxic gait, and paralysis of eye movements had been noted. The most likely findings in the brain are

(A) amyloid-containing neuritic plaques within cerebral cortex, amygdala, and hippocampus.
(B) degeneration of mamillary bodies and paramedian masses of gray matter.
(C) depigmentation of substantia nigra and locus ceruleus.
(D) diffuse cortical atrophy with hydrocephalus ex vacuo.
(E) multiple lacunar infarcts and progressive subcortical demyelination.

67. A 4-year-old girl has had multiple hospitalizations for pneumonia. Additionally, she is small for her age and has had symptoms of fat malabsorption. Her father refers to her as his "little potato chip" because she tastes salty when he kisses her. Chest radiograph demonstrates pulmonary infiltrates indicative of pneumonia. Which of the following is the most likely pathogen causing pulmonary infection in this patient?

(A) *Legionella pneumophila*
(B) *Haemophilus influenzae*
(C) *Pseudomonas aeruginosa*
(D) *Staphylococcus aureus*
(E) *Streptococcus pneumoniae*

68. A 55-year-old woman has cirrhosis. Twenty years ago she received a blood transfusion for profuse bleeding associated with a complication of childbirth. Shortly thereafter she had an acute disease diagnosed as non-A, non-B hepatitis. Throughout her lifetime, her alcohol consumption has been minimal. Which of the following viruses is most likely responsible for her past and current liver disease?

(A) Hepatitis A
(B) Hepatitis B
(C) Hepatitis C
(D) Hepatitis D
(E) Hepatitis E

69. A 65 year-old man has anemia, splenomegaly, and extramedullary hematopoiesis. He has experienced easy fatigability, weight loss, and weakness. Bone marrow biopsy reveals marked proliferation of fibrous tissue (myelofibrosis) consistent with agnogenic myeloid metaplasia. Which of the following is a characteristic finding in this disorder?

(A) Depletion of bone marrow megakaryocytes
(B) Teardrop-shaped erythrocytes
(C) Autosplenectomy
(D) Neoplastic plasma cells in the bone marrow
(E) Blast crisis in the peripheral blood

70. An autopsy is performed on a 35-year-old African-American man who died after a brief illness characterized by papilledema, severe hypertension, left ventricular hypertrophy and failure, and renal dysfunction. The most likely findings in the kidney are

(A) finely granular renal surface and hyaline arteriolosclerosis of afferent arterioles.
(B) swollen, hypercellular, "bloodless" glomeruli.
(C) nodular mesangial accumulations of basement membrane-like material and hyaline arteriolosclerosis of afferent and efferent arterioles.
(D) surface covered with multiple petechial hemorrhages, hyperplastic arteriolosclerosis, and necrotizing glomerulitis.
(E) swollen, pale kidneys and marked accumulation of lipid in convoluted tubules.

71. The most likely diagnosis in a 24-year-old woman with the nephrotic syndrome, progressive azotemia, and thickening of glomerular capillary loops apparent on light microscopy is

(A) Alport syndrome.
(B) diabetic nephropathy.
(C) focal segmental glomerulosclerosis.
(D) lipoid nephrosis.
(E) membranous glomerulonephritis.

72. A 23-year-old woman consults an obstetrician because she is hoping to become pregnant but is concerned about possible consequences of rubella infection. She received all of her childhood immunizations, but now she has been found to be negative for antibodies to rubella. The obstetrician administers rubella vaccination and advises her to return for an anti-rubella titer prior to becoming pregnant. Which of the following is true regarding congenital rubella infection?

(A) Associated fetal defects are limited to the cardiovascular system.
(B) The fetus is most vulnerable during the third trimester of pregnancy.
(C) The majority of cases of congenital heart disease are caused by rubella or other intrauterine infections.
(D) Patent ductus arteriosus and septal defects are the most frequent congenital cardiac abnormalities associated with rubella infection.
(E) A predominant IgG antibody response indicates recent primary infection.

73. A bone marrow aspiration from a 65-year-old man with long-standing profound anemia shows megaloblastic erythroid hyperplasia. Which of the following is the most likely diagnosis?

(A) Anemia of chronic disease
(B) Pelger–Huet anomaly
(C) Pernicious anemia
(D) Homozygous hemoglobin E
(E) Thalassemia

74. A 30-year-old woman has sudden blurring of vision in her right eye, paresthesias, and spasticity. CSF findings include oligoclonal bands on electrophoresis. Magnetic resonance imaging of the brain reveals T2 hyperintensities characteristic of demyelination in the paraventricular regions. Which of the following is a prominent characteristic of this patient's disorder?

(A) Axonal degeneration
(B) Optic nerve, brain stem, and paraventricular areas are favored sites
(C) Confined to the peripheral nervous system
(D) Associated with leukemia or lymphoma
(E) Caused by prions

75. A 65-year old man is evaluated for abdominal pain radiating through to the back, jaundice, anorexia, and recent weight loss. An additional likely finding is

(A) history of thorium dioxide (Thorotrast) exposure.
(B) increased AFP.
(C) migratory venous thrombosis.
(D) pancreatic calcification and pseudocyst formation.
(E) urine test negative for bilirubin.

76. A 25-year-old woman has recently been diagnosed with a suspicious pigmented skin lesion and is waiting for the results of a biopsy. She is concerned because she had heard that such lesions vary, with some being more serious than others. Which of the following pigmented lesions is most likely to metastasize early?

(A) Dysplastic nevus
(B) Nodular melanoma
(C) Pigmented nevus
(D) Juvenile melanoma
(E) Superficial spreading melanoma

77. A 27-year-old man who recently arrived in the United States from Central America is found to have hypochromic microcytic anemia. Which of the following is the most likely cause of this finding?

(A) Hookworm infestation
(B) Fish tapeworm infestation
(C) A strict vegetarian diet
(D) Prolonged use of the antiseizure medication phenytoin
(E) Anemia of chronic disease

78. A 10-month-old girl presents with recurrent pulmonary infections, steatorrhea, and failure to thrive. Measurement of which substance is the most appropriate procedure in this patient?

(A) Erythrocyte glucose-6-phosphate dehydrogenase (G6PD)
(B) Serum ceruloplasmin
(C) Serum β-lipoprotein
(D) Serum phenylalanine
(E) Sweat chloride

79. A pathologist examining a histologic preparation from an autopsy finds a lesion with abundant granulation tissue. This finding is most likely to be indicative of which of the following?

(A) Cat-scratch disease
(B) Foreign body reaction
(C) Histoplasmosis
(D) Tuberculosis
(E) Wound healing

80. A 17-year-old African-American girl recently had her ears pierced for the first time. She now presents to her primary care provider with the complaint of a large "tumor-like" growth in the immediate site of one of the piercings. This lesion is likely a

(A) benign fibrous histiocytoma.
(B) dermatofibrosarcoma protuberans.
(C) fibroepithelial polyp.
(D) keloid.
(E) xanthoma.

81. While being investigated for long-standing hypertension, a 55-year-old woman is found to have the following serum laboratory test values: normal creatinine, total protein, albumin, and globulin; increased calcium and alkaline phosphatase; and decreased phosphorus. These findings suggest the presence of

(A) carcinoma metastatic to bone.
(B) excessive dietary calcium intake.
(C) multiple myeloma.
(D) parathyroid adenoma.
(E) sarcoidosis.

82. A 20-year-old woman with episodic hypertension is found to have a marked increase in urinary VMA. Several close relatives have had vascular tumors of the eye and cysts of the liver, kidney, and pancreas. Which of the following familial syndromes is most likely?

(A) von Hippel-Lindau disease
(B) von Recklinghausen disease
(C) Marfan syndrome
(D) Familial hypercholesterolemia
(E) Tuberous sclerosis

83. A 60-year-old woman presents with fever, chills, dysuria, hematuria, and pain. She reports a long-standing history of use of phenacetin, acetaminophen, nonsteroidal anti-inflammatory drugs (NSAIDS), and aspirin. Abuse of these medications is associated with necrosis is which of the following sites?

(A) Basal ganglia
(B) Hilar lymph nodes
(C) Myocardium
(D) Renal papillae
(E) Splenic arterioles

84. A 3-month-old, apparently female infant is evaluated for ambiguous genitalia. The clitoris appears large, and there are palpable masses in the inguinal region. Further investigation reveals the presence of both ovarian and testicular tissue. Which of the following terms is used to describe these findings?

(A) Male pseudohermaphroditism
(B) Female pseudohermaphroditism
(C) True hermaphroditism
(D) Turner syndrome
(E) Klinefelter syndrome

85. A 62-year-old man is seen because of a change in bowel habits. A lesion similar to that illustrated below is resected from the sigmoid colon. The diagnosis is

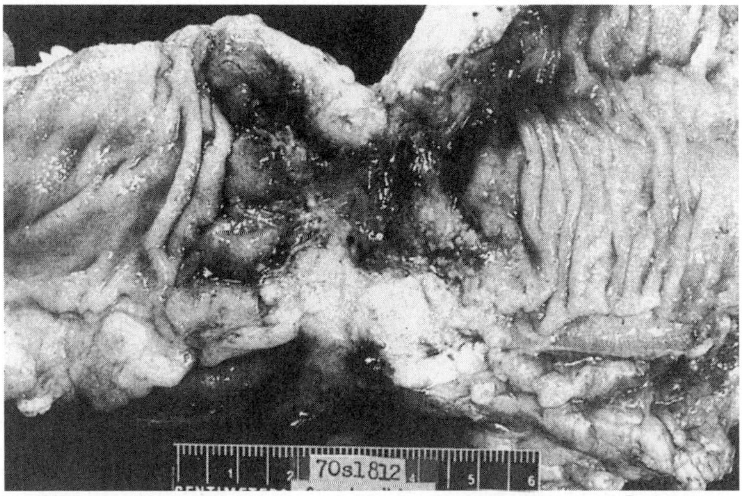

(Reprinted with permission from Golden A, Powell D, Jennings C: *Pathology: Understanding Human Disease,* 2nd ed. Baltimore, Williams & Wilkins, 1985, p 144.)

(A) adenocarcinoma.
(B) Crohn disease.
(C) non-Hodgkin lymphoma.
(D) pseudomembranous colitis.
(E) tubular adenoma.

86. A 23-year-old woman with systemic lupus erythrematosus (SLE) is placed on high doses of the steroid prednisone. Prednisone is a potent inhibitor of the enzyme phospholipase A_2, which normally functions in which of the following events?

(A) Cyclooxygenase pathway
(B) Liberation of arachidonic acid from membrane phospholipids
(C) Lipoxygenase pathway
(D) Synthesis of prostacyclin (PGI_2)
(E) Synthesis of thromboxane A_2 (TxA_2)

87. A 14-year-old girl dies after an illness characterized by progressive motor and mental deterioration. At autopsy, there is profound cortical atrophy, loss of white matter, and ventricular enlargement. Special studies indicate participation of a defective measles virus. Which of the following is the diagnosis?

(A) Creutzfeldt-Jakob disease
(B) Guillain-Barré syndrome
(C) Kuru
(D) Progressive multifocal leukoencephalopathy
(E) Subacute sclerosing panencephalitis

88. A 20-year-old man is hospitalized with fever, shaking chills, and widespread cutaneous hemorrhages. He complains of severe headache, and nuchal rigidity is noted on physical examination. Examination of the peripheral blood and CSF reveals gram-negative diplococci within neutrophils. A well-known complication of this disorder is hemorrhage into the

(A) adrenal cortex.
(B) anterior pituitary.
(C) brain stem.
(D) pancreas.
(E) subarachnoid space.

89. A 56-year-old man with a history of stable angina was seen in the emergency room one hour following the onset of unrelenting substernal pain not relieved by nitroglycerin. An electrocardiogram (ECG) revealed deep Q waves across the precordium, ST segment elevations, and inverted T waves. Serum levels of creatinine kinase MB (CK-MB) and cardiac troponin I (cTn-I) were within the normal range. What is the best explanation for these findings?

(A) Lactate dehydrogenase (LDH) should have been ordered rather than CK-MB and cTn-I.
(B) The diagnosis is acute myocardial infarction, and CK-MB and cTn-I were determined too early in the course of the disease.
(C) The diagnosis is unstable angina rather than acute myocardial infarction.
(D) The findings are indicative of a dissecting aneurysm (dissecting hematoma) of the aorta.
(E) CK-MB alone can be misleading, and more definitive information would have been expected from total CK determination.

90. A 60-year-old man with pancreatic cancer dies following a terminal episode that began 3 days earlier, characterized by generalized bleeding with oozing from intravenous infusion sites, widespread petechial and ecchymotic cutaneous bleeding, and intractable epistaxis. At autopsy, a glomerular change similar to that shown in the illustration was demonstrated. Prior to death, which of the following laboratory measures of blood coagulation would have shown a decrease in the reported value?

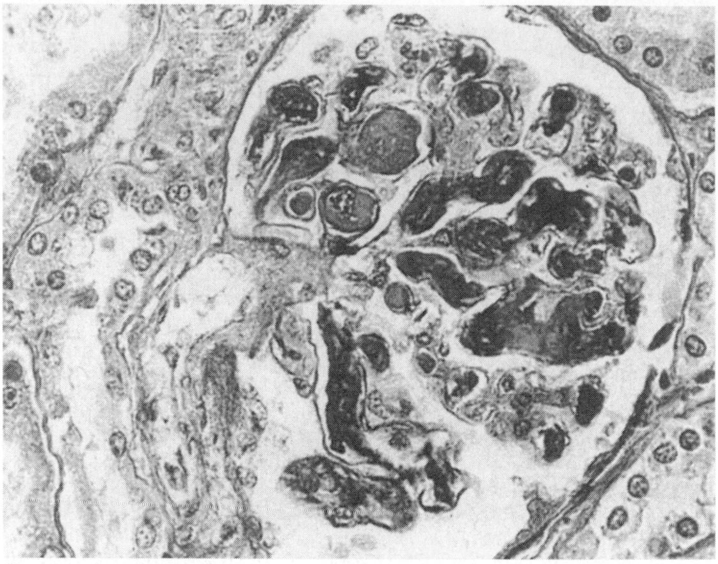

(Reprinted with permission from Golden A, Powell D, Jennings C: *Pathology: Understanding Human Disease,* 2nd ed. Baltimore, Williams & Wilkins, 1985, p 83.)

(A) Activated partial thromboplastin time
(B) Fibrin and fibrinogen degradation products
(C) Platelet count
(D) Prothrombin time
(E) Thrombin time

91. A 28-year-old man was evaluated for progressive weakness, weight loss, and anorexia. He was found to be hypotensive, and has generalized hyperpigmentation involving exposed surfaces of the skin, lips, and buccal mucosa. Which of the following laboratory findings is expected in this patient?

(A) Increased serum sodium
(B) Decreased serum potassium
(C) Increased serum glucose
(D) Decreased plasma cortisol not corrected by administration of adrenocorticotropic hormone (ACTH)
(E) Increased urinary 17-ketosteroids

92. A 35-year-old man whose father had died of Huntington disease has the onset of neurologic abnormalities that had been predicted earlier by genetic analysis. Changes in the distance between the heads of the two caudate nuclei by magnetic resonance imaging are consistent with atrophy of the caudate nucleus and putamen. Which of the following is an important characteristic of this disorder?

(A) Copper deposition in lenticular nuclei
(B) Early childhood onset most common
(C) Sphingomyelinase deficiency
(D) Substantia nigra depigmentation
(E) Trinucleotide repeat expansion

93. Membranous glomerulonephritis is found at autopsy in a 25-year-old woman who died in renal failure. Other autopsy findings include pleuritis, diffuse interstitial fibrosis of the lungs, concentric rings of collagen surrounding splenic arterioles, and warty vegetations of the mitral and tricuspid valves affecting the surfaces behind the cusps as well as the surfaces exposed to the forward flow of blood. Which of the following is an expected laboratory finding?

(A) Increased titer of antistreptolysin O (ASO)
(B) Lymphocytosis
(C) Peripheral rim pattern of antinuclear antibody fluorescence
(D) Positive blood cultures for *Streptococcus viridans*
(E) Serum antibodies reactive with glomerular and pulmonary alveolar basement membranes

94. A single nodule was resected from the peripheral portion of the right lower lobe of the lung of a 45-year-old woman. The microscopic findings were similar to those shown in the illustration. The diagnosis is

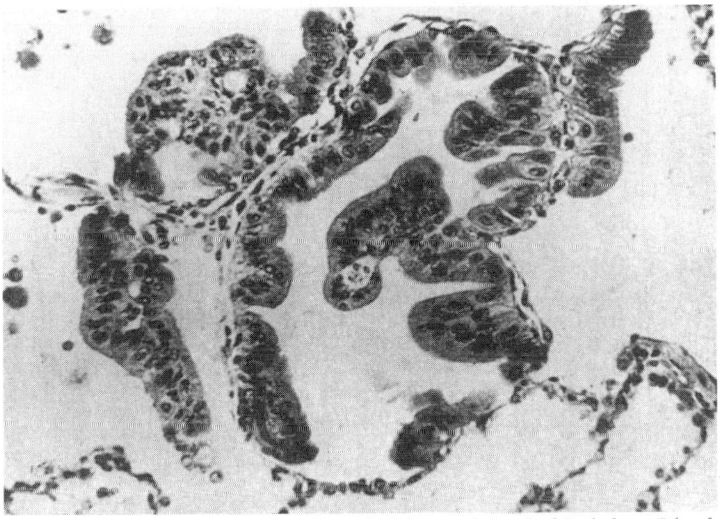

(Reprinted with permission from Rosai J: *Ackerman's Surgical Pathology,* 7th ed. St Louis, CV Mosby, 1989, p 301.)

(A) bronchioloalveolar carcinoma.
(B) carcinoid.
(C) mesothelioma.
(D) small cell carcinoma.
(E) squamous cell carcinoma.

95. A 54-year-old man presents with multiple recurrent peptic ulcers of the duodenum and the jejunum. Gastric acid secretion is refractory to proton pump inhibitors. These findings suggest an underlying

(A) adenocarcinoma of the pancreas.
(B) adenoma of the adrenal medulla.
(C) carcinoid of the jejunum.
(D) islet cell tumor of the pancreas.
(E) pheochromocytoma.

96. A 65-year-old man is seen for the recent onset of jaundice, weight loss, and anorexia. Abdominal examination reveals a distended, palpable gallbladder. Laboratory studies reveal conjugated hyperbilirubinemia, positive urine tests for bilirubin, and total absence of urobilinogen in the urine and stools. The probable diagnosis is

(A) adenocarcinoma of the pancreas.
(B) amebic abscess of the liver.
(C) hepatic vein thrombosis.
(D) hepatitis A infection.
(E) hereditary spherocytosis.

97. A 33-year-old woman presents with episodic palpitations, sweating, tremor, and a sense of apprehension. During these episodes, her blood pressure is markedly elevated. Which of the following laboratory tests is most likely to be of diagnostic significance?

(A) Serum serotonin
(B) Serum gastrin
(C) Urine VMA
(D) Urine cortisol
(E) Serum PTH

98. A 30-year-old woman dies following a prolonged period in a vegetative state that resulted from injuries sustained in a head-on auto collision 5 years earlier. An expected autopsy finding would be

(A) A cherry-red spot on the macula
(B) Asbestos bodies in the lung
(C) Autophagic granules in skeletal muscles
(D) Lewy bodies within neurons
(E) Mallory bodies within hepatocytes

99. A 5-year-old child in a refugee camp in sub-Saharan Africa is seen by a volunteer doctor in the camp, and is diagnosed as having severe protein-calorie malnutrition consistent with kwashiorkor. Which of the following is a characteristic of this disorder?

(A) Impaired apolipoprotein synthesis
(B) Increased fat storage in adipocytes
(C) More severe than marasmus
(D) Myocardial fatty change exceeds that in liver
(E) Precursor to cirrhosis

100. A 54-year-old man presents with a painless unilateral swelling just anterior to the ear. Biopsy of the mass suggests it is a pleomorphic adenoma, and he is scheduled for surgery to remove the mass. Which of the following is true of this tumor?

(A) Often recurs
(B) Is less prevalent than Warthin tumors of the salivary gland
(C) Totally resectable
(D) Results from mumps infection
(E) Often results in Horner syndrome

101. A 2-year-old girl with a history of repeated pulmonary infections is found to have elevated chloride in a sweat test. An additional expected finding is

(A) hypercalcemia.
(B) hypotension.
(C) increased metabolism.
(D) renal failure.
(E) steatorrhea.

102. A 36-year-old woman experiences a severe headache. Investigation including computed tomographic angiography (CTA) reveals a saccular outpouching of the anterior cerebral artery. Which of the following is a major characteristic of this type of vascular change?

(A) Occurs anywhere within branches of internal carotid artery
(B) Infrequent site of subarachnoid hemorrhage
(C) Middle meningeal artery most frequent location
(D) Usually a complication of severe atherosclerosis
(E) Often associated with polycystic kidney

103. A 56-year-old man has severe chest pain, and angiography demonstrates acute occlusion of the circumflex branch of the left coronary artery. Blood flow is successfully restored by percutaneous transluminal coronary angioplasty (PTCA) with stenting. During the period of cellular hypoxic injury, which of the following intracellular changes is likely to have occurred?

(A) Decreased calcium
(B) Decreased pH
(C) Decreased sodium
(D) Increased activity of Na^+K^+ pump
(E) Increased adenosine triphosphate (ATP)

104. A cystic ovarian mass was palpated in a 23-year-old woman. If X-ray films revealed calcifications in the mass, which of the following would be most likely?

(A) Teratoma
(B) Brenner tumor
(C) Mucinous cystadenocarcinoma
(D) Krukenberg tumor
(E) Choriocarcinoma

105. A 45-year-old woman presents with an insidious and progressive syndrome characterized by pain and tenderness in multiple joints, with joint stiffness on rising in the morning, and early afternoon fatigue and malaise. Joint involvement is symmetric, with the proximal interphalangeal and metacarpophalangeal joints especially involved. Physical examination reveals tenderness in nearly all inflamed joints. Which of the following laboratory abnormalities is most likely?

(A) Antibodies to double-stranded DNA
(B) IgM anti-IgG antibodies
(C) Urate crystals and neutrophils in synovial fluid
(D) Anti-DNAase B
(E) HLA-B27 antigen

106. A 35-year-old, HIV-positive man presents with productive cough, hemoptysis, fever, night sweats, weight loss, and anorexia. Chest radiograph demonstrates a cavitary lesion in the apex of the left lung. Sputum examination reveals acid-fast bacilli. The patient is diagnosed with tuberculosis, in which the classic histologic feature is granulomatous inflammation. The epithelioid cells and multinucleated giant cells of this form of chronic inflammation are derived from which of the following?

(A) Basophils
(B) CD4+ T lymphocytes
(C) Eosinophils
(D) Monocytes and macrophages
(E) Plasma cells

107. A 25-year-old woman is seen because of numbness and pain in her fingers and hands on exposure to cold. When either her hands or feet are very cold, they turn white and then blue. These changes are characteristic of which of the following?

(A) Buerger disease (thromboangiitis obliterans)
(B) Raynaud disease
(C) Wegener granulomatosis
(D) Kawasaki disease
(E) Takayasu arteritis

108. An 80-year-old woman on a "tea and toast" diet presents with bleeding gums, petechiae and easy bruising, and pain in her arms and legs. She states that she almost never eats fruits and vegetables. She is diagnosed with vitamin C deficiency. Which of the following is the basis of the clinical abnormalities that occur as a result of lack of vitamin C?

(A) Defective calcification of osteoid matrix
(B) Increased intestinal absorption of iron
(C) Defective hydroxylation of proline and lysine
(D) Increased proliferation of collagen and fibrous tissue
(E) Destruction of endothelial cells

109. A 65-year-old man presents with recurrent fever and painless cervical and supraclavicular lymphadenopathy. Biopsy and further studies reveal that the patient has Hodgkin disease at a stage that is usually associated with a very poor prognosis. Staging is based on which of the following?

(A) Cell of origin
(B) Degree of anaplasia
(C) Degree of differentiation of tumor cells
(D) Distribution and extent of disease
(E) Number of mitotic figures

110. A 3-year-old girl presents with dark precipitates along gingival margins, radiopaque deposits in the epiphyses of her bones, and urinary excretion of delta-aminolevulinic acid (delta-ALA). Her father states that they live in an old house that has chipped paint. The patient is diagnosed with lead toxicity. The child's blood would likely also have which of the following?

(A) Basophilic stippling of erythrocytes
(B) Schistocytes and helmet cells
(C) Increased osmotic fragility of erythrocytes
(D) Clumping of erythrocytes at temperatures below 30°C
(E) Macrocytes

111. A 60-year-old woman with uterine bleeding is found to have endometrial hyperplasia and an ovarian tumor. Which is the most likely ovarian tumor?

(A) Serous cystadenocarcinoma
(B) Krukenberg tumor
(C) Dysgerminoma
(D) Teratoma
(E) Granulosa cell tumor

112. An 18-year-old man presents with left knee pain he's had for several months. Knee radiograph demonstrates elevation of the periosteum of the bone, with areas of a "sunburst" appearance. What is the likely diagnosis?

(A) Osteochondroma
(B) Osteosarcoma
(C) Giant cell tumor
(D) Ewing sarcoma
(E) Chondrosarcoma

113. A pathologist examines an excisional biopsy specimen and confirms the working diagnostic impression of adenocarcinoma. Because of the nature of the tumor, he requests molecular diagnostic evaluation by the molecular pathology laboratory. Amplification of the *HER-2/neu* oncogene is demonstrated. This finding is a negative prognostic indicator in carcinoma of the

(A) adrenal.
(B) breast.
(C) kidney.
(D) stomach.
(E) thyroid.

114. A 35-year-old woman consults a gynecologist because she has postcoital vaginal bleeding. The Papanicolaou (Pap) smear is abnormal. Colposcopy and cervical biopsy lead to a diagnosis of carcinoma of the cervix. Which of the following is most characteristic of this disorder?

(A) Association with human papillomavirus (HPV) infection
(B) History of exogenous estrogen therapy
(C) Most common gynecologic malignancy
(D) Secretion of AFP
(E) Spontaneous regression following menopause

Questions 115 and 116

A male infant was seen for recurrent bacterial infections beginning at age 6 months.

115. Immunoglobulin assay reveals absent IgG. An additional expected finding is

(A) absence of germinal centers in the lymph nodes.
(B) autosomal recessive inheritance.
(C) decreased CD4+:CD8+ T lymphocyte ratio.
(D) defective leukocytic bacterial killing.
(E) impaired phagocytosis.

116. In this infant, the period of well-being for the first 6 months of life is best explained by

(A) antibacterial substances supplied by breast-feeding.
(B) deficient opsonization due to immaturity of complement synthesis.
(C) delayed responsiveness of lymphocytes to mitogenic stimuli.
(D) protection by maternal antibodies.
(E) need for a viral infection to trigger immune destruction of thymic tissue.

117. A diagnosis of acute hematogenous osteomyelitis is made in a 5-year-old boy who had presented with the sudden onset of a high fever. He had been limping and had had erythema, edema, and pain around his right knee for several days. Which of the following is true of this condition?

(A) It occurs with peak incidence in the elderly.
(B) It most commonly affects the iliac crests.
(C) Surgical incision and drainage is almost always required.
(D) It is most commonly caused by *Staphylococcus aureus*.
(E) It is more common in females.

118. A 60-year-old man presents with painless hematuria. Transurethral biopsy of the bladder is performed, and histologic evaluation demonstrates the presence of carcinoma of the urinary bladder. Which of the following is the most common type of carcinoma of the urinary bladder?

(A) Transitional cell carcinoma
(B) Squamous cell carcinoma
(C) Adenocarcinoma
(D) Clear cell carcinoma
(E) Small cell carcinoma

119. A 56-year-old man is seen in the emergency room because of the acute onset of severe crushing precordial chest pain that began on the golf course 1 hour earlier and has persisted until the time of admission. The ECG reveals precordial QS waves and elevated ST segments. Although normal at admission, both the serum creatine kinase MB (CK-MB) and troponin I (cTn-I) are significantly elevated 12 hours later. These changes are related to which type of necrosis?

(A) Caseous
(B) Coagulative
(C) Fat
(D) Gangrenous
(E) Liquefactive

120. A 68-year-old woman has fever, generalized lower abdominal pain, and bright red blood in the stools. The white blood cell count is 15,000/μL, with 85% segmented neutrophils. The most likely diagnosis is

(A) acute appendicitis.
(B) carcinoma of the rectum.
(C) Crohn disease.
(D) diverticulitis.
(E) tubular adenoma in sigmoid colon.

121. Which of the following is a predisposing factor in the pathogenesis of clear cell adenocarcinoma of the vagina?

(A) Excess estrogen stimulation
(B) Herpes simplex virus infection
(C) HPV infection
(D) In utero exposure to DES
(E) Oral contraceptive therapy

122. A 65-year-old man presents with urinary hesitancy, frequency, urgency, sensation of incomplete bladder emptying, and straining to start the urinary stream. Digital rectal examination is performed. Further workup reveals the diagnosis of nodular prostatic hyperplasia. Which of the following is an association of this disorder?

(A) Tends to arise in the peripheral zone of the prostatic glands
(B) An increase in serum prostate-specific antigen (PSA) may occur
(C) Low incidence in older men
(D) May frequently progress to bony osteoblastic metastases
(E) Often improves over time without intervention

123. A 50-year-old chronic alcoholic with jaundice and ascites secondary to known cirrhosis becomes disoriented and confused. Asterixis (flapping tremor) can be demonstrated. Which of the following features of his disease is most closely related to the change in mental status?

(A) Hypoalbuminemia
(B) Increased hepatic lymph formation
(C) Increased portal venous pressure
(D) Portal-systemic venous shunting
(E) Renal retention of sodium and water

124. In preparation for a stem cell transplant in a patient with leukemia, the oncologist considers the differential susceptibility of various tissues and cells to high-dose chemotherapy and lethal irradiation. So-called permanent cells are the least vulnerable to injury, but also have the least capacity to regenerate. Which of the following is a permanent cell?

(A) Bronchial epithelial cell
(B) Gastric mucosal cell
(C) Hepatocyte
(D) Hippocampal neuron
(E) Renal tubular cell

125. A 60-year-old man presents with the new onset of dyspnea, chest pain, cough, and weight loss. In the past, he had worked in construction, installing insulation in buildings. Chest radiograph shows a right-sided pleural effusion with marked pleural thickening and mass formation. A malignant neoplasm is demonstrated by biopsy. What is the most likely diagnosis?

(A) Small cell carcinoma
(B) Squamous cell carcinoma
(C) Mesothelioma
(D) Adenocarcinoma
(E) Carcinoid tumor

126. A 60-year-old man presents with chronic headache and personality changes since he had been in a car accident a month ago, during which he had suffered a whiplash neck injury. A CT scan of the head demonstrates a hyperdense crescentic region along the inner skull. Which of the following is the most likely diagnosis?

(A) Bruising of the brain substance of the cerebral hemisphere
(B) Enlargement of the cerebral ventricles
(C) Epidural hematoma
(D) Subdural hematoma
(E) Subarachnoid hemorrhage

127. A 50-year-old man is seen in the emergency room. He sustained a head injury after falling from a ladder. He had a brief period of loss of consciousness after the fall which then resolved. He now has headache, vomiting, and borderline state of consciousness. Emergency CT demonstrates a fracture in the temporoparietal area of the skull as well as a lens-shaped homogeneous density contained within the suture lines. Which of the following is the most likely diagnosis?

(A) Bruising of the brain substance of the cerebral hemisphere
(B) Enlargement of the cerebral ventricles
(C) Epidural hematoma
(D) Subdural hematoma
(E) Subarachnoid hemorrhage

128. A 55-year-old woman presents with "the worst headache of my life" and severe nausea. She states that the headache and nausea started suddenly several hours ago. A CSF tap reveals frank blood in the CSF. A CT scan of the head reveals diffuse hemorrhage over the surface of the brain. Which of the following is the most likely mechanism causing these findings?

(A) Laceration of the middle meningeal artery
(B) Laceration of the bridging veins
(C) Rupture of a berry aneurysm in the circle of Willis
(D) Rupture of a Charcot-Bouchard aneurysm
(E) Hypertensive intraparenchymal hemorrhage

129. An 8-year-old boy presents with irritability, vomiting, and gait ataxia. CT scan demonstrates a midline tumor of the cerebellum. Which of the following is the most likely diagnosis?

(A) Glioblastoma multiforme
(B) Medulloblastoma
(C) Meningioma
(D) Neurilemmoma (schwannoma)
(E) Oligodendroglioma

130. A 30-year-old woman presents with weakness and hyperreflexia of the left lower extremity. These symptoms had begun as mild weakness, but had slowly and progressively become more severe. A CT scan of the head reveals a well-defined right-sided parasagittal mass compressing (but not invading) the brain parenchyma. Which of the following is the most likely diagnosis?

(A) Glioblastoma multiforme
(B) Medulloblastoma
(C) Meningioma
(D) Neurilemmoma (schwannoma)
(E) Oligodendroglioma

131. An autopsy is performed on a 75-year-old man, who for the past several years had had a pill-rolling tremor in his hand, slowing of his movements, and muscle rigidity. Autopsy findings reveal depigmentation of the substantia nigra and locus ceruleus. Which of the following is the most likely diagnosis?

(A) Alzheimer disease
(B) Huntington disease
(C) Idiopathic Parkinson disease
(D) Myasthenia gravis
(E) Wernicke-Korsakoff syndrome

132. A 30-year-old woman presents with ptosis and severe generalized muscle weakness. Administration of edrophonium (an anticholinesterase) results in a rapid and dramatic recovery of muscle strength. Which of the following is the most likely diagnosis?

(A) Alzheimer disease
(B) Huntington disease
(C) Idiopathic Parkinson disease
(D) Myasthenia gravis
(E) Wernicke-Korsakoff syndrome

133. A 50-year-old man presents with a neurologic disorder that began with choreoathetoid movements and has progressed to dementia. Other family members have been similarly affected. A CT scan reveals atrophy of the caudate nucleus, resulting in the appearance of enlarged lateral ventricles. Which of the following is the most likely diagnosis?

(A) Alzheimer disease
(B) Huntington disease
(C) Idiopathic Parkinson disease
(D) Myasthenia gravis
(E) Wernicke-Korsakoff syndrome

134. A 45-year-old man with a history of chronic obstructive pulmonary disease (COPD) manifests marked clubbing and joint pain of the fingers. Radiographs demonstrate soft tissue swelling at the ends of his fingers and osteolysis of the terminal phalanges. Which of the following is the most likely diagnosis?

(A) Ankylosing spondylitis
(B) Hypertrophic osteoarthropathy
(C) Osteoarthritis
(D) Rheumatoid arthritis
(E) Felty syndrome

135. A 60-year-old woman with a 10-year history of severe rheumatoid arthritis presents with splenomegaly and neutropenia. Which of the following is the most likely diagnosis?

(A) Ankylosing spondylitis
(B) Hypertrophic osteoarthropathy
(C) Osteoarthritis
(D) Rheumatoid arthritis
(E) Felty syndrome

136. A 45-year-old man presents with breast enlargement, erectile dysfunction, and decreased libido. On physical examination, an intratesticular mass is palpated. Which of the following is the most likely diagnosis?

(A) Androblastoma (Sertoli cell tumor)
(B) Endodermal sinus tumor
(C) Mature teratoma
(D) Mixed germ cell tumor
(E) Seminoma

137. A 35-year-old man presents with a painless lump in his right testicle. Scrotal ultrasound reveals a homogeneous intratesticular mass. Histologic examination of the testicular mass tissue demonstrates morphology that closely resembles that of dysgerminoma of the ovary in women. Which of the following is the most likely diagnosis?

(A) Androblastoma (Sertoli cell tumor)
(B) Endodermal sinus tumor
(C) Mature teratoma
(D) Mixed germ cell tumor
(E) Seminoma

138. A 12-year-old boy presents with smoky brown-colored urine, oliguria, azotemia, and hypertension. After further tests, the patient is diagnosed with a nephritic syndrome. Which of the following is the most likely diagnosis?

(A) Renal amyloidosis
(B) Diabetic nephropathy
(C) Membranous glomerulonephritis
(D) Minimal change disease
(E) Poststreptococcal glomerulonephritis

139. A 65-year-old woman with a long-standing history of severe rheumatoid arthritis presents with proteinuria, hypertension, edema, and hypoalbuminemia. Which of the following is the most likely diagnosis?

(A) Renal amyloidosis
(B) Diabetic nephropathy
(C) Membranous glomerulonephritis
(D) Minimal change disease
(E) Poststreptococcal glomerulonephritis

140. A 60-year-old man presents with proteinuria, hypertension, edema, and hypoalbuminemia. Histologic findings in the glomeruli of his kidneys include mesangial accumulation of basement membrane-like material. Which of the following is the most likely diagnosis?

(A) Renal amyloidosis
(B) Diabetic nephropathy
(C) Membranous glomerulonephritis
(D) Minimal change disease
(E) Poststreptococcal glomerulonephritis

ANSWERS AND EXPLANATIONS

1. **The answer is C.** The laboratory abnormalities (increased serum calcium, parathyroid hormone, and alkaline phosphatase; and decreased serum phosphorus) are diagnostic of primary hyperparathyroidism, a well-known cause of hypercalcemia. One of the consequences of hypercalcemia (regardless of cause) is deposition of calcium salts in previously undamaged organs or tissues, a phenomenon known as metastatic calcification.

2. **The answer is D.** Nuclear pyknosis, along with karyorrhexis and karyolysis, is a sign of necrosis and is, of course, irreversible. Fatty change, formation of cell blebs or myelin figures, and swelling of the cell or of organelles are all reversible changes.

3. **The answer is C.** The fat embolism syndrome occurs 2 to 3 days after severe fracture injury and includes progressive central nervous system (CNS) dysfunction and severe respiratory insufficiency. Thrombocytopenia with petechial bleeding is common, and petechial hemorrhages can result from obstruction of the microvasculature by embolic fat droplets. Respiratory insufficiency may be due to injury to pulmonary microvessels with leakage of fluid into the alveoli, resulting in adult respiratory distress syndrome (ARDS).

4. **The answer is E.** Hemolytic disease of the newborn is a type II hypersensitivity reaction mediated by antibodies directed against intrinsic cell surface antigens (with complement-induced cell lysis). Modern management requires administration of IgG anti-Rh antibodies to the mother at the birth of a first Rh-positive child in order to avoid maternal sensitization. Another type of type II reaction is exemplified by the reaction of antibodies with cell-surface receptors, as occurs in Graves disease. Activation of sensitized CD4+ T cells with release of cytokines is descriptive of type IV cell-mediated reactions such as the delayed-type cell-mediated hypersensitivity exemplified by poison ivy dermatitis. "Graft- versus- neonate" is a fictitious condition, but transfusion-mediated transplant rejection is an ever-present danger when immunodeficient persons receive transfusions that contain immunocompetent precursor cells. IgE-mediated degranulation of mast cells and basophils underlies type I hypersensitivity reaction such as allergic asthma, hay fever, or anaphylaxis. Immune complex deposition with secondary inflammation occurs in generalized immune complex disorders such as systemic lupus erythematosus (SLE).

5. **The answer is A.** The scenario is strongly suggestive of infectious mononucleosis, a benign, self-limited lymphoproliferative disorder that is most often caused by Epstein-Barr virus (EBV) infection. However, the heterophil test for sheep red cell agglutinins is negative, and so-called heterophil-negative infectious mononucleosis is most often caused by cytomegalovirus (CMV).

6. **The answer is D.** The clinical behavior of neoplasms is the underlying basis for all other indicators that distinguish malignant from benign lesions. For example, some extremely well-differentiated, otherwise benign-appearing lesions are known to metastasize and thus are classified as malignant.

7. **The answer is A.** The combination of emphysema and hepatic cirrhosis in a young person with a family history of similarly affected family members is strongly suggestive of homozygous α_1-antitrypsin deficiency. In these instances the emphysema is usually panacinar in type.

8. **The answer is C.** Peptic ulcer of the duodenum is not a precursor lesion to carcinoma. The risk of malignant transformation in familial multiple polyposis approaches 100%. Colorectal villous adenomas undergo malignant change in about 30% of cases. There is a markedly increased incidence of colon cancer in long-standing cases of ulcerative colitis. The incidence of colon cancer is also increased in Crohn disease but to a lesser degree than in ulcerative colitis.

9. **The answer is E.** The history is suggestive of Paget disease of bone, which is also marked by bone pain, anterolateral bowing of long bones, and sometimes high-output heart failure. This disorder is complicated by osteosarcoma in about 1% of cases. Paget disease of bone should not be confused with Paget disease of the breast, which is closely associated with an underlying ductal carcinoma.

10. **The answer is D.** Although too nonspecific for initial diagnosis or screening, carcinoembryonic antigen (CEA) is useful for followup of cancer of the colon. Increased serum human chorionic gonadotropin (hCG) may be observed in normal pregnancy, hydatidiform mole, choriocarcinoma, and many testicular mixed germ cell tumors. Fetal neural tube defects are associated with increased levels of α-fetoprotein (AFP) in the mother. In addition, elevated levels of AFP (unrelated to pregnancy) may be associated with hepatocellular carcinoma, yolk sac (endodermal sinus) tumors, and some nonseminomatous germ cell tumors of the testes. Vanillylmandelic acid (VMA) is a marker for neuroblastoma and pheochromocytoma. Granulosa cell tumors and thecomas of the ovary characteristically produce estrogen.

11. **The answer is E.** Hypertrophic cardiomyopathy, a condition that is usually inherited as an autosomal dominant disorder, is often associated with sudden death in young athletes. The ventricular septum is especially involved, with protrusion into the left ventricular cavity (asymmetric septal hypertrophy), sometimes leading to left ventricular outflow tract obstruction.

12. **The answer is A.** In disseminated intravascular coagulation (DIC), widespread thrombosis activates the fibrinolytic system, with degradation of both fibrin and fibrinogen. Therefore, fibrin and fibrinogen degradation products are markedly increased. Since platelets are consumed, thrombocytopenia, not thrombocytosis, is an expected finding. In addition, the consumption of coagulation factors results in prolongation of the prothrombin time (PT), a measure of the extrinsic pathway of coagulation; the activated partial thromboplastin time (APTT), a measure of the intrinsic pathway of coagulation; and the thrombin time, a measure of fibrinogen concentration. The clinical history strongly suggests premature separation of the placenta (abruptio placentae), a well-known cause of DIC.

13. **The answer is C.** The clinical history is strongly suggestive of pyogenic meningitis, the most common form of meningitis in the newborn. The diagnosis is confirmed by abnormalities in the the cerebrospinal fluid (CSF). These findings include increased pressure, cloudy appearance, markedly increased cell count with numerous neutrophils, increased protein, and decreased glucose (a useful rule is that the normal CSF glucose concentration is about two-thirds that of the serum glucose).

14. **The answer is D.** Carbon tetrachloride (CCl_4) injury is the classic model of membrane injury incurred by free radical formation. In this instance, CCl_4 is converted to the active free radical CCl_3 in the smooth endoplasmic reticulum by the P450 system of mixed function oxidases.

15. **The answer is A.** GTPase activity, which is required for inactivation, is decreased in mutant ras (p21) proteins. This change is mediated by reduced responsiveness to GTPase-activating protein.

16. **The answer is B.** The clinical history is strongly suggestive of bacterial pneumonia. Pleural fluid from this patient would typically be an exudate rather than a transudate, and would be expected to be cloudy and contain many neutrophils. The fluid would also demonstrate reduced glucose, increased protein, and increased specific gravity.

17. The answer is E. The absence of both fetal kidneys leads to a decreased volume of amniotic fluid (oligohydramnios) because fetal urine is a major source of amniotic fluid. This leads to a group of secondary abnormalities, often including distorted facies and unilateral pulmonary hypoplasia. This sequence of events is referred to as the Potter progression. The other choices refer to a group of related syndromes often grouped together as the TORCH complex (produced by a group of organisms: ***T***oxoplasma, ***O***ther etiologies, ***R***ubella virus, ***C***ytomegalovirus, or ***H***erpes simplex virus; the "***O***ther" designation includes diverse viruses and the treponemal spirochete of syphilis). These infections are associated with a similar group of fetal abnormalities, including microcephaly, brain lesions with focal calcifications, and ocular and cardiac anomalies. Microcephaly is also a common feature of the fetal alcohol syndrome.

18. The answer is B. Splenomegaly occurs in children with sickle cell anemia, but repeated bouts of splenic infarction and fibrosis reduce the spleen to a fibrous remnant in adults (autosplenectomy). The other listed conditions are all well-known causes of splenomegaly.

19. The answer is D. Carcinoma of the urinary bladder, almost always transitional cell carcinoma, is associated with industrial exposure to aniline dyes such as β-naphthylamine, usually many years in the past. This type of cancer most often spreads by local extension to surrounding tissues. Hematogenous dissemination is a late finding. Exposure to aflatoxin is associated with hepatocellular carcinoma, and *Schistosoma haematobium* infection is associated with squamous cell bladder carcinoma, not transitional cell. Methyldopa is an association of bile duct cancer.

20. The answer is E. Pseudohypoparathyroidism is characterized by renal end-organ unresponsiveness to PTH and by shortened fourth and fifth metacarpals and metatarsals, short stature, and other skeletal abnormalities. These abnormalities are due to mutations in GNAS1, a G protein that mediates receptiveness to PTH and other hormones. Selective imprinting results in maternal inheritance of the end-organ unresponsiveness. The clinical findings mimic those of hypoparathyroidism, but PTH is most often normal or elevated.

21. The answer is C. Multiple myeloma often presents with diffuse demineralization of bone, even though punched-out lesions are more characteristic. Findings in this scenario that distinguish multiple myeloma from other conditions also characterized by bony demineralization include anemia, hypergammaglobulinemia, proteinuria, and normal (rather than increased) serum alkaline phosphatase.

22. The answer is C. Medullary carcinoma is characterized histologically by sheets of tumor cells in an amyloid-containing stroma. This neoplasm is a calcitonin-producing tumor derived from "C" cells of the thyroid. Medullary carcinoma can occur singly or as a component of multiple endocrine neoplasia (MEN) syndromes types IIa and IIb.

23. The answer is E. The most frequent cause of cardiac rupture is myocardial infarction. This complication, which often results in hemopericardium and cardiac tamponade, occurs with peak incidence within 4 to 10 days after infarction.

24. The answer is A. Henoch-Schönlein purpura is an IgA immune complex disease characterized by involvement of small vessels (venules, capillaries, arterioles) with multiple lesions, all about the same age, and is a form of hypersensitivity or leukocytoclastic vasculitis. The disorder may involve only the skin, presenting as palpable purpura, or it may involve a variety of other sites, including the glomeruli, gastrointestinal tract, lungs, or brain.

25. **The answer is B.** The vignette is suggestive of long-standing, late stage hereditary hemochromatosis, and the expected findings would include markedly increased serum iron and moderately reduced TIBC. This combination often results in almost 100% saturation of iron-binding capacity.

26. **The answer is B.** Alveolar hyaline membrane formation is a characteristic finding in the adult respiratory distress syndrome (ARDS). The common factor in ARDS is diffuse alveolar damage induced by a number of agents or conditions, one of which is septic shock. Other prominent causes include trauma, uremia, gastric aspiration, inhalation of chemical irritants, oxygen toxicity, *Mycoplasma* infection, and the severe acute respiratory syndrome (SARS).

27. **The answer is E.** The scenario is typical of neuroblastoma, the most frequently occurring tumor in infants less than 1 year of age. The tumor may occasionally undergo spontaneous differentiation to a benign ganglioneuroma. Marked amplification of N-*myc* is characteristic, and greater amplification is a negative prognostic indicator. Most neuroblastomas are peripheral, and the most frequent site of origin is the adrenal medulla or adjacent tissues. CNS neuroblastomas are less common, and most often involve the cerebral hemispheres. Origin in the posterior cranial fossa is rare. Catecholamine production is characteristic.

28. **The answer is D.** Disseminated histoplasmosis is characterized by widespread dissemination of macrophages filled with fungal yeast forms.

29. **The answer is C.** A linear pattern of glomerular immunofluorescence for IgG is found in Goodpasture syndrome, which is caused by antibodies that react with both glomerular and alveolar basement membranes.

30. **The answer is E.** Progressive somnolence leading to metabolic acidosis (low bicarbonate with significant anion gap), coma, and severe dehydration, often with prerenal azotemia, are all strongly suggestive of diabetic ketoacidosis. Expected findings in this condition include increased serum and urine glucose and ketones.

31. **The answer is D.** Folate deficiency leads to megaloblastic anemia. The red cells are macrocytic (increased MCV) and normochromic (increased MCHC). Since the thickened red cells appear more dense on peripheral blood smears, these cells are often erroneously thought to be hyperchromic; however, the mean corpuscular hemoglobin concentration (MCHC) is normal. An increased MCHC is found in hereditary spherocytosis, however. Hypochromic erythrocytes are typical of iron deficiency anemia, some cases of the anemia of chronic disease, and the thalassemias. Suppressed β-chain synthesis is characteristic of the β-thalassemias. Decreased susceptibility to malaria is associated with absence of the Duffy blood group antigen and with glucose-6-phosphate dehydrogenase (G6PD) deficiency.

32. **The answer is C.** In the first several hours after myocardial infarction, the most common cause of death is arrhythmia. Although evidence of acute coronary artery obstruction may be found, morphologic myocardial changes and serum myocardial marker protein elevations are most often delayed for several hours. A myocardial fibrotic scar is evidence of old prior myocardial infarction.

33. **The answer is E.** The clinical description is most consistent with infection with *Neisseria gonorrhoeae,* which is most often manifest in men as acute purulent urethritis. Without treatment, gonorrheal infection can extend to the prostate and seminal vesicles and sometimes to the epididymis. The testes are rarely involved.

34. **The answer is E.** Whipple disease, a systemic illness almost always involving the small intestine, is characterized morphologically by distinctive periodic acid Schiff (PAS)-positive macrophages within affected organs. On electron microscopy, the PAS-positive material is seen to consist of numerous bacillary forms of the gram-positive actinomycete *Tropheryma whippelii.* The disorder responds to a number of antibacterial agents, but without therapy the course is usually progressive and fatal.

35. **The answer is E.** von Willebrand disease (congenital deficiency of von Willebrand factor [vWF]) is characterized by defective platelet adhesion, resulting in a prolonged bleeding time even though the platelets are qualitatively and quantitatively normal. The APTT is also prolonged because of a secondary deficiency of factor VIII. Factor VIII normally circulates in a complex with vWF and is unstable when vWF is deficient.

36. **The answer is B.** Pleural and peritoneal mesotheliomas are associated with exposure to asbestos, and the apparent tumorigenic effect of asbestosis is markedly enhanced by cigarette smoking. Aflatoxin B_1 is associated with hepatocellular carcinoma. Clear cell adenocarcinoma of the vagina has been a hazard to daughters exposed during intrauterine life to diethylstilbestrol (DES) administered to their mothers to prevent spontaneous abortion. Ionizing radiation is associated with many cancers, including leukemias, breast cancer, and thyroid malignancies. β-Naphthylamine and other aniline dyes are associated with transitional cell carcinoma of the bladder.

37. **The answer is D.** The most important factor in the pathogenesis of endometrial carcinoma appears to be prolonged estrogen stimulation, such as that associated with estrogen therapy or estrogen-secreting tumors. Obesity and conditions associated with it, such as diabetes mellitus or hypertension, may contribute to hyperestrinism because estrone can be synthesized in peripheral fat cells. Arsenic exposure is associated with carcinomas of the lung and skin and with hepatic hemangiosarcoma. *BRCA* mutations are associated with breast and ovarian cancer. Endometriosis is not a neoplasm and has no relation to carcinoma of the endometrium. Sexual promiscuity is a risk factor for cervical cancer, not endometrial cancer.

38. **The answer is D.** During the first several hours of an inflammatory process, the predominant inflammatory cells are neutrophils. After 1 or 2 days, neutrophils are largely replaced by longer-lived monocytes–macrophages.

39. **The answer is B.** The vignette is consistent with a hematologic diagnosis of acute lymphoblastic leukemia, a condition that occurs with markedly increased incidence in association with Down syndrome.

40. **The answer is E.** Of the choices listed, only membranous glomerulonephritis is an immune complex disease.

41. **The answer is A.** The most common cause of a breast mass in women younger than age 25 is fibroadenoma. Characteristically, this benign tumor presents as a firm, rubbery, painless, well-circumscribed lesion.

42. **The answer is B.** The association of episodic headache, palpitation, and diaphoresis, along with severe hypertension and hyperglycemia, is most suggestive of a catecholamine-secreting pheochromocytoma. Other nondiabetic endocrine disorders associated with hyperglycemia include Cushing syndrome, either pituitary or adrenal, with hypersecretion of corticotropin or cortisol; acromegaly, with hypersecretion of growth hormone; and hyperthyroidism, with hypersecretion of thyroxine.

43. **The answer is E.** The VIPoma is an islet cell tumor of the pancreas that is associated with ***W***atery ***D***iarrhea, ***H***ypokalemia, and ***A***chlorhydria (WDHA syndrome or Verner-Morrison syndrome), all caused by the secretion of vasoactive intestinal peptide (VIP) by the tumor.

44. The answer is E. This is a classic case of acute pyelonephritis, an acute infection of the renal parenchyma. White cell casts in the urine are pathognomonic of acute pyelonephritis. Although microscopic hematuria is a frequent finding in acute pyelonephritis and other urinary tract infections, red cell casts are not seen since the glomeruli tend to be spared in renal infection. Red cell casts are a specific indicator of glomerular inflammation.

45. The answer is A. Congenital pyloric stenosis is an obstruction of the gastric outlet caused by hypertrophy of the pyloric muscularis. The hypertrophic muscle is often perceived as a palpable mass. The principal manifestation of this condition, more common in boys, is projectile vomiting, most often occurring in the first 2 weeks of life.

46. The answer is A. The combination of aortic diastolic murmur, "water-hammer" pulse, and wide pulse pressure is an indicator of aortic valve insufficiency. Although now rare in the United States, tertiary syphilis remains the most common cause of this abnormality in many parts of the world. Aneurysm of the ascending aorta commonly accompanies this valvular lesion. The other listed choices are all complications of atherosclerosis, which infrequently involves the ascending aorta.

47. The answer is C. The history is consistent with the ARDS. ARDS is a cause of severe life-threatening respiratory insufficiency and may be caused by a variety of etiologic agents, among them severe trauma such as a gunshot wound. The common feature, regardless of etiology, is diffuse alveolar damage.

48. The answer is B. The most frequent causes of mild anemia with hypochromia and microcytosis include iron deficiency anemia, the anemia of chronic disease, and β-thalassemia minor. In the latter, the diagnosis is confirmed by demonstrating increased concentration of hemoglobin A_2 and the characteristic complete blood count (CBC) findings of marked microcytosis, as evidenced by a very low mean corpuscular volume (MCV) with only moderate reduction of the hemoglobin and hematocrit. In iron deficiency anemia, serum iron is decreased, TIBC is increased, and storage iron is depleted, as indicated by decreased serum ferritin and absent bone marrow hemosiderin on Prussian blue stain. Additionally, a source of blood loss is often apparent. The anemia of chronic disease is most often normochromic and normocytic, but can be hypochromic and microcytic. In such cases, a decrease in TIBC and the presence of an obvious chronic disease are indicative of the cause of the anemia.

49. The answer is C. The description is that of lymphocyte depletion, the least frequently occurring form of Hodgkin lymphoma. It is marked by few lymphocytes, numerous Reed-Sternberg cells, and extensive necrosis and fibrosis. Lymphocyte depletion in Hodgkin lymphoma often presents in an advanced stage and has the poorest prognosis of the Hodgkin lymphoma variants. This variant is associated with EBV infection in the great majority of cases, and also is more common in persons infected with HIV.

50. The answer is B. The jaundice of hemolytic anemia is due to unconjugated hyperbilirubinemia. Because unconjugated bilirubin is not excreted into the urine, the type of jaundice is acholuric, jaundice without bilirubin pigment in the urine. In hemolytic anemia, haptoglobin is markedly decreased. Peripheral red cell destruction is mirrored by marrow erythroid hyperplasia with release of newly formed red cells into the peripheral blood, manifest as reticulocytosis.

51. The answer is D. Juvenile melanoma, or Spitz nevus, is a benign lesion that can be confused with malignant melanoma. Acanthosis nigricans is sometimes an indicator of visceral malignancy. Actinic keratosis is a premalignant epidermal lesion. Dysplastic nevus may transform into malignant melanoma. Xeroderma pigmentosum is associated with a markedly increased incidence of skin cancer caused by failure of DNA repair.

52. **The answer is B.** The clinical presentation is illustrative of acanthosis nigricans, a cutaneous lesion that is indicative of a visceral malignancy, such as carcinoma of the stomach, lung, breast, or uterus. Other associations of malignancy include migratory venous thrombosis, which is also associated with visceral malignancies; clubbing of the fingers, which may be associated with a number of disorders, including carcinoma of the lung; and mararantic endocarditis, which is associated with wasting diseases such as widespread cancer.

53. **The answer is B.** The clinical picture is that of alcoholic hepatitis, which is characterized by fatty change, focal liver cell necrosis, infiltrates of neutrophils, and intracytoplasmic hyaline inclusions referred to as Mallory bodies.

54. **The answer is D.** In spite of the somewhat atypical presentation, the histologic findings are typical of contact dermatitis, which is a classic example of T cell-mediated (type IV) hypersensitivity.

55. **The answer is A.** Adult polycystic kidney is frequently associated with berry aneurysm of the circle of Willis, often in association with cysts in the liver or pancreas.

56. **The answer is E.** The clinical picture strongly suggests a diagnosis of sarcoidosis. The granulomas of sarcoidosis are characteristically noncaseating. Sarcoidosis is a multisystem disorder. Common findings in this highly variable disorder include anergy to tuberculin, hypercalcemia, and broad-based polyclonal hypergammaglobulinemia.

57. **The answer is B.** The vignette describes an instance of traumatic fat necrosis, which must be distinguished from enzymatic fat necrosis. The description of amorphous basophilic material is indicative of calcification, and calcification of previous damaged tissue is termed dystrophic calcification. Dystrophic calcification must be distinguished from metastatic calcification, which occurs in the presence of hypercalcemia and affects nondamaged tissues.

58. **The answer is A.** A diet low in fiber and high in fat is believed to be a risk factor for the development of colon cancer. Both aflatoxin B_1 ingestion and hepatitis B infection are risk factors for hepatocellular carcinoma. *Helicobacter pylori* infection is associated with stomach cancer. Cancers of the mouth, tongue, and esophagus have a marked association with the combined abuse of tobacco and alcohol.

59. **The answer is E.** Small cell carcinoma of the lung is almost always metastatic at the time of initial diagnosis, and is thus poorly amenable to surgery. Despite morphologic differences, the bronchogenic carcinomas, including small cell carcinoma, all share a common endodermal origin. The location is most often central rather than peripheral, and there is a marked association with cigarette smoking. Paraneoplastic syndromes include inappropriate secretion of adrenocorticotropic hormone (ACTH) and ADH. Secretion of a protein with PTH-like activity is an association of squamous cell bronchogenic carcinoma.

60. **The answer is B.** C3b is an important opsonin. C3a and C5a (anaphylatoxins) mediate degranulation of mast cells and basophils. In addition, C5a is a potent chemotactic agent for neutrophils. C5b-9 is the membrane attack complex that mediates complement-induced cell lysis.

61. **The answer is D.** Chronic bronchitis, which is clearly linked to cigarette smoking, is defined as productive cough occurring during at least 3 consecutive months over at least 2 consecutive years.

62. **The answer is C.** Severe diarrhea, fever, and toxicity following broad-spectrum antibiotic therapy is likely due to pseudomembranous colitis. This disorder is caused by overgrowth of *Clostridium difficile,* a commensal microorganism indigenous to the bowel, and is marked morphologically by superficial mucosal erosions with overlying necrotic, loosely adherent mucosal debris. The clostridia remain intraluminal but secrete an enterotoxin that is responsible for the clinical and pathologic manifestations of the disorder.

63. **The answer is B.** The description of clear vacuoles displacing intact nuclei to the periphery is characteristic of fatty change (steatosis) of the liver. However, clear intracytoplasmic vacuolization of hepatocytes may be due to accumulations of water or glycogen, and sometimes special stains are required for confirmation of the nature of the vacuoles. In industrialized countries such as the United States, the most common cause of fatty change of the liver is alcoholism.

64. **The answer is B.** The patient has secondary hemostatic bleeding, which is characteristic of disorders of the coagulation pathway. Relatively common coagulation pathway disorders include classic hemophilia (factor VIII deficiency) and Christmas disease (factor IX deficiency). Both are disorders of the intrinsic pathway of coagulation, and are clinically indistinguishable one from the other except by specific factor assays. Disseminated intravascular coagulation (DIC) is characterized by widespread thrombosis and hemorrhage with both primary and secondary hemostatic bleeding. The other choices listed are characterized by primary hemostatic bleeding, which is manifest by punctate cutaneous hemorrhages and oozing from mucosal surfaces.

65. **The answer is A.** Association with certain human leukocyte antigen (HLA) types, autoantibodies, and increased incidence in persons with other autoimmune disorders are frequent occurrences in autoimmune disorders. In addition, Hashimoto thyroiditis is characterized by dense lymphocytic infiltrates with germinal center formation, striking morphologic evidence of immune cell (B lymphocyte) participation.

66. **The answer is B.** Sustained ethanol abuse and progressive dementia are strongly suggestive of the Wernicke-Korsakoff syndrome, which is due to thiamine deficiency, most often in association with chronic alcoholism. Clinical characteristics include the Wernicke triad (confusion, ataxia, and ophthalmoplegia) and often Korsakoff psychosis, characterized by memory loss and confabulation (making up stories in an attempt to hide the inability to remember). The morphologic counterparts of these changes include degeneration of the mamillary bodies and of paramedian masses of gray matter.

67. **The answer is C.** This patient has cystic fibrosis. Cystic fibrosis is an autosomal recessive disease caused by mutations in the CFTR gene, which encodes a protein that functions as a chloride channel. *Pseudomonas aeruginosa* is the most likely pathogen causing chronic pulmonary infection and pulmonary failure, and is the leading cause of death in patients with cystic fibrosis. *Pseudomonas aeruginosa* is also (after *S. aureus* and *E. coli*) the leading cause of nosocomial (hospital-acquired) infections and a frequent cause of death from burns.

68. **The answer is C.** The most frequent cause of transfusion-related hepatitis is hepatitis C virus infection. Hepatitis C virus is the most frequent cause of what was formerly termed non-A, non-B hepatitis.

69. **The answer is B.** Agnogenic (idiopathic) myeloid metaplasia is characterized by extensive non-neoplastic myelofibrosis and extramedullary hematopoiesis resulting in hepatosplenomegaly. Teardrop-shaped erythrocytes, as well as scattered nucleated red cells and granulocytic precursor cells, can be found in the peripheral blood smear. Although marrow myeloid (granulocytic) and erythroid precursor cells are depleted, megakaryocytes tend to be spared and even increased in number.

70. The answer is D. A rapidly fatal course with severe hypertension, left ventricular hypertrophy and failure, papilledema, and renal dysfunction is characteristic of malignant hypertension. This syndrome is most frequently seen in relatively young African-American men. The defining renal arteriolar lesion, malignant nephrosclerosis (hyperplastic arteriolosclerosis, fibrinoid necrosis, necrotizing arteriolitis), and the associated necrotizing glomerular lesion result in capillary rupture and the consequent "flea-bitten" kidney appearance due to petechial hemorrhages covering the surfaces of the kidneys.

71. The answer is E. The observation of thickened glomerular capillary loops apparent on light microscopy permits the diagnosis of membranous glomerulonephritis. This condition is most frequent in young women and is characterized clinically by the nephrotic syndrome and progressive azotemia.

72. The answer is D. Patent ductus arteriosus and septal defects are the most frequent congenital cardiac abnormalities associated with congenital rubella infection. However, defects are not limited to the cardiovascular system, and congenital infection can also lead to deafness and mental retardation. In addition, congenital rubella infection, along with other congenital intrauterine infections, accounts for only a small proportion of cases of congenital heart disease, the majority being of unknown cause. The most severe consequences occur as a result of infection during the first trimester of pregnancy. As with all infections, an IgM antibody response indicates recent primary infection.

73. The answer is C. The hallmark of the megaloblastic anemias is the finding of megaloblastic erythroid hyperplasia in the bone marrow; pernicious anemia is a megaloblastic anemia.

74. The answer is B. The clinical history is characteristic of multiple sclerosis, the most frequently occurring of the demyelinating diseases. Multiple sclerosis is characterized by destruction of myelin, with preservation of axons. The optic nerve, brain stem, and paraventricular areas are favored sites of demyelination. Other characteristics of note include multiple oligoclonal immunoglobulin bands on CSF electrophoresis, association with certain HLA haplotypes, and geographic distribution, with incidence increasing with distance away from the equator.

75. The answer is C. Carcinoma of the pancreas with common bile duct obstruction is strongly suggested by the clinical findings. Spontaneous migratory venous thrombosis with visceral neoplasms is known as the Trousseau sign or syndrome.

76. The answer is B. Nodular melanoma tends to expand vertically rather than horizontally, a phenomenon associated with a more aggressive course and a greater likelihood of metastasis. Among the malignant melanomas, nodular melanoma has the poorest prognosis.

77. The answer is A. Hypochromic microcytic anemia is most often associated with iron deficiency secondary to chronic blood loss. Hookworm infestation causes chronic blood loss and should not be confused with fish tapeworm infestation, which causes megaloblastic anemia. Folate deficiency with megaloblastic anemia can occur in severely malnourished persons (often alcoholics) or in association with increased demand for folate in pregnancy. Cobalamin (vitamin B_{12}) deficiency megaloblastic anemia can occur in pernicious anemia, in strict vegetarians (vitamin B_{12} is only found in foods of animal origin), and in association with surgically induced intestinal blind loops overgrown with microorganisms with high avidity for cobalamin. The anemia of chronic disease is most often normochromic and normocytic, but can be hypochromic and microcytic. Usually, signs and symptoms of the underlying chronic disease are evident.

78. **The answer is E.** In a pediatric patient, the combination of recurrent pulmonary infections and steatorrhea (presumably due to pancreatic insufficiency) is strongly suggestive of cystic fibrosis. This disorder is characterized by a generalized defect in the reabsorption of anions, leading to increased sweat chloride concentration, an important diagnostic indicator.

79. **The answer is E.** Granulation tissue is formed in healing wounds and consists of young fibroblasts and newly formed capillaries. Cat-scratch disease, foreign body reaction, histoplasmosis, and tuberculosis are all well-known causes of granulomatous inflammation and have nothing to do with granulation tissue.

80. **The answer is D.** A keloid is a result of excessive production of collagenous fibrous tissue and is characterized by a tumor-like scar consisting of dense bundles of structurally abnormal collagen. Keloids have a marked tendency to recur after resection. Propensity to keloid formation is markedly increased in persons of African lineage.

81. **The answer is D.** The combination of increased serum calcium and alkaline phosphatase along with decreased serum phosphorus is most consistent with primary hyperparathyroidism. The most frequent cause of this endocrine abnormality is a parathyroid adenoma. Decreased phosphorus would not be an expected finding in metastatic carcinoma. The normal serum proteins mitigate against multiple myeloma and sarcoidosis. Additionally, the alkaline phosphatase is usually normal in multiple myeloma. Hypercalcemia from increased intake of calcium (as in the milk-alkali syndrome) is usually unaccompanied by significant changes in phosphorus or alkaline phosphatase.

82. **The answer is A.** Von Hippel-Lindau disease is an autosomal dominant disorder characterized by multiple vascular tumors and multiple cysts of the liver, kidney, and pancreas. The renal cysts have a high potential for malignant transformation. Retinal and CNS hemangioblastomas are characteristic, as are pheochromocytomas.

83. **The answer is D.** Renal papillary necrosis is a well-known complication of chronic analgesic nephritis, which is caused by long-term abuse of phenacetin or its metabolite, acetaminophen, most often in combination with aspirin or a nonsteroidal anti-inflammatory drug (NSAID). Another major cause of renal papillary necrosis is diabetes mellitus. Phenacetin abuse is also associated with a markedly increased incidence of transitional cell carcinoma of the renal pelvis.

84. **The answer is C.** True hermaphroditism requires the presence of both ovarian and testicular tissue, as in this case. The karyotype is either XX (with translocation of at least part of the Y chromosome to an X chromosome or to an autosome) or a mosaicism such as XX/XXY.

85. **The answer is A.** The illustration demonstrates an adenocarcinoma diffusely infiltrating the wall of the colon, with marked constriction of the lumen and ulceration of the mucosa.

86. **The answer is B.** Phospholipase A_2 catalyzes the release of arachidonic acid from membrane phospholipids. Arachidonic acid metabolism then proceeds through two major pathways, the lipoxygenase and cyclooxygenase pathways. The lipoxygenase pathway yields HETE and leukotrienes. The cyclooxygenase pathway yields thromboxanes and prostaglandins. Prostacyclin (PGI_2) is synthesized in endothelial cells, and thromboxane A_2 (TxA_2) is synthesized in platelets. It should be noted that prednisone inhibits both the cyclooxygenase and lipoxygenase pathways by inhibiting the formation of precursors to each pathway.

87. **The answer is E.** Subacute sclerosing panencephalitis, one of the slow virus infections, is thought to be caused by persistent infection with a defective measles virus. The virus lacks the M component, a protein required for extracellular spread of the virus. This deficiency is thought to explain the slow nature of the infection.

88. **The answer is A.** The findings are characteristic of meningococcemia with meningococcal meningitis. A well-recognized complication of meningococcemia is the Waterhouse-Friderichsen syndrome, which is catastrophic adrenal insufficiency and vascular collapse caused by hemorrhagic necrosis of the adrenal cortex, often with associated DIC.

89. **The answer is B.** Persistent chest pain unrelieved by nitroglycerin and the abnormal electrocardiogram (ECG) findings are diagnostic of myocardial infarction (MI). It would be unusual to observe significant elevations of creatine kinase MB (CK-MB) and cardiac troponin I (cTn-I) as early as 1 hour following an MI. These markers rise in parallel and are weakly positive in about 6 hours and reach peak levels in about 10 to 15 hours following an MI. CK-MB returns to normal levels in 3 to 7 days, while cTn-I can remain elevated a week or longer.

90. **The answer is C.** The illustration demonstrates thrombotic obliteration of glomerular capillary loops and is typical of DIC. In DIC–sometimes termed consumption coagulopathy–coagulation factors, fibrinogen, and platelets are depleted by the widespread thrombotic process. Thus the coagulation assays (APPT, PT, and thrombin time) are prolonged and the platelet count is decreased. Increased fibrin and fibrinogen degradation products are sensitive indicators of DIC.

91. **The answer is D.** Primary adrenocortical deficiency (Addison disease), as distinguished from adrenal cortical insufficiency secondary to pituitary hypofunction, is indicated by the presence of pigmentation. Also, decreased plasma cortisol in Addison disease is unresponsive to adrenocorticotropic hormone (ACTH) administration. Progressive weakness and hypotension are strongly suggestive of adrenocortical deficiency regardless of cause, and other expected findings include decreased serum sodium, increased serum potassium, decreased serum glucose, and decreased urinary 17-ketosteroids.

92. **The answer is E.** Huntington disease results from an expansion of the CAG trinucleotide repeat within the *huntingtin* gene, which can be detected by restriction length polymorphism (RFLP) analysis. Unlike many autosomal dominant disorders, it manifests later in life, in the fourth to fifth decade of life. Deposition of copper in the lenticular nuclei occurs in Wilson disease. A deficiency of sphingomylenase results in some forms of Niemann-Pick disease. Loss of dopamine-producing neurons in the substantia nigra occurs in Parkinson disease.

93. **The answer is C.** The combination of membranous glomerulonephritis, pleuritis, and Libman-Sacks endocarditis (vegetations on both surfaces of the mitral or tricuspid valves) as well as proliferative splenic arteriolitis is characteristic of SLE. Diffuse interstitial pulmonary fibrosis also occurs in SLE. A variety of antinuclear antibodies (ANAs) are found; the most specific are antibodies to the Sm (Smith) antigen, antibodies to double-stranded DNA, and antibodies that result in a peripheral rim pattern of nuclear immunofluorescence.

94. **The answer is A.** In a typical well-differentiated bronchioloalveolar carcinoma, tumor cells line the walls of terminal air spaces, as shown in the illustration. When the tumor is localized to a single nodule, it is potentially curable by surgical resection.

95. **The answer is D.** The Zollinger-Ellison syndrome, characterized by markedly increased gastric acid production and intractable peptic ulcer, is caused by hypersecretion of a gastrin-producing islet cell tumor (gastrinoma).

96. **The answer is A.** Conjugated hyperbilirubinemia and positive urine tests for bilirubin are indicative of obstructive jaundice. The further finding of the complete absence of urine and stool urobilinogen indicates total common bile duct obstruction. Additionally, the palpable gallbladder (Courvoisier sign) strongly suggests that the etiology is a malignant tumor such as adenocarcinoma of the head of the pancreas.

97. **The answer is C.** Pheochromocytoma of the adrenal medulla (and its extra-adrenal counterpart paraganglioma) secretes the catecholamines epinephrine and norepinephrine. Increased urinary excretion of catecholamines or their metabolites metanephrine and VMA is a clinical indicator of this tumor.

98. **The answer is C.** Autophagic granules are intracytoplasmic vacuoles containing debris from degraded organelles such as mitochondria. They are especially prominent in cells that have become atrophic, such as skeletal muscle cells after prolonged immobilization.

99. **The answer is A.** Kwashiorkor is a form of protein-calorie malnutrition attributed to a relative lack of protein despite a diet relatively high in carbohydrates. Marasumus, in contrast, is more severe, and results from a major lack of calories from any source. Carbohydrate metabolites are converted to lipid, which is processed and stored by the liver. However, protein sources to serve as precursor amino acids for apolipoprotein synthesis are lacking. The result is hepatic fatty change, not cirrhosis.

100. **The answer is A.** The majority of salivary gland tumors occur in the parotid, and most are pleomorphic adenomas. This tumor most often presents as a painless mass just anterior to the ear. Due to its proximity to the facial nerve, it is often not completely resectable and therefore tends to recur. Mumps infection can lead to parotid swelling that is often bilateral and painful. Horner syndrome is a consequence of some lung tumors, not of salivary gland tumors.

101. **The answer is E.** Repeated pulmonary infections and a positive sweat test are characteristic of cystic fibrosis. In this condition, viscid secretions cause defective exocrine gland function. The lungs and pancreas are the most significant sites of involvement, and the disorder is marked by repeated bouts of pneumonia and by pancreatic failure with wasting and steatorrhea.

102. **The answer is E.** An increased incidence of berry aneurysm is associated with adult polycystic kidney. Berry aneurysm occurs at sites of discontinuity of the arterial media, most frequently at bifurcations of vessels of the circle of Willis. The most common locations are the junction of the anterior cerebral and anterior communicating arteries, the bifurcation of the middle cerebral artery, the junction of the internal carotid and posterior communicating arteries, and the junction of the basilar and posterior cerebral arteries. Berry aneurysm is the most frequent cause of subarachnoid hemorrhage, and there is no association with atherosclerosis.

103. **The answer is B.** Intracellular pH is decreased in severe hypoxic cell injury. This change is caused by mitochondrial damage, which in turn results in decreased oxidative phosphorylation and diminished adenosine triphosphate (ATP) synthesis. Decreased ATP stimulates glycolysis with lactate formation, thus resulting in decreased intracellular pH. Decreased ATP also diminishes the activity of the membrane-associated Na^+K^+ pump, allowing an influx of sodium and water. The final steps leading to cell death in severe hypoxic injury are associated with massive influx of extracellular calcium.

104. The answer is A. Calcification within a cystic ovarian tumor in a young woman is most characteristic of mature teratoma of the ovary, a benign lesion and the most frequently occurring ovarian tumor.

105. The answer is B. Symmetric polyarthritis with involvement of the proximal interphalangeal and metacarpophalangeal joints in a female patient are characteristics of rheumatoid arthritis. Rheumatoid factor, an IgM antibody directed against the Fc portion of IgG, is found in about 80% of affected individuals.

106. The answer is D. Both epithelioid cells and multinucleated giant cells are modified macrophages. A macrophage is a mononuclear phagocyte that has migrated into tissue.

107. The answer is B. Raynaud disease is cold-induced vasospasm of arterioles and small arteries, most often involving the fingers and sometimes the hands and feet. Young, otherwise healthy women are most often affected.

108. The answer is C. Vitamin C is required for hydroxylation of proline and lysine residues, which are required steps in collagen and osteoid matrix synthesis. Poor collagen formation contributes to impaired wound healing and fragility of capillary walls, which in turn leads to abnormal bleeding. Vitamin C also maintains the reduced state of metabolically active agents, such as iron and tetrahydrofolate. The maintenance of iron in its divalent ferrous form is required for intestinal iron absorption. Thus iron absorption is decreased, rather than increased, in vitamin C deficiency. Defective osteoid matrix formation occurs in vitamin C deficiency.

109. The answer is D. Staging is based on clinical evaluation of the distribution and extent of the disease process and is contrasted with grading, which is based on histopathologic evaluation of a malignant neoplasm.

110. The answer is A. Classic features of lead poisoning include dark precipitates forming a gingival lead line (composed of precipitated lead sulfide), radiopaque deposits in epiphyses, basophilic stippling of erythrocytes, increased urinary delta-ALA, and peripheral neuropathy and other CNS changes.

111. The answer is E. Granulosa cell tumors are sex cord-stromal tumors that typically secrete estrogen. For this reason, endometrial hyperplasia or endometrial carcinoma may be a concomitant finding in women diagnosed with a granulosa cell tumor.

112. The answer is B. The most common primary malignant neoplasm of bone is osteosarcoma. The classic radiographic findings are the Codman triangle (periosteal elevation by new bone formation) and the "sunburst" appearance (extension of tumor cells through the periosteum).

113. The answer is B. Amplification of the *HER-2/neu* oncogene is frequently observed in breast cancer, and an increased degree of amplification is thought to be a negative prognostic indicator.

114. The answer is A. Carcinoma of the cervix is associated with infection with certain serotypes of human papillomavirus (HPV). Other characteristics include a history of early sexual activity, squamous cell morphology, and frequent origin at the squamocolumnar junction. Leiomyomas (fibroids) may increase in size during pregnancy and decrease in size following menopause. Endometrial carcinoma is the most common gynecologic malignancy and is associated with hyperestrinism from estrogen therapy. Endodermal sinus (yolk sac) tumors produce α-fetoprotein.

115. **The answer is A.** The findings described are characteristic of congenital agammaglobulinemia of Bruton, an X-linked disorder characterized morphologically by agammaglobulinemia, absence of plasma cells, and absent or poorly defined germinal centers in the lymph nodes. Leukocyte functions, such as phagocytosis and bacterial killing, are unimpaired. T lymphocytes are unaffected.

116. **The answer is D.** Maternal antibodies provide passive immunization and protection from bacterial infection during the first months of life in children with congenital agammaglobulinemia.

117. **The answer is D.** Acute hematogenous osteomyelitis occurs with peak incidence in children, most commonly affects the metaphyses of long bones, and is more common in boys. In the acute stage, pyogenic osteomyelitis often resolves with antibiotic therapy. If the disorder is allowed to progress to necrosis and sequestrum formation, surgical intervention is usually required.

118. **The answer is A.** Transitional cell carcinoma is the most common tumor of the urinary collecting system and can occur in renal calyces, pelvis, ureter, or bladder.

119. **The answer is B.** Chest pain, ECG findings of QS waves with elevated ST segments, and elevated serum creatinine kinase MB (CK-MB) and troponin I (cTn-I) are diagnostic of acute myocardial infarction (MI). MI is the prototype of coagulative necrosis.

120. **The answer is D.** Generalized lower abdominal pain, bloody stools, and signs of acute inflammation in an older patient are classic findings in diverticulitis. Appendicitis and Crohn disease occur more often in younger persons, and bloody stools would not be expected. Signs of acute inflammation would not be expected in carcinoma of the rectum or in tubular adenoma.

121. **The answer is D.** Clear cell adenocarcinoma of the vagina is a rare malignant tumor that is markedly increased in incidence in daughters of women who received DES therapy during pregnancy.

122. **The answer is B.** An increase in prostate-specific antigen (PSA) may occur in both nodular prostatic hyperplasia and in carcinoma of the prostate. Both of these disorders have a peak incidence in elderly men, and nodular prostatic hyperplasia tends to arise in the central zone of prostatic glands.

123. **The answer is D.** Portal-systemic venous shunting leads to encephalopathy in end-stage cirrhosis. It also leads to esophageal varices, rectal hemorrhoids, and distention of periumbilical venous collaterals. Hypoalbuminemia, increased hepatic lymph formation, increased portal venous pressure, and renal retention of sodium and water all contribute to the development of ascities but have little to do with encephalopathy.

124. **The answer is D.** Neurons are permanent cells, and the classic teaching has been that neurons do not proliferate during adult life (recent evidence casts some doubt on this concept). Bronchial epithelial cells, gastric mucosal cells and skin epithelial cells are labile cells. Hepatocytes and renal tubular cells are stable cells. Both labile and stable cells are capable of proliferation and regeneration.

125. **The answer is C.** Exposure to asbestos (common in construction workers, shipyard workers, or people who have worked with insulation or fire safety materials) markedly predisposes to mesothelioma of the pleura or peritoneum and is also closely linked to bronchogenic carcinoma (especially in smokers).

126. **The answer is D.** Subdural hematoma can be acute (e.g., due to moderate head trauma) or chronic (e.g., due to whiplash). Subdural hematomas are caused by venous bleeding, most often from laceration of the bridging veins, which join the cerebral vessels to the venous sinuses within the dura. The classic computed tomography (CT) scan finding is formation of a "crescent" along the inner skull, which is due to subdural venous bleeding.

127. **The answer is C.** Epidural hematoma is most often caused by skull fracture with laceration of the branches of the middle meningeal artery. The classic CT scan finding is formation of a "lens-shaped" density contained within the suture lines of the skull.

128. **The answer is C.** Subarachnoid hemorrhage is most often caused by rupture of a berry aneurysm of the circle of Willis. Frank blood may be found in the CSF, and diffuse hemorrhage over the surface of the brain is due to subarachnoid bleeding.

129. **The answer is B.** Medulloblastoma, a highly malignant tumor, is one of the most frequently occurring malignancies of early childhood. The posterior cranial fossa is the most common site of this tumor. Other high-incidence tumors of early childhood include acute leukemia, Wilms tumor, and adrenal neuroblastoma.

130. **The answer is C.** Meningioma is a benign tumor of the meninges that is external to the brain and is therefore usually surgically resectable. Meningioma is the second most common primary intracranial neoplasm. This tumor causes a mass effect (a space-occupying defect) that physically compresses but does not invade brain parenchyma. Symptoms correlate with the location of the meningioma. For example, this patient's right-sided parasagittal meningioma caused slow and progressive left-sided lower extremity weakness.

131. **The answer is C.** Idiopathic Parkinson disease is manifest morphologically by depigmentation of cells of the substantia nigra and locus ceruleus.

132. **The answer is D.** Myasthenia gravis is an autoimmune disorder caused by autoantibodies to acetylcholine receptors of the neuromuscular junction. Dramatic improvement in muscle strength with an anticholinesterase agent such as edrophonium is a useful diagnostic sign.

133. **The answer is B.** Huntington disease, a disorder caused by an increased number of trinucleotide repeats, is manifest anatomically by progressive degeneration and atrophy of the caudate nucleus, putamen, and frontal cortex. The caudate nucleus normally bulges convexly into the lateral ventricles; thus atrophy of the caudate nucleus results in the appearance of "bat-wing-shaped" or enlarged lateral ventricles.

134. **The answer is B.** Hypertrophic osteoarthropathy, manifest as clubbing of the fingers and associated periostitis of the distal radius and ulna, is associated with chronic lung disease, cyanotic heart disease, and other systemic disorders.

135. **The answer is E.** Felty syndrome is the combination of splenomegaly, neutropenia, and rheumatoid arthritis.

136. **The answer is A.** Androblastoma (Sertoli cell tumor), a nongerm cell tumor derived from the sex cord, is most often benign. These tumors, along with Leydig (interstitial) cell tumors, may be hormone-producing, sometimes elaborating estrogens and presenting in males with gynecomastia and other feminizing effects.

137. **The answer is E.** Seminoma, a germ cell tumor of the testis with peak incidence in the mid-30s age group, is analogous to (and histologically closely resembles) dysgerminoma of the ovary.

138. **The answer is E.** The prototype of the nephritic syndrome is poststreptococcal glomerulonephritis.

139. **The answer is A.** Renal amyloidosis can occur in both primary and secondary amyloidosis. In the latter, the most frequently occurring underlying illness is rheumatoid arthritis.

140. **The answer is B.** Diabetic nephropathy is marked by diffuse or nodular mesangial accumulations of glycosylated basement membrane-like material.

Index

B

C

D

I

J

K

L

M

N

T

U